ADAPTED PHYSICAL EDUCATION IN THE MAINSTREAM

SECOND EDITION

BRYANT J. CRATTY
*UNIVERSITY OF CALIFORNIA,
LOS ANGELES*

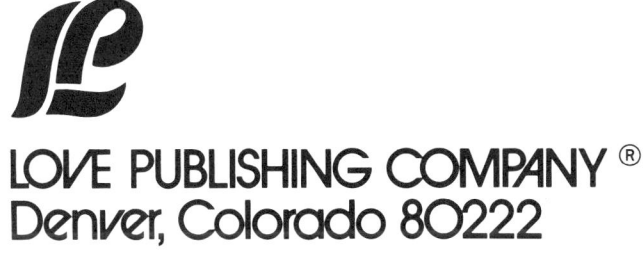

LOVE PUBLISHING COMPANY ®
Denver, Colorado 80222

dedicated to the memory of

Astrid Jessy Kiphard

daughter of Ingrid & Ernst

Library of Congress Catalog Card Number 86-82896

Copyright © 1989 Love Publishing Company
Printed in the U.S.A.
ISBN 0-89108-130-5

Contents

II Sensory Impairments

III Behavioral and Learning Disorders

Preface

This second edition was written with several thoughts in mind. First, it was intended to update information concerning the exceptionalities normally dealt with in physical education classes, as well as to survey contemporary information concerning teaching and therapeutic strategies employed with various handicapped groups.

The first edition met with broad approval and was translated into several languages, including Japanese. Thus, this second edition presents broad guidelines applicable in cultural environments in addition to that of the United States. It does not dwell obsessively upon laws governing special and adapted physical education applicable only in the United States. These are covered for the most part in chapter 2.

Further, this edition focuses upon application of research data. It is not a text overburdened with medical terms and concepts, although these are covered adequately for the reader's understanding. The range and depth of information also exclude some of the material often found in adapted physical education tests that I think is more appropriately found in books dealing with teaching methods for elementary physical education. In essence, this book combines practical and theoretical information. Principles accompany specific suggestions on how to improve fitness, deal effectively with the various handicapping conditions, develop motor skills, utilize games in learning, teach specific skills, and other ways to enhance the child's total well-being.

New material in this edition includes a chapter on infant stimulation, containing information that may well be used with severely handicapped and delayed older individuals as well. The new chapters on hyperactivity and awkwardness are useful additions to the literature in general, and to this book in particular. Other chapters, including those on tests and measurement, the various exceptionalities, and legislation, have undergone extensive revision and rewriting and have been updated using the most contemporary resources available.

This book has been organized into several sections. The first, consisting of chapters 1-5, provides a framework and introduction for readers who are interested in a career in adapted physical education as well as those who are likely to need this kind of background as they deal with special children in regular education settings. These chapters cover theoretical foundations, individualized education programs, testing and measurement, and teaching principles.

The chapters in Sections II, III, IV, V, and VI cover specific handicapping conditions. Each of these chapters in general follows a format of first providing an overview of the condition, including definitions, incidence and prevalence, classifications, and characteristics of that population. Each chapter concludes with specific principles and suggestions in applying physical programming and services.

Section II, Sensory Impairments, covers the blind and visually impaired, the deaf and hard of hearing. Section III addresses behavioral and learning disorders including learning disabilities, emotional disturbances, mental retardation, and speech and language impairments—along with their specific implications for physical education.

In Section IV problems of the central nervous system and neuromotor difficulties are covered. These discussions include attention to awkward children and those with cerebral palsy, progressive degenerative diseases, epilepsy, and muscular dystrophy. Section V, Fitness and Structural Problems, discusses obesity, posture, and body build, as well as the more traditional topics of orthopedic impairments and arthritis. Section VI is devoted to cardiovascular, pulmonary, and metabolic problems, including chronic heart conditions, hemophilia, sickle cell amenia, asthma, and juvenile diabetes.

Section VII discusses specific practical interventions, including infant stimulation programs, hyperactivity and impulsivity, and explains how rhythm, dance, and music can be used, as well as tumbling, locomotion, aquatics, and various exercises, as effective therapies. The final chapter presents physically oriented games that can be used to further cognitive learning.

The writing and research time devoted to this text uncovered several trends, reflected both in the research literature and in the everyday ways in which physical educators operate. Trends include increased emphases on fitness and exercise for special populations, as well as infant stimulation programs and those for the lower functioning handicapped populations. Trends in the field also include the diminuation of children in special schools as mainstreaming increasingly is placing them within the public schools. This results in a lower functioning population to be dealt with in classes that were formerly more homogenous in nature and the dispersion of special needs youngsters within normal populations—a situation that makes virtually every physical educator a special and adapted physical educator for at least some part of the school day.

This latter trend requires that *every* physical educator be at least a part-time adapted physical educator. Thus, information like that contained in this book, and in courses it supports, is becoming a must for physical educators in training—many of whom entered the profession originally planning to teach only more proficient youngsters.

The material in this book, I hope, will be helpful in supporting and maintaining special youngsters in physical activities that will serve them well as they live in the real world.

B.J.C.

ACKNOWLEDGMENTS

I would like to thank several people who helped me during preparation of this text. Mr. Shoftner and Mrs. Efron, administrators of the Francis Blend School for the Visually Handicapped in Los Angeles, were my hosts for several filming and picture-taking sessions. Moreover, Rose Engle, principal of the Sven Lokrantz School for the Handicapped, helped me greatly with new photos, as did her physical education staff. Mr. Stanley Love, president of Love Publishing Company, was supportive as usual, along with his staff. They have been helpful to me when writing this and other books dealing with physical education and sports.

The New Challenges of Physical Education

1 Introduction and Overview

Ever since the dawn of recorded history, physical activity has been recognized as a helpful adjunct to improvement of the human condition. The form and intensity of this activity have varied over the centuries, but the presence of physical education and recreation in programs of medicine has remained almost constant. The practitioners have ranged from physicians to educators to charlatans.

This history of special physical activities for special children ranges from exercises prescribed by the early Greek, Roman, and Arabian doctors to medical gymnastics that emerged in Europe during the 1700s. Still more recently, terms such as sensory-motor and perceptual-motor training, movement education, sensory integration, and adapted physical education denote special schools of thought relative to the manner in which motor tasks may contribute to people's physical, emotional, social, and even academic betterment.

The focus in this chapter, and in the book, is not on the past but instead on the present and future. For it could be argued that at no other period in history are members of the public and educators of special children more willing to accept substantial and well conceived programs of special physical education for special children.

LEGISLATION

Legislative trends, mirroring social conscience, have made the formulation of sound guidelines and programs of special education imperative. In the United States, current legislation clearly states that specially designed programs of physical education are necessary parts of the total remedial thrust directed toward children and adults with special needs. Thus, physical educators and other specialists in motor development should feel the challenge to produce special programs that make sense, to develop achievable objectives, and to formulate and use assessment tools that not only do their job but also afford clear insights for both professionals and parents as to what is and is not possible to achieve through programs of special education.

Current legislation veers away from a medical model for remediation of the handicapped. Rather, an educational model has been called for—one that clearly delineates how children are to be assessed as "different" and how various "delivery services" should meet those children's needs. Educators, whether working with classroom activities or movement activities, have become more accountable for program outcomes than was true in the past. Although laws do not make it illegal to fail to meet stated objectives, moral imperatives surrounding the achievement of written objectives are likely to be felt by both administrators and teachers.

Legislation has imposed other professional obligations on those dealing in adapted physical education. In the past, communication between adapted teachers and other professionals (doctors, psychologists, paramedical personnel) has been present, but their efforts at communication often were less than fruitful, and at times their conferences were informal and brief. The law now mandates formal meetings between and among professionals, who not only must talk to each other in language they all understand but at the same time must be monitored and understood by an attentive, highly interested set of parents! Thus, physical educators must bring to these meetings the jargon learned in college physical education courses and must understand some of the language heard in the corridors of hospitals, at meetings of special educators, and in the offices of social workers and psychiatrists. Thus, legislation imposes specific assignments and challenges on workers in movement activities:

—to formulate achievable objectives and then to be held accountable for their achievement, and

—to integrate program, thinking, and language into a total effort joined by other professionals in education, medicine, psychology, and social work.

Physical educators now need a grounding in the theory and "language" of exceptional children, as well as specific strategies and techniques that will bring movement services in nonabrasive and useful ways to youthful clients.

Finally, physical education teachers no longer can work unmonitored in their gymnasiums and athletic fields. More and more they are exposed to questions of the sometimes naive but always intense parents who, with legal support, may want to know just *what* objectives are planned, *why* things are being done to reach these objectives, *what* the expected outcomes may be, and exactly *when* these goals may be realized. Furthermore, parents have the legal right to constantly review programs and to aid in formulating additional objectives. Physical education teachers must deal in goals, activities, and objectives that are highly visible to parents, fellow professionals, and the children and youth themselves!

The scrutiny that has been alluded to should have a salutary effect on program development and implementation if (a) professionals are to emerge from college and university programs well trained not only in theory but also in meaningful laboratory experiences with "real children"; (b) school districts and the public itself are willing to finance facilities, equipment, and personnel in ways that will bring optimum services to those clamoring for them; and (c) those presently in the field are flexible enough to seek change and betterment, not only in their personal backgrounds and theoretical understanding but also in the methodologies they bring to the children and youth they serve.

Achieving objectives, however, is not always easy. An initial stumbling block is to determine just who special children are in populations of so-called normal children. Who are the ones who must be singled out and provided with special services? Just how handicapped must children be, and in what facet of their physical or mental make-up, before individual attention is accorded them? Into what categories should these children be placed administratively after being identified? Most important, what tools are available to identify children who are different? After children are identified, how must they be dealt with? What exact form must services take?

This book concentrates on children whose behaviors and capacities make them both different and disadvantaged in relation to normally functioning children and youth. Although definitions arrived at by Dunn (1973) include rather broad references to children who "differ from the average" and who require "special ancillary services" to achieve levels commensurate with their respective abilities and Kirk's (1972) definition similarly might include emotionally, physically, and intellectually superior children, the meaning of legislation in

The Education for all Handicapped Children Act (Public Law 94-142) is quite specific in its language. It focuses efforts on children who are *deficient* and different, not superior and different. PL 94-142 quite clearly mentions that adapted physical education must constitute part of the services available to special children. Both general and regular physical education services must be provided to special children, with the general services "specially designed, if necessary." Further, "each handicapped child must be afforded the opportunity to participate in regular physical education programs available to the nonhandicapped children."

In section 121a.4 of this same law, the components of physical education for special children are clearly spelled out to include "special physical education, adapted physical education, and motor development, means for development of physical and motor fitness, fundamental skills and patterns, body mechanics, individual and group games and sports, skills to include intramural and lifetime sports, and dance and movement education." Section 121a.225 clearly delineates the specifications for each child's individualized education program (IEP). (These guidelines and their implications will be discussed in the next chapter.)

Thus, the legal and moral mandate seems clear: All special children must be served with appropriate physical education. But the implementation suggested by this seemingly simple tenet is not easily accomplished. These children first must be located and identified. Means for getting them into appropriate special or regular programs, or a combination of both, must be provided. Most difficult, the law states clearly that services provided must be the "least restrictive" to the child's progress. Thus, placement of children with reference to physical education is a constant challenge—one that requires assessment and continual reevaluation, as well as adjustments over time by both teachers and administrators.

INCIDENCE AND PREVALENCE

Legal documents relative to special education and services usually group children into neat categories. As mentioned, PL 94-142 defines the deaf, blind, physically handicapped, and so forth. In the real world, however, astute professionals realize that children's abilities lie on a continuum, many times approximating the curve of normal distribution. In the case of physical handicaps, this is true. Some "handicapped" children have minimal motor problems and function reasonably well with compensations in many of the school's activities. The number of these children has been estimated to range from 8% to 15%. Still another 20% to 30% of children in regular schools may evidence what has been termed "neurological soft signs," or subtle problems, such as minor indices of incoordination or wearing glasses.

If one collects large numbers of scores reflecting human abilities and characteristics (height and weight, for example), the scores tend to arrange themselves in the following manner.[1] The majority (over 68%) is clustered around the average, with a decreasing number of scores at the extremes. Statisticians have assigned *standard deviations* (SDs) to groups of scores that extend from the mean in either direction, with 1 standard deviation occurring as the line depicting the scores changes from convex to concave.

---

1. A mathematician first noted this distribution when collecting the heights and weights of soldiers in Napoleon's armies in the late 1700s.

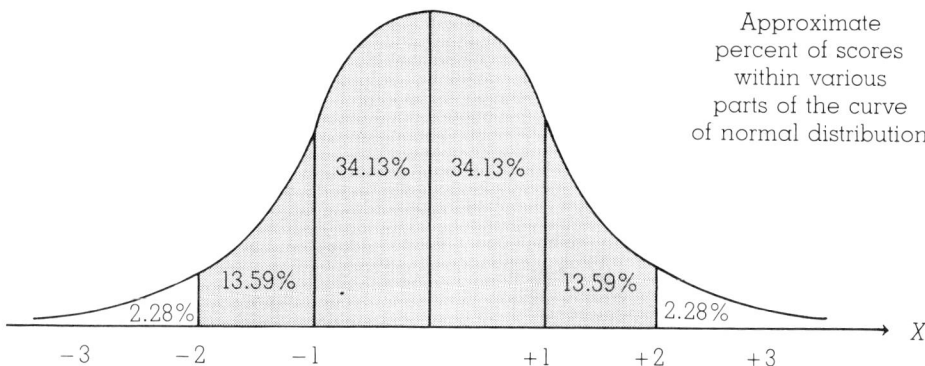

Approximate
percent of scores
within various
parts of the curve
of normal distribution

34.13%   34.13%

13.59%   13.59%

2.28%   2.28%

-3 -2 -1 $+1$ $+2$ $+3$ X

This general notion has been used in several ways to reflect and at times to identify people and populations whose differences are great enough to warrant special labels, as well as special attention in the form of educational programs. For example, test scores on the Wechsler Intelligence Scale for Children that are more than 2 standard deviations below the average have come to denote mild retardation, while scores on the same test that are below 3 standard deviations (a score of about 50) signify moderate mental retardation. Conversely, gifted children must score more than 2 standard deviations *above* the mean (on the Wechsler as well as the Stanford-Binet).

Reference to this curve and the notion of standard deviations from the average or mean are met throughout the book and have relevance for understanding how the abilities and characteristics of various handicapped groups differ from the "average" curve of normal distribution. For example, many physical abilities of the moderately retarded are, on the average, about 1 standard deviation below the mean of similar scores obtained from "normal" populations. In another context, the fitness scores of a group of blind children may tend to be more than 1 standard deviation below the mean of scores obtained from sighted youngsters. The same is true when comparing running and throwing scores of blind and sighted populations.

One should consider carefully *why* such differences exist. In truth, the differences are often the result of differences in programs available, as well as opportunities available to the handicapped, rather than simply a result of the handicapping condition itself. With adequate physical education programming, the fitness and the performance scores of retarded children often approximate those of children with average intelligence. The same differences may be reduced through adequate programming for blind and deaf populations.

A further impediment to the exact categorization and placement of groups of special children is the fact that many children with a given problem (e.g., blindness) also possess other abnormalities. Blind children, for example, may evidence neurological impairments by incoordination associated with the deficiency in behavior by which they are *mainly* classified. An unknown but considerable percentage of children with moderate motor problems who have an average or above average IQ also evidence some degree of emotional instability. Their frustration in games and in trying to write and print can lead to behavioral problems that require attention.

Thus, when working with a given child, a variety of services is likely to be needed. The "label" placed on a child may be a reflection of the most obvious problem rather than a true and comprehensive identification of the entire spectrum of the handicapping condition.

WHO IS HANDICAPPED AND IN NEED OF SPECIAL SERVICES?

Public Law 94-142 contains definitions of categories of students eligible for special education services (including adapted physical education), as synopsized in Table 1.1. In addition, Public Law 95-602, signed in 1978, changes the meaning of *developmental disability*. That label now encompasses mental retardation, cerebral palsy, autism, and epilepsy, among other disabilities. State councils are established to define the needs of developmentally disabled citizens.

HISTORY AND BACKGROUND—A WORLDWIDE VIEW

Exercises believed to have medical value may be found within the historical writings of many countries of the world. The culture of ancient (and modern) China contains exercise rituals that combine both spiritual and physical components of the human personality. These rituals, still practiced by many each morning in the parks of Chinese cities (see chapter

TABLE 1.1   Categories of Handicapping Conditions and Their Definitions

Label	Definition
Mentally Retarded (MR)	Significantly subaverage intellectual functioning, including deficits in adaptive behaviors, adversely affecting child's educational performance.
Orthopedically Impaired (OI)	Severe structural impairment adversely affecting educational performance. Includes congenital anomalies caused by disease, as well as impairments from other causes.
Speech Impaired (SI)	A communication disorder such as stuttering, impaired articulation, language impairment or voice impairment, which adversely affects educational performance.
Seriously Emotionally Disturbed (ED)	Inability to learn, which cannot be explained by intellectual, sensory, or health factors. Inability to build or maintain satisfactory interpersonal relationships with peers and teachers. Inappropriate types of behavior or feelings under normal circumstances. General pervasive mood of depression or tendency to develop physical symptoms or fears associated with personal or school problems. Includes schizophrenic and autistic children.
Visually Handicapped (VH)	Visual impairment that, even with correction, adversely affects educational performance. Includes both partially seeing and blind children.
Deaf (D)	A hearing impairment so severe that child is impaired in processing linguistic information through hearing, with or without amplification, which adversely affects educational performance.

26), continue to contribute to the flexibility and bodily vigor of middle-aged and older Chinese people.

More recently during the 1800s, European systems of medical gymnastics arose, particularly in Germany and Sweden. The Swedish system of medical gymnastics instigated by Ling contained a series of "natural" movements meant to improve a number of bodily functions including digestion and functioning of the heart and lungs. This form of graceful exercise, in part, has evolved into modern rhythmic gymnastics—now an asthetic competitive sport for women worldwide.

Early programs of physical education in the United States, both in the last century and in the first part of 1900s, were medically based. The leaders were university physicians who usually were in charge of health inspections and body improvement. The programs of vigorous exercise they proposed (a) were intended for "normal" children in an effort to improve their health and vigor, and (b) excluded extensive reference to social-emotional objectives that might be derived from physical activities and vigorous exercise. Thus, the justification for physical education during this period was the prevention of illness and disease and was directed toward the improvement of normal youngsters.

1930s-1950s

Expanded views of education, in general proposed by educational philosophers—notably *John Dewey*—based at Columbia University, began to find their way into physical education programs. *Rosalind Cassidy* and others began to influence teacher education philoso-

Table 1.1 Continued

Label	Definition
Hard of Hearing (HH)	A hearing impairment, permanent or fluctuating, that affects educational performance, but which is not included under definition of "deaf."
Deaf-Blind (DB)	Concomitant hearing and visual impairments, the combination of which causes such severe communication and other developmental and educational problems that they cannot be accommodated in special education programs solely for deaf or blind children.
Other Health Impaired (OHI)	Limited strength, vitality or alertness, due to chronic problems, such as heart condition, tuberculosis, rheumatic fever, nephritis, asthma, sickle cell anemia, hemophilia, epilepsy, lead poisoning, leukemia, or diabetes, which adversely affects educational performance.
Specific Learning Disability (LD)	A disorder in one or more psychological processes including understanding or using language, spoken or written, which may manifest itself in an imperfect ability to listen, think, speak, read, write, spell, or do mathematical calculations.
Multihandicapped	Concomitant impairments, the combination of which causes such severe educational problems that they cannot be accommodated in special education programs solely for one of the impairments. Does not include deaf-blind children but can include the retarded-blind, retarded-orthopedically impaired, and similar combinations.

phies and programs in physical education through writings incorporating more of a social-psychological approach to the formulation of objectives. Student-based curriculum decisions were advocated, replacing the stiffer, traditional, authoritarian-led games and exercises of earlier decades with more flexible programs and a wider range of activities.

The previous decades had seen "the battle of the systems," in which advocates of various programs of dance, formal exercise, and games emanating from various European cultures had come together. Now programs in the United States accommodated a number of components including games, formal exercise programs, physical ability and fitness testing, as well as dance and rhythms.

One of these components began to evolve into what was termed *corrective physical education* during the 1930s to the 1950s. Special classes were composed of youngsters identified as needing help in improving their vigor and posture. The children, screened from normal populations, usually were exposed either to group or individually designed programs of exercises in classes that often were smaller than those within the regular program. Asthmatics, and sometimes youngsters with heart conditions, were placed in these classes.

Most of the emphasis was upon posture. Some school districts even had beauty-contest-like posture competitions to select the boy and girl with the best "bearing" from each school. Having poor posture was an onus indeed, and those youngsters were banished to the "posture" or "corrective" physical class and teacher.

Teacher preparation curricula during this period usually contained one "correct" physical education course. Farsighted people, however, were beginning to ascertain that special populations had special physical activity needs. *Charles Buell,* for example, began to formulate programs and write texts designed for physical education for the blind in the 1950s, reflecting his work at the Berkeley School for the Blind. Educators of the deaf in similar residential programs likewise began to encourage sports programs for the hearing impaired following World War II (see chapters 6 and 7). For the most part, however, regular school programs did not include the broad range of children now served by special physical education services.

1960s

Trends away from the placement of handicapped children in residential schools led increasingly to these youngsters' entering the public school system. More and more programs dealing in special physical education began to emerge in schools specifically targeted for various handicapping conditions and found in larger school districts.

Additionally during these years a growing amount of research information became available delineating the nature of the physical abilities and fitness of special groups of children and youth. This data base made it apparent that many handicapped populations needed better physical education programs, and with establishment of these programs, improvement of the physical qualities of many handicapped groups could be expected. For example, one study (Cratty, 1967) showed that if educationally handicapped and retarded children were not afforded good physical activity programs, their fitness and vigor tended to drop during later childhood and early adolescence. *Lawrence Rarick,* among others, also began to study the physical qualities in special populations. Down syndrome youngsters were given special attention in these investigations.

In 1966 the Bureau of Education for the Handicapped in the U.S. Office of Education began to fund grants involving the training of special physical educators, as well as allocating monies that supported special demonstration and research projects.[2] These projects signaled the merger of physical education and special education at the national level.

Also during the 1960s two other trends and events gave impetus to special physical education. First, the *National Wheelchair Basketball Association*, founded in 1949, greatly expanded its program; and other, similar organizations reflecting an interest in sports participation for the handicapped grew in strength and numbers. Second, in 1968 the *Special Olympics* movement was started as the Joseph P. Kennedy Jr. Foundation, and leaders within the recreation department in Chicago, began to see a need for competitive sports programming for mentally retarded youngsters and adults. The program now encompasses thousands of youngsters and adults, with participation by many countries of the world, signifying that it is truly an Olympic movement of international proportions.

The 1970s, 1980s, and Beyond

During the 1970s and 1980s adapted physical education programs grew in number and quality. Their expansion and change paralleled growth and change in special education itself. Teacher education programs, stimulated in part by federal sponsorship, began to expand, and curricula began to contain more than one course in how to deal physically with special youngsters. More than one physical education program enabled undergraduate students to place their main emphasis upon physical education for the handicapped. More and more graduate student theses reflected an interest in how physical activity interacted with various handicapping conditions. These studies provided an additional data base for those interested in programmatic improvements.

Perhaps most useful to adapted physical education was the inception of the *Adapted Physical Activity Quarterly* in 1984. This journal provides a periodical pertinent to the specific needs of adapted physical educators, complementing journals directed toward a specific handicapped group (e.g., *American Journal of Mental Deficiency*) and those dealing with teaching the handicapped (e.g., *Teaching Exceptional Children*).

The 1980s also saw a powerful and expansive trend toward sports for the handicapped on the international level. The Scientific Congress held prior to the 1984 Olympics contained a special section dealing with sport and physical activity for the handicapped. Seven sports organizations for the handicapped met criteria for membership by the U.S. Olympic Committee under the U.S. Amateur Sports Act (PL 95-606). These include (a) the National Wheelchair Athletic Association, (b) Special Olympics, (c) U.S. Association for Blind Athletes, (d) American Athletic Association for the Deaf (whose deaf Olympics in 1985 was a hallmark event), (e) National Handicapped Sports and Recreation Association, and (f) U.S. Amputee Athletic Association.

The Olympic year of 1984 saw two events for the disabled in the "regular" Olympics and also the International Games for the Disabled held in Nassau County, New York, and in England (Stoke Mandeville). Over 1,500 blind, cerebral palsied, and amputeed athletes from over 50 countries competed in this event. More than 1,000,000 retarded persons around the world compete in various Special Olympic events each year. Individuals are busy col-

---

2. This office is now called the Office of Special Education Programs (SEP).

lecting basic research data intended to make these events even more useful and memorable in the future. This expansion of sports for the handicapped holds important implications for those who plan and conduct school-based programs containing motor activities for special children.

Contemporary Perspectives

Modern adapted physical education programs are broadly based and multidisciplinary in nature. The data upon which they rest are composed of information obtained from (a) special education in general and the teaching of special subgroups in particular, (b) basic medical and psychological information focused on specific abnormalities, and (c) information obtained from and directly related to adapted physical education itself.

The program content, and thus the preparation of teachers for the program, should contain provisions for gaining proficiencies in (and teaching) sports skills, improving fitness and vigor levels, and improving basic movement qualities, as well as opportunities for rhythmic and dance experiences. Likewise, the objectives of adapted physical education should be broadly conceived. These objectives are:

—the improvement of basic motor and physical qualities, including abilities necessary to move with precision, force, and endurance.
—the opportunity to maintain existing physical qualities.
—maintaining and improving the self-concept and other psychosocial qualities.
—improvement of children's self-perceptions of their opportunities to participate in a variety of contexts including dance, sport, and recreational environments.

An imperative quality needed by adapted physical educators and those who train and supervise them is *flexibility*. Varied approaches are necessary when implementing services in the 1980s and beyond. Children in special schools will likely be more severely handicapped than their more able peers, who have been mainstreamed in regular schools. The tendency to mainstream special children has created a situation in which fewer and fewer children with similar handicapping conditions are likely to be contained within one school environment. This has resulted in more and more special children being served by regular physical education teachers who, like their counterparts in classrooms, must bring special sensitivities to situations that are complex at best and overpowering at worst.

ROLES AND INTERACTIONS

Physical educators have several roles. Some of these roles and interactions are prescribed by law; others are up to the discretion of the P.E. teacher or are set by school district policy. In general, teachers have had to assume more expansive roles in recent years, and the range of people with whom they must interact also has expanded in the 1970s and 1980s.

Roles

Some of the roles a teacher of adapted physical education assumes are those traditionally held by all teachers of special children. Others are unique to the practice of adapted physical education. These include:

1. *Evaluation*. The P.E. teacher is involved in three chronological stages in the assessment process:
   (a) *finding* children who have special movement needs, including a district-wide screening, usually conducted at the beginning of the year, initiated by a parent, teacher, or through district policy;
   (b) initial *data collection* for a pre-IEP meeting, and parent contact for their consent;
   (c) *periodic updates* illuminating a child's progress prior to and as the result of further IEP meetings.

   The teacher-evaluator should be familiar with the types of tests available, such as normed versus criterion-referenced (see chapter 3) and be sensitive to the social ecology of the testing environment. Moreover, the teacher should be a professional interpreter of test results, including the ability to interpret results in ways that will be useful in formulating an IEP. This interpretive function should be able to be transmitted effectively both in written form and verbally in coherent explanations that can be understood by parents and others at IEP meetings.

2. *Prescriptive teaching*. The teaching role assumes that the physical educator possesses competencies in several areas including:
   (a) an awareness of and the ability to apply basic knowledge of motor development and motor learning;
   (b) the ability to translate knowledge of special needs of handicapped children into programmatic operations, strategies, and outcomes;
   (c) knowledge about equipment typically used in physical education, as well as facilities, devices, and equipment unique to special education and to adapted physical education for special children;
   (d) specific awareness of legislation and policies affecting special education in general and adapted physical education in particular, including provisions of the IEP;
   (e) the ability to apply effective learning principles in providing an effective teaching environment.

   Provisions must be made for motivation at high levels and for a social-emotional climate compatible with effective learning. Provisions also should be made for teachers' continuous self-evaluation. This may be done in an informal way, but formal provisions for self-evaluation are better, including the use of feedback from observing colleagues as well as from pupils themselves.

3. *Counseling*. Effective adapted teachers often must function in counseling roles. A number of people may interact with the P.E. teacher in this role, including:
   (a) *other teachers*. The P.E. teacher may have to interpret program content and goals to the classroom teacher(s) of children served in physical education. The P.E. teacher may have to understand and point out how similar teaching strategies and behaviors in two settings (gymnasium and classroom) interact and are compatible. Two-way communication in this professional interaction should contribute to the P.E. teacher's understanding of the individual needs of youngsters to which both the classroom teacher and the P.E. teacher are exposed.

(b) *parents.* Frequently, P.E. teachers are called upon to interpret to parents the meaning of program content, results of assessment procedures, and even the various models and theories that impact on adapted physical education. At times these interactions are formal, as prescribed by district policy or law; at other times the counseling may be informal and brief. In any case, P.E. teachers should be aware of the impact their counseling efforts may have upon parents and seek to present information in simple, nonthreatening terms. Sometimes, formulating phrases that may be used later in an informal counseling setting is helpful. Careless verbal communication during these sessions can have devastating effects on the emotional rapport between teacher and parent and upon the parent himself or herself. The teacher should be aware of the highly charged nature of parental feelings about their "special" children and avoid heightening these already volatile feelings.

(c) *youngsters.* Traditionally, all teachers have counseling functions in the educational lives of their pupils. Often, however, P.E. teachers have to fulfill rather unique counseling roles. Youngsters who are handicapped often look to their physical education teacher for specific information concerning the manner in which their limitations may translate into physical activity and recreational skills. At times they may bring up specific personal problems independent of the physical education setting. Teachers should carefully consider which personal problems may be discussed in a brief informal talk and which require the immediate professional attention of a counselor, psychiatrist, or psychologist. The physical educator should work closely with school counselors as well as counseling personnel outside the school.

4. *Community relations.* The role the P.E. teacher takes in the community may be mutually enriching. The teacher may become better informed of the community's needs and special interests. Members of the community, including individuals and groups (service clubs, etc.), on the other hand, may become better able to understand and aid programs for the handicapped in the community. Because of their unique roles in formulating special athletic events and the like, physical educators tend to have more opportunities for community involvement than do other teachers. This is a role that the P.E. teacher should seek when it is useful and should fulfill in a professional manner. Among the interactions adapted teachers might have with the community are:

(a) program needs, as presented in a speech to a service club in the community;

(b) fund-raising efforts, jointly coordinated between school and community groups;

(c) parent groups representing the handicapped groups, who may need special help in understanding the physical needs of their children and assistance in formulating ways to work with their youngsters at home;

(d) involvement with two or more community groups interacting in useful ways to provide resources for the handicapped (for example, a parent group and a community service group may be brought together in fund-raising efforts to provide new physical education equipment for the school).

Overall, the various roles overlap in the daily efforts of a physical educator. A child needs effective teaching and during that teaching asks a question that calls for the teacher's

counseling skills. A parental conference may be scheduled to provide assessment information, as well as more general information that again may require counseling skills. An effectively taught lesson may attract the attention of a visiting community group, which in
turn requests the physical educator to provide specific information about program content
and goals at its next luncheon meeting.

Professional Interactions

The P.E. teacher works in an environment with many professionals including classroom
teachers, curriculum supervisors, administrators, and school counselors. The physical
educator also comes in contact with specialists who are not of as immediate importance
as the classroom teacher. These include recreational specialists (therapeutic recreational
specialists, developmental specialists) as well as physical and occupational therapists, optometrists, and physicians.[3] Several of these specialists—among them, medical personnel—act
as professional advisors and support personnel for the physical educator. Others, who may
be viewed more as "teammates," might include physical and occupational therapists and
those interested in recreation for the handicapped. And parents and families sometimes
are overlooked as members of the team in providing the best possible services for their
children.

When dealing with these specialists, the P.E. teacher must bring into focus several
concepts: (a) knowledge of how each of the specialties views itself—its unique area of competence, and (b) how each specialty overlaps and is separate from the roles and services
the physical educator provides. A brief description of some of these specialties and their
relationships to adapted physical education and P.E. teachers follows.

Recreational Specialists   Two sub-disciplines of interest to the physical educator within
the rather broad discipline of recreation are *therapeutic recreation* and *community recreation*. In general, recreational specialists take a broader view and provide a wider range
of services than do physical educators. *Therapeutic recreational specialists* try through
recreation to bring about desirable physical, emotional, or social changes in people, including the handicapped. They may use art, music, camping, and horticulture in addition
to the sports found in adapted physical education programs. *Community recreation specialists*
draw upon a broad range of community resources to enhance the leisure time of all citizens.
Handicapped citizens and the aged often are included in their services, but they tend to
focus on the entire population of a community, the physically able as well as the disabled.
Community recreation specialists sometimes help the handicapped bridge the gap between
supervised living situations and independent living when such transitions are called for.

The role of the physical educator is more like that of the therapeutic recreational
specialist than the community recreational leader. The therapeutic recreational specialist,
however, incorporates a broader range of tools and services than does the physical educator
and enters more aspects of the client's life than generally is true of the physical educator.
Recreational specialists utilize the arts, drama, and the like more frequently than do physical

---

3. The list could well be extended to also include social workers, chiropractors, massage specialists, lay coaches
in the community, and so on.

educators. Recreational specialists (particularly therapeutic recreation personnel), however, often work with physical educators in parts of their programs that focus upon physical activity, fitness, and sports skills.

Physical Therapists   Physical therapists have a background in applied kinesiology and various neuromotor pathologies. They are educated to provide services emanating from various modalities including ultrasonics, massage, functional training, and the use of heat, cold, and water. (Two systems of physical therapy are reviewed in chapter 5.) In general, physical therapists who are well grounded provide individually tailored services, under the direction of a physician, to (a) post-operative cases in which muscles and actions need strengthening, (b) developmentally delayed children and youth, including the cerebral palsied, and (c) post-accident cases and post-trauma situations involving spinal cord injuries.

Physical therapists are broadening their philosophy. Within the last decades they have begun to view patients as social-emotional as well as muscular beings. Treatment often focuses upon larger muscle groups, with a particular emphasis on helping clients gain adequate locomotor skills.

Physical educators come in contact with physical therapists frequently. Some differences and similarities in the two professions are:

- Physical therapists more often work with individuals on a one-to-one basis, directing their attention at reeducation and recovery of specific muscle groups. Physical educators, on the other hand, more often work with groups and focus upon functional recreational and sports skills—often skills needed as youngsters interact within game contexts. Increasingly, however, physical educators are working on a one-to-one basis with special children.
- Physical therapists are not always trained in the nature of various behavioral disturbances but, rather, their education deals with the complexities of pathological neuromotor conditions and their remediation. In contrast, P.E. teachers with training in adapted physical education have been introduced to various behavioral disturbances, including emotional disorders, speech-language problems, and sensory conditions that limit people. Thus, most P.E. teachers deal with a broader range of client problems than physical therapists do.
- Traditionally the physical therapist focuses upon large-muscle skills including those that contribute to sitting, standing, and walking. The P.E. teacher, on the other hand, often must teach fine-motor skills including the hand-eye coordination needed when catching and throwing balls.

The P.E. teacher and the physical therapist often come together when both are dealing with developmental problems in children and youth. It is incumbent upon the P.E. teacher to (a) understand the general aims of the physical therapist when both are working with the same individuals, (b) with the guidance of the therapist, provide activities that will enhance therapy, and (c) avoid activities that detract from the physical therapist's efforts. For example, if the therapist is working to overcome the scissoring of a cerebral palsied child (see chapter 13), the physical educator should avoid activities that require vigorous work by the muscles that bring the legs together in a crossing manner (leg-assisted rope-climbing, the elementary backstroke, or other swimming strokes requiring a ''frog-kick'' action).

Occupational Therapists   Occupational therapists work developmentally in useful ways with youngsters, and employ some strategies similar to those used by physical educators. Often their backgrounds include more work in neuropathology and attention to the various modalities than is true of physical educators, however. Occupational therapy traditionally has focused on fine-motor skills, particularly those that involve vocational activities and those that contribute to daily living. These daily living skills might include dressing, grooming, and eating skills. When working on these efforts, the physical educator and the occupational therapist are likely to come together to work with the same child.

Occupational therapists also help in the introduction and use of various assistive equipment often needed by the handicapped. These devices may help a handicapped patient hold a spoon when eating, for example, or turn the pages of a book while reading. The roles of occupational therapy have expanded in recent decades to include all activity areas in which humans function, including work, play, and self-care skills.

According to PL 94-142, occupational therapy consists of "improving or restoring functions impaired or lost through illness, injury, or deprivation." Restoring of independent functions of daily living also are mentioned in that law as a function of occupational therapists. Finally, the law makes note of functions of interest to physical educators who work with younger children. It states that occupational therapy is concerned with "preventing, through early intervention, initial or further impairment or loss of function."

Of note to physical educators is a movement within occupational therapy that has spawned interest in *sensory integration*. Although at this writing the movement is losing some popularity within the profession, the services that sensory integration therapy purports to provide within handicapped groups closely resemble the goals that physical education teachers list and voice (see chapter 4). Thus, physical educators should become aware of those within the profession of occupational therapy who practice this type of therapy and have a professional and emotional investment in its outcomes.

Developmental Specialists   The label "developmental specialist" is often used informally, but several states of the union designate this specialty. These people frequently are found in tax-supported facilities helping parents of "suspect" infants and children to obtain remedial services. Their background may consist of a B.S. degree with a specialty in child development or a 2-year certificate from a community college. They focus upon a broad range of developmental problems—motor, social, psychological, and linguistic. For the most part, they deal with younger children, from birth to middle and late childhood.

Corrective Therapists   The corrective therapist often is found in a hospital setting. At times, adapted physical educators hold certificates in corrective therapy. The services of a corrective therapist, however, are not substitutes for adapted physical education services.

Dance Therapists   Dance therapists have backgrounds in the use of dance in rehabilitation or habilitation of the physically and sensorially handicapped, emotionally disturbed, and retarded. Their specialty may be interwoven with traditionally applied adapted physical education with excellent results. The preparation of dance therapists usually involves clinical experience together with classes in dance methodology and theory. Often they possess a Master's degree, and their ability to work with the severely emotionally disturbed can be an asset in a residential setting.

Optometrists   Within the past decade numerous developmentally oriented optometrists have offered services similar to those in adapted physical education classes. They often are from an *optometric extension program*, initially inspired by the writings of Gerald Getman and others who advocated the use of visual training (see chapter 5). Although some of these optometrists are expansive in their claims for visual training, others work in more conservative ways, helping with hand-eye coordination, for example, when a child's visual system seems to dominate and disrupt motor coordination, particularly printing and writing efforts.

A well grounded optometrist can work with physical educators to help them to understand how a child's visual-motor function may disrupt the ability to catch and throw balls, for example. At times both the physical education teacher and the optometrist are confronted with reeducation of the hand-eye, or foot-eye, coordination of a child who recently has undergone surgery to correct a "wandering eye."

Medical Doctors   Many interventions at the disposal of physical educators should be employed only with the consent and permission of a child's physician. Medical records must be consulted prior to working with any handicapped individual. Moreover, developmentally oriented doctors specializing in infancy, or adolescence, can be important helpers in remedial efforts of a physical educator. Physicians can advise physical educators what to avoid, as well as what exercise loads and tolerances handicapped individuals and groups can withstand. Although some perceive their role only as diagnosticians, many physicians recently are taking more active roles in the continuing supervision and follow-up efforts that reflect an interest in remedial-educative functions after they have diagnosed and assessed a child. Physical educators will find that some physicians (or situations) permit them more thorough medical conferences and support than other physicians (and situations).

Physical educators who, through design or carelessness, overlook or ignore medical advice pertinent to the children in their classes, do so at their professional and legal peril. Moreover, medical information that is needed should be sought prior to application of both moderate and vigorous programs of physical activity. In the absence of medical information, youngsters with special needs should be subjected to minimal stress involving passive recreational activities until the necessary medical data and information are obtained.

Psychologists   Psychologists of several types influence the adapted physical education program. Usually a school-based psychologist has had some role in the assignment of children to special classes, particularly if their problems appear to be emotional or educational in nature. Furthermore, psychological assessments usually contain drawing tests, indices that may result in a child being referred to a physical educator (or other motor specialist) for a more thorough evaluation of motor competencies, including gross motor skills.

Additionally, psychologists may follow the progress of children in the charge of a physical educator. The P.E. teacher may confer with a psychologist about a particular child, to learn how better to deal with problems that arise in class. Moreover, the psychologist may enlist the physical educator for aid with a child who is emotionally disturbed or has a behavior problem.

Parents and Family Members During the past 25 years I have evaluated between 2,500 and 3,000 neurologically impaired children at the university. During these evaluations I encourage my students to observe from a viewing room containing a one-way mirror. Also in this room are the parents of the children being tested. The experience for the students can be vivid, not primarily because they see an awkward child being tested but, rather, because they observe and listen to the reactions of the parents as *they* observe the testing, and they are permitted to attend the parent-teacher discussions that follow.

In this way the attending students are made acutely aware that handicapped children are not isolates but, rather, are critical and often central figures in a social system of varying degrees of complexity. Physical education teachers working with handicapped children should similarly realize that a handicapped child is a discrete and single "piece" of a usually complex social system composed of parents, friends, relatives, and peers. Thus, the behaviors that students evidence have served them reasonably well with other power figures and constitute strategies, circumventions, and devices that these important others have reinforced.

Some have suggested that the birth of an obviously handicapped child marks the psychological death of the perfect offspring the parents envisioned when they first began to discuss the pregnancy. A normal child is something the mother symbolically presents to the father, and the one they both in turn offer to their parents, the child's grandparents. When the infant is obviously flawed in some way, these social interactions can be traumatic. Moreover, the degree to which an infant is obviously handicapped at birth or its handicapping condition is gradually revealed during the months and years after birth permeates the family's initial and long-term feelings about the child.

In the 1960s and 1970s numerous studies addressed parent-child interactions in which the children were handicapped. Initially in the life of young handicapped children, distortions begin to appear in their relationships with one or both parents. Blind children do not return the smiles of their parents; deaf children do not echo the murmurings of their parents. Thus, an early and usually disturbing dissonance begins to appear in the social systems of families of the handicapped.

Parents of handicapped children differ along several dimensions relative to their feelings and interactions with their offspring. For example, in terms of acceptance, (a) some intellectually and emotionally accept the handicapping condition; (b) some intellectually acknowledge the problem but emotionally do not accept it; and (c) some reject, both intellectually and emotionally, the possibility that something is wrong.

Because of the social dissonance, parents may operate on at least two levels when seeking therapy and help for their child. At one level, they operationally try to do what is best; at another level they somehow may feel uncomfortable or even threatened when the sought-for help seems to make a positive difference. Their guilt or need for the child's dependence sometimes are better served when the condition is permitted to go uncorrected.

Thus, parents' feelings about their handicapped child undergo distortions—which is understandable. Parents may overprotect the child in loving—or in subtle, nonloving—ways. Overfeeding a retarded child is looked on by some psychiatrists as a subtle, hostile "mothering" act, to cite one example. Eheart (1982) found that mothers tend to dominate their retarded youngster and to produce children who are less likely to initiate social and motor behavior.

Clearly, the handicapped child represents a stress to the social system (i.e., the family) that he or she enters. The data indicate that such stress either strengthens the system (the parents pull together to help the child through this trauma) or causes the system to break down (divorce rates are relatively high in these families).

Grandparents are a consequential component in the social aura surrounding the handicapped child. At times they emotionally and intellectually reject the premise that anything is wrong with a child who represents their immortality on earth; at other times they act as valuable caretakers of the child, often supplying transportation to therapeutic sessions and even therapy itself to children who may be rejected to varying degrees by their parents.

Moreover, the family often contains normal peers who suffer some degree of deprivation of parental time and resources siphoned off for their less able sibling. This kind of deprivation may cause emotional problems in brothers and sisters of handicapped children that actually are more severe than the handicapped sibling experiences.

Physical education teachers, with proper guidance, can educate an older brother or sister to help a younger, less able sibling with the acquisition of physical skills. Knowledge of the nature of the family constellation, plus some time spent with brothers and sisters of the handicapped, may turn a negative, tension-filled social interaction into a positive, supportive one, as the more able siblings teach the less able sibling skills such as throwing and catching a ball.

With proper training and understanding, parents, too, can be important therapists/ physical educators, for at least two reasons: (a) They spend a considerable amount of time with their charges, usually more than anyone else in the child's life; (b) they arrive in the child's life first—and it has been continually demonstrated that early intervention pays greater dividends in improvement than do later interventions (Connolly, Morgan, Russell, & Richardson, 1980). One study, for example, found that mothers serve as effective therapists with young Down children (McInerney, McLaughlin, & Truhllicka, 1982).

Furthermore, parent involvement in obesity programs for retarded adolescents has been shown to be effective (Jackson & Thornbecke, 1982). In this latter program important parent understandings of how nutrition influences obesity resulted in a significant weight loss among both retarded adolescents and young adults.

Physical education teachers would do well to consider several ways of proceeding with parents who ask how they can help. With children who are 4 years of age and younger, parents should be encouraged to participate in workshops in which they are taught to work on a one-to-one basis with the child. After an initial meeting in which they have been given general and theoretical information, the child should accompany them to many of the sessions. With older children the parents also are helpful as volunteers but not usually when working with their own children. For the most part, older children already have received so many punishments and rewards from their own parents that parental reinforcers may not be vivid and useful. Too, parental tensions often interfere with the therapy. Children usually perceive that parents care too much when they perform or fail to perform a requested act. Parental anxiety heightens children's fears, which in turn feed back to the parents in a never ending chain of less than desirable behavioral events.

Classroom teachers or physical education teachers who want to help handicapped children should become sensitive to and aware of the nature of the family circumstances in which the child or youth has been functioning. This information, plus sensitivity to the total situation and taking time to counsel and aid parents and other siblings in interactions with their less able family member, may benefit all concerned.

Summarized, several principles should be considered by physical education teachers in interaction with parents and families:

1. Teachers should make every effort to determine both the obvious and the subtle feelings that exist within the family constellation relative to the handicapped child. This should not always be carried out in a direct manner but may at times be ascertained with the help of a clinical psychologist or other professional who has been dealing with the child and family.

2. Teachers should not be accusative or otherwise taken aback if they find that the feelings family members have about the child are distorted and involve some guilt or rejection of the child.

3. Many parents may be productively enlisted in the motor therapy of their own children or as aides with other children. Often, working as an aide helps parents place the problems of their own children in a more realistic context.

4. Other family members, including siblings and grandparents, with proper counseling, may be useful adjuncts to remedial motor processes. This should be considered a bonus, not an imperative family obligation.

5. When teachers are working with distractable and hard-to-manage children and youths, parents should be kept at a distance most of the time. Parents should be permitted to observe the therapy and program content without their children seeing them.

For the most part, a great deal of parental guilt and other distortions may be reduced if parents are given a realistic picture of the child's problems and progress relative to motor development and are armed with helpful and productive strategies and exercises with which to aid in the remedial process.

Figure 1.1 graphically presents the discussed information sources and service-givers in relation to the physical educator. The individuals listed in the blocks above and under the physical educator are sources of information about youngster(s). Those in the blocks on line with the physical educator are both information sources and service providers.

DELIVERY OF SERVICES

The mandate of PL 94-142 is to identify handicapped children in a community and to devise individualized programs for remediation that will impose the least restrictive learning environment on the child. This identification process —the crux of the matter—is dealt with in chapter 3. At this point we will consider in a rather global way just how services, including adapted physical education, may be delivered to those children and youth.

Models have been formulated reflecting the variety of ways in which educational services may be offered to atypical children. These services range from inclusion of the child in a regular classroom, to provision of special services and tutoring in a regular school, to confinement in a state hospital with other children evidencing a similar (and usually profound) disability.

Figure 1.1   Information Sources and Service Providers

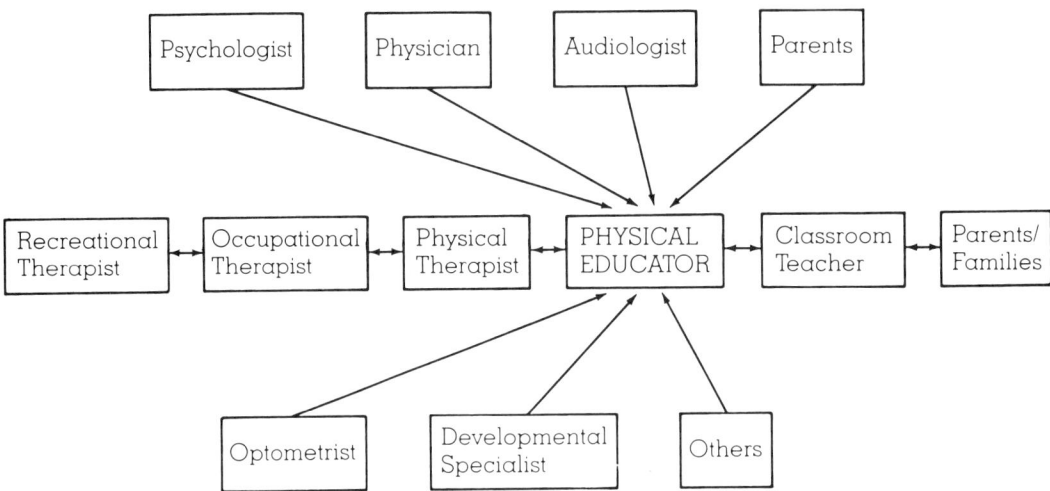

Deno's (1970) cascade system of special education services (Figure 1.2) is one model from which a range of possible services to the special child is projected. The tapered design of the cascade indicates the considerable difference in numbers of students involved at the different levels and calls attention to the fact that the system serves as a diagnostic filter. The most specialized facilities are likely needed by the fewest children on a long-term basis. This organizational model can be applied to development of adapted physical education services for all types of disabilities. Projecting physical education services within each of the seven levels of the model results in the following:

Level I

If the handicapped child functions normally in the regular physical education class, little or no aid may be given by the physical educator, other than periodic consultant services if requested or needed.

Level II

If the child is in a regular classroom, particularly if the child is physically handicapped, the physical education teacher has the job of providing specific services to the child and to others in the school with specific handicaps that permit grouping in a special class. The least restrictive environment provision of the law seems to mean that a handicapped child (perhaps confined to a wheelchair) may be more restricted if forced to play an inactive role in a regular physical education class in which relays are being run than if that child is permitted to exercise actively in a special physical education class. (Section VII of this book presents types of activities suitable for physically handicapped students.)

Level III

The physical education teacher may take handicapped children, in groups of either moderate-ly handicapped or obviously handicapped, into special classes once each day. The concept

Figure 1.2 Deno's Cascade System of Special Education Service

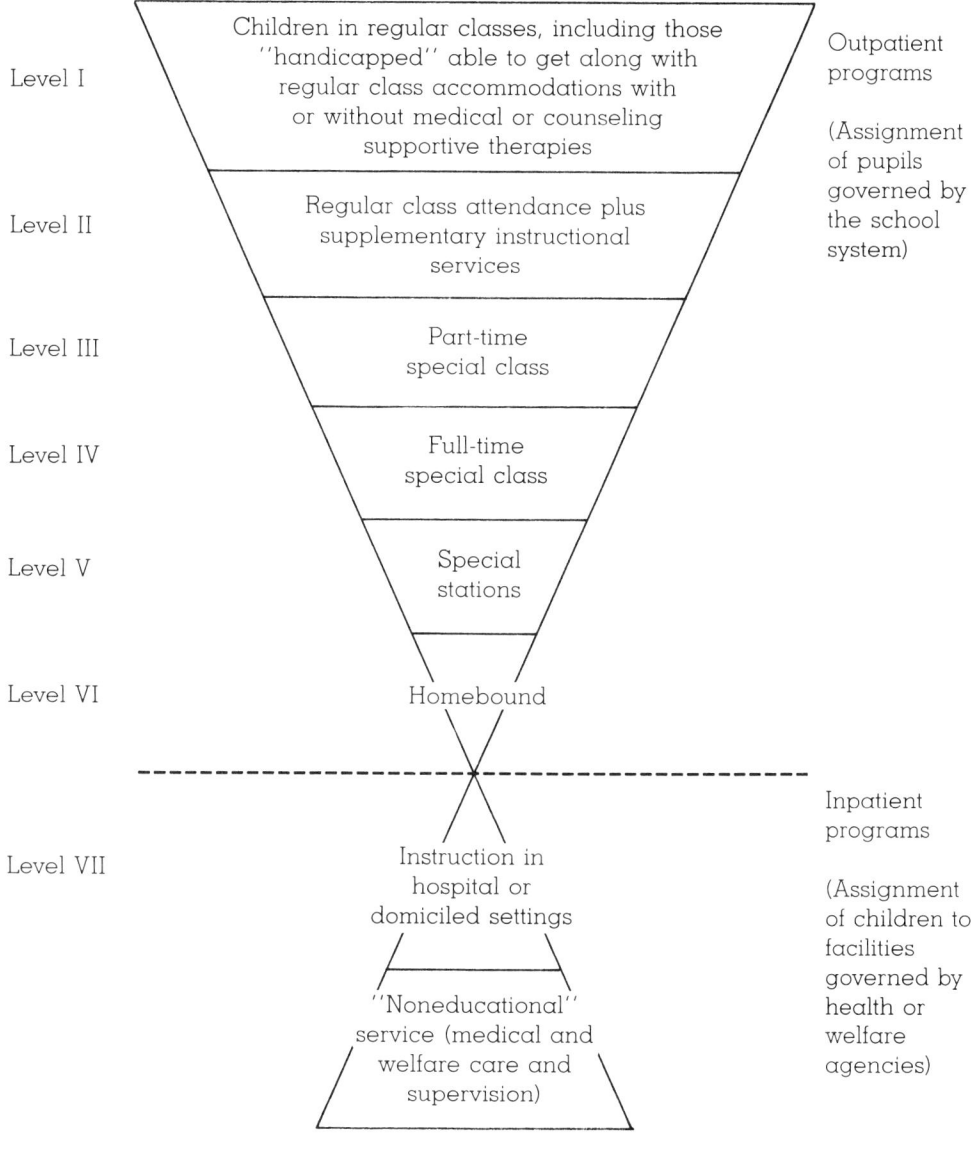

Level I — Children in regular classes, including those "handicapped" able to get along with regular class accommodations with or without medical or counseling supportive therapies

Level II — Regular class attendance plus supplementary instructional services

Level III — Part-time special class

Level IV — Full-time special class

Level V — Special stations

Level VI — Homebound

Level VII — Instruction in hospital or domiciled settings

"Noneducational" service (medical and welfare care and supervision)

Outpatient programs

(Assignment of pupils governed by the school system)

Inpatient programs

(Assignment of children to facilities governed by health or welfare agencies)

From E. Deno, 1970, "Special Education as Development Capital," *Exceptional Children, 37*(3), 229-237. Reprinted by permission.

of least restrictive environment may be specific to the functions a child is expected to exhibit within each portion of the school program rather than a measure of the child's performance in meeting the demands of a regular restricted school program as an amorphous, undifferentiated whole.

Level IV

Adapted physical educators function in roles in special schools and as offshoots of special classes, as indicated in Level III.

Level V

Special stations may be provided within a school, to which children may be assigned for help in the development of skills, fitness, and the like.

Level VI

Homebound children may receive services from a physical education specialist. Services may include: (a) initial evaluation to set achievable objectives and tasks for the home teacher and parent to work on with the child; (b) periodic assessments and readjustment of goals and sequences to be worked on; (c) conferences with one or both parents to cover principles and content of motor development programs, including sports skills, self-care skills, and fitness improvement and maintenance.

Level VII

Inpatient programs may or may not have the services of a physical education specialist to (a) work directly with the patients, or (b) provide inservice education for staff members who do contact patients. Evaluative and reevaluative services relative to motor fitness and development should be part of the job of the physical education specialist assigned to such units.

TRENDS

Contemporary trends important to physical education and educators include: (a) a growing research base, along with journals that present that research to scholars and practitioners; (b) an expansion at both national and international levels of sports for various handicapped groups including those with spinal cord injuries, cerebral palsy, and sensory impairments, as well as those who are motorically less capable, including the cerebral palsied. Competitions each year are in the hundreds, and competitors are in the millions.

Modern adapted physical education draws from the medical sciences and special education, as well as from knowledge about motor activity, motor learning, and motor development, in order to provide more and more comprehensive and useful services to children and youth with special needs. Professional colleagues from the therapies (physical, recreational, and occupational), as well as from the medical profession and psychology, provide information and inspiration to physical educators today. Program objectives in adapted physical education now incorporate ways to provide rhythmic-dance experience and the means to improve recreational and sports skills, as well as to improve and maintain the more basic physical attributes of strength/power, fitness, and accuracy of movement.

Finally, P.E. teachers—similar to those in other helping professions—are now placing special emphasis on improving social-emotional qualities among those partaking in their programs. Enhancing youngsters' self-concept is listed as an objective of equal worth to that of improving muscular endurance and fitness. Along with these objectives, the P.E. teacher is increasingly called upon to provide able assessments and to interpret these assessments in both formal and informal ways to classroom teachers, other professionals, and parents of those they serve.

SUMMARY

The evolution of modern adapted physical education has undergone several stages. Historical beginnings can be traced back to therapeutic exercises practiced within ancient cultures. The more contemporary trends have their roots in the last century, when forms of therapeutic gymnastics were introduced in countries of Western Europe. In the United States the flowering of adapted physical education has taken place only within the last 20 years, as youngsters with handicapping conditions became exposed to special efforts, spurred by federal legislation, to improve their physical welfare.

Those who may require special services include—in addition to the physically and sensorially impaired—the mentally retarded, learning disabled, and emotionally/behaviorally disordered, as they present unique problems that require individualized attention. Adapted special education services may be delivered in a number of different settings to youngsters ranging from very mildly handicapped to those with profound disabilities. Most often, the adapted physical educator or regular physical education teacher sees them in a regular school mainstreamed class containing mostly "normal" students.

In serving handicapped students, the physical educator interacts with a number of supportive professionals from other disciplines including medicine, psychology, counseling, physical and recreational therapy, and optometry, in addition to the obvious involvement of classroom teachers. Parents and families come into the picture and can provide a great deal of insight, information, and even volunteer assistance; in turn, they require the physical educator's support and feedback. Continual assessment and reassessment of a child's progress is required, the results of which are used to modify and update the student's individualized program.

REFERENCES

Connolly B., Morgan S., Russell, F.F., & Richardson B. (1980). Early intervention with Downs syndrome. *Physical Therapy, 60*, 1405-1408.

Cratty, B.J. (1967). *Perceptual and motor attributes of mentally retarded children and youth.* Los Angeles: Los Angeles County Mental Retardation Services Bureau.

Deno, E. (1970). Special education as developmental capital. *Exceptional Children, 37*(3), 229-237.

Dunn, L.M. (1973). *Exceptional children in the schools* (2nd ed.). New York: Holt, Rinehart & Winston.

Eheart, B.K. (1982). Mother-child interactions with nonretarded and mentally retarded pre-schoolers. *American Journal of Mental Deficiency, 87,* 20-25.

Jackson, H.J., & Thornbecke, P.J. (1982). Treating obesity of mentally retarded adolescents and adults. *American Journal of Mental Deficiency, 87*, 302-308.

Kirk, S.A. (1972). *Educating exceptional children* (2nd ed.). Boston: Houghton Mifflin.

McInerney, M.F., McLaughlin, T.F., & Truhllicka, M. (1982). Increasing eye-contact and instruction following behavior with a three-year-old Downs syndrome child with parents as therapists. *Journal for Special Educators, 18*, 71-80.

ADDITIONAL REFERENCES

Gearheart, B.R., & Weishahn, M.W. (1976). *The handicapped child in the regular classroom.* St. Louis: C.V. Mosby.

Jordan J.B. (1976). *Exceptional child education at the Bicentennial: A parade of progress.* Reston, VA: Council for Exceptional Children.

Spicker, H.H., Anastasiow, N.H., & Hodges, W.L. (Eds.). (1976). *Children with special needs: Early development and education.* Minneapolis: University of Minnesota, Leadership Training Institute, Special Education.

QUESTIONS FOR DISCUSSION

1. What are the roles outlined for physical educators in this chapter? What role(s) might you have more problems with? How might you overcome these problems? With what role(s) might you find yourself more compatible? Why?

2. How do the roles and strategies of the physical education teacher differ from those of the occupational therapist? The physical therapist?

3. What kinds of services for the handicapped are you most familiar with? What kinds have you not seen or heard of before?

4. Within which level of the model for service delivery do you see yourself personally, either now or when you complete your educational program?

5. What forces and conditions within your community have possibly influenced the incidence of various handicapping conditions? (Obtain data that may support your assumptions.)

6. How might physical education teachers' perceptions of personal role differ from educator to educator? How might these differences be reflected in the content of the offerings they present to handicapped children? In the evaluation tools they use?

7. With what other professionals might the physical educator consult and work? Which of these specialists have objectives closest to those of the physical educator? Which specialists perform only ancillary consultant functions relative to the work of the physical educator? With what specialists might a physical educator have more communication problems? How might these problems be avoided?

STUDENT PROJECTS

1. Interview individuals in your community who are physical education teachers. What are their specific duties?

2. Find out how special services for enhancing movement functions are delivered to handicapped youth in your community, and design a model to improve the delivery system if the present operating model is less than adequate.

3. Visit a treatment complex in which more than one specialist is delivering motor development services to a special population. Discuss with the professionals how they may perceive roles that may conflict or may be congruent.

4. Survey the literature in special education to learn how movement capacities have been addressed in the past.

5. Survey the historical literature in therapeutic recreation, special medical exercises, and physical education in general for trends throughout the century that have contributed to present practices and attitudes about special remedial physical education for handicapped children and youth.

6. List contemporary trends and issues pertinent to physical education teachers, individually. Then discuss them in a group.

RESOURCES

Adapted Physical Activity Quarterly
Human Kinetics Publications
Champaign, IL 61820

Council for Exceptional Children
1920 Association Dr.
Reston, VA 22091

Exceptional Education Quarterly
Aspen Systems Corp.
1600 Research Blvd.
Rockville, MD 20850

Minnesota Outward Bound School
  (Courses for the Handicapped)
308 Walker Ave.
South Wayzata, MN 55291

National Foundation/March of Dimes
1275 Mamaroneck Ave.
White Plains, NY 10605

Rehabilitation International USA
20 W. 40th St.
New York, NY 10018

2 Laws, Trends, and Individual Programs

The ways in which adapted physical education programs in the United States are, and must be, conducted in the last two decades of this century are the result of national trends, expanding philosophies, and laws dating back to the 1950s. During the late 1950s both the private and public sectors began spending an increased amount of money on support services for the handicapped. Expenditures were directed at, among others, speech pathology, psychiatric and psychological counseling, vocational training and placement, physical and occupational therapy, and more comprehensive educational programs including remedial physical education. This expansion of services brought about an awareness that meaningful changes could be elicited in children and youth who needed help and that multidisciplinary approaches are needed when working with a single child; special school placement is not enough.

Moreover, civil rights legislation beginning in the 1950s and expanding in the 1960s provided further impetus to the notion that equal opportunities should be extended to all within American society—to all races and ethnic groups, as well as to all who were somehow "special" and in need of enrichment and help. By the end of the 1970s, legislation had established the principle of nonrestrictive placement of handicapped children in educational programs. Throwing off the notion that "different" children and youth should be cloistered either in remote residential schools or in separate day schools, enlightened changes in philosophy, court rulings, and laws decreed that handicapped youngsters should be permitted and prepared to interact with their more fortunate peers from early in their educational and social lives. In 1971, for example, the principle of "least drastic educational placement" was seen in the ruling of *Mills v. Board of Education of the District of Columbia*. It implied that if a child might be placed in two or more educational settings, that child should be placed in as normal a setting as possible—one in which little interference with normal educational growth would likely take place.

EDUCATION FOR ALL HANDICAPPED CHILDREN ACT

In 1975 the Education for All Handicapped Children Act (PL 94-142) firmly established the principle that handicapped children could be placed in special classes and environments only when a regular class (plus special auxiliary services) would not meet their needs. Passage of PL 94-142 further established detailed principles and guidelines for programs for the handicapped that had an impact more powerful than any previous educational, legal, or historical event in American special education. This law not only expanded and made more specific the principle of the least restrictive environment but also presented in detail the guidelines for how individualized education programs (IEPs), for those found to have special needs, should be formulated, agreed upon, and carried out.

Least Restrictive Environments

The following points relative to the concept of least restrictive environment are of critical importance:

1. A handicapped child, even if given a precise label, must be thought of in a flexible manner when planning that child's educational program.

2. Placement of a child may not be fixed and immutable but, rather, temporary and, upon review, modifiable. The desirable goal is to move the child upward into programs that more and more resemble those of normal children.

3. The needs of a given handicapped child may be highly varied, and thus individualized programs containing both regular and special services may be combined to provide a least restrictive educational setting.

4. Even though PL 94-142 seems to indicate that moving a child upward (with reference to Deno's model in chapter 1) into facilities and educational settings habituated by normal children is desirable, a child with a problem may find certain "normal" situations (or components of situations) *more restrictive* to educational and emotional well-being than special situations and programs for that child's development.

For example, children in a wheelchair, when taking physical education with physically normal youngsters, may find themselves placed in a highly restrictive situation in which they cannot participate. Thus, those children may be better served in a less restrictive manner—by being provided special equipment, program content, and instructional services with other similarly handicapped children. During another part of the day, those same children may be served best educationally by receiving their academic lessons in a regular school classroom.

Children or young adults also may be served best in the least restrictive manner if their placement is altered at various times during a school year. For example, a profoundly deaf youth might be placed for a few months in a class of normally hearing youngsters, after which he or she might again be best served by returning to a class or school for the hard of hearing. Further, the most involved children in a handicapped group may not be the ones who necessarily profit least or most from a change in placement but, rather, those who are emotionally or academically suited to changes in either direction.

Over time, therefore, children may be moved from more to less restrictive environments as their needs warrant. Implied in this concept is the idea that the abilities of handicapped children are not "carved in stone." Positive changes may occur—modifications of emotional fiber and academic competencies, as well as physical and linguistic abilities that periodically demand (a) a review of progress and evaluation of current status, (b) frequent reassessment of what least restrictive environment means for a particular child at a particular point in time, and (c) possible modifications in the type of services that may produce optimum progress in the future.

Recent Trends

During the past 10 years implementation of these procedures has had identifiable effects upon special education in general. Demands by parents for early intervention have tended to decrease needs for future services. A marked reduction has occurred in handicapped people residing in state residential institutions. Only about 7% of the handicapped population is now being educated in special schools, and those who remain in those schools tend to rank lower on developmental scales.

Parents are taking a more formal role in the education of their special children. Informed parents are becoming more and more critical and evaluative of IEP meetings and tend to monitor their child's progress more closely. Moreover, they carefully prepare themselves for IEP meetings in ways more useful than in the past. Special publications (Mori, 1983) are appearing to help parents in their roles as partners in educating their child and for their part in formulating IEPs.

Some people are beginning to question whether an overemphasis upon mainstreaming is not in reality producing *more* restrictive environments for some students than was true within more traditional settings for education of the handicapped. Finally, a tendency to decategorize children and reduce labeling (e.g., mentally retarded, emotionally disturbed) sometimes comes in conflict with carefully worded laws for implementation of programs for the handicapped. The legislation requires categorization and labeling for the primary purpose of determining who is eligible for special services and appropriating the necessary funds.

Implications of the Legislation

Numerous implications for administrators of programs of adapted physical education, as well as for physical educators, have arisen from the least restrictive environment portion of PL 94-142. Some of these implications are philosophical; others are operational. It is not incumbent on physical education teachers to interpret subtle nuances of the law and formulate the manner in which it is operationalized by the school district. But it is the obligation of physical education teachers of special children to *understand* the principles involved and to have an *awareness* of the options that may arise from these principles. Some of the more important implications are:

1. Physical educators (or administrators) should be able to provide a *range of services* including direct work with occupants of institutions who may not have had any physical education in the past and provision of special classes and resources for children who are physically different and enter a regular school for the first time. Services also should encompass consultation with administrators, classroom teachers, classroom aides, and the like. This consultation may take the form of demonstration workshops, provision of books and materials, and direct or indirect evaluation and assessment, as well as direct work with children.

2. Physical educators should be aware of, and use hard evaluative evidence to make others aware of, the *heterogeneity* of physical capacities and abilities of special children. All children labeled moderately or mildly mentally retarded are not alike when exposed to opportunities to participate in games and physical fitness exercises or folk dances. All those who work with the children should be made aware of the diversity of physical capacities, as well as the differences in emotionality, that influence the quality and quantity of their participation in various components of physical education programs. Most important, these differences should be accommodated through individualized physical education programs for single children and special sub-groups of children.

3. Physical educators should be present, if possible, at all meetings and hearings in which the educational placement of special children is discussed. PL 94-142 specifies that physical education is to be included as a distinct and imperative service. Thus, the input of physical educators should be included in decisions that are made.

4. Discussions and consultations should be preceded by valid and thorough assessments of the recreational and physical needs of special children conducted by physical education teachers together with other specialists concerned with motor development. Occupational and physical therapists, for example, should determine in advance what components of the child's physical development might be their special purview relative to both testing and programming.

Thus, the concept of least restrictive environment, though seemingly expressed in simple words, in reality implies rather complex planning and professional operations. Physical education teachers should understand the flexibility and complexities the concept implies, and be prepared to bring their professional expertise to bear on implementation of the concept, as reflected in programming for special children.

INDIVIDUALIZED EDUCATION PROGRAMS

Perhaps the most important concept contained in legislation influencing special education is the individualized education program (IEP). Teachers and administrators for years have paid lip service to the ideas of planning program objectives related to the needs of both special and normal children. But the law brought about several mandatory and distinct changes that bear directly on the professional demeanor of school personnel.

These differences, related to the IEP, included the following:

1. For the first time, formal parent participation was required in planning goals and objectives for the child. Goals and objectives have to be approved by the children's parents.

2. Mandatory and formal conferences were provided for. Once a child has been designated handicapped, a conference must be held within 30 days, wherein the proposed individual program is discussed by the professionals involved and the parents, and the child, if appropriate.

3. Assessment procedures are needed and required. Prior to the first formal conference, the school district is obligated to identify handicapped children and assess them thoroughly. Members of the assessment team should be present at the initial conference, when the IEP is planned.

School districts have a degree of latitude as to how to institute, formalize, and implement the IEP for each handicapped child. The law, however, *does* specify that the program shall include:

—statements reflecting the child's present level of educational performance, together with statements reflecting short-term instructional objectives, as well as annual goals.
—statements indicating the specific special education and related services to be provided to the child and the extent to which the child will be able to participate in the regular educational program.

—projected time schedules containing the dates on which services will be begun and their anticipated duration.

—the objective criteria and evaluative procedures on which it is decided whether the short-term instructional objectives are being achieved.

The law is quite clear in stating that short- and long-term objectives must be formulated and agreed on. Program implementation and assessment procedures must be clearly spelled out. The law, however, does not hold the district or its personnel liable if goals for educational improvement are not met. The lawmakers were sagacious enough to realize that establishment of goals, as well as means for their achievement, does not guarantee success, given the unpredictable manner in which human behavior may or may not change under even the most advantageous educational circumstances.

Mandates of the IEP

Some of the specific mandates that the school district must abide by are listed below.

- Before the child is evaluated, the parents or guardians must be fully informed and give their consent to testing procedures applied to their child. This process is known as *informed consent*. If a child's problem is discovered through normally applied mass testing, this informed consent process need not be carried out. In most cases, however, identification of problems through mass physical education testing should be followed up by obtaining informed consent and then applying more thorough testing procedures.
- Testing must be completed within 35 school days after receiving written consent from parents or guardians. During this period a meeting date for the IEP meeting must be set.
- Testing procedures must be presented in the language constituting the child's usual method of communication. Moreover, testing procedures should not discriminate either racially or culturally. The physical education teacher thus must consider how or if the testing tool used might reflect racial or cultural qualities other than the motor abilities tested for.
- Test procedures must be valid for the specific purpose for which they are used. Additionally, the performance measured must be specific to the child's educational needs. The validity issue is more clearcut, based upon scientific evidence discussed elsewhere, but the second part of this principle is subject to interpretation. For example, a medical problem alone may not provide justification for referral for adapted physical education services.

  A boy having epilepsy that is under control, for example, might well be placed within a normal physical education setting, whereas another child with moderate clumsiness preventing adequate physical interactions with peers at play might be placed in adapted physical education. In the latter case, despite the absence of any traditional medical diagnosis, the child's testing and placement provide reason enough for adapted physical education services. In the case of the epileptic boy, the medical diagnosis in itself is not reason enough for his placement and special physical education services.

- The law states that the decision for placement and planning the IEP must be based upon evidence formed after evaluation by a *multidisciplinary team*. Clarified in an interpretation of the PL 94-142 mandate by the U.S. Office of Education in 1980, the four options of physical education for a child with special needs are: (a) a regular physical education class, (b) a regular physical education class with modifications, (c) a separate class, such as an adapted physical education class, or (d) a physical education class in a separate facility, such as one within a school for the handicapped.

    Moreover, placement must be based on assessment of a child's *motor performance*, not on the child's educational classification. A student placed in a regular P.E. class requires no IEP. When a child is placed in a modified class, the modifications must be described in the IEP. Students grouped in separate classes or in a special school class for adapted physical education must have IEPs for physical education.

- Parents or guardians have the right to obtain a separate and independent evaluation of their child by a qualified examiner independent of the educational agency formulating the IEP. Thus, those who initially evaluate the motor competencies (and problems) of suspect children must be well qualified, thorough, and comprehensive. Often the P.E. teacher is the professional who first gathers evidence of motor dysfunction, obtained in an ancillary way by other professionals (psychologists, physicians, and the like). At times the adapted teacher may refer a child to others after motor testing.

- Parents or guardians must consent to any changes in the child's identification, assessment, or placement. The parents must approve any placement relative to adapted physical education.

The IEP and Physical Education

Implications of the IEP for physical education teachers are:

1. Physical education teachers should take a direct role in the *assessment* of children's psychomotor competencies, including fitness levels, physical skills, motor abilities, and game skills. This assessment also might include manipulative skills, self-care abilities, and even handwriting and printing competencies, if the background of the physical education teacher permits it and these ancillary parts of motor assessment are not integrated into developmental evaluations performed by other professionals.

2. Physical education teachers should aid in the formulation of reasonable and attainable *short- and long-range goals* for inclusion in the IEP. This goal setting assumes that the background of physical educators is adequate to ascertain developmentally what can be reasonably expected in improvement over 3-month, 6-month, and 1-year periods. Physical educators should be capable of properly dividing components of the children's psychomotor behaviors into discrete and understandable components. Examples of skill assessment, as well as reasonable goals, are found in chapter 3.

Despite the fact that the school district and, by inference, the teacher is not liable for the child's failure to attain goals stated on the IEP, the mere inclusion of various objectives

In summary, from an operational standpoint the sequential steps in developing an IEP are:

—obtaining parental consent.
—evaluating the child.
—reviewing services available to meet the assessed needs.
—presenting data and program needs, previously discussed and collected, at an IEP conference.
—preparing a written plan.
—disseminating the plan to all who will participate in the child's educational program.
—continually monitoring the student's performance.
—evaluating student progress toward initially formulated goals. During this evaluation overall effectiveness of the IEP is assessed and decisions are made about any modifications that may be needed, including additional services, if necessary. These reevaluations must be carried out annually but usually are done more often. Decisions about further IEP conferences also are made at this time.

More detailed information on writing and implementing IEPs is found in many sources, including Deno and Mirkin (1980), Deno, Mirkin, and Wesson (1984), Lovitt (1980), and Torres (1979).

implies that the goals are valid and capable of being achieved over the time period(s) specified. To create and maintain harmony and unity of purpose in the group of professionals and parents involved, physical educators and others concerned with formulating objectives should arrive at identifiable goals that are likely to be attained with reasonable effort (on the part of the children and the teachers).

3. Physical education teachers have the responsibility for delineating *delivery service* that will lead toward achievement of psychomotor goals and for stating in what way they will either offer directly or supervise those who offer services to the child. The physical educator may be responsible for making clear to members of the IEP conference just where services will be offered, at what level (special class, individual basis, regular physical education program, home exercises, etc.) they will be offered, and the nature, as well as the quality, of the personnel and facilities available to initiate and carry out these services.

4. Physical educators should stand ready to meet with personnel and parents in further informal or formal *conferences* to explain what goals have or have not been met and why, and to carry out further appraisals of the children's movement attributes so that goals and delivery services can be modified if necessary. Recommendations for further placement relative to providing physical education services should emanate from the physical education teacher.

Long-Range Goals   The physical education teacher, with the help of others, is required to formulate both long-range and short-term goals. Moreover, the P.E. teacher is required to state how much time will be required to reach these goals. For the most part, long-range goals are a reflection of the overall nature of the program available within the administrative unit. Therefore, long-range goals may involve formulating which components of a physical program will be utilized and thus are available to the youngster. By their very nature, long-range goals are less precise than short-term objectives, which in addition address the precise behaviors or skills to be taught or changed.

A long-range goal might consist of teaching the child a simplified form of volleyball (one that involves catching and rethrowing the ball, for example). Another goal might be to introduce the child to rudimentary aquatics, involving water familiarization, basic floating positions, and initial stroke mechanics. If the program is comprehensive enough, a third goal might be to teach the child basic rhythmics using simple dance movements and simple percussion instruments. *Long-range goals reflect a year's plan.* Short-term behavioral objectives are intended to reflect more specific developmental tasks.

Long- and short-term goals interlace to present a blueprint for the year's program. Short-term objectives are placed within general components of the program reflecting long-range goals.

Short-Term Objectives   When formulating the "motor" portion of a youngster's IEP, the P.E. teacher is faced with a responsibility that requires specific, precise, and professional action. Several principles are inherent, including (a) measurability of objectives, (b) precision of objectives, (c) comprehensiveness of objectives, (d) reasonable steps in goals setting, and (e) matching objectives with program content, evaluative tools, and test components.

Measurability   Objectives on the IEP must be measurable in terms and units that are apparent to all. This is not to say that somewhat subjective qualities, such as an improvement in attitudes toward physical education, might not be included. But if that objective is included, the means to evaluate attitude should be stated in the pre- and post-evaluative program.

Thus, an objective stating that a child "will be taught to run with better form" is not acceptable. But if three or four stages in running form are specified and may be reliably scored by two independent observers, an objective that the child "shall become able to run with an appropriate cross-extension pattern involving the opposition of arm and leg-knee action" would be acceptable.

For the most part, however, measures of "form" are not as amenable to inclusion in an IEP as are measurements of the *results* of actions. These more measurable objectives could include:

1. Progresses from 4 to 6 push-ups using good form.
2. Is able to throw an 8"-diameter rubber playground ball 4 of 5 times to another child 10 feet away so that it is catchable.
3. Can make 3 "baskets" in a garbage can placed 5 feet away.
4. Can go through an entire lesson without evidencing angry physical or verbal behavior toward others in the class.
5. Can pass a simple, verbally applied test of 4 basic rules of basketball [list rules].

Precision   The principle of precision is closely aligned with measurability. Precision implies that an objective should be stated so that all (including lay members) can understand and agree upon what is being stated. Vague terms such as "improvement over time" or "evidences more cooperation" or perhaps "becomes better able to play" should be avoided. Rather, the objectives should be precise, as in the following alternatives to the amorphous phrases listed.

Improvement statements should specify improvements of *what*. For example: "The child should improve in dribbling from the ability to dribble a ball while standing to becoming able to walk and dribble at the same time, for 15 feet."

"Evidences cooperation" can be made more precise by stating the *specific behaviors, when, where, and with whom*. For example: "The child should become able to cooperate with one other child in a 2-on-2 game of basketball for a period of 20 minutes with no significant arguments with the teammate or competitors."

"Becomes better able to play" should be expanded and modified to include *playing what, using what skills, in what ways*. For example: "The child becomes better able to play dodge-ball by achieving the ability to (a) move laterally to the left and right easily and smoothly, without crossing the feet, for a distance of 15 feet in either direction, and (b) becomes able to throw and hit a target (person) 5 feet high at a 15-foot distance."

Comprehensiveness   The principle of comprehensiveness implies that a reasonable number of motor objectives should be included. When contributing to an IEP, physical educators often proceed too conservatively and fail to include a reasonable number and range of objectives—objectives that in reality have a reasonable chance of being reached, given the program content to which the youngster will be exposed.

Factor analyses of motor abilities of both normal and atypical youngsters indicate that 6 to 8 independent physical qualities comprise total "movement personalities," and these might be included in a program intended to help children move better. These could include tasks involving (a) hand-eye coordination, (b) trunk strength, (c) agility involving movement of the total body, (d) arm-shoulder strength and/or speed, (e) precise finger dexterity, (f) balancing of various kinds, both moving (dynamic) and stable (static—e.g., posturing on one foot). These are exclusive of social-emotional goals, self-control, and other possible qualities that might result from application of a physical education program.

Physical educators who list only one "safe" and restricted objective (e.g., "Child becomes able to move a wall pulley 8 times using a 10-lb. weight) might examine the program make-up, for indeed the program may be highly restrictive in nature. Playing a game and not requiring the exhibition of three or even more abilities, for example, is not likely. Including three movement objectives, however, might be a reasonable contribution of the physical educator to the IEP.

Reasonable Steps   This is perhaps one of the most important principles to follow when formulating IEP objectives. It implies that the steps should be gradual and well within the child's ability to accomplish and the teacher's purview to teach. Though laws, of course, do not *require* objectives be reached, everyone concerned will be happier if they are! Therefore, the P.E. teacher should be well equipped with knowledge of the small increments in motor development/performance that underlie each developmental stage or task. In this way, a small but significant gain may be listed in the IEP and the youngster has a reasonable chance of accomplishing the objectives.

For example, a child who can jump (2-foot take-off and landing) but who cannot hop (1-foot take-off and same-foot land) might not be expected to suddenly gain the ability to hop within a 3- to 6-month period. Instead, the intermediate stage of accomplishing an "unsupported step" might be listed as an objective (taking off with one foot, a non-support stage, and landing on the opposite foot). An even more gradual improvement would consist of taking an unsupported step from a raised (6"-high) surface to a lower-level surface.

Or a child who can do a one-footed skip might not become able to accomplish a "true" two-footed skip in a relatively short time period. Instead, a supported two-footed skip, in which the youngster holds onto a support while simply repeating the movement patterns of the feet in a skipping rhythm without attempting the whole movement and balance involved, might be a reasonable objective.

As another example, exhibiting finger dexterity might entail first a finger opposition task (touching each finger in order to the thumb of the same hand), in which the teacher guides each finger into the correct placement to the thumb, then a stage in which the child guides one or two fingers to their correct placement, rather than the objective of accomplishing this task completely unaided. In a similar way, ball catching, throwing, and other movement tasks may be broken down into precise, discrete stages.

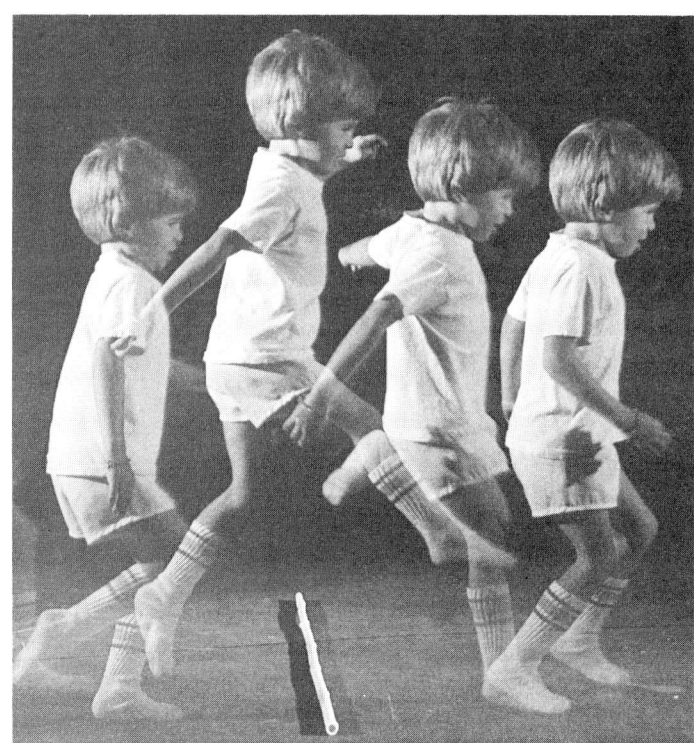

An intermediate step between one-foot hopping and two-foot (simultaneous) jumping is an unsupported step.

Reprinted from *Perceptual and Motor Development in Infants and Children* (3rd ed.) by B.J. Cratty, with permission of the publisher, Prentice-Hall

The physical educator runs no danger of overanalyzing tasks—particularly when formulating IEP objectives for more severely involved populations. Formulating objectives that consist of too large a leap forward only frustrates those interested in the content of the IEP and the progress of the child.

Matching Objectives to Program Content and Evaluative Tools   The careful matching of stated objectives to program content and feasible evaluative tools and tasks would seem an obvious principle—one that would be violated infrequently. All too often, however, this matching may not take place. Failure to match objectives with the program content and evaluation tasks may have the following outcomes:

- When stated objectives are not expansive enough and do not truly resemble program content, the quality of the program is not reflected in the stated objectives. The teacher-administrator shortchanges himself or herself. Often, more is happening in a program than the teacher involved realizes. When formulating objectives, care should be taken to analyze program content thoroughly.
- Conversely, if objectives stated are not provided for in the program, they probably will not be realized. For example, an "improvement in self-concept" goal often is stated, but the program offers no specific steps to improve the child's concept of his or her physical self. Provision for such improvement could be built in to a program by (a) exposing the child frequently to objective evidence of improvement, and (b) giving parents opportunities to observe, understand, and assess their child's progress so that their positive social feedback will contribute to the child's self-image.
- Finally, if program content is not adequately tested/evaluated, the quality of the program will not be apparent to all. The above stated self-concept objective, for example, should be accompanied by available tests of self-concept to determine whether improvement in this social-emotional quality actually has taken place.

Forms/Records   Figure 2.1 gives sample pages from forms typical of those employed to record the IEP and other data pertinent to formulating and executing a youngster's individualized education program. Forms vary from district to district, but these three contain essential information to comply with existing federal laws.

Form A-1 contains the child's personal data, together with results of evaluations, conducted by experts, on general health, vision, hearing, academic ability, social-emotional status, speech/language skills, and motor abilities. This information is accompanied by a notation indicating into what classification (type of disability) the child falls.

The second form, A-2, lists the personnel present for the IEP meeting and allows for the required parent approval/disapproval. It also gives general recommendations, as outcomes of the meeting, from vocational education, physical education, classroom education, psychiatric-psychological counseling, physical therapist, speech-language specialists, and others, as appropriate.

Figure 2.1 The IEP: Three Examples

Form A-1

Name _HOCH, PAUL LEWIS_ Birthdate _11/9/80_

Address _1210 SALTAIR_ Home Language _ENGLISH_

Type of Meeting _____

Initial ☑ Review ☐
Review, 3 yr assessment ☐

School _LINCOLN_ Teacher _SALTZER_

Evaluation Levels of Performance

☑1. Health _PRONE TO ALLERGIES_

☑2. Vision _20/20 RIGHT EYE   20/40 CORRECTED TO 20/20 LEFT_

☑3. Hearing _NORMAL_

☑4. Academic Ability/Levels _SLOW TO GRASP CONCEPTS ; WORKS BEST SM. GROUP_

☑5. Social-Emotional _HAS DEFICIENCIES IN SOCIAL RELATIONSHIPS_

☑6. Speech/Language _IMMATURITY IN SPEECH AND LANGUAGE_

☑7. Motor Abilities _OVERALL MOTOR ACHIEVEMENT > 5 YEARS_

☑8. Others _AUDITORY PERCEPTION: ITPA: AE I. 5.0 II. 5.2_
III. 4.0 IV. 3.9 V. 4.5

Eligibility for services/person with special needs

MEETS ELIGIBILITY REQUIREMENTS: EH — STATE OF
CALIFORNIA

Certificates Sought, Overall Goals

NONE SOUGHT IMMEDIATELY · HIGH SCHOOL
GRADUATION CERTIFICATE POSSIBLE

Figure 2.1 Continued

Form A-2

Individualized Education Program for <u>HOCH, PAUL</u>   <u>11/9/80</u>
Name of student   birthdate

Date of IEP <u>2/6/87</u>   Place <u>LINCOLN SCHOOL</u>

Participants: (Names, signatures, dates)

Administrator/Designee <u>L.B. PALMALES ·L·B· Palamales 2/6/87</u>

Teachers: <u>MARY SUE SMITH   Mary Sue Smith 2/6/87</u>

Others/Specialists/Specialties
<u>PAUL SCHIFFREN ADAPTED PE   PS 2/6/87</u>
<u>NELLIS RANKIN   ED. PSYCH.   NR 2/6/87</u>

Parents: _____

Decisions (check one)   I attended and approve   ☑

                        I was notified and could not attend,   ☐
                        reviewed IEP and approve

                        I disagree with IEP:
                        Evaluations (which?)   ☐ _____
                        Placement/setting   ☐ _____
                        Instruction/services (which?)   ☐ _____

<u>Brenda Hoch 2/6/87</u>   I wish to schedule an informal   ☐
Parent Signature/date   meeting to resolve problems

                        I wish to initiate a due process   ☐
                        hearing.

General Recommendations

Vocational Education	Physical Education	Classroom Education
NONE NOW – EX.	SPECIAL ADAPTED	12 STUDENT EH
CERT. IND. SHOP	PE – 3 HRS./WK.	CLASS
CRAFTS PROGRAM		

Other Special Services:

Psychiatric-Psychological Counseling	P-T	Speech-Language	Other
1 HR./WK. –	NO PT	2 HRS./WK.	2 HRS./WK.
GROUP COUNSELING		SPEECH/PATH.	REMEDIAL READING

Recommendations for Follow-ups re: Placement

_____

_____

Figure 2.1 Continued

Form A-3

Pupil Name _HOCH, PAUL_   Date of Meeting _2/6/87_

Annual Long-Range Goals and Short-Term Objectives

Instructional Areas Responsible Personnel	Short-Term Objectives	Evaluation Criteria

1. Instr. Area: _SP. CLASS_
    Goal: _PHONIC WORD ATTACK SKILLS_
 	
Responsible Personnel _MR_
beg. date _2/7_ end date _____
	a. _KNOW VOWEL SOUNDS_
	b. _HARD CONSONANT SOUNDS_
	c. _WORD ATTACK SKILLS AT 1ST GRADE LEVEL_
		Observation ☐
		Formal Test
		(which) _MET READING TEST_
		date achieved_____
		  not achieved _____

2. Instr. Area: _SP. CLASS_
    Goal: _SOCIAL – SELF-CONTROL SKILLS_
 	
Responsible Personnel _MR_
beg. date _2/7_ end date _____
	a. _KEEPS SEAT FOR 20 MIN._
	b. _SHARES MATERIALS W/ CLASSMATE_
	c. _____
		Observation ☑
		Formal Test
		(which) _____
		date achieved_____
		  not achieved _____

3. Instr. Area: _SPEECH–LANG._
    Goal: _IMPROVE ARTICULA-TION OF SELECTED SOUNDS_
Responsible Personnel _NR_
beg. date _2/7_ end date _____
	a. _ARTICULATES SH, PH,-CH-_
	b. _"THANK YOU" WITH CLARITY_
	c. _FORMULATES SOCIAL GREETINGS WITH EYE CONTACT_
		Observation ☑
		Formal Test
		(which) _____
		date achieved_____
		  not achieved _____

4. Instr. Area: _ADAPT. PE_
    Goal: _IMPROVE BASIC MOTOR SKILLS_
 	
Responsible Personnel _PS_
beg. date _2/7_ end date _____
	a. _LEARNS UNSUPPORTED STEP_
	b. _CATCHES BOUNCED BALL (8"dia.) 5 TIMES OF 7_
	c. _WALKS 10'4" BALANCE BEAM W/ALTERNATED STEPS_
		Observation ☑
		Formal Test
		(which) _____
		date achieved_____
		  not achieved _____

The final form, A-3, indicates more specific goals for the forthcoming program. Both long-range goals and short-term objectives are listed, along with how each specific objective is going to be tested and when the retest (or observation) is to take place. As indicated previously, the short-term objectives are specific and precise, and they suggest achievable steps forward.

SUMMARY

Current U.S. policies and legislation containing guidelines for educational programming of the handicapped arose from laws, attitudes, and philosophies generated during the 1960s and 1970s. Promises to minorities for equal rights were reflected a few years later in laws governing education and treatment of the handicapped.

Policies influencing educational programming include the concept of *least restrictive environment*. This involves optimum educational placement for all handicapped pupils in programs intended to maximize their opportunities and exposure to society at as early an age as deemed feasible. Moreover, these policies dictate precise and visible educational planning based on the individualized education program. The IEP requires participation by teachers, parent, administrators, and specialists, in developing long-range goals and short-term objectives and timelines projected for the child to attain these. Each program must be approved by all those involved. The IEP also is subject to frequent and regular review.

In this decade and the ones that will follow, continued adherence to these concepts requires professionals to maintain precise and valid programs of evaluation, along with carefully considered activities pointing toward achievement of goals that are reasonable and clearly spelled out. Writing short-term objectives in the IEP involves the principles of measurability, precision, and comprehensiveness. Moreover, these objectives should be written in ways that permit gradual steps of improvement. Goals, program content, and components of testing batteries should be in congruence.

REFERENCES

Deno, S.L., & Mirkin, P.K. (1980). Data based IEP development: An approach to substantive compliance. *Teaching Exceptional Children, 12*, 92-97.

Deno, S.L., Mirkin, P.K., & Wesson, C. (1984). How to write effective data-based IEP's. *Teaching Exceptional Children, 16*, 99-104.

Lovitt, T.C. (1980). *Writing and implementing an IEP: A step-by-step plan.* Belmont, CA: Pitman Learning.

Mori, A.A. (1983). *Families of children with special needs.* Rockville, MD: Aspen Systems Corp.

Torres, S. (Ed). (1979). *A primer on individualized education programs for handicapped children.* Reston, VA: Foundation for Exceptional Children.

ADDITIONAL REFERENCES

Nelson, C.M., Gast, D.L., & Trout, D.D. (1979). A charting system for monitoring student performance on instructional progress. *Journal of Special Education Technology, 3*, 43-49.

Price, M., & Goodman, L. (1980). Individualized educational programs: A cost study. *Exceptional Children, 46*, 446-454.

QUESTIONS FOR DISCUSSION

1. How did history seem to prepare the way for passage of PL 94-142? What problems arise in its implementation? Do you see a need for any future legislation to facilitate the physical education of handicapped students?

2. What are some possible problems and conflicts between professionals during the initial IEP meeting? What steps might be taken to reduce these differences?

3. How might parents be prepared for their participation in formulating IEPs? What might be the physical educator's role in working with parents?

4. How might physical educators facilitate the goal-setting process in formulating reasonable expectations for improving movement capacities in students?

STUDENT PROJECTS

1. Research the laws in your state reflecting the federal legislation described in this chapter. Did your state laws precede or follow enactment of the federal legislation?

2. Interview a principal or special education director and ascertain how PL 94-142 is being implemented. Discuss problems that occur in implementing the law.

3. Inspect an IEP form being used in a public school. In what ways does it reflect local (state, county, city) laws, and in what ways does it reflect the federal laws described in this chapter?

4. Interview, on two separate occasions, two parents of two handicapped children. Contrast their feelings and understanding of legislation affecting the education of their children. Does the type of disability seem to influence their attitudes and knowledge of the mandated role of the schools?

5. Keep a 1-week diary of what a physical education teacher of mainstreamed handicapped students does with his or her school-related time. This may be done through interview or by visiting the educator daily for 1 week (or once a week for 5 weeks). List the ways, and the amount of time, in which legislation influences his or her time.

3 Evaluation: A Vital Process

Educators throughout the world advocate the precise evaluation of abilities and progress made by children in the schools. Among the numerous theoretical and practical objectives and dimensions of testing are to:

—obtain an indication of present status.
—aid in the formulation of program objectives.
—determine the degree to which the objectives have been carried out, as reflected in student progress.
—give administrators an idea of teacher effectiveness.
—help teachers assess themselves in a valid manner.
—aid the instructor in perceiving slight changes in the behavior of difficult-to-educate children.
—help all concerned bring about modification in program content.

The philosophy undergirding how and what tests should be given to assess qualities important to an adapted physical education program should rest on a broad base of principles formulated for the entire school district. Recently an assessment tool was developed to encompass broad principles and reflect the needs of the school district relative to adapted physical education (Sherrill & Megginson, 1984). The Survey of Adapted Physical Education Needs (SAPEN) contains 50 items, divided into five areas reflecting (a) the significance of physical education in the district, (b) assessment and placement of children relative to the IEP, (c) instruction and programming, (d) personnel, and (e) other considerations. This field-tested assessment tool appears to be a reliable and useful means of ascertaining the overall relationship of an adapted physical education program to a school district's needs and philosophy.

The required individualized education program for the handicapped obviously places additional responsibility on evaluators. Thus, the physical educator, as well as others on the evaluation team, should be prepared not only to select and administer appropriate measures but also to justify and explain the measuring instruments to parents and others, including administrators and those taking part in the IEP conference, which may include the child or youth involved.

GUIDELINES FOR SELECTING TESTS

Extreme care should be taken in selecting tests from among the many evaluative instruments available—not only to satisfy appropriate technical standards (to be discussed later) but also to assure that the components of the testing program are (a) economical of the time and energy of the child and tester, (b) appropriate to the level of the child's development, both physical and emotional, and most important (c) adequate enough to be included in subsequent programming arrangements. To test for *something* implies rather emphatically that *something* is capable of being changed—or at least a change in that quality may be worked toward.

At times the tests selected influence placement of children in adapted physical education programs. Broadhead and Church (1984), for example, demonstrated how placement decisions might differ depending upon the motor test(s) selected for use with mentally retarded children. Some so-called normed motor tests may be more difficult than others, and thus a significant number of children may be misclassified unless care is taken in both test selection and interpretation of assessment results.

Therefore, when selecting testing instruments, adapted or special physical educators of the handicapped should keep in mind the large number of possible combinations of goals toward which children might work. These may include:

—obvious and real changes in physical capacities, recreational skills, and motor development.
—moderate changes in physical development brought about with the help of paramedical personnel.
—maintenance of physical capacities through involvement in recreational activities.
—improvement in self-concept through exposure to physical activities in the face of rather formidable obstacles to the modification of measurable physical capacities.
—improvement in attention span, general alertness, and responsiveness to simple or complex stimuli.
—development of self-care skills.
—improvement of children's social–emotional behaviors in the adapted physical education class.

The testing instruments should be appropriate to the testability of the child, as well as to the general nature of the child's apparent physical abilities and capacities. In the case of children evidencing moderate awkwardness, the tests may include content that resembles that of assessments administered to normal children. In the case of those more severely physically handicapped, situation-specific checklists might be employed from which a range of simple recreational skills (e.g., holding a ball in the lap) might be selected and administered to the population. Finally, scales that resemble those administered to normal young children or infants are sometimes helpful. These instruments are appropriate both for young suspect infants and for older children or young adults who might be labeled severely or profoundly handicapped.

Another dimension of a physical testing program is the precision of the instrument being used. The instrument's precision often reflects the quality of background of the tester. When surveying large populations, it is sometimes expedient, however, to first administer a rather crude checklist of developmentally appropriate tasks, by age, on which children are scored on a pass-fail basis. Following administration of this less precise instrument, children failing a given percentage of the items (usually items expected to be passed by about 80% of the population represented by those tested) then may be exposed to a more individualistic testing program. This second testing level more exactly confirms results of the checklist and suggests materials and content that are appropriate for the child's IEP.

Still another important consideration in formulating a testing philosophy and selecting tests is to determine how broad a range of tests might be assigned to the physical educator. In districts whose special services entail the time of many professionals, physical educators' assessment chores should be confined to those directly related to the more obvious components of their programs, including tests of physical fitness, recreational and sports skills, and basic motor capacities, involving balance, agility, and the like. In addition, physical education teachers should be familiar with evaluation instruments that assess self-concept, attention span, and hand-eye coordination as reflected in printing and writing effort, because these qualities are inherent in physical education goals and objectives.

Three major dimensions of any testing program, as illustrated in Figure 3.1, are *precision,* the *qualities* to be assessed, and *who* is to do the testing. Numerous other considerations are important, too, including the *time* required for testing, as well as the testers' *experience*, reflected in how well the overall program and individual testing instruments are interpreted.

PRACTICAL CONSIDERATIONS

Testability

Several technical and practical aspects apply to testing the physical abilities of the handicapped. For example, educators should first ascertain how testable the clients are. Elkin and Friedman (1967) devised five levels of cooperability:

1. Failure to respond to tester in a situation in which the child's motivation presumably is high.
2. Minimal response to tester within the same situation.
3. Imitation of tester in a simple task.
4. Compliance with simple verbal instructions given by tester.
5. Obeying tester's complex verbal instructions concerning test administration.

Comments relative to the child's testability, with reference to this scale, should accompany evaluation data obtained during a testing session to add depth and understanding to the objective measures obtained.

Some classifications of youngsters obviously pose more testing challenges than others entering an adapted physical education program. Even in the case of profoundly and severely retarded children, however, motor test scores can be obtained. Tomporowski and Ellis (1984), for example, described how they prepared individuals who were labeled profoundly and severely retarded for motor testing. They used *modeling* techniques (the severely retarded were models for the profoundly retarded) and *physical guidance* (prompts). Overall they found that some (but not all) of the clients they attempted to assess became more testable as a result of interventions imposed.

Figure 3.1 Dimensions of the Evaluation Process

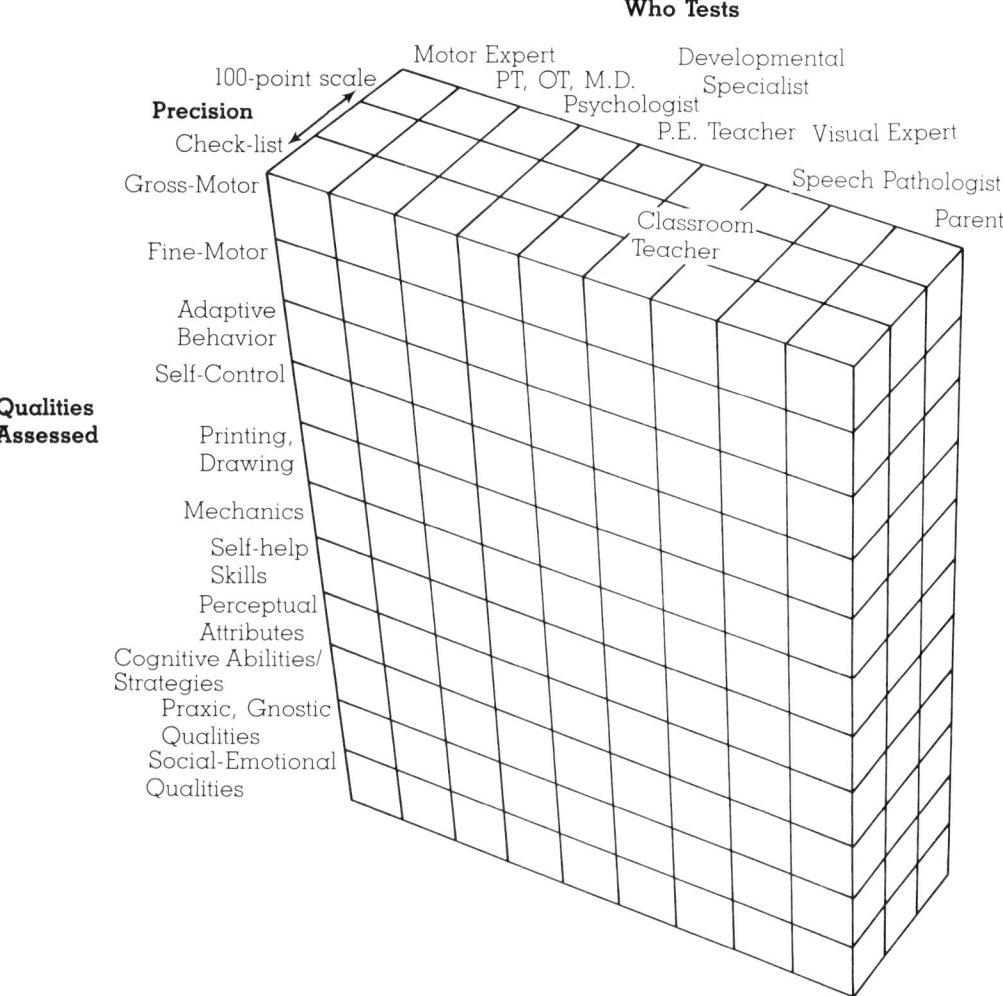

Time and Space

Of critical importance is the time—and thus the monies—allotted for testing physical capacities. Sometimes a program of perceptual-motor improvement has not gotten under-way in a school district until just before or after Christmas vacation, because of the extensive testing program that began with the school year in early September! In general, a testing program that takes more than 10%-15% of the total program time is excessive. Additionally, it should be decided how often physical progress should be reevaluated. Generally school districts reevaluate children every 12-14 weeks, thus affording three evaluations per year.

The space allotted for testing is also important. Although educators often try to screen children in large groups, the results are less than satisfactory. Testing of physical competencies, like academic competencies and psychological parameters, should be done in a quiet, secluded setting so that results will be uncontaminated by noise or the distractions of others.

TYPES OF TESTS

When assessing various characteristics of special people and populations, several types of tests may be employed. These can be divided into the two broad categories of (a) standarized, normed tests, and (b) criterion-referenced tests. Some tests are a combination of more than one type. In any case, each is used for specific purposes, and each type of test has both strengths and drawbacks.

Normed Tests

A normed and standardized test is often the type that professionals interested in testing status and change in human performance qualities first think of. These tests generally form the central core of an assessment program by P.E. teachers. Just because a test is presented and published as normed and standardized, however, does not mean that it is acceptable. Indeed, tests that purport to precisely measure various motor performance skills often lack important technical and practical qualities. If tests lack these qualities, the scores emanating from them are difficult to interpret, making their use questionable. The technical and practical qualities that these tests should possess are discussed in the following pages.

Norms   Finding tests whose norms, or averages, are appropriate to the measurement of individual differences in populations of handicapped children is difficult because the concept and label of "normed" contrasts with the concept of "different/special/limited" that applies to handicapped children. Although, for example, a modification of the AAHPERD battery has declared norms for the retarded, one might well ask, "What percent of the retarded upon whom the test normed evidenced neurological problems limiting motor coordination?" Similar problems arise when using instruments that have been "normed" with limited numbers of the blind, the deaf, and other small groups whose make-up and individual characteristics are often unknown.

Nevertheless, norms based upon large numbers of so-called average children are often of use when contrasting children with moderate coordination problems to average or above-average youngsters they must compete within a regular school setting. In this case, the child evaluated may be correctly identified as differing a given amount (e.g., 6 months, a year or more) from the average child upon whom the test has been based. But, sadly, few well normed tests of motor ability are based upon the scores of a vast number of children from ages 5 to 12 years. When formulating such instruments, thousands of scores are needed so that when differences in age and sex, for example, are included, a sufficient number of scores remains in the sub-groups identified (e.g., boys of 6, girls of 10).

Thus, great caution must be taken when comparing the scores obtained from an evaluation of any atypical youngster with norms (either those based upon "normals" or those based upon a "typical" population purportedly representing the youngster's exceptionality). Perhaps at no other time are the tester's abilities to interpret called upon more strongly than when comparing precise and objective test scores obtained from a single child or a small group of handicapped children to "norms."

Several instruments hold promise for the evaluation of various categories of special children. Henderson's revision of Stott's test (Stott, Moyes, & Henderson, 1984), for example, provides a tool for measuring moderate motor clumsiness. Most useful in this latest revision are provisions for observing and noting various social and cognitive qualities (e.g., "coping styles") the child may bring to the testing situation. And Hughes' test, recently normed on 1,260 subjects, provides nine task areas in which to evaluate the motor abilities of children 5-12 years of age (Hughes & Riley, 1981).

Various historical revisions of the Oseretsky (1948) test, including that by Bruininks (1978), often are used to assess special populations. This latter instrument, however, contains no ball skills, concentrating rather on items reflecting hand-eye coordination and manipulation. Also of possible use is a short form of the Bruininks test formulated by Beitel and Mead (1980).

Tests useful to physical education teachers have been surveyed in a recent monograph by Werder and Kalakian (1985). Current tests have been surveyed also in chapter 13 of Cratty (1986). And one of the best surveys and evaluations of early infant scales may be found in chapters 4-7 of Osofsky (1979). Other suggestions for tests applicable to special groups are found where appropriate in the remainder of this book.

Reliability In common speech, reliability refers to the extent one can depend upon something or someone. People are considered reliable if they keep their word and they show up to work when they say they will. Reliability of a test, however, implies concepts involving some degree of precision and statistical verification. *Reliability is the degree to which the test* (or testers) *is consistent in obtaining similar scores from a similar group of children.* Essentially, a reliable test will tend to rank a group of children in roughly the same order (from most to least able) from day to day, from one test administration to the next.

Reliability measures are expressed in correlation coefficients. A perfectly reliable test perfectly ranks children the same from day to day (or from administration to administration), resulting in a correlation of +1.00, which indicates a perfect concordance between the ranking of a group of children on one day (or test administration) and the ranking the second time.

Reliability can reflect how reliable any number of things are within the testing context. For example, one can obtain a correlation that expresses how closely two observer-testers agree when watching the same children perform. This is known as inter-tester reliability; their agreement should be fairly high if they have previously agreed upon how a test is to be administered and scored. Obtaining inter-tester (or observer) reliability on less precise observational measures is more difficult, but inter-observer reliability should be in the range of 70%-80%.

Depending on how well it is explained, the test itself may reduce or heighten the reliability of measures obtained or how closely two observers-testers agree when scoring clients with the instrument. And qualities inherent in the test may be difficult to reliably evaluate. Measures of kinesthesis (the position sense), for example, are easily altered, depending upon just-prior positions held, and measures of precise motor acts are easily disturbed by stresses, the changing arousal levels of those tested, and similar circumstances.

Essentially, the correlation coefficient expresses the percentage of variation resulting from a comparison between score rankings after the test's first and second administration. As mentioned, a perfect correspondence results in a correlation of +1.0. Less predictability between the two testings (or reflection of what is called the "common variance") is expressed in lower and lower correlation coefficients. The common variance is computed by taking the *square* of the correlation coefficient obtained (when test and retest scores are contrasted) and changing it to a percent.

The following indicates the common variance when correlations of less than +1.0 are obtained either in a test–retest situation or when the scores obtained at the same time by two testers (inter-tester reliability) are contrasted:

.9 = 81%	.5 = 25%
.8 = 64%	.4 = 16%
.7 = 49%	.3 = 9%
.6 = 36%	.2 = 4%

Less than 50% of the common variance (reflecting similarity in ranking) is obtained with a correlation of .7 on a test–retest basis. This indicates that over half (51% to be exact) of individual variance on the second administration of a test bears no relationship to how the individuals ranked the first time the test was given!

Test *consistency* is a concept similar to reliability but refers to reliability over time. Thus, a motor (or intelligence) test readministered after 6 months may result in a test-retest correlation of well under +.5 or +.6 and still constitute a reliable testing instrument.

A scientifically normed test cannot claim validity (that it essentially is a measure of *something*, or some quality) unless it first is ascertained as reliable. That is, the test has to be measuring *something consistently* before making any claims that it is measuring something in a valid way.

More and more physical educators have become concerned about the reliability of their observations and of the scores obtained from various instruments they are employing to assess motor qualities of the handicapped. Harris (Harris, Haley, Tada, & Swanson, 1984), for example, surveyed the inter-observer reliability when two and three observers observed movement qualities, including reflexes and voluntary movements, in infants. They found that in the traditional items on the various infant scales, reliability ranged from "fair" to "good," with greater reliability when three, rather than two, observers were involved.

Likewise, Ulrich and Wise (1985) found that observational measures obtained from 10 subjects by 10-20 observers were reasonably reliable. The skills included running, galloping, hopping, skipping, throwing, and kicking. Each skill was evaluated on a 3- to 4-level qualitative scale.

Validity   *Validity refers to the extent to which a test really tests the qualities it purports to measure.* Generally, the validity of a test is ascertained by comparing its results with the results obtained on a similar test of the same qualities for which validity already has been established. Again, a correlation of +.7 or above seems adequate.

Validity of motor tests may be ascertained by simply observing the results and deciding that the test has *face validity.* That is, the stability with which the child can posture on one foot might be arbitrarily said to have face validity, insofar as this type of task involves the child's orientation to gravity under some stress and, thus, constitutes balance.

Another way to ascertain validity is to compare the average scores of two groups that already have been separated (perhaps through clinical observations) as different in the quality (qualities) purportedly evaluated by the test. For example, a test that purportedly evaluates physical awkwardness in children might be contrasted in two groups that previously have been designated by observing teachers or motor experts as awkward or as "normal."

An associated concept is termed *construct validity.* Scientifically well prepared instruments have been based upon factor analyses to ensure that (a) each test is highly representative of an important movement quality and (b) each test is evaluating a separate and independent trait or quality. This second reason is important when considering the principle of *efficiency.* Large test batteries containing more than one test evaluating the same quality sometimes have been applied to handicapped populations.[1]

Factor analyses essentially are correlations of correlations that result in clusters or groups of tests that together evaluate some quality. Each test, however, does not represent that quality to the same degree. The degree or representation of the quality is represented by a number termed a *factor loading,* which is a correlation between each test and a common quality that apparently is contained to varying degrees in all the tests within a particular group or cluster. An example of this type of cluster, indicating factor loadings, is:

Factor II (hand-eye coordination)

.60   Pursuit rotor performance
.50   Figure drawing
.40   Finger opposition
.30   Target throwing (ball)

In the above case the test that should be selected for a larger battery of motor ability testing, and most representative of this quality, should be "pursuit rotor performance." Other tests of the battery should be selected in a similar way. Proceeding in this manner to formulate a battery of tests, the battery then is said to be factor-pure; each test in the battery is testing a separate and independent quality. The Fleishman (1965) tests of physical fitness constitute a prime example of a battery based upon factor analyses—and one that is factor-pure. Unfortunately, the age range of this battery is 10-14 years and does not apply to children in the younger age groups.

Unfortunately, motor ability tests formulated by using factor analytic techniques are rare. Their scarcity results from the reality that they are time consuming and expensive to develop. Factor analyses should begin with numerous tests, from which a fewer number

---

1. I was once introduced to a testing program applied to adult cerebral palsied individuals in a workshop setting. The test battery, compiled by a psychologist, took 3 days to administer and contained only tests of manual abilities. In truth, manual abilities contain about six factors or qualities; thus, six tests taking an hour or less to administer would have been sufficient.

of factors, traits, or qualities is extracted. Hundreds of subjects are needed, and sometimes more than one analysis, using more than one combination of tests, is necessary. This adds to the expense.

To further complicate the picture, different numbers and patterns of qualities or factors emerge when conducting factor analyses of abilities within groups of children and youth at various ages and developmental levels. Fewer factors usually are present when tests of younger or developmentally less advanced children are surveyed. As one ascends the developmental or age scale, more factors or specific qualities emerge from larger groups of tests. Figure 3.2 illustrates the comparison.

This picture of factor change as a function of age or development strongly suggests that more precise batteries should be applied to older, more able children, to comprehensively survey all their motor ability traits, than to younger, or developmentally more delayed, populations. Moreover, programming content may be more complex, containing more components, when devising work for more able or older youngsters than when working with less able or younger clients.[2]

Criterion-Referenced Tests

Criterion-referenced tests reflect established developmental points for "average children," but have obtained no norms for the test instrument itself. Because these instruments do not compare handicapped chidren to normal children, they are highly useful in assessing special children. Criterion-referenced tests form an important part of a total assessment program that also contains carefully collected behavioral observations and data from normed/standardized instruments. Their quality depends upon the expertise of the individual who formulates the instrument.

Figure 3.2   Comparison of Motor Qualities of Younger and Older Children

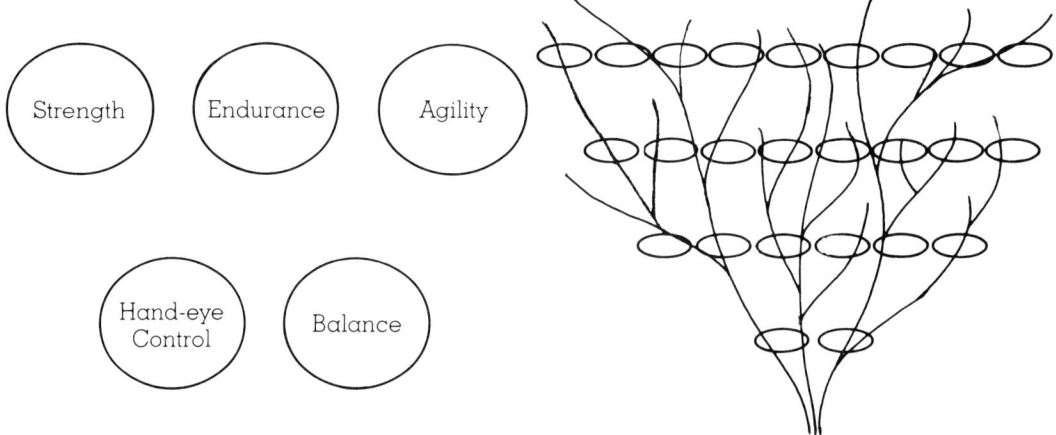

---

2. Further discussion of the rationale behind this tendency may be found in chapter 1 of B.J. Cratty, *Perceptual and Motor Development in Infants and Children* (3rd ed.) Englewood Cliffs, NJ: Prentice-Hall.

Often, these tests appear in the form of checklists of behaviors that are appropriate at a given age or month in development. They are among tools frequently used to assess early developmental milestones (e.g., the Koontz Developmental Survey). Thus they are appropriate for evaluating younger children, as well as for assessing the severely developmentally disabled. The Koontz survey includes not only desirable stages of behavior for children during the first years and months of life but also contains useful teaching strategies matched to the various milestones described (Koontz, 1974).

Perhaps one of the more comprehensive criterion-referenced assessment programs was developed in the early 1970s by the Santa Cruz County School District with the help of a federal grant and monies from the State of California.[3] This program contains 59 different groups of behaviors, which have been divided into sub-steps totaling 2,400 in all. The 59 groups, containing what are termed *behavioral strands*, present exact definitions of the behaviors within each strand. The program is designed for a wide variety of special needs students, and many of the groups contain items appropriate for consideration by P.E. teachers and others interested in promoting motor development.

Some of the items included are the self-care skills of feeding/eating, dressing, toileting, and the like, and specific motor groups covering visual-motor and gross motor skills. The adaptive behaviors group contains manipulative tasks involving objects (e.g., "plays games with another person").

The VORT program covers a wide variety of behaviors including ethical conduct (honesty), as well as academic tasks including math. Detailed sections deal with language-speech, and pre-language task-functions. Other sections include rhythm/music and spatial orientation skills of the blind. Physical education teachers dealing with nonambulatory youngsters will benefit from a survey of items contained in the "wheechair use" category.

Among other recent criterion-referenced instruments that have appeared is that by Noller and Ingrisano (1984). Incorporating 192 items from over 15 instruments, they produced a test that scores motor ability, qualitatively as well as quantitatively. They employ a 3-point scale (scoring children from 0-2 on each of the items). Like many of this type, this scale is used to evaluate infant functioning.

Two examples of criterion-referenced items for specific qualities are given below, and others are found throughout the book.

Attentional Qualities

1. Complete inattention—active
   Must be held to be physically present for lesson; no eye contact or other evidence of attention to lesson.
2. Complete inattention—passive
   Will stand or sit in place but with no eye contact or apparent awareness.
3. Hyperactive types
   a. *Locomotor movement,* plus visual attention and manually busy.
   b. *Movement of total body,* but child knows what is going on some of the time.
   c. *Manual activity constant* while standing, seated, or when *any* objects are present to be manipulated.

---

3. The Santa Cruz Special Education Management System (SEMS), VORT Corp., P.O. Box 11132, Palo Alto, CA 94306.

    d. *Passive, visual distractibility*—child appears cooperative, but visual attention precludes optimum learning.

4. Close and general attention
    a. Fair general attention, but brief close attention.
    b. Good general attention, and fair close attention.
    c. Good general attention, and good close attention for age and maturity.

5. Overattention, perseveration
    a. Continually perseverates in most situations and tasks.
    b. Periodically tends to perseverate, gets stuck on a task for too long.
    c. Relatively flexible in changing from task to task.
    d. Changes from task to task appropriately with no signs of perseveration.

Labels of maturity expressed as the child plays also may be evaluated using a criterion-referenced checklist, as follows.

Levels of Play Behavior C

1. Autistic behavior level—little awareness of self and environment.
2. Unoccupied behavior level—some awareness of environment, but lack of interaction.
3. Independent play level—isolated play.
4. Observing behavior level—sustained observation, but no direct interaction with another child.
5. Parallel play level—works with another child, but is not directly stimulated by another child.
6. Attempted interactional level—attempts to work with one or other child.
7. Associative play—uses same materials, but interacts infrequently.
8. Cooperative play level—plays directly with others, throws ball to another child.

"Homemade" Instruments Criterion-referenced tests are often formulated by administrators or by teachers of adapted physical education. These "homemade" instruments can be highly useful when the test formulator's background is broad and deep. A criterion-referenced instrument sometimes is blended or combined with criteria specific to the situation or environment of the population served by a school district.

Situationally Specific Instruments Often the most useful tool that can be applied within a setting containing children with special needs is a checklist of tasks and behaviors that relate directly to the environment in which the youngster works, plays, and studies. Using such a checklist, highly visible tasks that are pertinent and imperative to a youngster's progress through a typical day may be listed and assessed. At times the tasks are broken down into sub-stages. For example, washing the hands may be divided into the sub-stages of turning on the correct faucet, picking up and using the soap, drying the hands, and so on. The Nihara scale (Nihara, Foster, Shellhaas, & Leland, 1969) is one that contains a breakdown of these and other self-care skills.

At other times tasks useful within the child's room or play-recreational setting may be listed, observed, and checked off when a youngster successfully completes each item. This latter kind of situationally specific checklist might contain the following:

1. Can open the classroom door unaided, and with care and caution.
2. Can move a chair from one place to another in the class without disrupting others.
3. Can step up with both feet to the lower rung of the playground jungle-gym without fear and with safety.

These instruments have high validity relative to the specific needs of individual children. They also are motivating, insofar as children can perceive direct relationships between checks (stars) earned and concrete accomplishments each day. A situationally specific checklist, however, is not highly generalizable. A checklist obtained within one environment may be of little value in another environment. Those who interpret the scale also must be familiar with the child's work and play areas in order to correctly determine present conditions and future needs.

These instruments thus contain high *face validity.* They are most useful, however, when supplemented with other types of measures including normed tests and other criterion-referenced assessment tools.

"Mixed" Instruments

Some evaluation instruments may be within more than one category. For example, the Denver Developmental Screening Test (Frankenburg, Dodds, & Fandal, 1975) is both a normed test and a checklist. Scores of several thousand children were used to formulate this assessment/survey tool. More precise than most checklists, it indicates at what ages what percent of children can accomplish a listed task. After each child is tested, a vertical line is drawn, passing through the test from top to bottom, at the point of the youngster's chronological age. Using this line as a reference point, judgments are made as to performance levels met within four categories: language, personal-social, gross-motor, and fine-motor. Figure 3.3 shows the format of the Survey, along with a detail illustrating the behavior "walks well." The bar indicates at what age 25%, 50%, 75%, and 90% of children (based on the norms) may be expected to accomplish the behavior listed within the bar. For example, 50% of children can be expected to walk well by the age of 12 months.

SCOPE OF EVALUATION

Programs of evaluation compiled by physical education teachers differ in scope. These differences are partly attributable to other professionals interested in movement qualities of the children served, including physical and occupational therapists, pediatricians, psychologists, and so forth. And the scope and delimitations placed on the testing program are partially governed by self-perceptions of the physical education teacher. Some, for example, are well versed in manual skills and skills testing, so they naturally use instruments of that nature in their work-ups. Others may utilize self-concept tests (particularly those

Figure 3.3 Denver Developmental Screening Test

Format

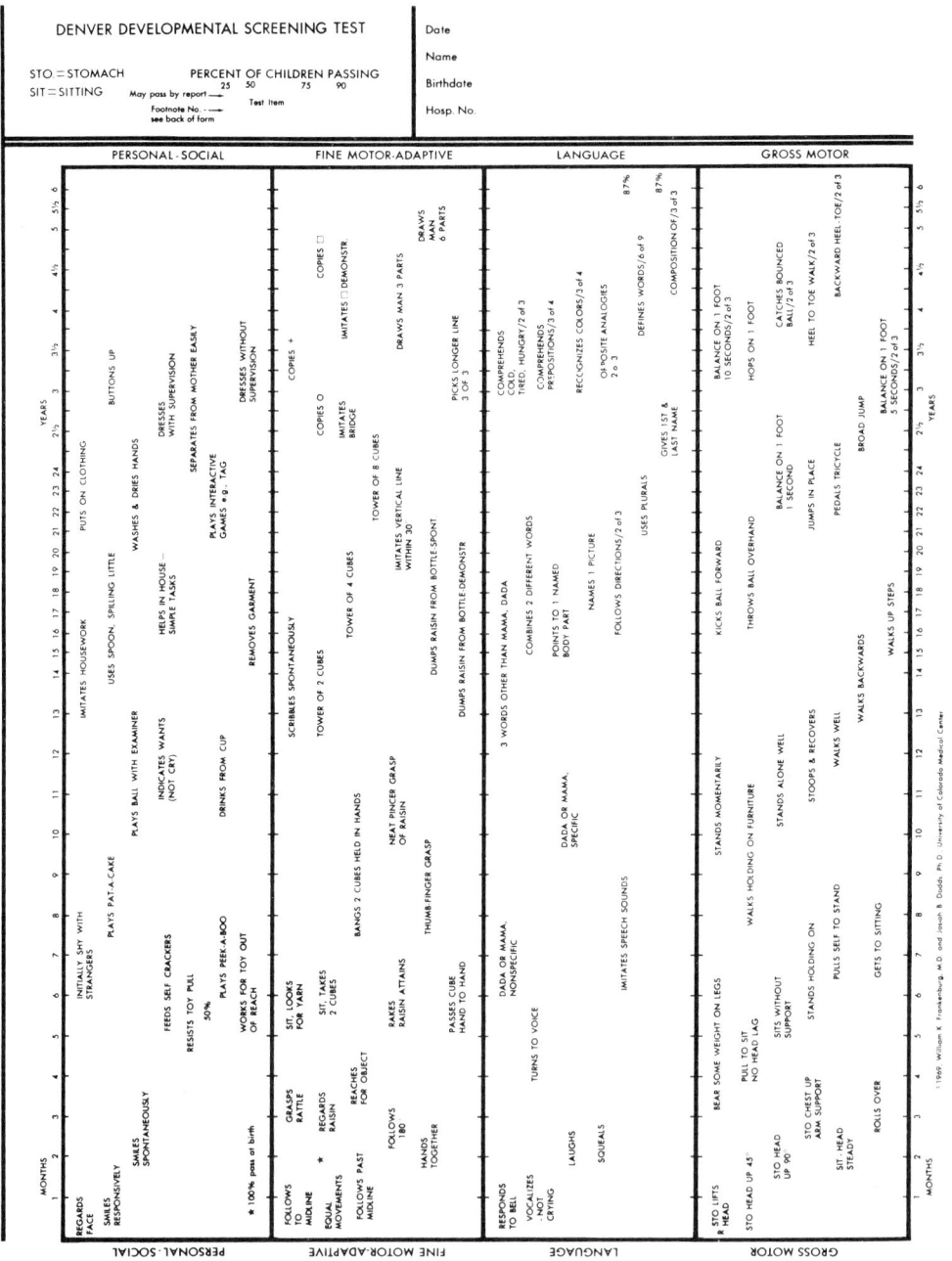

Note. From *Denver Developmental Screening Test* by W.K. Frankenburg, J.B. Dodds, and A. Fandal, 1975, Denver: Ladoca Publishing Foundation. Used by permission.

Figure 3.3 Continued

Detail

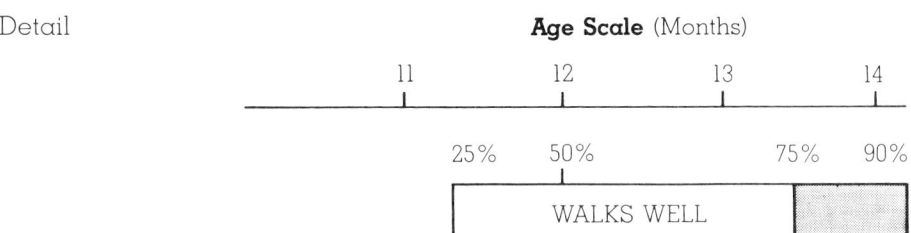

dealing with the child's body image and physical capabilities) or measures of self-control that might include a motor act (e.g., "Move as slowly as you can").

Harter and her colleague at the University of Denver have produced a two-level self-concept instrument (Harter & Pike, 1984). It is a projective test in which children are asked to respond to pictures of children in performance situations. This test has been suggested for possible use by physical educators (Weiss, 1984). The Piers-Harris test (Piers & Harris, 1965) is also helpful within this context. A useful test of motor planning ability has been developed by Cornish (1980). And the recently developed behavioral-observational method of ascertaining whether a relaxed state has been achieved in children holds great promise indeed (Brandon, Eason, & Smith, 1986).

When formulating and applying various testing procedures and instruments, physical educators sometimes tend to stretch too far beyond their backgrounds. These well meaning and often energetic individuals receive encouragement from brief essays in adapted physical education texts, and perhaps from weekend workshops given by developmentally oriented optometrists or enthusiastic sensory-integration therapists, to evaluate qualities in which they are not well versed. Their assessments, then, include "reflex testing," "visual-perceptual" assessments, and the like, for which they have not been thoroughly trained. By stretching beyond the well formulated motor content of the course curricula to which they were exposed in undergraduate and graduate programs, they may be taking professional risks and inviting complications. By being too expansive in what they think they can test—and, most important, what test behavior information they can correctly *interpret*—this kind of "test everything" attitude may even result in legal encounters.

As an example, some believe that since they are able to evaluate what has been termed *perceptual-motor* behaviors, they may detach "motor" from that hyphenated term, add "visual," and thus be able to evaluate visual-perceptual behaviors—and even move past that to the testing of vision itself. Visual testing—or any kind of information suggesting that visual-perceptual behaviors are being tested—may anger parents because they know the source of the information and question its validity. Or it may suggest to unsophisticated parents that their child's vision has been tested and found adequate when in reality it isn't, or prove alarming if a negative evaluation suggests a problem with the youngster's visual system when the only problem lies with the tester and tools employed in its evaluation. These two situations illustrate what is called either a *false positive*—that everything is all right when, in truth, it is not—or a *false negative*—a pronouncement of a problem when one does not exist.

Visual testing is best left to visually sophisticated professionals such as a well prepared optometrist (who can correctly assess both mild and severe visual problems) or an ophthalmologist (a physician specializing in the eyes and vision). P.E. teachers, as is true of all classroom teachers, should be sensitive to signs suggesting referral to one of these professionals when a child displays suspect behaviors such as squinting, turning the head to one side to obtain a good visual field, consistently evidencing playground behaviors that indicate poor depth perception, ball interception, or a limited visual field.

Physical education specialists might become interested in infant reflexes, or in the pathological reflexes exhibited by various handicapped groups.[4] At this time, however, it is highly questionable whether teachers of adapted physical education should make reference to reflex activity (the persistence of unwanted reflexes in the make-up of the cerebral palsied child, for example) when evaluating and programming children. Each motorically handicapped child with excess tonus displays a highly individualistic pattern of reflex and normal activity.

Understanding how this complex, but slightly out-of-tune, orchestra of muscles plays within an individual child is best left to those who are qualified in this kind of assessment and programming. Pediatric neurologists are well grounded in the nature of cerebral palsy, and the background of physical therapists includes theoretical, as well as practical and applied, neuropathology. Despite encouragement from writers of some texts of adapted physical education, adapted teachers should stay within the framework of their background and work in concert with therapists and physicians who are better qualified to deal with the complex interactions of reflex and normal activity possessed by many who are motorically handicapped.

Similar cautions apply in evaluating sensory-tactile awareness. Tactile insensitivity can be a critical sign of neuropathology, in which assessment, and most of all, interpretation, is best left to the neurologist. This is not to say, though, that the physical education teacher should not be aware of various motorical ineptitudes such as in hemiplegic youngsters, or those with spina bifida.

PUTTING IT ALL TOGETHER

Building a comprehensive and useful evaluation program seems to require knowledge of test construction as a science, as well as thoughts about how a group of tests might work in a practical situation and at an applied level. Essentially the test builder must consider "what's out there" as a cafeteria from which a selection of appropriate items may be selected. The best testing program generally contains a variety of instruments, ranging from at least one well normed motor ability test, containing a number of appropriate movement qualities, to less precise tools in the form of criterion-referenced and situationally specific checklists reflecting daily observations, common problem areas, and what seems practical and useful in a given situation.

Sophistication increasingly is attained by test developers and those attempting to objectify motor behaviors of atypical persons. Scales for the deaf-blind, such as the Callier-

---

4. A survey of normal infant reflexes whose persistence indicates pathology may be found in chapter 5 of *Perceptual and Motor Development in Infants and Children* (3rd ed.) by B.J. Cratty, 1986, Englewood Cliffs, NJ: Prentice-Hall.

Azuza (Stillman, 1982) are appearing—illustrating that even difficult-to-test populations are being given some attention. Ellison, Browning, Larson, and Denny (1983) have developed ways to score what was formerly a rather subjective clinical instrument intended to evaluate the interactions of reflexes and voluntary behaviors in suspect infants (Milani-Comparetti & Gidoni, 1965, 1967).

Of equal importance to selecting instruments is determining what instruments may be easily and accurately interpreted to others, including parents, who are interested in evaluation and outcomes. This aspect of testing is closely linked to the background, biases, and experience of the tester and should be given careful consideration.

Practical limitations of time, money, personnel, and space often sabotage the best intentions of those who construct evaluation programs for the handicapped. They often spend more time assessing their charges than they do presenting them with developmentally useful tasks within the program content itself. Testing programs that take more than 20%–30% of the budget and more than 10%–15% of the available programming time are suspect.

From a wide range of various types of tests, each containing numerous items, a selection must be made in compiling a comprehensive evaluation program suitable for a given situation in a given school or district. Those choices are more complex today because schools may be called upon to assess groups and qualities not historically evaluated. The infant population is one example. Here, tests might include the Denver Developmental Screening Test (Frankenburg et al., 1975), the Gesell (1940), or perhaps the Bayley (1984) scale.

Maybe social maturity, or changes in maturity, are to be evaluated. In this case, items from various scales of social maturity, such as Doll's (1985), may be useful. In addition, severely retarded individuals now are included within educational mandates. Self-care skills, for example, might be evaluated using the Nihara scale (Nihara et al., 1969), and gross-motor items and awareness could be exposed to the scales developed by Ruth Webb (1968, 1969).

Further, the manner in which a child copes with various tests and test items is being observed and recorded. And, finally, there is a growing trend to evaluate various subtle movement qualities in more detail. These (as discussed in chapter 12) include motor planning and associated movements (Connolly & Stratton, 1968), general hyper- or hypotonus, asymmetries, and other less obvious facets of the child's "action personality" (Williams, Fisher, & Trisch, 1983; Davis, 1984).

SUMMARY

Evaluative processes are imperative in the operation of an adapted physical program. Legally mandated, they must begin with tools that fit the overall role of adapted physical education within a school district's philosophical orientation and program. In evaluating an individual child, several types of instruments might be combined into a total program of assessment. The tools available include instruments that are *normed* (which should be both reliable and valid) and *criterion-referenced* (composed of scores reflecting norms gleaned from the literature rather than specifically for the instrument itself).

Physical education teachers should consider (a) the skills and abilities that they feel competent to test and interpret, and (b) ancillary qualities such as self-concept, self-control, attention, visual-perceptual, and tactile-sensory. In testing these qualities, the P.E. teacher should recognize his or her own limitations and readily refer the child to other professionals who are best qualified to assess these areas.

The uses of test information are many and include: (a) determining the "starting places" of students and formulating programs accordingly, (b) evaluating whether the program is meeting stated objectives, and, if not, adjusting it, and (c) helping staff members evaluate their own abilities.

In general, the number of abilities to be tested may differ depending upon the maturity and ability level of the population tested. Higher functioning youngsters (or older ones) exhibit a more diverse group of abilities than do lower functioning children (or younger ones).

Assessment programs should contain provisions for evaluating *all* the objectives for the program, as well as all program components. Lack of congruence between stated objectives, evaluative criteria, and program components could result in disappointment and frustration on the part of teachers, youngsters, and parents of the children involved.

REFERENCES

Bayley, N. (1984). *Bayley scales of infant development.* New York: Psychological Corp.

Beitel, P.A., & Mcad, B.J. (1980). Bruininks-Oseretsky test of motor proficiency: A viable measure for 3-5 year old children. *Perceptual & Motor Skills, 51,* 919-923.

Brandon, J.E., Eason, R.L., & Smith, T.L. (1986). Behavioral relaxation training and motor performance of learning disabled children with hyperactive behaviors. *Adapted Physical Activity Quarterly, 3,* 67-68.

Broadhead, G.D., & Church, G.E. (1984). Influence of test selection on physical education placement of mentally retarded children. *Adapted Physical Activity Quarterly, 1,* 112-117.

Bruininks, R.H. (1978). *Bruininks-Oseretsky test of motor proficiency.* Circle Pines, MN: American Guidance Service.

Connolly, K., & Stratton, P. (1968). Developmental changes in associated movements. *Developmental Medicine & Child Neurology, 10,* 49-56.

Cornish, S.V. (1980). Development of a test of motor planning ability. *Physical Therapy, 60,* 1129-1132.

Cratty, B.J. (1986). *Perceptual and motor development of infants and children* (3rd ed.). Englewood Cliffs, NJ: Prentice-Hall.

Davis, W.E. (1984). Motor ability assessment of populations with handicapping conditions: Challenging basic assumptions. *Adapted Physical Activity Quarterly, 1,* 125-140.

Doll, E.A. (1985). *Vineland social maturity scale.* Circle Pines, MN: American Guidance Service.

Elkin, E.G., & Friedman, E. (1967). *Development of basic motor abilities tests for retardates: A feasibility study.* Washington, DC: American Institute for Research.

Ellison, P., Browning, C.A., Larson, B., & Denny, J. (1983). Development of a scoring system for the Milani-Comparetti and abnormalities in infancy. *Physical Therapy, 63,* 1414-1423.

Fleishman, E.W. (1965). *The measurement of physical fitness.* Englewood Cliffs, NJ: Prentice-Hall.

Frankenburg, W.K., Dodds, J.B., & Fandal, A. (1975). *The Denver developmental screening test.* Denver: Ladoca Publishing Foundation.

Gesell, A.L. (1940). *The first five years of a child's life.* New York: Harper & Row.

Harris, S.R., Haley, S.M., Tada, W.L., & Swanson, M.W. (1984). Reliability of observational measures of the movement assessment of infants. *Physical Therapy, 64,* 471-475.

Harter, S., & Pike, R.G. (1984). *The pictorial scale of perceived competencies and acceptance for children*. Denver: University of Denver, Dept. of Psychology. (Monograph).

Hughes, J.E. (1979). *Manual for the Hughes basic motor assessment*. Boulder: University of Colorado.

Hughes, J.E., & Riley, A. (1981). Basic gross motor assessment: Tool for use with children having minor motor dysfunction. *Physical Therapy, 61*, 503-511.

Koontz, C.C. (1974). *Koontz developmental program*. Los Angeles: Western Psychological Services.

Milani-Comparetti, A., & Gidoni, E.A. (1965). Routine developmental examination in normal and retarded children. *Developmental Medicine & Child Neurology, 9*, 631-638.

Milani-Comparetti, A., & Gidoni, E.A. (1967). Pattern analysis of motor development and its disorders. *Developmental Medicine & Child Neurology, 11*, 625-630.

Nihara, K., Foster, R., Shellhaas, M., & Leland, H. (1969). *Adaptive behavior scales*. Washington, DC: American Association of Mental Deficiency.

Noller, K., & Ingrisano, D. (1984). Cross-sectional study of gross and fine motor development. *Physical Therapy, 64*, 308-313.

Oseretsky, N.A. (1948). A metric scale for studying the motor capacity of children. *Journal of Clinical Psychology, 12*, 37-47.

Osofsky, J.F. (1979). *Handbook of infant development*. New York: John Wiley & Sons.

Piers, E. & Harris, D. *Children's self-concept scale*. Nashville, TN: Counselor Recordings & Tests.

Sherrill, C., & Megginson, N. (1984). A needs assessment instrument for local school district use in adapted physical education. *Adapted Physical Activity Quarterly, 1*, 147-157.

Stillman, R. (1982). *Callier-Azusa scale*. Dallas: Callier Center for Communication Disorders.

Stott, D.H., Moyes, F.A., & Henderson, S.E. (1984). *Test of motor impairment: Henderson revision*. Guelph, Ontario: Educational Publications Ltd.

Tomporowski, P.D., & Ellis, N.R. (1984). Preparing severely and profoundly mentally retarded adults for tests of motor fitness. *Adapted Physical Activity Quarterly, 1*, 158-163.

Ulrich, D.A., & Wise, S.L. (1985). Reliability of scores obtained with objectives-based motor skill assessment instrument. *Adapted Physical Actively Quarterly, 2*, 125-131.

Webb, R.C. (1968). Sensory-motor training of the profoundly retarded. *American Journal of Mental Deficiency, 74*, 28-35.

Webb, R.C. (1969). *AMP index* (7th ed.). Glenwood, IA: State Hospital.

Weiss, M.R. (1984). Review of the Harter scale of perceived competencies. *Adapted Physical Activity Quarterly, 1*, 337-339.

Werder, J.K., & Kalakian, L.H. (1985). *Assessments in adapted physical education* (p. 126). Minneapolis: Burgess.

Williams, H.G., Fisher, J.M., & Trisch, L.E.R. (1983). Descriptive analysis of static posture control in 4, 6, and 8 year old normal and motorically awkward children. *American Journal of Physical Medicine, 62*, 126-132.

ADDITIONAL REFERENCES

David, K.S. (1985). Motor sequencing strategies in school-aged children. *Physical Therapy, 65*, 883-889.

Henderson, S.E., & Stott, D.H. (1977). Finding the clumsy child: Genesis of a test of motor impairment. *Journal of Human Movement Studies, 3*, 38-48.

QUESTIONS FOR DISCUSSION

1. What factors should be taken into consideration when formulating a testing philosophy?

2. What problems might be encountered when looking for well normed tests for movement qualities of both normal and handicapped children and youth? How may these problems be overcome?

3. What does reliability of a test mean? Validity? May a test be reliable and not valid? Valid and not reliable? Explain.

4. What does construct validity, or factor purity, mean? What practical considerations may be hindered if construct validity is not present in a test?

5. What advantages and disadvantages does a criterion-referenced test have?

6. What might a situation-specific testing instrument consist of? With what kinds of handicapped groups might such tests be employed? What may be the strengths and weaknesses of such an evaluation tool?

7. Why might the sub-tests selected for a battery of motor performance tests be modified after an interview with a child's parent prior to an IEP meeting?

8. What interview data concerning a handicapped child's play behavior might be relevant prior to the IEP meeting? What items might be placed on a checklist for parents in a pre-IEP meeting interview?

9. How might a test be too precise for practical purposes? In what ways might a test be too imprecise to give useful outcomes? Give examples of test content or scoring procedures to illustrate your answers.

STUDENT PROJECTS

1. Observe the motor testing of a handicapped child or youth by a physical education teacher. In what ways might you improve the testing content or procedures? What tests might you add or leave out of the battery administered?

2. Seek permission from a pediatric neurologist to observe the neurological evaluation of a suspect infant, child, or adolescent. Prepare yourself for this observation by consulting appropriate literature.

3. From a survey of the literature, formulate a valid and useful battery of six to eight sub-tests to administer to a population of normal children in a regular elementary school in an effort to identify those with minimal to moderate movement disorders. Devise subjective cut-off criteria (What constitutes passing on your sub-tests? How many sub-tests must an individual child fail to be included in your program?).

4. What advantages and disadvantages do checklists have in comparison with more precise instruments in the evaluation of various movement qualities? Formulate your own checklist, observe a child at play, and fill it out. Contrast your results with the teacher's perception of the same child's movement abilities.

5. Interview a physical education teacher to discuss the nature of evaluation instruments used in the school. What conditions does the teacher perceive to either facilitate or impede the evaluation program? How might the situation be improved?

4 Teaching Roles and Strategies

Perhaps never before have both physical education teachers and those in academic classrooms faced greater challenges. The concept of *least restrictive environment,* expounded in Public Law 94-l42, has encouraged school districts to integrate more and more youngsters with special needs into regular classrooms and schools. These special children then find their way into physical education classes populated with vigorous, adroit, average and above-average physical performers who may pose special problems to both the integrated child and the presiding teacher.

For the most part, integration into regular school settings is based upon academic considerations rather than upon the physical education needs of children who are different. Thus, some children may feel comfortable and accepted within one part of the school program—the classroom—but feel inadequate or worse in physically oriented activities. I recently received a phone call from the mother of a little girl with spina bifida, who with anguish in her voice explained that although her daughter benefited greatly from exposure to classroom experiences that stimulated her intellectual abilities, recesses and physical education periods were highly stressful.

NEW CHALLENGES

Not only is mainstreaming creating unique problems for physical educators, but even greater challenges must be met when dealing with handicapped children who are "left behind." Classes and schools contain more and more low functioning youngsters. Needless to say, teachers are becoming more and more challenged when working with youngsters who exhibit more than one problem behavior.

Moreover, teachers of physical education who have had little or no special training in dealing with various handicapped groups now must cope with a blind youngster, one who is deaf, or one with an exotic or rare physical abnormality. Regular physical education teachers are confronting the same challenges as classroom teachers of children who have special needs and are integrated into regular school settings. Sometimes these teachers cope well and keep the "ship" of education on a sound footing, but at other times classroom and physical education problems rock the "boat" of educational progress.

These challenges, encountered by both classroom and physical education teachers when confronted with special children, have led to several outcomes. The teacher's knowledge must stretch and expand, and sometimes this can be stressful. A recent longitudinal study (De Paepe, French, & Lavay, 1985), for example, described symptoms reflecting teacher burnout in adapted physical education teachers. Among their recommendations to help dispel this problem are to relate closely to other staff members, participate in professional meetings, exercise, and set realistic goals for themselves and their programs.

P.E. teachers in these new and often stressful settings often are required to expand their duties. Adams and Younger (1984) have described the *counseling* role in which a physical education teacher must engage. They pointed out that this counseling function not only serves students better, but it also enables teachers to relate better to their associates and colleagues.

These new roles and functions are subserved by individual attitudes on the part of both adapted and regular physical education teachers. Teacher attitudes, negative or positive, may contribute or detract from the difficult jobs these professional workers face when working with the handicapped. Rizzo (1984) pointed out that some children may be more accepted in special classes, or as special students in regular classes, than others. He found that learning disabled children were more accepted than were those who were physically handicapped. Teachers in the higher grades were less accepting of special needs children in their midst than were teachers of younger children.

Physical education teachers must deal with special children in a complex social-emotional surrounding. The class may have a number of normal children along with the usual number of children in the schools who have behavior problems. In addition, the teacher may have to deal with one or more childen who have other types of handicaps. The forces within the integrated physical education class will be discussed next, together with methods that may help teachers effectively deal with problems that are likely to arise.

THE MAINSTREAMED PHYSICAL EDUCATION CLASS

Historically society has reacted in many ways to the presence and needs of handicapped children and youth. The pendulum tends to swing from extreme to extreme when programs are developed (De Pauw, 1986). At this writing several children in the Angeles Unified School District regular setting have spinal cord injuries that require them to remain in a portable respirator 24 hours a day. It is not difficult to understand how these children might create special problems and raise the anxieties of administrators and teachers as they are wheeled to the playground and placed next to the vigorous actions (and thrown balls) of their classmates at play.

Educators and other observers who write about the advantages and disadvantages of mainstreaming give several arguments for and against the mainstreaming concept. One argument of proponents is that schools must expose handicapped individuals to regular settings in order for them to succeed in the normal world. At the same time, the normal populace must be educated about the manifestations of handicaps. Moreover, specific skills may be enhanced when a child with a problem is placed and accepted within a normal school setting (Gottlieb, 1981). For example, the rate of social interactions increases among severely retarded youngsters when they are placed in regular school settings (Brinker, 1985). And language use often is enhanced in children who are language deficient when they are exposed to a normal language environment (Knox, 1983).

On the other side of the coin are critics of mainstreaming and its outcomes. For the most part, however, those expressing reservations about this trend seem to believe in the practice philosophically but urge caution and care in its implementation (Retish, 1982). These critics point out that mainstreaming may not work well because of inadequate teacher preparation and inadequate preparation of the normal youngsters prior to including children with special needs in the classroom.

Physical educators should prepare themselves, their students, and their environments carefully before receiving a youngster with special needs into their classes. They must:

—be armed with special knowledge about the medical, emotional-social, physical, and sensory nature of the conditions of youngsters added to their class.
—carry out specific efforts and operations to prepare regular class members to receive a specific child.
—acquire special interpersonal skills in preparation for adding a child who has a problem (acquiring a few signs for use with the hearing impaired is one example).
—become equipped with a new set of teaching methods and techniques appropriate to managing, encouraging, and nurturing the special youngster.

Pupil Attitudes

Attitudes of the special and regular youngsters in the class may interact in ways that are not always positive. Exceptional children sometimes possess feelings of powerlessness, coupled with self-hate, that may emerge in the form of negativism or aggression (Gans, 1984). The teacher (as well as classmates) has to be aware of these possibilities, and the teacher must be prepared to set behavioral limits when a handicapped child enters the class.

Of equal importance are the attitudes and feelings of class members who are to interact with a special child. At times regular class members may have negative attitudes initially, but these often change to positive ones over time (Westerfelt & Turnbull, 1980). Or an attitude of unqualified acceptance of a handicapped classmate may change to more realistically reflect their feelings about a specific handicapped classmate (Eason & Schuler, 1979).

Various intervention programs may help promote positive, realistic attitudes. These programs should include:

—opportunities for increased exposure to the handicapped.
—opportunities to ask questions, and have them answered, about a given handicap.
—emphasis on the similarities rather than the differences between handicapped and nonhandicapped people.
—opportunities for normal children to simulate conditions experienced by the handicapped, such as using crutches or a blindfold (DeWar, 1982).

The current literature is reflecting the instigation and operation of peer-guide programs intended to help handicapped children interact and be integrated within a normal physical education setting. Folio and Norman (1981), for example, have described how children in upper elementary grades were trained to aid younger handicapped children in a physical education setting. Even younger children have been used as peer-guides in mainstreaming the handicapped in physical education settings. Cecconi and Rothenberg (1980) have written about how first-grade children have been employed successfully in programs with the cerebral palsied.

Even difficult-to-understand autistic children have been helped by better functioning peers (Campbell, Scaturro, & Lickson, 1983). In this latter program the peer-helpers were armed with a set of 10 guidelines, including information about how to reward specific

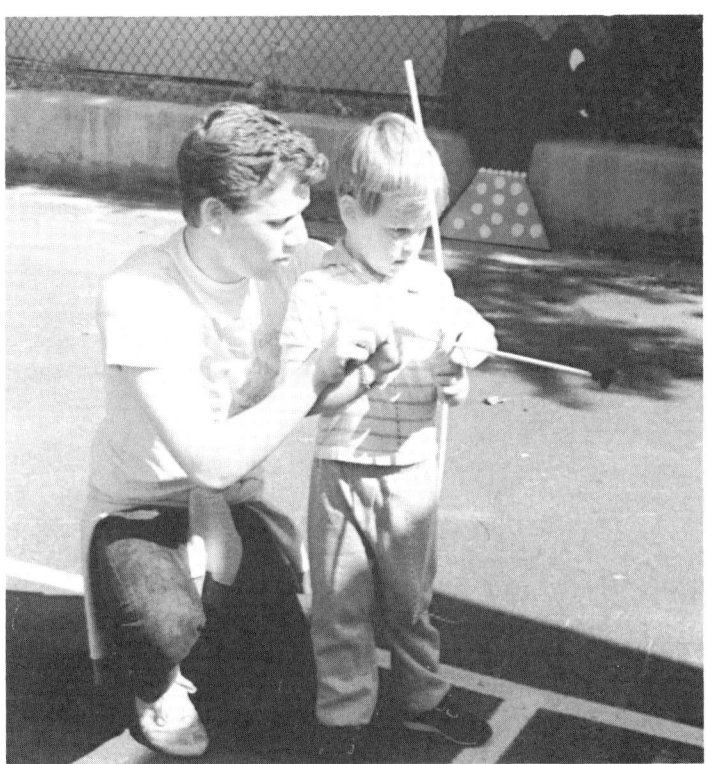

Peer-helpers can be an important part of mainstreaming in physical education.

Courtesy, Special Education Branch, Los Angeles City Schools

behaviors and ignore unwanted behaviors, directions for simple, direct verbal communication, and instruction on how to act as a correct model for useful behaviors.

The concept of peer-helpers seems extremely useful. This kind of educated peer, backed by a program that prepares all class members for inclusion of a special person, produces conditions that seem to optimize the physical education experience for a handicapped youngster in an integrated setting.

Special Techniques and Methods

Regardless of whether college or prior preparation has included work in dealing with the handicapped, the physical educator must bring special skills, attitudes, methods, and operations to a setting that includes one or more handicapped youngsters. Without these skills, exceptional children may be made to feel more helpless, especially if the teacher subtly implies that a task is not accomplishable because of a child's lack of ability (Raber & Weisz, 1981). The statement, "This task is too hard for you . . . let's try an easier one" is not as helpful as, "If you try just a little harder, you'll be able to do it!" The second phrase conveys that with effort, over which the child has some control, he or she will prevail.

The former phrase, indicating that low ability is somehow "locked-in," perpetuates the feelings of inadequacy that many handicapped youngsters possess.

Some other special techniques are discussed in the following pages. They include behavior modification; quantity, pacing, and sequencing of information; transfer of learning; thinking strategies; touching and "therapy hands."

Behavior Modification   Professionals familiar with this methodology almost seem to draw themselves into two armed camps—one including those for whom all things may be learned via the principles of Skinner, and a second group, usually cognitive theorists or humanistic psychologists, that decries behavior modification methods as inhuman, ignoring the intellect. I believe that a thorough understanding of the principles and practices of behavior modification is critical for teachers of physical education for the handicapped.

Recent literature abounds with studies depicting how behavior modification techniques have contributed in positive ways to the skill development of various atypical children and youth. For example, Hester (1981) has shown how basic locomotor behaviors of a profoundly retarded child were improved with a well applied schedule of reinforcement. Relaxation and various useful locomotor behaviors may be instilled in cerebral palsied patients through behavior modification (Hill, 1985).

Survey articles recently have emphasized the importance of understanding behavior modification techniques for those teaching special children in physical education (Dunn & Fredericks, 1985), as well as physical therapists (Gouvier & Richards, 1985). These techniques are particularly important for physical educators who are attempting to integrate children with behavioral-emotional problems into physical education classes. Heltma and Vogler (1985) have demonstrated how punishments such as loss of free time can effectively reduce the time children are not attending to the task at hand. In this investigation, on-task time improved from 44% to 70% using this kind of "punishment."

Advantages   Behavior modification techniques have certain advantages:

1. They teach us the desirability of carefully analyzing sub-sequences and approximating small steps toward the performance of an obviously useful task—either a sports skill or a self-care activity involving motor competencies.

2. If carefully applied with appropriate rewards given at correct times with a well analyzed task, positive changes do occur.

3. Behavioral modification is never absent in a teaching context. Social rewards and punishments ensue constantly between teacher and student, with both tending to change the other through their obvious and subtle behaviors. Thus, to say that "I don't believe in behavior mod" is a superficial observation and statement.

Disadvantages   Offering extrinsic rewards in a program intended to modify the behavior of exceptional children, however, has drawbacks. At times the best planned program of behavioral modification can somehow misfire. Some if its disadvantages are:

1. Individuals being rewarded—particularly the severely handicapped—simply may not connect the offered inducement with the behavior, or segment of a behavior, they have just performed.

2. Instructors offering rewards may not do so at the proper times and in the proper ways. The reward may be offered too frequently for behavior that has shown no change. Or a social reward (a constant smile) may lose its reinforcing qualities because of its constant availability ("You're doing fine!").

3. What instructors or teachers see as rewarding may not be perceived as rewarding by students. Both must be in accord as to what truly rewards and punishes. For example, emotionally disturbed children sometimes perceive compliments as punishments rather than the rewards teachers intend them to be.

4. Students whose behavior instructors are attempting to modify may not perceive improvement and change in the same way the teacher does. Teachers may not be sensitive to slight changes that occur as children struggle to acquire complex skills. On the other hand, children may not believe they are improving and may be surprised when a reward is offered for what they perceive as little or no change in their actual behavior.

5. Free-play situations or sports competitions in which children may be freely and vigorously engaged may be disrupted with the insertion of external rewards. The child may feel more rewarded in just doing the activity (intrinsic reward).

Quantity, Pacing, and Sequencing of Information   Many of the handicapped are
not good information processors; they are not able to handle large quantities of information at the same time. Some categories of the handicapped are behind their normal peers in assimilating and decoding verbal as well as visual information.

The platitude "talk slowly" is perhaps an obvious one. But with some handicapped youngsters, one not only must talk slowly but, if some manual guidance is not more effective, also extend relatively limited bits of information to the child at any given moment, gradually adding information as the child's actions confirm that the first parts of the message have been received and properly translated into task performance.

Teachers of the handicapped should be prepared to repeat instructions patiently, change instructions from modality to modality (tactile, visual, verbal), and at the same time modify the amount of information in all modalities. Teachers who speak rapidly should be made aware of it, as was an instructor in my program. His rapid-fire delivery of instructions to the hapless children with whom he was attempting to work made him incomprehensible, both to them and to the supervisors listening to the lesson.

Recent work on short-term memory indicates that following completion of a movement, learners often need time to monitor the feel of the movement itself prior to response from an external source. Children with a problem similarly need time to assimilate kinesthetic awareness of the movement pattern just completed before heaping more information on a perhaps limited channel capacity.

Studies that my students and I have conducted over the past 10 years clearly show that the pace of a demonstration, and the quantity of information it contains, is important when teaching physical skills to average as well as atypical children (Cratty, 1978; Cratty & Gibson, 1985; Cratty & Samoy, 1984). In general, the amount of motor information that can be processed and repeated by a normal child is about two "bits" less than the child's age. That is, a 5-year-old, when given three movements to chain together (presented one per second) usually can manage to repeat three (two less than the age of 5). Similarly, an average

7-year-old child usually can process five pieces of motor information given in sequence at the same pace (one per second). These data were obtained from average youngsters.

In other investigations we have found that mentally retarded youngsters are not as able to process the same amount of pieces of visually demonstrated motor information (Cratty, Forero, Cornell, & Omata, 1985). Thus, care should be taken to reduce the amount of information given to children who obviously are deficient in information processing capacities.

The limitations many atypical youngsters have relative to information processing suggest that limited parts of a task should be presented at a time. Usually a *part method* of teaching is recommended, because pure-part learning is seldom effective. That is, a child, if given five parts separately, has difficulty chaining them together into a whole. Usually a progressive method works better, wherein a single (usually first) part of a skill is learned, then a second added to the first and learned, then both practiced together. This continues, with a third part added, and so on, until the entire skill is acquired.

This progressive, part method may be applied in two ways: (a) The chaining may occur from the beginning of the skill; or (b) the chaining may be initiated by putting together the parts at the end and moving backward. This *backward chaining* method at times has been found to be more effective than the usual *forward chaining*. In a bowling task studied by Hsu and Dunn (1984), for example, moderately retarded individuals learned best by backward chaining (reverse chaining) techniques.

A *whole method* may be effective, when used with *prompts*, for children who are normal as well as those who are expected to have difficulty with skill acquisition. The program outlined by Gold (1983) is both interesting and effective. First, Gold suggests that tasks (usually self-care and household tasks) be carefully analyzed and broken down into sub-stages. Scrambling an egg, for example, is broken into 37 steps. Next the learner is taken through the entire process and exposed to three types of prompts: (a) verbal ("try another way" or perhaps "stir it"), (b) gestural/modeling (a tap in a given direction or perhaps touching or tapping the object to be used—a fork or an egg), and (c) physical (manipulating the limb or hand in reaching for an implement).

The goal in this type of program is to gradually remove the amount as well as the type of prompts as the individual begins to take over from the teacher. Although Gold's program focuses primarily on manipulative, household and self-care skills, these same principles may be applied to teaching sports skills and other large-muscle activities of interest to the physical educator.

Transfer of Learning   Transfering learning to tasks at home, on the playground, and in all of life is desirable. This requires careful planning. For effective learning and transfer to take place, many transferable tasks should be presented to an atypical child. If, for example, a child is to learn the names of and differences between the left and right hands, many left-right actions must be introduced, and many games should be played. When studying motor skill transfer in retarded boys, Portella (1982) found that practicing variations of a skill produced better transfer than practicing only one specific way to do a task.

Another way to elicit transfer is to help a child form cognitive bridges of understanding between the two tasks in which transfer is desired. The child should understand why a given training task is being used and to what task it is expected to transfer, or help. Transfer should not be left to chance. Conditions that optimize transfer must be carefully planned.

Thinking Strategies   Studies with normal youngsters, and with others attempting to learn skills, have asked the learners to record their thoughts as they repeatedly attempt a sometimes difficult action (e.g., tennis serve). Research of this kind indicates that learners themselves not only talk to themselves about corrections to be made on subsequent trials but also usually concentrate on a single correction at a time rather than trying to rectify several perceived movement problems at the same time. Teachers of physical education should be sensitive to this kind of finding and (a) attempt to ascertain what correction the learner may have in mind, (b) determine whether that correction is appropriate, (c) reinforce the learner with an awareness of the single correction they both may agree on, and (d) offer helpful feedback in terms of a single simple, easy-to-understand correction of the just completed movement, skill, or task.

Various handicapped groups have been shown to be able to instruct themselves in various physical skills. For example, Gonella, Hale, Ionta, and Perry (1981) demonstrated that children using videotape demonstrations could teach themselves a 3-point crutch gait. Emphasis in this kind of conceptual training was placed on initial stages of learning the task, as cognitive aspects of skills learning have been demonstrated to be most important during this phase (Fleishman & Hempel, 1954).

A clear-cut trend of importance to those working with atypical youngsters incorporates the use of mental strategies and *metacognition*. In this approach to teaching physical skills, emphasis is placed upon how children think about the skill and also how children are able to analyze and think about their own thought processes. Even normal youngsters seldom begin to analyze how they are learning, remembering, and dealing with tasks much before age 7 (Flavell, 1979). Atypical youngsters need more help in this important kind of planning behavior. Chapter 26 suggests ways in which this quality may be improved through the use of cognitive behavioral therapy.

Touching and Therapy Hands   Good physical education teachers of the handicapped are able to work effectively in many modalities, including clear *verbal* explanations and *visual* demonstrations of what is wanted. An often slighted approach to working with the handicapped is the use of *touch* and manual guidance to mold children's bodies and limbs to the desired positions. Not all handicapped children quickly grasp an action upon being lectured to, even with visual demonstration. The demonstrated action (particularly for students with motor planning problems) may be too complex for them—especially with tasks that require multiple or sustained movements. Likewise, a lecture is often lost on normal children, much less children with some kind of perceptual or cognitive handicap.

The incredible variety of behaviors and feelings that can emanate from the human hand can be channeled as a guide for action by physical education teachers. The concept of *therapy hands* suggests that good manual assistance requires children to sense the appropriate sub-actions of the movement themselves rather than being carried through the movement by the therapist. Teachers with good therapy hands do not permit a child walking a balance beam to clutch strongly at their arms while traversing the equipment, for then the therapist, not the child, is doing the action. Rather, therapists or physical education teachers should discourage undue grasping by the child or, alternatively, reduce the difficulty of the task so that the child's muscular patterns become the ones that are critical in executing the task (e.g., lowering the beam, widening it, or permitting the child to walk a line on the floor instead).

Thus, when manually guiding children, physical education teachers should be aware than many children will be unable to master the skill if *not* guided through it. But overly directive guidance, in which the instructor's actions and muscles play a major role in replicating the movement through the muscles of the children, may simply fatigue the teacher rather than instill the feel of movement in the children.

Touch can be a highly effective reward. A pat on the shoulder or back is often more effective than the frequently heard "that's good." Touch can convey something deeper, particularly to someone who is not accustomed to a great quantity or quality of rewards from others.

Class Size and Class Composition

Too many children with exaggerated problems simply cannot be directed and held on focus by even the most patient and able teacher. Children who are highly emotionally disturbed, are distractible, or evidence multiple sensory and motor problems should not be dealt with in large groups. At times, even one teacher with one child—seemingly an ideal ratio—is still not the correct formula. Distractible children sometimes feel less pressure and work best when placed in groups of three or four. In this arrangement they may relax more.

Formulating teacher-pupil ratios, either for classes composed only of handicapped children or for mainstreamed classes, is not a valid or useful undertaking. Rather, a somewhat rare quality called *common sense* should be called into play. Observations should be made about the nature of the children, both normal and atypical, as well as the emotional and professional make-up of the teacher. When combined and analyzed, these variables, together with available space and equipment, should reveal in an appropriate class size—one that permits each student to experience productive physical activity.

Several principles should be kept in mind when determining class size and environment.

1. When working with distractible children, a reasonably *distraction-free environment* is usually preferable. Partitions separating children into smaller groups and screening them from auditory and visual distractions may be helpful.

2. When working with perceptually or developmentally handicapped youngsters in large spaces, *visual reference points*—squares or circles arranged in symmetrical rows— may help youngsters orient themselves spatially and take part in meaningful exercises, games, and skill development activities.

3. Classes of certain sizes may present problems that classes of other sizes do not. For example, a class of three children might produce a two-on-one coalition, a "ganging up" of two children on the third. In a class of four, children can be separated into two even groups of two children each should controversy or strife arise. Thus, an *optimum class size* is desirable.

4. Each class, large or small, constitutes a unique psychosocial entity in and of itself. Allport (1924) ago first wrote about *synality*, or personality, a group quality separate and

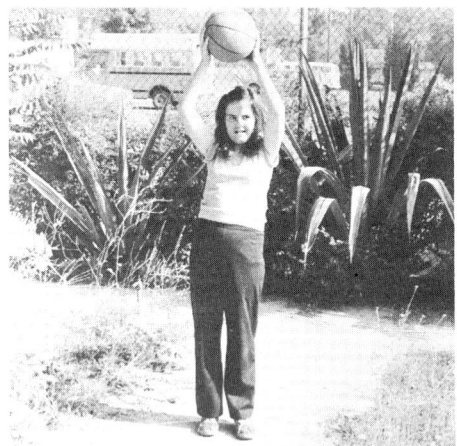

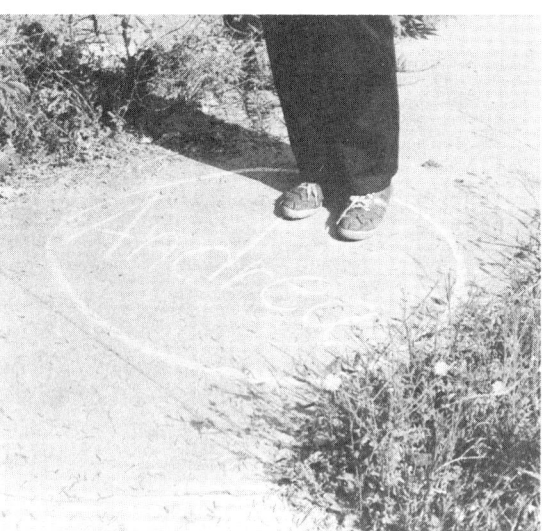

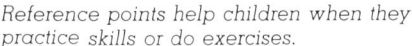
Reference points help children when they practice skills or do exercises.

Courtesy, Special Education Branch, Los Angeles City Schools

apart from the sum of the personalities of each member. Thus, any grouping of special children for physical activity may present surprises and difficulties. A group that seems to function well may suddenly blow up socially when a new, perhaps abrasive, child is added to it. Entrants may bring with them social vibrations that are out of tune with the harmonious social music played in the group prior to their inclusion. The reverse also may occur. After removing a single child, a poorly functioning group may reflect a group personality of productivity and tranquility. Sensitive physical education teachers should be open to the obvious and subtle social-psychological factor that inevitably resides in groups and should make adjustments if the situation is intolerable.

TEACHING MODELS

In addition to the specific teaching principles and strategies discussed, physical education teachers should be familiar with broader, more global models of teaching. These models represent operational descriptions of various philosophical viewpoints about education, the nature of children, and how learning may best take place. One of the most useful of these models was proposed in the late 1960s and early 1970s by Muska Mosston (1968, 1972). He focused upon the importance of who is in control within the teaching/learning environment. As had been true among industrial psychologists studying employee-employer interactions, Mosston wrestled with the difficult question of how much freedom learners should be given versus how much control and authority the teacher/authority figure should exert.

His solution emerged in a model for teaching that contained varying degrees of control for the teacher. He proposed a ''spectrum of teaching styles'' ranging from a teacher-dominated "command mode" to modes that were more flexible and permitted decision making by the youngsters. His rationale contained several basic tenets that are appropriate to the teaching of special children:

1. The best learning takes place when the learner is able to make decisions about components of the educational process.

2. The means, or thought processes, through which children are led (or are permitted to engage in) are more important than immediate and practical outcomes. Emphasis should be placed upon *thought*—what Mosston termed "mediating" behavior—in both physical activity and academic lessons.

3. Decision making shifted to the learner should proceed in a step-by-step manner, from the time teacher and pupil are confronted with each other, to evaluation decisions after completing the lessons, to the final period.

This model has been reviewed elsewhere (Cratty, 1985) and combined with other ideas including the exposure of children to various opportunities to engage in cognitive processes. Influenced by his ideas, some of Mosston's students (e.g., Morris, 1976) have proposed highly innovative ways to design games and programs of physical activity.

Prior to program planning, physical education teachers would do well to consider this and similar models. In doing so, problems of control, teacher-student interactions, and similar behavioral aspects of programming may be dealt with in productive ways. Chapter 5 explores several models in some detail.

SUMMARY

Adapted physical education teachers and physical education teachers dealing with regular and special youngsters now face challenges that seldom have been equalled. Accommodation to special populations, either in a heterogeneous or homogeneous setting, entails a number of special considerations and teaching behaviors. Some of these are enumerated here.

1. Special provisions have to be made when integrating a special youngster into a regular physical education setting. These must take into account the emotional and academic nature of the class and each member in it. Identification and training of special peer-guides can be an important aid to integration. Also, class members may be helped to understand the problems of handicapped classmates through various simulations (e.g., by using blindfolds or crutches).

2. Teachers confronted with special youngsters should arm themselves with a number of skills and attitudes. These may range from learning signs with which to communicate to the deaf, to knowledge appropriate in understanding specific conditions such as asthma, diabetes, epilepsy, or various manifestations of emotional disorders.

3. Adapted and regular physical education teachers should understand and apply principles of behavior modification, including rewards and punishments. An awareness of these principles should help the teacher become better able to analyze and break down tasks into components small enough for special children to master.

4. Teachers of special children should be aware of the limited information processing capacities of many handicapped children and extend smaller chunks of carefully selected information to these pupils than to typical populations.

5. Models and demonstrations, as well as physical prompts (therapy hands) should be utilized appropriately. These teaching techniques should be geared to the unique needs and characteristics of the special child with whom one is dealing.

6. Variables including classroom space and distractions should be carefully considered. An area that is too large or contains too many distractions is likely to sabotage even the best teaching efforts.

7. The physical education teacher should be aware of various models of teaching appropriate to special children. One of the more useful models represents an effort to sort out the problem of how much authority to exert in the teaching/learning situation (Mosston, 1972).

REFERENCES

Adams, G., & Younger, T. (1984). Personal perspectives on counseling in adapted physical education. *Adapted Physical Activity Quarterly, 1*, 185-193.

Allport, G. (1924). *Social psychology.* Boston: Houghton Mifflin.

Brinker, R.P. (1985). Interactions between severely mentally retarded students and other students in integrated and segregated public school settings. *American Journal of Mental Deficiency, 89*, 587-594.

Campbell, A., Scaturro, J., & Lickson, J. (1983). Peer tutors help autistic students enter mainstream. *Teaching Exceptional Children, 15*, 64-69.

Cecconi, C.M., & Rothenberg, S.P. (1980). Model instructional program for mainstreaming handicapped children. *Physical Therapy, 60*, 1022-1025.

Cratty, B.J. (1978). Motor planning behaviors in kindergarden children: A pilot study. *Motorik, 1*, 13-18.

Cratty, B.J. (1985). *Active learning* (2nd ed.). Englewood Cliffs, NJ: Prentice-Hall.

Cratty, B.J., Forero, N., Cornell, S., & Omata, C. (1985). *A comparison of motor planning abilities in normal, deaf and retarded children.* Unpublished manuscript.

Cratty, B.J., & Gibson, S. (1985). Bewegungsplanung (Praxie), bewegungs-impulsivitat und aufmerksamkeit bei kindern im kindergartenalter. (Motor planning and impulsivity in kindergarden children). *Motorik, 8*, 51-57.

Cratty, B.J., & Samoy, L. (1984). Ein vergleisch praxischer verhaltensweisen bei sjahringen kindern [A study of motor planning behavior in young children]. *Motorik, 7*, 52-57.

De Paepe, J., French, R., & Lavay, B. (1985). Burnout symptoms experienced among special physical educators: A descriptive longitudinal study. *Adapted Physical Activity Quarterly, 2*, 189-196.

De Pauw, K.P. (1986). Toward progressive inclusion and acceptance: Implications for physical education. *Adapted Physical Activity Quarterly, 3*, 1-5.

DeWar, R.L. (1982). Peer acceptance of handicapped students. *Teaching Exceptional Children, 14*, 188-192.

Dunn, J.M., & Fredericks, H.D.B. (1985). The utilizations of behavior management in mainstreaming in physical education. *Adapted Physical Activity Quarterly, 2*, 338-346.

Eason, J., & Schuler, J. (1979). *Changes in school attitudes toward disability following the integration of handicapped children.* Minneapolis: University of Minnesota, Dept. of Physical Medicine. (Monograph)

Flavell, J.H. (1979). Meta-cognition and cognitive monitoring. *American Psychologist, 34*, 906-911.

Fleishman, E.A., & Hempel, W.F. (1954). Changes in the factor structure of a complex psychomotor test as a function of practice. *Psychometrika, 19*, 239-254.

Folio, M.R., & Norman, A. (1981). Toward more success in mainstreaming: A peer-teacher approach to physical education. *Teaching Exceptional Children, 13*, 110-114.

Gans, J. (1984). Hate in the rehabilitation setting. *Archives of Physical Medicine & Rehabilitation, 64*, 176-179.

Gold, M.W. (1983). *Try another way.* Champaign, IL: Research Press.

Gonella, C., Hale, G., Ionta, M., & Perry, J.C. (1981). Self-instructions in a perceptual-motor skill. *Physical Therapy, 61*, 177-184.

Gottleib, J. (1981). Mainstreaming: Fulfilling a promise. *American Journal of Mental Deficiency, 86*, 115-126.

Gouvier, W.D., & Richards. J.S. (1985). Behavior modification in physical therapy. *Archives of Physical & Mental Rehabilitation, 66*, 113-117.

Heltma, K., & Vogler, E.W. (1985). Effects of an individual contingency program on behaviorally disordered students in physical education. *Adapted Physical Activity Quarterly, 2*, 127-135.

Hester, S.B. (1981). Effects of behavioral modification on the standing and walking deficiencies of a profoundly retarded child. *Physical Therapy, 61*, 907-909.

Hill, L.D. (1985). Contributions of behavioral modification to cerebral palsy habilitation. *Physical Therapy, 65*, 341-344.

Hsu, P.-Y., & Dunn, J.M. (1984). Comparing reverse and forward chaining instructional methods on a motor task with moderately retarded individuals. *Adapted Physical Activity Quarterly, 1*, 240-246.

Knox, M. (1983). Changes in the frequency of language use by Down's syndrome children interacting with non-retarded peers. *Education & Training of the Mentally Retarded, 35*, 185-190.

Morris, D. (1976). *Learning new ways to play games.* Minneapolis: Burgess.

Mosston, M. (1968). *Teaching physical education.* Belmont, CA: Wadsworth.

Mosston, M. (1972). *From command to discovery.* Minneapolis: Burgess.

Portella, D. (1982). Motor schema formation by EMR boys. *American Journal of Mental Deficiency, 87*, 164-172.

Raber, S.M., & Weisz, J. (1981). Teacher feedback to mentally retarded and non-retarded children. *American Journal of Mental Deficiency, 86*, 148-156.

Retish, P.M. (1982). Mainstreaming in the secondary schools: What price? *Journal for Special Educators, 18*, 46-48.

Rizzo, T.L. (1984). Attitudes of physical educators toward teaching handicapped pupils. *Adapted Physical Activity Quarterly, 2*, 267-274.

Westerfelt, V.D., & Turnbull, A.P. (1980). Children's attitude toward physically handicapped peers and intervention approaches for change. *Physical Therapy, 60*, 896-900.

ADDITIONAL REFERENCES

Craft, D.H., & Hogan, P.I. (1985). Development of self-concept and self-efficacy: Considerations for mainstreaming. *Adapted Physical Activity Quarterly, 2*, 320-327.

Rarick, G.L., & Beuter, A.C. (1985). Mainstreamed mentally retarded children. *Adapted Physical Activity Quarterly, 2*, 227-282.

Rider, R.A. (1980). Mainstreaming moderately retarded children in the elementary school physical education program. *Teaching Exceptional Children*, *12*, 150-153.

Smoot, S.L. (1985). Exercise programs for mainstreamed handicapped students. *Teaching Exceptional Children*, *35*, 262-266.

QUESTIONS FOR DISCUSSION

1. How might you break down the behavior of putting on a jacket into parts as small as possible for the behavioral modification schedule of a moderately retarded 5-year-old? What are the problems inherent in teaching a child this age this kind of task?

2. In your experience, what have been the best rewards to use in working with either typical or atypical youngsters in situations involving physical activity?

3. What does "good therapy hands" mean? Give examples of "good" versus "poor" therapy hands.

STUDENT PROJECTS

1. Visit a class in which motor activities are being taught. Evaluate how the class is taught, relative to size-space considerations, teacher behavior, and class composition. How would you change the situation to provide optimum teaching and learning?

2. Devise (a) a program that breaks down a motor learning task into its smallest components, or (b) a program that facilitates transfer of learning from one situation to another.

5 Theories and Models About Movement Activities

Writings of the first physicians in India, China, the Arab nations and, later, Greece and Rome contained prescriptions for exercises that, when combined with surgical procedures and the administration of herbs, were intended to dispel bad vapors associated with diseases or perhaps hasten recovery from a debilitating condition or operation. A history of the use of therapeutic exercise may be found in Licht's (1965) book, as well as others.

In the early 1880s the first experimental psychologists in Germany, the United States, and England began to explore the manner in which simple sensory and sensory-motor tasks might be indicative of intelligence. Although their efforts to predict intelligence from measures of kinesthesis, reaction time, and the like did not prove fruitful, their work represents some of the first objective attempts to pair movement with intelligence.

Clinicians in the late 1700 in France and other countries of Western Europe paired their first efforts to aid the handicapped—including the deaf, emotionally disturbed, and retarded—with sensory-motor tasks. When working with the legendary Wild Boy of Aveyron, *Itard* and *Seguin* attempted to instill speech, as well as spelling and mathematics concepts, in him, using games and tasks involving motor activity. The educational movement, spawned by the efforts of Maria *Montessori*, a physician in the slums of Rome around the turn of the century, leaned heavily on concrete experiences, including various balancing and manipulative movement tasks.

Many of the models most pertinent to readers of this book arose during and after World War II. *Kabat*, a physician, formulated his system of *proprioceptive neuromuscular facilitation* as a result of working with the war-injured in California. Following the War, the systems of *Getman, Kephart, Doman-Delacato,* and others received widespread attention.

Physical education teachers of special children should gain a thorough grasp of the rationale, program content, and expected outcomes of some of the these models for several reasons. Parents often come to the teacher for interpretation of what they have heard or read about the benefits of specific systems for their children. In response, teachers should be able to advise parents on the worth of the system or direct parents to literature that might help them judge the validity of the system themselves. The manuals and books promoting a particular approach are not always objective.

Teachers should, when possible, coordinate program content and efforts in the same direction as practitioners who are working with a child. For example, if physical therapists are employing one of the systems to prevent a child from scissoring the legs when attempting to walk, the physical education teacher should not require the same child to walk a narrow line, as that exercise is likely to make the condition more pronounced.

Models have to be carefully interpreted by professionals in movement-related services. This scrutiny is particularly important when considering the models that suggest that changes in academic, perceptual, or cognitive-intellectual abilities will occur as a result of movement tasks. In the following pages, theories and models of several types are described briefly. These include perceptual-motor theories, recapitulation theories, models blending cognition and action, and models that underlie traditional therapy methods.

PERCEPTUAL-MOTOR THEORIES

The premise that movement behavior both antedates and positively influences later perceptual and intellectual behavior undergirds perceptual-motor and sensory-motor theories. This broad classification can be divided according to two sub-theory categories: (a) those that rely on tasks combining visual and movement activities, and (b) those that rely primarily on movement tasks and include independent visual training.

Proponents of perceptual-motor theories assume that perceptual functions that underlie academic learning have a movement basis. Further, it usually is hypothesized that (a) physical awkwardness, when corrected, will elicit positive changes in classroom learning, and (b) enhancing the movement abilities of average children likely will heighten classroom learning potentials.

Among the most prominent of the writers espousing perceptual-motor theories were Gerald *Getman* and Newell *Kephart*. Their publications in the 1950s aroused widespread interest, and the popularity of various perceptual-motor activities was heightened in school programs for both average and below-average children and youth.

Getman, an optometrist, described a variety of tasks involving visual-motor integration, as well as those involving "pure" visual judgments, in his monograph *How to Develop Your Child's Intelligence* (Getman, 1952; Getman & Kane, 1957). Tasks based upon Getman's ideas currently are practiced in the offices of many optometrists throughout the United States. This type of visual training is intended to aid the hand-eye coordination needed in printing and writing, as well as visual-perceptual qualities that these clinicians believe undergird reading and other academic subjects.[1]

The book by Newell Kephart (1960) titled *The Slow Learner in the Classroom* also attracted a wide audience of parents, educators, and related professionals. Like other perceptual-motor theorists, Kephart proposed that motor learning was the basis of *all* learning, including reading. The several tasks he presented in his original book were expanded in subsequent publications. Generally, Kephart's tasks involved more movement than visual-motor activity, in contrast to Getman's program suggestions.

Like others espousing various movement models, Kephart formulated an evaluative instrument to assess the progress of children exposed to his program. The Purdue Perceptual-Motor Survey, published with co-author Roach, contains 21 sub-tests, scored on a 1-4 basis (Roach & Kephart, 1966). This battery of tests, including those designed to evaluate balance, drawing, muscular fitness, body-image, and other qualities, received widespread acceptance by teachers and others who engaged in perceptual-motor education programs during the 1960s and 1970s.

These and similar perceptual-motor models proposed by Barsch (1967) and others were highly popular because they seemed to promote a lot of transfer as the result of a relatively few movement or visual-motor tasks. Essentially, as Figure 5.1 illustrates, they might be classified as *broad transfer* theories. The broad transfer model implies a greater payoff for efforts expended by therapists and teachers than is true of the narrow-transfer model. This may explain why this model was, and still is, so popular. The question remains, however, whether broad transfer really occurs between a relatively few key training tasks and a longer list of objectives that one wishes the child to reach.

---

1. Many more optometrists include visual training tasks in an effort to rectify various *visual* problems, independent of possible transfer to academic learning.

Figure 5.1 Broad Transfer Width Model

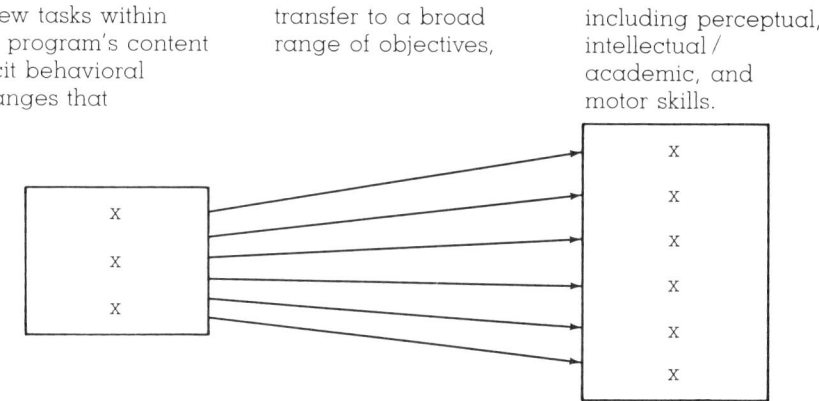

A few tasks within the program's content elicit behavioral changes that

transfer to a broad range of objectives,

including perceptual, intellectual / academic, and motor skills.

In contrast, *narrow transfer*, as illustrated in Figure 5.2, involves symptom-specific training in which a list of objects is formulated and evaluative tasks are applied and then matched with program content. In that way, children with apparent visual-perceptual, auditory-perceptual, and specific motor problems are presented with programs containing content that corresponds to the exact qualities in need of help or enrichment. This model requires a broad, deep background in the ability areas on which the program is focused.

Scholarly evaluation of the effects of perceptual-motor programs may be classified into three basic phases. *First,* those examining them wrote general reviews based upon what was known about transfer of training, motor abilities, and the academic abilities these programs purported to change. Many of the reviewers were critical of the possible program outcomes (Cratty, 1968).

Second, as more and more studies were made of the possible effects, the reviews focused on data obtained directly from perceptual-motor programs. These also were critical of possible outcomes of the program, as well as the quality of the research. Specific objections

Figure 5.2 Narrow Transfer Width Model

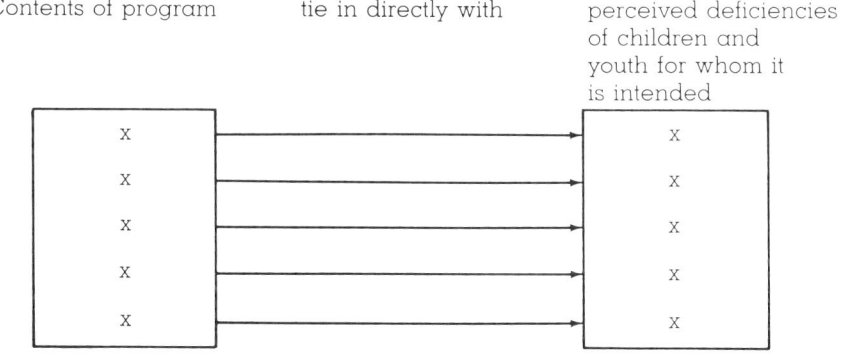

Contents of program

tie in directly with

perceived deficiencies of children and youth for whom it is intended

centered on the lack of sufficient control groups, the absence of adequate statistical treatment of the data, and inadequate descriptions of the subjects involved (Hebbelinck et al., 1968; Meyers & Hammill, 1976).

Third—and perhaps most devastating to the perceptual-motor models—meta-analyses appeared. These were essentially surveys of the data obtained from studies of the methods, which were treated and analyzed rather thoroughly. In one of the more ambitious of these surveys, Kavale and Mattson (1983) analyzed the data from 14,000 children represented by 180 studies. They found that the effects on reading and other academic skills not only were negligible but, further, that (a) specific help in reading would have produced far better results, and (b) the perceptual-motor programs did not produce significant changes even in the *motor qualities* apparently embedded in the training tasks. This latter finding suggests the need to carefully construct programs that purport to produce change in coordination, independent of what other fallout is expected.

Like the other models described in this chapter, this perceptual-motor approach has had both negative and positive effects. On the positive side, many special educators began to take a close look at the motor personalities and abilities of children and youth in their charge. On the negative side of the ledger, however, many children needing competent, specific help in reading and other academic skills have been denied the help, and instead given a watered down and not very effective program in physical education.

RECAPITULATION THEORIES

Recapitulation theories are not exclusive to programs of physical activity. They are found in the pages of philosophy books, which propose that the development of children in some ways reflects how the race evolved from more primitive beginnings. In motor activity programs this reasoning has been attached to notions about developmental neurology and translated into programs containing sensory and motor experiences designed to somehow "fill in" neural, and thus behavioral, deficiencies.

Because models based on these theories suggest activities that purport to influence the central nervous system in direct ways, the problems their proponents claim will be changed are literally without end. After all, if one changes the central nervous system, and all behavior is controlled by this system, will not all kinds of problem behaviors become modified (Delacato, 1964; Doman, 1960)?

Doman-Delacato

The earliest of the recapitulation models was proposed by a Philadelphia group composed of Dr. Carl *Delacato*, with a degree in school administration, and the *Doman* brothers, one a medical doctor. Beginning with self-published monographs in the 1950s, their publications and ideas caught hold, with help from the media, in the early 1960s and became widely applied by parents of atypical children and other interested lay people and educators.

The basic premise was that, if one practiced a range of simple and basic motor activities that in general resemble the evolutionary-like movements of our prehuman ancestors, one would be training both lower and higher portions of the brain and as a result, particularly in handicapped children, produce positive changes in other function levels purportedly controlled by the brain. The brain was envisioned as a composite of horizontal layers—the midbrain, pons, medulla, cortex, and neurocortex—with qualities reflecting hemispheric dominance. Various animal-like movements such as crawling, creeping, and cross-patterned walking (usually guided by therapists) were suggested.

What is referred to by the Doman-Delacato groups as *patterning* also is used, in which clients are placed on their stomachs and their heads turned while arm and leg movements are guided in what is called a *tonic neck reflex* position. This is considered a primitive action believed to remediate relatively basic functions mediated by the lower part of the brain stem.

In this therapy program one-eyed and one-handed activities also are encouraged to promote what is termed *hemispheric dominance*, which is considered a higher function unique to humans. Through the recommended activities it is believed more difficult functions, including reading and language, are enhanced.

Although it was initially widely accepted, by the middle of the 1960s some began to doubt the model's basic premises and promised outcomes. Following research by Glass (1967), Robbins and Glass (1968), and others, as well as inspection of professional groups in several countries, critical statements were made by organizations such as the American Academy for Cerebral Palsy, the American Academy of Physical Medicine, the American Congress of Rehabilitation Medicine, and various organizations in Canada representing disabled and retarded children and children with learning disabilities. These statements claimed that the method was without merit and chided those who promised cures without proper scientific documentation.

By the 1970s the method was not held in high repute. Although some continued to research its possible efficacy (Neeman, Ross, McCann, Menolascino, & Heal, 1974), the research was also criticized for methodological shortcomings (Zigler & Seitz, 1975). In an article published in the *Journal of the American Medical Association*, Freeman (1967) summarized objections that were expressed most frequently by professional individuals and groups. These included statistical defects in the reported studies and in the testing instruments; the rigidity of the method, which excludes a wide variety of universal child-rearing practices and possibly damages children's potential; the assumption that the methods treat the brain; and the forceful prevention of self-motivated activities by children.

Like the programs of Getman and Kephart, however, the Doman-Delacato program probably had mixed effects. Many parents were given relatively useless straws at which to grasp. But others, expanding the practices suggested by the Philadelphia group, began to at least try to remediate problems of the more severely brain damaged with an expanded list of techniques (Edgar, 1970; Edgar, Ball, McIntyre, & Shotwell, 1969). Physical educators who are asked about possible outcomes of this methodology would be well advised to direct inquirers to some of the pertinent literature so that they might inspect the possible outcomes before devoting a considerable amount of time, money, or energy to these methodologies.

Sensory Integration

In the middle and late 1950s an occupational therapist, A. Jean *Ayres*, began publishing work reflecting an interest in the improvement of motor functions. After obtaining a doctorate in educational psychology at the University of Southern California in 1961, her interests expanded to include development of a therapeutic method focused on improving what she termed sensory integration. Accompanying this was the formulation of a test battery called the Southern California Sensory Integration Test. She later formulated a second instrument called the Southern California Post-rotary Nystagmus Test.

Several basic premises underlie the Ayres approach, as described in her many writings from 1968 to the present.

1. So-called higher neural activity, including cortical function, does not operate independently of more primitive portions of the nervous system, including parts of the brain stem and reticular formation.

2. Exposing children to three types of activities purportedly will stimulate and involve portions of the brain stem. These include (a) *tactile* stimulation, usually administered via battery-operated rotating brushes mounted on a handle; (b) *vestibular* stimulation, including rotation of the child and rocking movements in a hammock or within an inner tube; and (c) motor activity, or *kinesthetic* stimulation, usually given while children attempt to propel themselves on a low scooterboard device up ramps and around obstacles in a graded sequence of tasks.

3. Stimulation of the brain stem through the activities described will exert a positive effect on the higher brain centers, which in turn will exert positive influences on a variety of motor and academic tasks, reflecting improved sensory integration.

As in the theories described previously, Ayres is advocating an approach that is not symptom-specific but, rather, one in which relatively few types of motor and sensory experiences are believed to generate improvement in a wide variety of perceptual, motor, and academic attributes and operations. Activities are hypothesized to go directly to the central nervous system, first influencing brain stem structures, which in turn will exert positive influences on higher centers. Moreover, the idea of improving sensory integration suggests that virtually all behavior will be positively changed. After all, most behaviors combine two or more senses.

Given its central effects and the somewhat vague but promising notion of integrating the senses, zealous colleagues in occupational therapy and others not surprisingly began to turn their attention to an incredible variety of abnormal behaviors using the methods described. Sensory integration therapists have focused upon developmentally delayed children (Kanter, Clark, Allen, & Chase, 1976), learning disabled children (Ottenbacher, 1980), persons lacking language (Ayres & Mailloux, 1981), cerebral palsied children (Ayres, 1977), those with visual problems (Ottenbacher, Watson, Short, & Biderman, 1979), low-achieving college students (Angelo, 1980), blind adults (Baker-Nobles & Bink, 1979), autistic children (Ayres & Tickle, 1980), and mentally retarded adults (Shuer, Clark, & Azen, 1980). Indeed, one might pause and reflect upon why other professionals in medicine, education, and related disciplines should continue their apparently hopeless work when sensory integration therapy can answer so many needs!

A primary criterion that Ayres believes is indicative of the degree to which a child's senses are apparently integrated involves *post-rotary nystagmus* (Ottenbacher, 1980)—the duration of jerky eye movements after stopping a child who has been spun around. Essentially it is believed that children who show an excess of this phenomenon have poor sensory integration, and diminuation of this effect reflects an improvement in sensory integration.[2] Reflecting an interest in this criterion, Ayres has developed a post-rotary nystagmus test that purportedly evaluates this visual-motor effect.

The assertion that the duration of post-rotational nystagmus is indicative of basic motor, sensory, or sensory-motor dysfunction has been questioned by many recent researchers. Potter and Silverman (1984), for example, while finding more post-rotational nystagmus in the deaf than in hearing persons, failed to find any significant correlation between the duration of these eye movements and balance problems in this same population.

Others also have been more critical of the rationale underlying the methods, the quality of research that has cascaded forth, and the test of sensory integration that Dr. Ayres has produced. Those reviewing the test for the *Buros Mental Measurement Yearbook* have pronounced the instrument to be based upon a rationale between neurological and educational criteria that are "impossible to locate" (Reed, 1978). This same reviewer suggested that the four research studies upon which the test is based consisted of "too many tests given to too few subjects." In a similar review Westman (1978) stated that the "norms are of questionable value. . ." and validity data are "virtually nonexistent."

In an "open letter to an occupational therapist," physician Robert J. Lerer (1981) noted that many therapists engage in well meaning evaluations and therapy based upon notions about sensory integration. After reviewing the data from many studies, he concluded that, among other things:

> There is not valid, convincing proof in the limited studies conducted thus far to indicate that this treatment [sensory-integration therapy] has directly remediated or helped anyone with a learning disorder of any kind. Every piece of research published offers only anecdotal, non-scientific, or poorly controlled material from which reasonable conclusions cannot be drawn. . . . I can find absolutely no solid basis for sensory integrative therapy to be used on any child in this country. (pp. 3-4)

Also, the methods may result in counter-productive effects when applied to special populations. Unique stress seems to occur when children are exposed to spinning and other techniques intended to stimulate the vestibular receptors in the inner ear and presumably the brain stem. Some children may experience nausea and even mild to severe seizures, under these conditions (Bhatara, Clark, & Arnold, 1978). Kanter, Clark, Atkinson, and Paulson (1982), however, pointed out that the vestibular stimulation apparently essential to this method did not produce seizures in a seizure-prone population exposed to this form of therapy.

Typical of both perceptual-motor theorists and those espousing a recapitulation model, the language and labels in the writings of Ayres often are confusing and confounding. For example, in one article Dr. Ayres (1977) stated that "sensory integrative therapy is designed to enhance sensory-integration rather than neuromuscular coordination!" (exclamation point mine). Further, in more than one investigation, subjects seem carefully selected to enhance

---

2. It is interesting to note that studies in the *American Journal of Occupational Therapy* (Ottenbacher, 1980; Ottenbacher, Watson, & Short, 1979) all professed positive clinical results, while a carefully designed "blind" study in *Developmental Medicine and Child Neurology* exploring these methods (Sellick & Over, 1980) resulted in non-supportive findings.

the possible positive effects of the therapy. To be fair, Ayres has often suggested that only a child with sensory integration problems can be helped academically with exposure to her methods (Ayres, 1968).

The effectiveness of sensory integrative therapy has been compared with more traditional motor developmental approaches. Jenkins, Fewell, and Harris (1983), for example, used two groups of moderately and mildly retarded preschoolers in this type of comparison. They found that the effects of the two methods were similar, but sensory integrative therapy, using occupational therapists, was more costly (per student) than more straightforward and traditional approaches.

Vestibular stimulation has been, and continues to be, an important part of programs designed for the stimulation of suspect infants and others with neuromotor problems (Ottenbacher, 1983). Insisting that vestibular stimulation is somehow a clear-cut road to improving a variety of learning disabilities, sensory losses, and even emotional problems, however, appears to be extremely optimistic, if not misleading, based upon the currently available data.

The writings of Dr. Ayres possibly, even probably, have useful clinical methods, including tactile stimulation, to be applied to the severely handicapped. Overall, though, the promises held for sensory integration therapy are not reflected in the clinical-descriptive research presently available. It may be a useful clinical tool, but only in the hands of one who is prepared to obtain additional data and can carefully interpret the results. When asked about the validity of these methods, physical educators might direct the questioner to data-based literature and current reviews of sensory integration, some of which are found in the reference listings at the end of this chapter.

COGNITIVE APPROACHES

Several types of movement-oriented theories and models are grounded in a cognitive approach to the stimulation of thought and academic accomplishments. Essentially these models are based upon the presumption that "intelligence is the basis of intelligence" rather than the premise of an imperative action basis to the emergence of intelligence.[3] Writers formulating these cognitive models suggest that to stimulate thought and improve academic abilities through movement, one must devise movement tasks and situations that in direct and obvious ways provide opportunities for children to think, make decisions, and practice the same academic exercises found in traditional classroom settings.

When writing about his spectrum of teaching styles, Muska Mosston has proposed that teaching and learning will produce motivated, creatively independent thought on the part of children, to the degree to which the learners (children) are able to make decisions about educational content and process (Mosston, 1972). His writings include examples of how a teacher may lead a child through independent discovery-learning by changing from an authoritarian leader to one who lets children have an important decision-making function within the educational setting. Research results exploring the influence and impact of this approach to teaching suggest that positive changes may be elicited in children's self-

---

3. A developmental model that contrasts with the traditional notion of Piaget's theory about an active basis of intelligence may be found in *Perceptual and Motor Development in Infants and Children* (3rd ed.) by B.J. Cratty, 1986, Englewood Cliffs, NJ: Prentice-Hall.

concept, sports skills, social helping skills, and creativity (Godbout, Brunelle, & Tousignant, 1983; Goldberger, Gerney, & Chamberlain, 1982; Mancini, Cheffers, & Zaichkowsky, 1976; Martinek, Zaichkowsky, & Cheffers, 1977; Schempp, Cheffers, & Zaichkowsky, 1983; Toole & Arink, 1982).

Other professionals in this area have taken a pathway less laden with social/philosophical theory and have simply produced activities that combine movement with thought, academic skills, and various social skills and attitudes. Their claims, while less expansive than those adhering to a perceptual-motor or a recapitulation theory, generally are supported by the available literature. James Humphrey (1966; Humphrey & Sullivan, 1970), for example, encouraged classroom teachers to engage in games that would reflect concepts and operations found in science, reading, and associated subject areas.

I have also provided a long list of movement activities that purportedly enhance academic skills, social awareness, language-communication tasks, and other imperative developmental tasks (e.g., Cratty, 1968, 1972, 1975, 1978, 1980, 1985). The premise is that movement will aid thought and academics because a high quality of task-attention may be elicited when moving and thinking, and thoughts and academic operations, when translated into action, afford immediate and vivid feedback about students' quality and progress. Some movement activities are found in chapter 32.

In one investigation of the efficacy of these methods, conducted within central-city schools in Los Angeles, the results were encouraging. As can be seen from Figure 5.3, an approach to learning that combined movement and academic content was superior to tutoring in a passive (classroom) setting or to simply engaging in more physical education each day.

Other research of learning and memory in general, as well as of the specific effects of an academically oriented movement program, is similarly supportive of these methods. For example, Levin (1976) and Saltz and Donnenwerth–Nolan (1981) found that memory is enhanced to the degree to which action is combined with visual-cognitive skills. Additional studies of my own specific methods generally have yielded positive and encouraging findings (Cratty & Martin, 1971; Thornburg & Fisher, 1970; Van Osdol, Johnson, & Geiger, 1974). Indeed, this action approach to learning has been extended into a variety of subject matter areas including high school physics (Johns, 1971) and foreign languages (Asher, 1969), as well as various other classroom skills (Grabbard & Shea, 1979; Hendrickson & Muehl, 1962; Humphrey, 1966; Ross, 1970).

Theorists of this persuasion do not make the remarkable claims of perceptual-motor and recapitulation theorists relative to the transferability of activities contained in their proposed programs. Instead, the cognitive models hypothesize rather narrow transfer width and focus on straightforward, obvious academic learning exercises such as spelling, reading, and mathematical operations and concepts. Similarly, these theorists do not recommend that their methods replace traditional classroom activities and teaching. Rather, they propose that action-based tasks should be used as helpful adjuncts to learning experiences traditionally found in our nation's schools.[4]

---

4. A theoretical model combining Mosston's notions of decision shifting to elicit freedom of thought, together with operations designed by Cratty to encourage various cognitive operations, may be found in *Active Learning* (2nd ed.) by B.J. Cratty, 1985, Englewood Cliffs, NJ: Prentice-Hall.

Figure 5.3 Effects of Learning Games Upon Letter Recognition

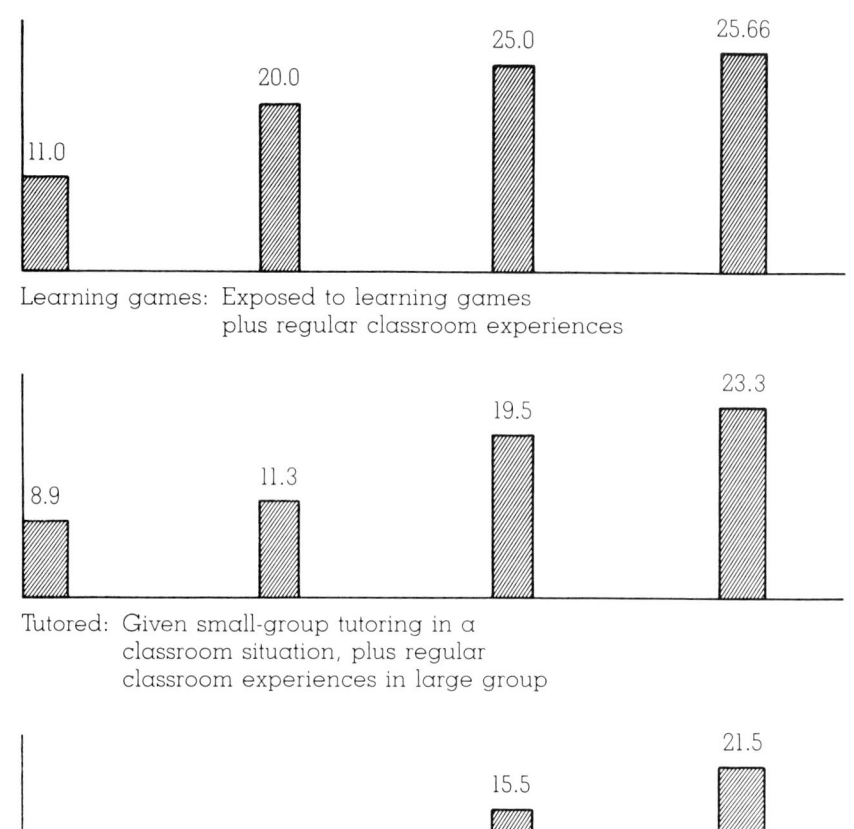

Learning games: Exposed to learning games
plus regular classroom experiences

Tutored: Given small-group tutoring in a
classroom situation, plus regular
classroom experiences in large group

P.E.: Given regular classroom activities with
the addition of physical education

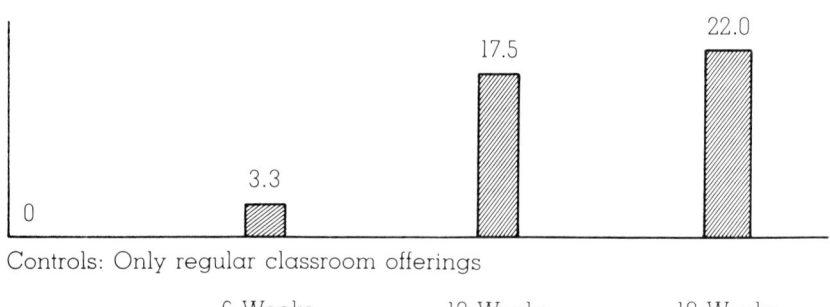

Controls: Only regular classroom offerings

6 Weeks   12 Weeks   18 Weeks

Note. From *Physical Expressions of Intelligence* by B.J. Cratty, 1972, Englewood Cliffs, NJ: Prentice-Hall. Used by permission.

MODELS FOR CHANGING MOVEMENT QUALITIES

The models discussed previously do not necessarily impact heavily upon physical education—nor should they. Many believe that adapted physical education should focus primarily upon improving skill, fitness, and associated physical parameters of atypical clients. The models that follow are used within traditional therapy settings, as well as in adapted programs. They focus on improving movement by using movement! Nothing magical or academic is implied in their practice. Physical education can have no more worthy aim than to help handicapped children and youth maintain and improve their physical capacities. The methods described next have that intent.

The three approaches to movement development selected for review are among those most widely used, in combination with the therapist's own ideas and methodologies. They have been included to provide a superficial familiarity with the basic rationales and some of the terminology used with these models. The inadequately trained are *not* encouraged to attempt to apply these approaches.

The Bobath Method

One of the more respected approaches to improving movement attributes in more severely involved children and youth, particularly those afflicted with cerebral palsy, was developed by an English physician, Karl *Bobath*, and his wife, a therapist. The approach is comprehensive, combining careful adherence to two main principles: (a) gradually leading the individual through normal sequences of motor development with repetitive exposures to normal functions, and (b) inhibiting unwanted and disruptive reflexes that prevent the assumption of adequate voluntary control (Bobath & Bobath, 1972).

Thorough application of the methodology requires a good background in brain function, developmental neurology, and motor development, including reflexology, as well as exposure to a certified course given by the Bobaths or one of their designated representatives. They advocate the following:

1. Infants suspected of having cerebral palsy should be dealt with early in life—preferably by the 6th month—before excessive muscular tonus has begun to appear and during the time when neural patterns may be more easily influenced and changed.

2. Early assessment should take into consideration individual differences in the extent and specific locations of neuromuscular abnormalities. The Bobaths' writings present, in detail, methodologies for carrying out early evaluations of this type.

3. Most important, only by changing children's abnormal postural patterns can an abnormal outflow of excitation be reduced, and thus developmentally normal movement patterns initiated and practiced. Through molding various postures, managed at key points in the body (head, shoulders, hips), unwanted reflex patterns are momentarily terminated. During this hiatus, children's normal movements may be encouraged. Also, through repetitive practice of this kind, children will begin to gradually reduce unwanted reflexes that inhibit voluntary movement and assume more and more voluntary control of their body and its parts.

When attempting to inhibit unwanted reflexes, the primary considerations are:

1. To reduce hypertonus, rigidity, or spasticity, therapists should carefully use graded force, taking care not to increase tonus by causing children to struggle and resist therapy.

2. Normal patterns have to be gradually introduced, in selected locations of the body and not in too many areas at the same time. This implies that children may be overloaded with too much new voluntary motor information.

3. Assistance in reducing spasticity should begin at points in the body where hypertonus is the least.

4. Patients should be aided not only in gaining gradual control over their voluntary movements, but also in suppressing unwanted, involuntary reflexes.

The Bobath method, and variations used by modern therapists, should be constantly reexamined. As new data regarding neurological and neuro-motor functioning become available, the model undoubtedly will be updated, refined, and modified. Kershner (1981) has suggested that an *interactive systems approach* is a more valid model of neuro-motor functioning than is the specific developmental approach advocated by the Bobaths.

Proprioceptive Neuromuscular Facilitation (Kabat)

Like the Bobaths' method, the proprioceptive neuromuscular facilitation (PNF) method developed by Kabat and advanced by his therapists, Knott and Voss (1968), rests on principles dictated by normal motor development (see Kabat & Knott, 1953). The treatments differ as to the specific methodologies employed, but Kabat has suggested the following principles:

1. Normal motor development is the basis for understanding how abnormal development may be changed.

2. Stress must be used in the therapy to promote learning, maturation, and capacities for exploring the environment.

3. Early motor development not only is permeated by reflexes but also is inseparable from sensory input.

4. Early motor behaviors are characterized by spontaneous rhythmical movements, carried out through full ranges and extremes of flexions and extensions, and these movements become increasingly selective and task-specific as maturation occurs.

This final principle forms the basis for a unique component of this therapy: *Basic qualities of human motion often are expressed in spiral and diagonal patterns.* That is, a movement may combine flexion and extension with abduction and adduction, with external *or* internal rotation. A developmentally delayed or disabled child, a post-stroke patient, or perhaps a post-operative patient are led through a sequence of movements that combine flexion and extension with rotation at the joints involved.

These complex spiral-shaped movements are first assisted by the therapist, and then, after some control is gained, patients try to take over from the therapist. Finally, resistance is added to the movement, with facilitative stress instigated by the therapist's tone of voice. A soft tone purportedly elicits less effort; a louder tone promotes more vigorous responses.

PNF techniques recently have been contrasted to both ballistic and static stretching in the production of increased range of motion. Although the PNF approach was determined to be slightly better, the authors (Sady, Wortman, & Blanke, 1982) emphasized that their results were not conclusive. Thus, as is often the case, clear-cut answers as to which therapy technique is best are difficult to come by.

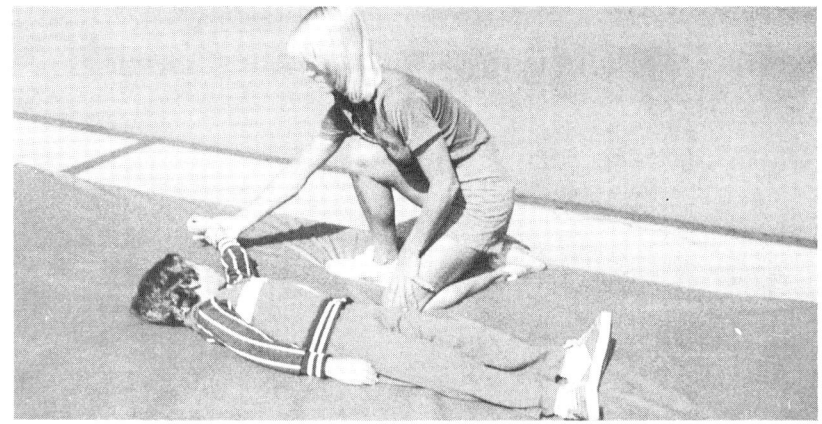

*One sequence of
spiral movements
in Kabat's PNF
method is assisted
by the therapist.*

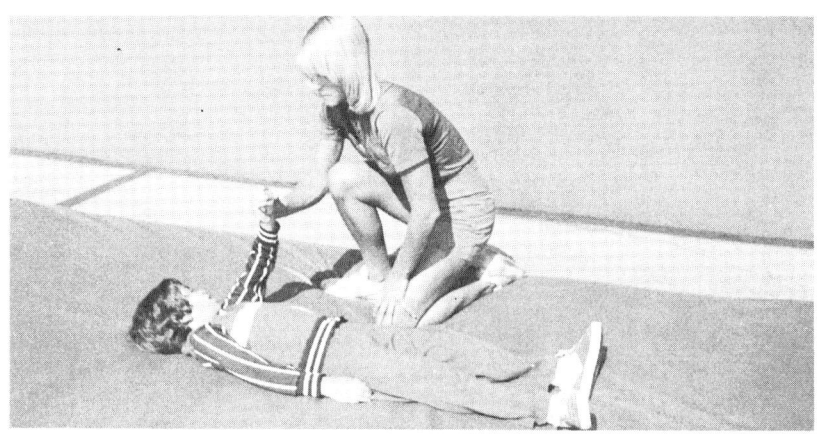

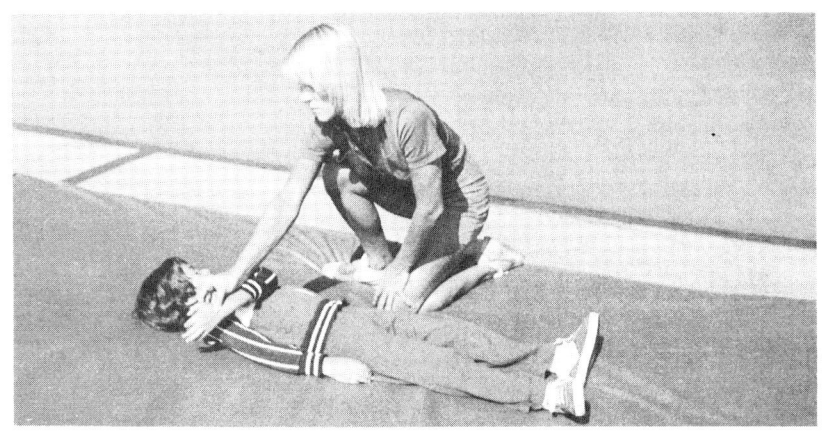

In any case, this methodology is widely used, and at times some components are combined with methods proposed by the Bobaths and others. Like the Bobath method, a knowledge of normal development is needed. The "quality" of the therapist's hands, through which is felt the resistance and cooperation of the client, is a major factor. If maladroitly applied, this method not only does not help individuals but also has been known to cause physical harm. Thus, physical education teachers should not try to emulate the pattern inherent in the PNF method but should try instead to understand what short-term and long-term goals the therapists practicing it have set for the individuals with whom they may both be working.

A Developmental Approach

The previous two methodologies are designed for more physically handicapped children, youth and adults—usually those with various kinds and degrees of cerebral palsy, as well as stroke patients, post-operative clients, and traumatic brain injury patients. These methods should be practiced by therapists thoroughly grounded in their application—not by uninitiated but interested educators.

A developmental approach used by educators attempting to change a variety of behaviors essentially assumes that (a) *all* children and youth go through roughly the same series of developmental tasks; the differences lie in the *time* during which the tasks may be encountered and mastered; and (b) to aid developmentally delayed children or youth, one should identify just *where* on one or more levels the individuals presently function and then attempt to take them further by presenting tasks that are developmentally just ahead of their present levels.

The success of this method depends on educators' detailed knowledge of the stages and sub-stages in the development area in which they are dealing and how artfully they can encourage students to move ahead in the various developmental channels. Section VII incorporates discussion of the manner in which motor capacities emerge within several developmental channels. In fact, most of the text contains suggestions that fall within this general developmental model.

Effective application of the two previously stated assumptions is facilitated to the degree to which physical education teachers keep in mind the following principles:

1. Children do not develop, even motorically, along a single channel; rather, concomitant areas of development emerge, often simultaneously. Children learn to sit and balance, for example, at the same time they are gaining manipulative skills. Thus, effective developmental motor therapy often involves the simultaneous involvement of more than one sequence of tasks.

2. Developing children (a) may evidence behaviors that are somehow out of the established developmental sequence, and (b) inevitably, at some given time, a variety of behaviors that are not congruent. For example, during a single day children may evidence a variety of manipulative behaviors, some of which might be designated immature and others precise and advanced. The same may be true in activities reflecting control of the larger muscle groups.

3. To elicit maximum change, teachers not only should seek to stress children moderately by presenting them with slightly advanced tasks in a given continuum but also permit children to obtain a foundation of motor and emotional successes by repeatedly practicing tasks they already have acquired. In this way, moderately stressful (difficult) activities that are introduced later are more likely to be accepted and practiced with some effort.

4. In working with older children or those who are developmentally more able, success likely will be achieved by exposure to a wider variety of tasks than those presented to younger, less able children. Factor analytic studies indicate that with increased age a more complicated factor structure of motor abilities emerges—and thus a more task-specific approach to improvement of motor capacities should be employed (Rarick & Dobbins, 1975).

Research illustrating motor changes in atypical, as well as normal, children as a result of this approach is, perhaps surprisingly, not plentiful. Nevertheless, research does suggest that a task-specific approach to the development of motor capacities is fruitful (Brekke, Burke, Landry, & Schaney, 1976; Hebbelinck, 1968; Rarick & Dobbins, 1975; Werner, 1974).

SUMMARY

Physical educators must interpret various theories about movement to other educators and parents and also incorporate in their own teaching the best practices from the various models. This chapter introduced the more popular theories about uses of movement with both normal children and special children and youth. Primary concepts include the idea of transfer. Narrow transfer width relates program objectives to specific child deficits (symptom-specific). In contrast, some theorists suggest that by practicing a relatively few movement tasks, transfer will occur to a larger number of motor, perceptual, and often intellectual and academic attributes (broad transfer).

Theories can be classified as (a) *perceptual-motor* or *sensory-motor*—the intent of which usually is to encourage development of perceptual and academic attributes by exposing children to various movement tasks and kinds of sensory stimulation; (b) *recapitulation* theories—the intent of which is to somehow fill in neurological development of children or youth by having them practice various sensory and sensory-motor tasks that not only reflect normal child development but also recapitulate the more primitive behaviors typical of human's primate ancestry; and (c) *cognitive* theories—in which movement is paired in precise ways with opportunities for children and youth to think about their motor experiences in an effort to improve thought and academic abilities. A final theory—most applicable to *adapted* physical education—seeks to improve movement attributes of the handicapped by exposing them to movement tasks themselves! The Bobath method and Kabat's proprioceptive neuromuscular facilitation (PNF) method combine various principles based on normal motor development. Many therapists base their techniques on these methodologies.

The developmental approach, which is generally the theme in this text, assumes that (a) the client is not severely disabled; (b) the movement specialist is not a physical or occupational therapist, but one well versed in developmental sequences, as reflected in movement behaviors; and (c) exposure to various kinds of movement tasks, selected in careful sequence, will help motorically deficient children and youth improve.

REFERENCES

Angelo, J.K.B. (1980). Effects of sensory integration treatment on the low achieving college student. *American Journal of Occupational Therapy, 34,* 671-675.

Asher, J.J. (1969). The total physical response technique of learning. *Journal of Special Education, 3,* 45-52.

Ayres, A.J. (1968). Sensory integrative processes and neuro-psychological learning disability. *Learning Disorders, 3,* 41-58.

Ayres, A.J. (1977). Effect of sensory integrative therapy on the coordination of children with choreoathetoid movements. *American Journal of Occupational Therapy, 35,* 383-390.

Ayres, A.J., & Mailloux, Z. (1981). Influence of sensory integration procedures on language development. *American Journal of Occupational Therapy, 35,* 383-390.

Ayres, A.J., & Tickle, L.S. (1980). Hyper-responsivity to touch and vestibular stimuli as a predictor of positive response to sensory integration procedures by autistic children. *American Journal of Occupational Therapy, 34,* 375-381.

Baker-Nobles, L., & Bink, M.P. (1979). Sensory integration in the rehabilitation of blind adults. *American Journal of Occupational Therapy, 33,* 559-564.

Barsch, R.H. (1967). Achieving perceptual motor efficiency: A space oriented approach to learning (Vol. 1). Seattle: Special Child Publications.

Bhatara, V., Clark, D.L., & Arnold, L.E. (1978). Behavioral and nystagmus response of a hyperkinetic child to vestibular stimulation. *American Journal of Occupational Therapy, 32,* 311-316.

Bobath, K., & Bobath, R. (1972). Cerebral palsy diagnosis and assessment and neurodevelopmental approach to treatment. In P.H. Pearson & C.E. Williams (Eds.), *Physical therapy services in developmental disabilities.* Springfield, IL: Charles C Thomas.

Brekke, B., Burke, J., Landry, R., & Schaney, Z. (1976). Effects of a perceptual-motor training program on kindergarten children. *Perceptual & Motor Skills, 43,* 428-430.

Cratty, B.J. (1968). *Perceptual-motor behavior and educational processes.* Springfield, IL: Charles C Thomas.

Cratty, B.J. (1972). *Physical expressions of intelligence.* Englewood Cliffs, NJ: Prentice-Hall.

Cratty, B.J. (1975). *Teaching about human behavior through active games.* Englewood Cliffs, NJ: Prentice Hall.

Cratty, B.J. (1978). *Intelligence in action.* Englewood Cliffs, NJ: Prentice-Hall.

Cratty, B.J. (1980). *Coding games.* Denver: Love Publishing.

Cratty, B.J. (1985). *Active learning* (2nd ed.). Englewood Cliffs, NJ: Prentice-Hall.

Cratty, B.J. (1986). *Perceptual and motor development in infants and children* (2nd ed.). Englewood Cliffs, NJ: Prentice-Hall.

Cratty, B.J., & Martin, Sister M.M. (1971). *The effects of learning games upon children with learning difficulties.* Los Angeles: UCLA, Dept. of Kinesiology. (Monograph)

Delacato, C.H. (1964). *The diagnosis and treatment of speech and reading problems.* Springfield, IL: Charles C Thomas.

Doman, R.J. (1960). Children with severe brain injuries, neurological organization in terms of mobility. *Journal of the American Medical Association, 174,* 257-262.

Edgar, C.L. (1970). The adaptation of perceptual-motor training techniques to the profoundly retarded. In *Some educational implications of movement.* Seattle: Special Child Publications.

Edgar, C.L., Ball, T., McIntyre, R.B., & Shotwell, A.M. (1969). Effects of sensory-motor training on adaptive behavior. *American Journal of Mental Deficiency, 73,* 713-720.

Freeman, R. (1967). Controversy over "patterning" as a treatment for brain damage in children. *Journal of the American Medical Association, 202*, 385-388.

Getman, G.N. (1952). *How to develop your child's intelligence: A research publication.* Luverne, MN: G.N. Getman.

Getman, G.N., & Kane, E.R. (1957). *The physiology of readiness: An action program for the development of perception for children.* Minneapolis: P.A.S.S.

Glass, G.V.A. (1967). *A critique of experiments on the role of neurological organization in reading performance.* Champaign, IL: University of Illinois, Center for Instructional Research and Curriculum Evaluation.

Godbout, P., Brunelle, J., & Tousignant, M. (1983). Academic learning time in elementary and secondary physical education classes. *Research Quarterly for Exercise & Sport, 54*, 11-19.

Goldberger, M., Gerney, P., & Chamberlain, J. (1982). The effects of three styles of teaching on the psychomotor performance and social skill development of fifth grade children. *Research Quarterly for Exercise & Sport, 53*, 116-124.

Grabbard, C.P., & Shea, C.H. (1979). Influence of movement activities on shape recognition and retention. *Perceptual & Motor Skills, 48*, 116-118.

Hebbelinck, M., et al. (1968, September). *A multidisciplinary longitudinal growth study: Introduction of the Project LLEGS.* Proceedings of the 21st World Congress of Sports Medicine, Brasilia.

Hendrickson, L.N., & Muehl, S. (1962). The effects of attention and motor response pre-training on learning to discriminate b, d, in kindergarten children. *Journal of Educational Psychology, 53*, 236-241.

Humphrey, J.H. (1966). An exploratory study of active games in learning of number concepts by first grade boys and girls. *Perceptual & Motor Skills, 23*, 819-822.

Humphrey, J.H., & Sullivan, D.D. (1970). *Teaching slow learners through active games.* Springfield, IL: Charles C Thomas.

Jenkins, J.R., Fewell, R., & Harris, S.R. (1983). Comparison of sensory integrative therapy and motor programming. *American Journal of Mental Deficiency, 88*, 221-224.

Johns, R.N. (1971). Gymnasium physics. *Physics Teacher, 9*, 23-27.

Kabat, H., & Knott, M. (1953). Proprioceptive facilitation techniques for treatment of paralysis. *Physical Therapy Review, 33*, 53-64.

Kanter, R.M., Clark, D.L., Allen, L.C., & Chase, M.F. (1976). Effects of vestibular stimulation on nystagmus response and motor performance in the developmentally delayed infant. *Physical Therapy, 56*, 414-421.

Kanter, R.M., Clark, D.L., Atkinson, J., & Paulson, G. (1982). Effects of vestibular stimulation on seizure-prone children (an EEG study). *Physical Therapy, 62*, 16-17.

Kavale, K., & Mattson, P.D. (1983). One jumped off the balance beam: Meta-analysis of perceptual-motor training. *Journal of Learning Disabilities, 16*, 165-173.

Kephart, N.C. (1960). *The slow learner in the classroom.* Columbus, OH: Charles E. Merrill.

Kershner, E.A. (1981). Reevaluating the theoretical model underlying the neurodevelopmental theory. *Physical Therapy, 61*, 1035-1040.

Knott, M., & Voss, D.C. (1968). *Proprioceptive neuromotor facilitation: Patterns and techniques* (2nd ed.). New York: Harper & Row/Hoeber Medical Division.

Lerer, R.J. (1981). An open letter to a therapist. *Journal of Learning Disabilities, 14*, 3-4.

Levin, J.R. (1976). What have we learned about maximizing what children learn? In J.R. Levin & L.L. Allen (Eds.), *Cognitive learning in children.* New York: Academic Press.

Licht, S. (1965). History (ch. 13). In S. Licht (Ed.), *Therapeutic exercise* (2nd ed.) (pp. 426-471). Baltimore: Waring Press.

Mancini, V., Cheffers, J., & Zaichkowsky, L. (1976). Decisionmaking in elementary school children: Effects on attitudes and interactions. *Research Quarterly, 47,* 80-85.

Martinek, T.J., Zaichkowski, L.D., & Cheffers, J.T.F. (1977). Decisionmaking in elementary age children: Effects on motor skills and self-concept. *Research Quarterly, 47,* 349-357.

Meyers, P.L., & Hammill, D.D. (1976). The perceptual motor systems (ch.9). In P.L. Meyers & D.D. Hammill (Eds.), *Methods of learning disorders* (2nd ed.). New York: John Wiley & Sons.

Mosston, M. (1972). *From command to discovery.* Minneapolis: Burgess.

Neeman, R., Ross, P., McCann, B.M., Menolascino, A., & Heal, L.W. (1974). Experimental evaluation of sensorimotor patterning used with mentally retarded children. *American Journal of Mental Deficiency, 79,* 372-384.

Ottenbacher, K. (1980). Excessive postrotary nystagmus duration in learning disabled children. *American Journal of Occupational Therapy, 34,* 40-44.

Ottenbacher, K. (1983). Developmental implications of clinically applied vestibular stimulation. *Physical Therapy, 63,* 338-341.

Ottenbacher, K., Watson, P.J., Short, M.A., & Biderman, M.D. (1979). Nystagmus and ocular fixation difficulties in learning disabled children. *American Journal of Occupational Therapy, 33,* 717-721.

Potter, C.N., & Silverman, L.N. (1984). Characteristics of vestibular functions in deaf children. *Physical Therapy, 64,* 1071-1075.

Rarick, G.L., & Dobbins, D.A. (1975). Basic components in the motor performance of children from six to nine years of age. *Medicine & Science in Sports, 7,* 105-110.

Reed, H. (1978). Review of the Southern California Sensory Integration Test. In O.K. Buros (Ed.), *Eighth mental measurement yearbook* (pp. 874-876). Highland Park, NJ: Gryphon Press.

Roach, E.G., & Kephart, N.C. (1966). *The Purdue perceptual-motor survey.* Columbus, OH: Charles E. Merrill.

Robbins, M.P., & Glass, G.V. (1968). The Doman-Delacato rationale: A critical analysis. In J. Hellmuth (Ed.), *Educational therapy* (Vol. 2). Seattle: Special Child Publications.

Ross, D. (1970). Incidental learning of number concepts in small group games. *American Journal of Mental Deficiency, 48,* 718-725.

Sady, F.P., Worthman, M., & Blanke, D. (1982). Flexibility training: Ballistic, static, or proprioceptive neuromuscular facilitation? *Archives of Physical Medicine & Rehabilitation, 63,* 261-263.

Saltz, E., & Donnenwerth-Nolan, S. (1981). Does motoric imagery facilitate memory for sentences? A selective interference test. *Journal of Verbal Learning & Verbal Behavior, 20,* 323-332.

Sellick, K.J., & Over, J. (1980). Effects of vestibular stimulation on motor development of cerebral-palsied children. *Developmental Medicine & Child Neurology, 22,* 476-483.

Schempp, P.G., Cheffers, J.T.F., & Zaichkowsky, L.D. (1983). Influence of decisionmaking on attitudes, creativity, motor skills, and self-concept in elementary children. *Research Quarterly for Exercise & Sport, 54,* 183-189.

Shuer, J., Clark, F., & Azen, S.P. (1980). Vestibular function in mildly mentally retarded adults. *American Journal of Occupational Therapy, 34,* 664-670.

Thornburg, K.R., & Fisher, V.L. (1970). Discrimination of 2-d letters by children after play with 2- or 3-dimensional letter forms. *Perceptual & Motor Skills, 30,* 979-986.

Toole, T., & Arink, E.A. (1982). Movement education: Its effect on motor skill performance. *Research Quarterly for Exercise & Sport, 53,* 156-162.

Van Osdol, R.M., Johnson, D.M., & Geiger, L. (1974). The effects of total body movement on reading achievement. *Australian Journal of Mental Retardation, 3,* 16-19.

Werner, P. (1974). Education of selected movement patterns of preschool children. *Perceptual & Motor Skills, 39,* 795-798.

Westman, A.S. (1978). Review of the Southern California Sensory Integration Test. In O.K. Buros (Ed.), *Eighth mental measurement yearbook.* Highland Park, NJ: Gryphon Press.

Zigler, E., & Seitz, V. (1975). On "An experimental evaluation of sensorimotor patterning," a critique. *American Journal of Mental Deficiency, 79,* 483-492.

ADDITIONAL REFERENCES

Ayres, A.J. (1954). Ontogenetic principles in the development of arm and hand functions. *American Journal of Occupational Therapy, 8,* 18-23.

Ayres, A.J. (1960). Occupational therapy for motor disorders resulting from impairment of the central nervous system. *Rehabilitation Literature, 21,* 302-310.

Ayres, A.J. (1964). Tactile functions: Their relation to hyperactive and perceptual motor behavior. *American Journal of Occupational Therapy, 13,* 135-138.

Ayres, A.J. (1968). Reading—A product of sensory integrative processes: Perception and reading (Proceedings of the 12th Annual Convention). *Occupational Therapy, 12*(4).

Ayres, A.J. (1980). *Sensory integration and the child.* Los Angeles: Western Psychological Services.

Cratty, B.J. (1981). Sensory motor theories and practices: An overview. In R. Walk & H. Pick (Eds.), *Intersensory perception and sensory integration* (pp. 345-369). New York: Plenum.

QUESTIONS FOR DISCUSSION

1. Contrast the model presented by Kephart with that of Getman. Contrast the model of Ayres with that of Kabat. What are the similarities and differences between the various theories in each of the categories described in this chapter?

2. Are you aware of other theories that relate movement to improvement in movement or other attributes of children and youth? How would you classify these other theories?

3. Have you ever seen a program reflecting the Delacato approach or the ideas of Jean Ayres? If so, what was the nature of the activities employed? For whom? What were the objectives for those conducting the program?

4. What is the primary premise of the cognitive theorists? What is their goal(s) when offering a movement program?

5. Can you give an example of an activity or sequence of activities reflecting a developmental approach? Have you ever seen this approach employed well? Badly? What principles might be followed to ensure the application of this theory in optimal ways?

STUDENT PROJECTS

1. Review some of the research articles evaluating one of the programs described in this chapter. What is your assessment of the article? Did the findings support or fail to support the assumptions made by the individual proposing the model being tested? What research is needed in this area?

2. Observe a program based on the ideas of one of the theorists reviewed. What was the emotional tone of the session you watched? What was the practitioner's background? What kind of group was being served? What objectives did the practitioner have in mind when applying the methods you watched?

3. Without any prior information concerning the theory on which it is based, watch a movement program, noting its contents. Following your observation(s), attempt to ascertain what theorist has influenced the practitioner you watched. Next, talk to the practitioner you observed to determine whether the assumptions you formulated about the underlying model were those of the practitioner.

4. Drawing from each theory, and after further reading, attempt to formulate three programs: (a) one that will best serve the movement needs of an awkward child; (b) one that will best serve the needs of a child with obvious cerebral palsy; and (c) one that will improve the intellectual functioning of a moderately retarded child.

5. Attend a meeting at which parents are being informed about the nature of a movement program to be conducted in a school. Attempt to ascertain the theoretical base of proponents of the program. Do you agree with the assumptions of the program designers?

6. Interview one or more physical therapists to learn what model, if any, they follow when administering therapy. Try to find out the nature of the system that was in highest repute at the therapy school they attended; whether they adopted this system, in whole or in part, or formulated their own eclectic systems when working with clients; and whether they modify the system and techniques when working with various types of clients.

6 Visual Impairments

The lay public has always viewed blindness as a rather dramatic and compelling condition. Public attitudes in the United States during the past 150 years have spawned innumerable special schools and programs, hundreds of publications, and intriguing mechanical devices for individuals lacking sight. Many articles and books deal with physical education for the blind. Charles Buell (1983) has listed 23 books and 88 articles on physical education for the blind alone. An even more extensive bibliography could be compiled for work with postures, manneristic behaviors, and mobility of the blind—all qualities dealt with by special education teachers and physical education teachers employing movement tasks.

Despite this attention, the prevalence of visual impairment in children is low. Estimates place the number of visually impaired children in the United States as about 1 in every 1,000 school-age children in the country (NSPB, 1980). Thus, it is an infrequently encountered handicapping condition among children and youth and is becoming largely a problem of the aged. About two thirds of the legally blind persons in the United States are over age 65.

BACKGROUND AND HISTORY

Perhaps no other group of exceptional children has been exposed longer to programs of physical education than have blind children in the United States. One of the three schools for the blind in existence between 1830 and 1833, the Perkins Institute in Boston, made special provisions for physical education. Its director, Dr. *Samuel Gridley Howe*, an early advocate of health and physical education, instituted a vigorous program of "exercise in the open air" for his charges. "Never check [discourage] the motions of the blind," Howe wrote. Howe also recognized the necessity for treatment of what he believed were physical manifestations of nervousness, or the rhythmic blindisms he observed in his students. This topic is covered in more detail later in the chapter.

Within the next decades facilities at the Perkins mansion in Boston were expanded to include a gymnasium and a bowling alley. In other parts of the United States, a general revival of physical culture, reflecting both German and Swedish systems of physical education, was manifested in the expanding system of residential schools for the blind (and often for the deaf *and* blind) that were established in most states by the 1900s.

After the turn of the century, the movement toward team sports also began to take root in programs for blind children and youth. Modified programs of football, baseball, and basketball (using sound cues when a basket was scored) were established for visually handicapped youngsters. At times competitions—usually wrestling—were arranged with seeing youngsters.

The National Athletic Association of Schools for the Blind was organized in 1908 to formulate rules primarily affecting track and field. Although the association was disbanded in 1953, by the 1950s competitions in a variety of sports had been formulated by administrators and physical educators in schools for the blind. For example, in 1938 the game of buzzer baseball was invented for the blind on the West Coast. Using base paths of wood 3 feet wide, the bases were wired with electric buzzers controlled by the umpire. This game and other "sound" variations on standard games are discussed later in the chapter.

In 1920 an important milestone in motor development of the blind was reached: The first nurseries for blind infants were founded. These institutions taught the importance of directed play to enable visually impaired young children to achieve physical normality. More and more, educators of the blind have come to realize the importance of early intervention in the enrichment of motor development of young blind children.

Experts now tend to agree that physical activities with normal children are beneficial and safe for most blind and visually impaired individuals (Winnick, 1985). And attitudes of the blind toward physical activity are largely positive (Sherrill, Rainbolt, & Erwin, 1984). Despite these generally positive attitudes, however, most blind students in public schools are not participating in vigorous physical education programs with their sighted peers. And community recreational programs often are not viewed as positively as carefully planned and structured physical education programs in the schools. Most blind persons surveyed in a recent poll opined that their lack of participation in community recreation programs was related directly to their handicap (Sherrill et al., 1984).

The outcomes of vigorous activity for blind youths and adults are positive. Weitzman (1985), for example, found an increase in self-esteem, independence, motivation, confidence, and pride that translated into improved mobility scores when blind adults were exposed to walking and aerobic exercise classes. Others have reported positive changes in the psycho-emotional qualities important to happy living when blind people were encouraged to participate in physical education programs (Sherrill et al., 1984).

Blind youngsters also have been found to benefit physically from participation in physical education programs. But programs of activity must be sustained throughout the school years on a continuing basis. As is true with normal children, fitness programs during the school year, if not continued throughout the summer months, result in lowered fitness levels among visually impaired and young blind populations (Di Natale, Lee, Ward, & Shepard, 1985).

DEFINITIONS AND CLASSIFICATIONS

The visually handicapped are classified in various ways. For example, two broad classifications are (a) the *adventitiously* blind—those blinded through an accident or pathological condition after birth, and (b) the *congenitally* blind. If blindness occurs within the first 5 years of life, however, adventitiously and congenitally blind individuals possess similar conceptual and perceptual systems, as they mature, relative to the reality of their world.

The blind also may be classified according to how their vision is adversely affected:

1. Defects of *visual acuity* usually are measured using the Snellen chart and are expressed as a fraction. For example, 20/200 means that the defective eye can see at 20 feet what the normal eye can see at 200 feet.

2. Restriction of *field of vision* may be manifested in two ways: (a) *peripheral vision* may be restricted while central vision remains intact, and (b) the eye may have a scotoma—a spot without vision within the center of the field of vision.

3. Defects of *color vision* relate to discrimination of three qualities of color—hue, saturation, and brightness. In rare cases of total color blindness, all colors are seen as shades of gray, black, and white; most color blindness, however, is partial.

For practical purposes, visual acuity is the most pertinent factor when considering physical education teaching strategies and program components for blind or partially sighted children and youth. The following classifications may appear on a student's visual evaluation record:

1. Legal blindness usually is considered 20/200 or less in the better eye with correcting lenses, or central visual acuity of more than 20/200 if there is a peripheral field defect in which the widest diameter of the visual field subtends an angular distance of no more than 20°.

2. Travel vision involves the ability to see at 5 to 10 feet what those with normal vision see at 200 feet (5/200 to 10/200).

3. Motion perception (3/200 to 5/200) is the ability to detect motion at this low level and involves how much illumination is present as well as the differences between illumination of the object in motion and the background.

4. Less than 3/200 light perception permits the individual to distinguish strong light at a distance of about 3 feet from the eye, but other, less well illuminated objects cannot be seen even at short distances from the face.

5. Lack of vision is the inability to recognize a strong light shining directly into the eye.

Most data indicate that about 75% of all children and youth termed blind possess some vision, and thus may be classified as visually impaired.

CAUSES OF VISUAL IMPAIRMENT

The causes of childhood blindness are many, and they vary according to age. For example, one of the leading causes of blindness in infants was virtually eliminated in the 1950s when *retrolental fibroplasia* (literally, the formation of fibrous tissue behind the lens) was found to result from administering oxygen at too high pressure in the incubators of premature infants. The pressure resulted in inflammation of the peripheral part of the retina and subsequent degeneration and detachment of the retina. Victims of this condition are now in their 30s and older, so they no longer constitute a great percentage of the school-age blind.

Rubella epidemics, occurring in the 1960s and periodically every 6 or 7 years in various parts of the U.S., also can produce blindness in infants at birth. The condition usually is just one manifestation of multiple handicaps—not infrequently hearing loss, motor problems, and retardation.

A few blind children suffer from detached retinas and *retinitis*, and conditions of the eyeball itself also contribute to blindness in the young—infantile *glaucoma*, hardening of the eyeballs, *albinism*, or inherited small eyeballs. *Microphthalmus*, the absence of one or both eyes, contributes only a small percentage to those blind from birth.

About 9.5% of blindness in children results from defects in the nervous system including, for the most part, the optic nerve. Damage to the optic nerve, or to parts of the brain that control vision, though not frequent, can result in partial blindness.

Furthermore, the partially sighted may reflect damage to various parts of the nervous system, including the cranial nerves that mediate vision. These conditions include:

1. *Scotomas*, blind areas in various portions of the visual field.

2. *Diplopia*, double vision, often accompanied by compensatory tilting of the head. Dizziness sometimes is present.

3. *Ptosis*, or dropped eyelid, caused by weakness of the superior levator muscles. Vision, however, may be clear.

4. *Nystagmus*, or rhythmic, rapid movements of the eyes, which may or may not be accompanied by problems with visual acuity.

Figure 6.1 illustrates the parts of the eye.

CHARACTERISTICS OF THE BLIND AND VISUALLY IMPAIRED

Making overall assumptions about the mental, physical, emotional, and social characteristics of any population as diverse as the blind and partially sighted is fraught with peril. Nevertheless, some probabilities relative to how visually handicapped children and youth function academically and socially are worthy of consideration.

Figure 6.1   Parts of the Eye

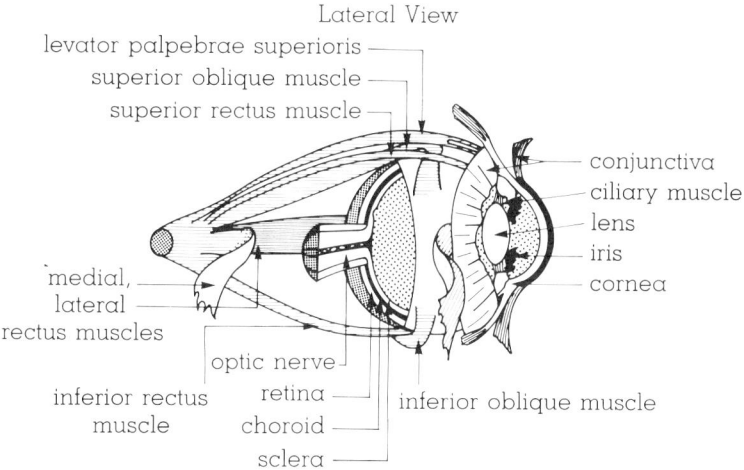

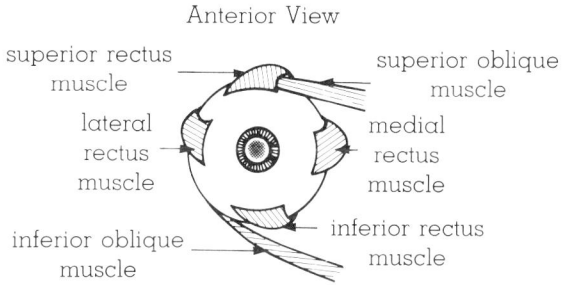

Intellectual Characteristics

Lowenfeld (1971) made an important point prior to his thorough review of the literature on psychological problems of the blind: Differences in blind youngsters, conceptually and perceptually, hinge on two interacting factors—the *age of onset* of blindness, and *extent of vision loss*, partial or total. He proposed a five-part categorization of children by extent and age of onset:

1. Total blindness, congenital or acquired before age 5.
2. Total blindness acquired after age 5.
3. Partial blindness, congenital.
4. Partial sight, congenital.
5. Partial sight, acquired.

Children who are blind or who lose their sight early in life must depend totally on the acquisition of concepts and perceptions through the other senses. Those who become blind later in life, or whose sight is partial, perceive the visual world in an entirely different way.

For example, the totally blind or children whose sight failed before they can remember cannot deal intellectually with objects that are very large (the sun, the moon, mountains), those that are very small (ants, dust), or those that are fragile and delicate (butterflies, flowers). The blind, while usually busy with their hands inspecting objects, lack the sensory apparatus (the eyes) to unify their perceptions of large or complex objects. With experience, however, they learn how to "expand their tactual space," to inspect a chair, for example, rapidly with both hands, and construct a perceptual whole of the experience.

Objects in motion, such as another child running, are also difficult for blind children to comprehend. This has been blamed for the awkwardness sometimes seen in blind children who have not had the opportunity to see their peers run and jump and throw and thus have not been able to copy these movements as have their sighted friends.

A multitude of "sighted words" (e.g., shiny, looking, falling, space), while heard and used by the blind, often have meanings different from those attached to them by the sighted. Colors are a mystery to the totally blind. They usually understand that colors are attributes often attached to certain things and objects (e.g., the grass is green, the sky is blue), but they have no idea what those qualities stand for.

The tactile and auditory senses of the blind have long been studied to support the supposition these are heightened as a result of (a) their frequent use, and (b) the fact that vision does not interfere with their use. For the most part, however, the blind have not been found to be superior to the sighted in gaining information from the other senses, unless a considerable amount of experience and learning have taken place. Object detection via finite sound cues, for example, is as good in the sighted (blindfolded) as it is in the blind, until the latter reach their late teens. Thus, physical education teachers should not expect some kind of magic awareness on the part of their visually handicapped charges. Rather, partially seeing or blind children should be afforded a lot of movement, tactile experiences, and conceptual information about the ideas and objects encountered in physical education classes.

Many studies have been done on the intellectual levels and characteristics of blind youngsters. For the most part, carefully constructed tests, different in part from those used with the sighted, indicate that (a) as a group, the blind may be verbally as able as the sighted, but (b) blind children's experiences and concepts may be less integrated than those of the sighted, and (c) blind children deal best with experiences that are concrete and not abstract in nature—things they can touch, hold, and otherwise manipulate with their remaining senses. For reasons that are obscure, some groups of blind children, including those inflicted with retinoblastoma, evidence superior intelligence, while other sub-populations of blind children—for example, those evidencing congenital anophthalmia (lack of eye structure formation)—in most, but not all, cases have additional developmental handicaps, including retardation.

Congenitally blind children cannot learn to speak by imitating the lip and mouth movements of their peers, so their speech development is delayed in comparison to seeing children. Likewise, blind children, being unable to conceptualize about the multitude of sighted terms permeating human speech, may use words inappropriately.

A summary of the work on differences in speech and communicative behavior between blind and seeing children suggests that:

—blind youngsters use fewer lip movements when speaking.
—appropriate facial expressions do not always accompany emotion-laden sentences and words.
—the blind show less vocal variety and speech inflection when communicating and often speak at a slower rate than do sighted persons.
—some blind persons speak louder than do sighted persons. At times this tendency is extreme and has been labeled a "broadcast voice." (The reason for this characteristic will be discussed later in the chapter.)

Social-Emotional Characteristics

Many studies have been done about perceptions of the sighted toward the blind, and additional work has been carried out to determine how the blind perceive *they* are perceived by the sighted. Most theories of social-emotional development in normal children take into account how they are dealt with by close members of their society. That blind youngsters' emotional make-up depends to a large extent on the amount of pity they feel emanating from important others who surround them is not surprising.

The blind believe that the sighted perceive the blind as naive and lacking in understanding of blind people—most of which has been confirmed by research. The degree to which these feelings, particularly from their parents, influence the blind plays a critical role in the formation of their self-concept and emotional make-up. Early work by Sommers (1944), as well as more recent work, discusses this subject in depth. For the most part, it has been demonstrated that the parents of blind children are often in great conflict, struggling to reconcile feelings of devotion, disappointment over having an imperfect child, and repulsion at the condition—all of which are feelings that are difficult to repress.

According to Sommers, the manner in which parents deal with these conflicting feelings determines to a large degree the adjustive behaviors of blind adolescents. Parental compensations range from "wholesome" to "hypercompensatory, through denial, defensive, and withdrawal reactions." Thus, teachers of blind adolescents might do well to: (a) attempt to determine the manner in which the parents are, and have been, dealing with the condition of their offspring, and then (b) show compassion for the blind child's emotional state at the time of contact with physical education teachers and programs. Because physical education teachers enter children's lives rather late, the forces that mold personality already have been brought to bear on the youngsters. Therefore, tolerance is a more realistic approach than frustration because the children or youth are not always well adjusted and attempts to apply "instant psychiatry" on the playground may be aborted.

The inability to communicate through gestures may result in a young child's escaping into self-absorbing activities. Thus, emphasis in recent years has been placed on early enrichment of communicative behaviors. Rowland (1984) studied the effects of mothers' stimulating their infant's communication by placing their mouths on the cheeks of their offspring in efforts to reach them vocally. Music therapy (Steele & Crawford, 1982) and pillows containing tactile images (Kronheim, 1985) also are used to stimulate the early development of blind infants. These "learning pillows" are tied directly to stories read to the child, encouraging imagery.

Overall, the forces bearing on blind youngsters may result in a type of psychological isolation that produces perceptual rigidity, as well as anxiety about the present and the future. Most able blind adolescents dwell a lot on their future vocations and professions and question their chances for success in maintaining themselves throughout life.

New trends in special education in which the blind are now found more often among the sighted could help to dissipate some of this emotional and perceptual rigidity. Teachers who interact with these youngsters should take gradual steps to introduce varied but nonthreatening experiences that will help reduce anxiety and the lack of flexibility previously directed toward this sub-population.

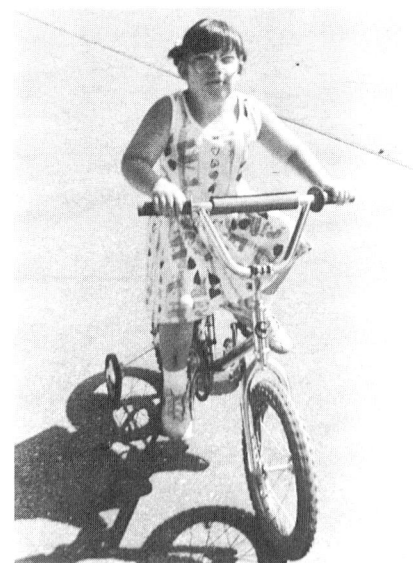

Training wheels help this visually impaired youngster achieve independence on her bike.

Courtesy, Special Education Branch, Los Angeles City Schools

Movement Characteristics

Obviously of critical importance to physical education teachers of special children are the movement characteristics of children with poor or absent vision. Superficial observations of blind children reveal a "movement picture" at variance with that of the sighted. The visually impaired exhibit behaviors that at times seem incongruous.

The children or youth, particularly if they are in an unfamiliar environment or one in which they feel threatened, tend to remain in one place longer than the sighted. But while keeping a relatively stable position, they often engage in rocking, rhythmic, and purposeless mannerisms similar to those seen in other atypical groups including the emotionally disturbed and retarded. In contrast to their fidgety and aimless movements, their facial expressions tend to be relatively bland and immobile. Their bodies suddenly, and for no apparent reason, may become limp as they slump in their chairs or against a wall. Movement of the partially sighted may introduce additional variety as they tilt their heads to one side or lift their chins to obtain what information they can from their environment. Other children may wave their fingers in front of their eyes or rub their eye sockets in ways that appear injurious. The kaleidoscopic variety of mannerisms and movement behaviors of visually impaired persons, even while they are apparently at rest, can be surprising to the uninitiated.

These behaviors and movement capacities have been studied for several decades. Manneristic behaviors, for example, caught the attention of Samuel Gridley Howe almost 150 years ago as he formulated the first physical education programs for the blind in the U.S. After World War II, programs of exercise and fitness for the blind multiplied and produced data reflecting their reactions to the stress of physical exercise.

Three movement qualities of the blind will be briefly surveyed: motor skill and performance, posture, and manneristic behaviors and blindisms. Physical education teachers will not likely deal fully with all of these behaviors. They may and should seek help from classroom teachers, as well as available school psychologists, when attempting to modify some of these behaviors. At the same time, they should remember that the blind, as all children, exhibit marked individual differences in movement preferences and motor capacities. Physical education teachers will be successful to the degree to which they construct highly individualistic programs for the children or youth with whom they are dealing. All visually handicapped and blind youngsters do not possess all of the movement characteristics and abnormalities discussed, and characteristics that youths do exhibit are uniquely their own, for they usually have had no models to copy!

Motor Skills and Performance   The motor skill and performance data obtained from blind or visually impaired youngsters show them to be inferior, in many tasks, to the sighted. One project that compared the fitness of blind and visually handicapped youth to the fitness of normal youngsters consisted of measures of throwing for distance, standing broad jump, tests of muscular strength of the upper limbs, and measures of body composition, endurance, agility, and balance. The study included 694 partially sighted and blind youths 10 to 17 years of age (Winnick & Short, 1982; Winnick, 1985).

Running was required in three of the events/tasks evaluated: a shuttle run, a 50-yard dash, and a long-distance run. Some of the blind subjects employed a sighted guide; others used a guidewire; and the partially sighted ran unassisted. As expected, scores posted by the blind and visually handicapped youngsters on these running tasks were significantly below the scores on the same events by normal youngsters. Moreover, the skin-fold measures of body composition, as well as softball throw scores recorded by the visually impaired and blind, were not as good as scores posted by normal subjects and by auditorily impaired subjects in the same investigation.

Thus, actions involving vigorous movement in space, including throwing and running, appear to be severely limited in blind youngsters. Also, the lack of vigorous actions seemed to be reflected in the scores of participants who had more obese body builds in contrast to normal youngsters of the same age (based upon skin-fold measures).

Results of these and other studies over the years suggest that lack of experience may be an important factor limiting the motor abilities and fitness levels of blind and visually handicapped youngsters. In an interesting study conducted in my laboratory (Williams, 1969) comparing the physical abilities of identical twin 13-year-old girls, the sighted twin out-threw her blind sibling 53 feet to 13 feet. Still, it is difficult to determine whether the apparently inferior motor skill and fitness scores recorded by the blind are attributable to

Filled space between hand-holds helps blind children begin to use climbing apparatus; later they can proceed to regular climbing apparatus with space between hand-holds.

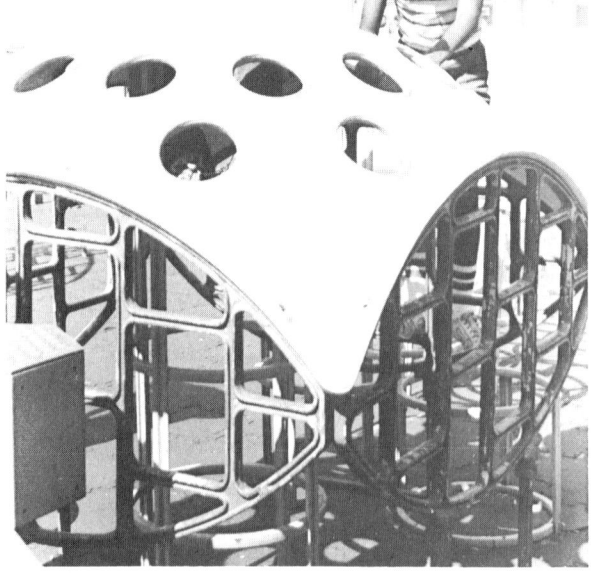

Courtesy, Special Education Branch, Los Angeles City Schools

(a) differences in experience, (b) differences in incentives gained by seeing others attempt the same tasks, (c) differences in opportunities to model appropriate skill patterns, or (d) possible neurological impairment that influences motor functioning among certain blind children. This latter reason often invalidates any so-called physical performance norms obtained from various atypical populations, including the emotionally disturbed and retarded. For practical purposes, when testing and programming for the blind, one should, with the help of a pediatric neurologist, separate children whose motor functioning seems intact from those exhibiting organically based physical awkwardness.

Buell's (1983) text contains norms for the AAHPER fitness test for both partially seeing and blind youngsters. These averages should be used only as rough guidelines. Most helpful when working with a few blind children or an individual blind child is to *construct evaluation goals that permit them to compare their performances with their own prior efforts rather than spurious norms.*

Posture   The static posture of the blind often appears unaesthetic to the sighted. Despite the fact that blind children may conceptually know what "stand up straight" means or be able to identify all body parts and muscle groups that contribute to an erect seated or standing posture, sometimes partially sighted or blind youngsters suddenly and inexplicably slump in their chairs or become limp while in a standing position. These behaviors indicate the difference between the youths' perceptions of their body and its ability to maintain an erect and rigid position and their ability to conceptualize their body image. Some blind children and youth suffering from general hypotonia simply get tired of maintaining an upright stance and slump into various floppy positions.

Because poor posture, particularly head posture, may become a social liability to blind children, it should be addressed by all educators who come in contact with these children— particularly the physical educator. Methods of combating this problem include (a) exercising the antigravity muscle groups and informing children which muscles to tighten (hips, leg extensors, back extensors, trapezius in the upper back and neck, etc.) to effect an upright position; (b) permitting children to "braille" either people or mannequins to ascertain what "good" versus "poor" posture consists of; and (c) informing blind youth of the social importance of "looking" at persons to whom they are speaking and maintaining the accepted posturing of the head and neck in social situations.

Posture and emotions may be closely related. A monograph by Siegel (1966) treats the subject of posture in the blind and delineates ways to deal with poor posture.

Manneristic Behaviors   The random, apparently pointless, rhythmic behaviors of the blind have long been noted by educators observing these children and youth. Often called *blindisms,* the more recent term *manneristic behaviors* was coined for these movements, as it became increasingly clear that they are not confined exclusively to the blind but appear in populations of the emotionally disturbed and retarded as well. Despite the concern and observations about these behaviors, however, relatively few attempts have been made to definitively classify and ameliorate them. Some of the specific mannerisms, and reasons advanced for their onset and perpetuation, are:

—eye rubbing (oculodigital behavior), which apparently can trigger some stimulation to the occipital areas and lead to self-initiation of internal visual "pictures."

—rocking motions of the body and rhythmic movements of the arms and hands, triggered by boredom and the need for self-stimulation in the absence of environmental stimulation. (Some observers have noted, however, that these behaviors occur both when children are apparently bored and when they become agitated and excited over an impending event or task.)

—fluttering and any of the other physical manifestations mentioned, as a substitute for physical activity. The compulsive foot tapping sometimes seen among sighted people when they are kept waiting is an analogous nervous affectation.

In a penetrating study Eichel (1979) classified behaviors into manageable types. She reasoned that, prior to attempting to reduce their occurrence, one should try to formulate a plan for enumerating and classifying them. Using observational methods and time sampling techniques, manneristic behaviors were broken down into five categories involving parts of the body: the face, head, hands and arms, trunk and whole body, and legs and feet. Moreover, she attempted to quantify various qualities of these rhythmic movements and rate them as to intensity, direction, and synchronization.

Based on 113 observations of 30 children ages 18 months to 11 years, which yielded 466 incidents of manneristic behavior, she found that most children showed one dominant and unique mannerism, with a consistent pattern of secondary mannerisms. Most mannerisms (72%) were of moderate intensity and often involved rocking along with hand-eye mannerisms (15%). Next in frequency were dominant mannerisms involving hitting and slapping. The children observed seldom evidenced simultaneous mannerisms but instead exhibited them one at a time in serial fashion. No significant differences were found in manneristic behaviors involving the hands and eyes of the visually impaired as compared with the totally blind. Inter-observer reliability was high, exceeding 80% of the agreement on most qualities and mannerisms classified and scored.

Manneristic behaviors in the blind are related positively to degree of blindness; the totally blind are more likely to exhibit them than are the partially sighted. Moreover, more intelligent blind children are less likely to exhibit manneristic behaviors than those with below average levels of intelligence. Manneristic behaviors also are more often seen in children and youth who have additional handicaps, including emotional disturbance (Jan, Freeman, & Scott, 1977; Chapman, 1978). Further, children having close emotional and physical contact with their mothers tend to exhibit fewer of these self-involved behaviors (Willis, 1979).

It is generally agreed that manneristic behaviors are not desirable, as they exaggerate differences between the blind and the sighted, are not socially accepted by the sighted, and often prevent blind youth from taking part in meaningful educational, physical, and intellectual experiences. Among the remedial strategies are (a) substituting appropriate behaviors (e.g., crafts) when the mannerism appears; (b) providing gentle to severe reminders to refrain from their use; (c) giving rewards for increased periods of time during which the mannerisms are absent, and punishments when the mannerisms appear. Often, however, when one mannerism is reduced or eliminated, it is replaced by another. Therefore, these techniques have been subjected to experimental scrutiny.

A study by Sklar and Rampulla (1973), using one subject, attempted to eliminate inappropriate hand-clapping by rewarding tokens and verbal praise when the clapping stopped. The 20-year-old subject's teacher, as well as her peers, participated in the study and helped her successfully eliminate the clapping behavior, permitting more meaningful classroom participation.

Strategies to eliminate or reduce manneristic behaviors in the blind should be carefully applied—particularly by physical education teachers. The causes of these compulsive and persistent movements in any given child or youth are not well known and the individual may require psychological or psychiatric counseling. Subtle reminders, with perhaps a guiding and gentle touch, may help reduce them, particularly when the mannerisms interfere with normal physical education activities or inhibit learning a new skill. Most of the time a blind child who exhibits mannerisms and who is reasonably emotionally stable will react appropriately when quietly asked to cease it and given something meaningful to accomplish.

Medical and Psychological Characteristics and Considerations

Prior to working with blind youngsters in any class, instructors should become thoroughly aware of their unique medical characteristics and needs. Any possibility that a jarring action would injure an already damaged retina, for example, should be clearly indicated on the child's medical record. If records do not exist, thorough work-ups should be done or physical education teachers should stop working with the children. Blind youngsters may have various other disorders such as cardiovascular problems, a tendency toward seizures, or other potentially dangerous conditions that may be triggered by the stress of a single vigorous act, the excitement of a game, or fatigue brought on by endurance activities.

Of similar importance are psychological considerations for the well-being of visually impaired and blind students when they are placed in what they may perceive as a moderately to highly threatening environment. Sighted students should be thoroughly grounded in the characteristics, both personal and physical, of these classmates. Children in the class should be "on the lookout" for signs of undue stress, mild seizure, or other signs of discomfort emanating from blind or partially sighted youth.

MOTOR IMPROVEMENT

Presently, one can ascertain two major objectives and directions relative to the physical welfare and motor development of blind infants, children, and youth: (a) early intervention programs for young blind and partially sighted youngsters in an effort to reach them during their formative months; and (b) thoughtfully directed movement experiences in educating important spatial concepts in visually handicapped and blind youngsters. These programs are exemplified by vigorous, yet modified physical education and sports programs for the blind, as discussed in the fine book on physical education by Charles Buell (1983), who is visually impaired himself.

Early Motor Development and Intervention

Although special physical education teachers of blind youngsters (or of classes in which blind and sighted children may be mixed) do not often deal directly with children younger than 4 or 5 years of age, they *do* have to face symptoms of blindness reflected in delayed motor development of blind children in middle childhood or later. Because so much of the physical behavior of normal infants is instigated by visually perceived objects or people, blind infants are behind their sighted peers in various aspects of physical development. Prehension of blind infants usually is delayed, and they evidence what are called "blind hands"—hands held high and apart at each shoulder, arms flexed, with fingers on each hand moving independently of each other and many times apparently not in reaction to any object that may be present. Blind infants do not reach out with these seemingly ineffectual appendages because they "see" no reason to do so.

Movements prior to and including walking also are delayed. In turning over they evidence a delay of several weeks to several months, and in creeping they may lag at least 10 months behind the average sighted infant (Davidson & Simmons, 1984). Blind children many times do not walk until near the end of their second year. The apparent lack of stimuli to move, reach for, crawl toward, or walk to something visual and tangible blocks or delays the onset of these normal movements. According to Fraiberg (1977), blind infants lack external "lures" that impel sighted infants to reach out and to travel throughout their environment. This disinclination to move often results in lags in locomotor development.

In perhaps one of the best conceived research studies dealing with handicapped children, Fraiberg (1968), when suddenly confronted with similar and "blunted" movements in 27 blind infants and children, noted some of the conditions alluded to above. Moreover, she began to see similarities in the posturings, rockings, and immobility of blind infants brought to her and her colleagues in their role as consultants to the Family Service Society of New Orleans. In the years that followed, through careful research, observations, and intervention, they not only documented the status of congenitally blind infants but also developed guidelines for helpful change (Fraiberg, Smith, & Adelson, 1969; Fraiberg, 1971).

Their work, observations, interventions, and results are contained in an important text (Fraiberg, 1977). Although it cannot be adequately summarized here, the approach in essence was to aid blind infants in perceiving that things were out there if the neonate would just reach out or move toward them.

Fraiberg's interventions for remediating the "blind hands" phenomenon were tasks devised to encourage infants to converge their hands at the midline of the body to grasp bottles, noisy stabiles hung over the crib, and the like. Locomotive and creeping behaviors were instigated by helping children experience "sound-reach" and to "reach on sound"—to react positively to sounds representing objects placed just out of their reach when they were postured in a creeping, sitting, or standing position. Careful evaluation of the effects of these intervention programs, using "sound lures" as well as midline tasks for the stimulation of prehension, were positive and encouraging.

The primary point of this chronicle of the Fraiberg program is that too few blind children have been subjected to such knowledgeable interventions as this. Thus, as blind children arrive at school at ages 4 to 6, they also may lack vigorous exploratory behaviors manifested in the upper limbs and be reluctant to display expansive locomotor behaviors. Physical educators should strive to be as creative as the Fraiberg group in formulating sound lures and other incentives that encourage vigorous exploratory and recreational movements in their older blind charges.

New technical aids are being applied to the early education of blind youngsters. The *sonicguide* reflects high-frequency waves off objects and passes these waves into earphones, which usually are placed in helmets or bands around a child's head. Children exposed to this aid during their first year of life have exhibited reaching and swiping behaviors similar to those of sighted infants. This type of aid can help the child identify the presence and distance of important other people (Ferrell, 1980). Electronic aids are also discussed by Warren and Strelow (1985). With thorough training, children become able to engage in confident, independent locomotion and to safely pass around objects. Other positive outcomes reported include a lessening of stereotypic mannerisms and an improvement in the child's spatial concepts—the concepts of up/down, under/above, and the like.

Spatial Education

Lacking efficient space receptors, blind persons are dependent on other senses to learn about space—the processing and interpretation of sounds, touches, and information gained from their movements. Most important, what they *think* about this information tends to unify and help them form useful impressions of themselves, others, objects, and their total environment.

In the 1940s, 1950s, and 1960s various research programs in the United States and abroad explored the manner in which blind people learned about space, the ways in which they seemed to sense the presence of objects and walls when approaching them, and the accuracy with which they could move in simple and complex ways through rooms in their homes, schools, and work places, as well as through their total neighborhood.

The discovery was made in the late 1940s that the blind detected obstacles through subtle sound cues in the form of echoes emanating from objects (and open places in walls), produced by the noises present in most life situations. In the 1960s I carried out research at UCLA on the accuracy with which the blind could move in space when asked to (a) walk straight for a distance, (b) return to a point after being led away, (c) detect gradients, as well as left-right tilt, in pathways, and (d) make precise facing movements—i.e., execute 90°, 180°, and 360° turns (Cratty, 1968).

Drawing upon this information, subsequent studies with blind children revealed that real and significant changes could be elicited in a number of spatial concepts and tasks reflecting ideas about space. For example, the body image of blind children ages 4.5 to 12 years was found to improve as the result of training using a mannequin with movable limbs.

Another study, by Carl Peterson (1968), found that facing movement accuracy, as well as the tendency of children to veer from a straight line, could be improved with twice-weekly training sessions. Correcting the veering tendency was accomplished by permitting the children to "braille" a flexible wire (overlying a small grid) that had been bent to conform to the pathway the children had just walked.

These and similar studies have indicated that spatial concepts in blind children and youth can be improved through the use of movement and tactile experiences, coupled with encouragement to conceptualize about the spatial dimensions of their world. Teachers of physical education, when confronted with blind students, should (a) gain an awareness of how much the children know about their bodies and about extensions in their space field, and (b) afford them helpful experiences, both directly in and ancillary to regular physical education tasks, to aid their ideas about space. Sometimes physical education teachers can work in useful ways with mobility trainers, if available.

Overall, the research suggests that four types of spatial education should accompany general education for the visually handicapped. These should overlap and be offered at different stages.

1. *Body image training* (from birth to late childhood or adolescence). This training should begin with subtle tactile experiences, during which the infant is touched and permitted to roll and contact objects, continuing, as the child becomes verbal, with identification of body parts and body movements, accompanied by a variety of movement experiences. Research with children has indicated that concepts in this sub-stage appear in four major phases: (a) concepts involving body planes, body parts, and body movements—parts of the face, front, back, side, etc.; (b) left-right discriminations—left and right limbs, etc., and "place an object to your left," etc.; (c) complex judgments about body-object relationships—"Move so that your left side is nearest the wall," parts of limbs, thigh, etc.; and (d) moving into another person's reference system—"Where is my left shoulder? Touch it," etc. A monograph by Cratty and Sams (1968) contains a detailed breakdown of the difficulty of various tasks within these four sub-sections.

2. *Dynamic spatial orientation* (from onset of walking to adulthood). This second part of spatial education consists of tasks that encourage children to make judgments about space while moving in space. Walking a line and returning to a starting point is a simple example of a task within this category. Learning the shape of base paths and the location of bases in a "sound" baseball game is an example of a more complex task. Making accurate one-quarter, one-half, and complete turns are still other examples of tasks in which mobility trainers, classroom teachers, and physical education teachers might cooperate.

Using various techniques described in *Movement and Spatial Awareness in Blind Children and Youth* (Cratty, 1971), the "obstacle sense" can be trained.

3. *Tactile exploration of maps and models* (from middle childhood to adulthood).

4. *Mobility training* (from middle childhood to adulthood).

The final two parts of the spatial education program may be instituted in intellectually normal and emotionally stable individuals in middle childhood. These two items consist of simple map reading and tactile exploration of environments through the use of scale models of structures in the school or other environments in which the blind person must operate. Mobility training involves teaching the "long cane" technique. This should be done by competent educators with an advanced degree in education of the blind and in mobility training specifically.

Several scales and assessment instruments have been developed to evaluate the extent to which blind children have acquired spatial concepts and a vocabulary about space, including an instrument with which to evaluate body image (Cratty & Sams, 1968). This device, like others, suffers from a lack of sufficient normative data and from technical problems related to test construction. The Kephart scale (Kephart & Kephart, 1973), for example, was designed to measure body and environmental concepts and used 86 children between the ages of 5 and 7, all of whom were totally blind or who had light perception. The Kephart scale, however, has been criticized for the absence of evidence of reliability and validity.

A test was formulated by Boehm (1971) to evaluate basic spatial concepts in visually impaired children from kindergarten to second grade. Although the test is apparently reliable, more data attesting to its validity would seem to be called for. The most promising test of spatial concepts in blind children was developed by Hill (1981). It was designed to evaluate a variety of selected spatial concepts in children from ages 6 to 14 by means of 75 items divided into three sections. Many of the spatial concepts evaluated must be demonstrated by the children via movements (inside, outside, on top of, etc.).

PROGRAMMING GUIDELINES AND PRINCIPLES

Traditionally, blind individuals have participated in wrestling and track-and-field competitions, in which extensive inter-school meets have been organized. But now the variety of programs in which blind and partially sighted students may be participating is much wider and more varied. Virtually no recreational activity is closed to them. They can even participate, with modifications, in difficult sports such as skiing, ice skating, football, and soccer.

Schools for the blind established in most states of the U.S. by the turn of the century had physical education programs designed exclusively for the blind and visually impaired. These programs, while still in existence, were largely replaced by special physical education classes in regular schools. Even more recently one or a few blind or partially sighted youngsters have been included in physical education classes for the sighted. Needless to say, the various situations call for teaching strategies, equipment, facilities, and game modifications that meet the needs of these students.

Perhaps the best and most comprehensive source for games and sports for blind youngsters is the text by Buell (1983). In general, partially sighted youngsters participate reasonably well in sports, even in ball games. At times "sound balls," in which a noise source has been embedded, are helpful. Both totally blind and partially blind children can participate in base games if a sound source (e.g., another child hitting a tin can) is provided at each base. Archery and golf also may be adapted for the blind, using sounds as cues. Running races is possible with the help of hand-railings or waist-high ropes strung along the course. I witnessed a marathon in which a blind runner periodically changed sighted guides who ran in front of him. With modifications, a cane can be made to grip the curbing of a regulation running track, permitting solitary blind runners to engage in cardiovascular fitness activities.

The blind particularly seem to enjoy tumbling and other gymnastic activities. If tasks are properly sequenced and reasonable safeguards are established, the exhilaration of moving on mats, apparatus, and even through the air may be enjoyed by both totally blind and partially sighted children.

Outdoor activity and play areas are most usable if the surfaces vary in texture and composition. In this way blind children can gain cues to the sizes of the field, its conformation, and its boundary—such as a gravel running track. Cement surfaces should have easily felt boundaries, perhaps of grass or rough asphalt.

When mainstreaming blind or partially sighted youngsters, they should be provided with constant, reliable companions from among sighted members of the class. These peer guides should be mature and dependable. Consistency in attendance and behavior is para-

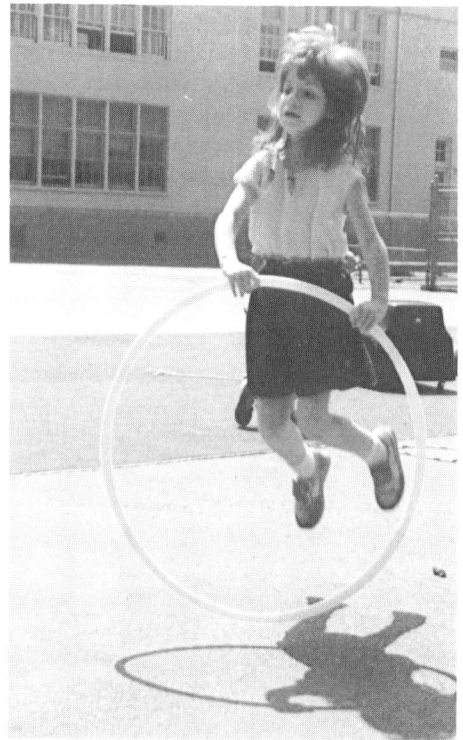

The hula-hoop presents a rigid and predictable pathway as a blind girl "jumps rope."

Courtesy, Special Education Branch, Los Angeles City Schools

mount, for the blind (as is true with other exceptional groups) do best when the time schedules to which they are exposed, as well as the objects and people that confront them, are predictable and consistent.

Principles that student guides should follow when working with blind or partially sighted youngsters include the following:

1. While not being overprotective, student guides should show reasonable concern about encountering the unexpected. Nothing is more irritating to blind persons than encountering difficulties that might have been easily avoided if they had been warned or aided by a sighted person standing by. Sighted observers often remain silent in an effort to not offend the blind or to erroneously aid them in gaining confidence by leaving them "on their own." This tendency to watch instead of to assist is inappropriate and not appreciated by blind people.

2. Peer helpers should lead their blind companions by offering their elbow and walking *ahead* of the sightless youngsters. The blind do not like to be led by being held out in front of their sighted companions like a "fish on a hook," as an irritated blind man once described it to me. The blind want the sighted to meet obstacles such as stairs first, and by feeling changes in the posture of the guide, the blind can adjust accordingly.

3. Blind youngsters always should be anchored socially. That is, sightless children should be told who is present and what is happening. Blind youngsters sometimes develop what has been called a "broadcast voice," overly loud speech, caused by not always knowing who, if anyone, is present to listen to them and hear their requests. To be talking and suddenly realize no one is present is disconcerting.

4. When appropriate, blind youngsters should be physically anchored and spatially oriented. Sightless youngsters should be seated or placed so that their hands are touching a chair, table, or some object that gives them some stability. In larger areas children should be told what cues are present in all parts of the spatial area. This kind of orientation is aided by making a small cardboard model of the gymnasium (or other area) showing doors, sides containing windows, and so on. Similar models can be made of other physical education and school facilities. If peers see that blind or partially sighted youngsters are becoming disoriented or otherwise confused, they should help their charges "square off"—bring them to a known location and point out what is to their front, their left, and their right— prior to beginning activities again.

Evaluation of the blind and deaf-blind during their early months of life is possible using standard infant development scales like that designed by Nancy Bayley (1984). Also, specific scales have been developed to evaluate the early motor development of this subpopulation of youngsters (Stillman, 1978).

Blind youngsters—particularly those with partial sight—can do more than one might expect in physical education classes for the sighted. Adhering to some of the above guidelines will optimize their participation. And their level of participation and activity can even be an inspiration to sighted members of a physical education class.

SUMMARY

The literature reflects how abilities important to the blind and visually impaired may be enhanced through movement—their movement through space, their posture, and their social behaviors. Studies by the Fraibergs dealing with enhancement of motor abilities of blind infants through sensory-motor experiences are helpful. Other work suggests that special body-image training techniques can enhance the lives of visually impaired individuals. And Eichel's work holds promise for the reduction of distracting rhythmic, manneristic behaviors. New technological aids also are useful.

Physical educators working with paritally sighted or blind youngsters may make use of sound balls and other auditory experiences to extend to these youngsters movement experiences usually reserved for the sighted. Recreational activities including skiing, mountain climbing, and the like are being taken up by blind children and adolescents. At times blindness, coupled with decreased activity, results in an unfit young adult. This chain of events may be reversed if younger blind children are encouraged to move vigorously and are given reasons for doing so.

Blind youngsters who are placed in regular physical education classes may benefit from sighted peer helpers. These individuals should be given special training in the psychological and social implications of blindness, together with helpful and useful ways to be of service to their sightless classmates.

REFERENCES

Bayley, N. (1984). *Bayley scales of infant development*. New York: Psychological Corp.

Boehm, A.E. (1971). *Boehm test of basic concepts: Test manual*. New York: Psychological Corp.

Buell, C.G. (1983). *Physical education for blind children* (2nd ed.). Springfield, IL: Charles C Thomas.

Chapman, E. (1978). *Visually handicapped children and young people*. Boston: Routledge & Kegan Paul.

Cratty, B.J. (1968, April). The development of perceptual motor abilities in blind children and adolescents. *New Outlook for the Blind*, pp. 191-195.

Cratty, B.J. (1971). *Movement and spatial awareness in blind children and youth*. Springfield, IL: Charles C Thomas.

Cratty, B.J., & Sams, T.A. (1968). *The body image of blind children*. New York: American Foundation for the Blind.

Davidson, I.F., & Simmons, J.N. (1984). Mediating the environment for young blind children: A conceptualization. *Journal of Visual Impairment & Blindness, 78*, 251-255.

Di Natale, J., Lee, M., Ward, G., & Shepard, P. (1985). Loss of physical condition in sightless adolescents during a summer vacation. *Adapted Physical Activity Quarterly, 2*, 144-150.

Eichel, V. (1979). A taxonomy for mannerisms of blind children. *Journal of Visual Impairment & Blindness, 73*, 167-178.

Ferrell, K.A. (1980). Can infants use sonicguide? Two years experience of Project VIEW! *Journal of Visual Impairment & Blindness, 74*, 209-220.

Fraiberg, S. (1968). Parallel and divergent patterns in blind and sighted infants. *Psychoanalytic Study of the Child, 23*, 264-300.

Fraiberg, S. (1971). Intervention in infancy: A program for blind infants. *Journal of the American Academy of Child Psychiatry, 10*(3), 381-405.

Fraiberg, S. (1977). *Insights from the blind: Developmental studies of blind children*. New York: Basic Books.

Fraiberg, S., Smith, M., & Adelson, E. (1969). An educational program for blind infants. *Journal of Special Education, 3*(2), 121-139.

Hill, E.W. (1981). *Hill performance test on selected positional concepts*. Chicago: Stoelting Co.

Jan, J., Freeman, R., & Scott, E. (1977). *Visual impairments in children and adolescents*. New York: Grune & Stratton.

Kephart, J., & Kephart, C.P. (1973). *The Kephart scale*. Unpublished document, Florida School for the Deaf and Blind.

Kronheim, J.K. (1985). Home-grown toys: The learning pillows. *Journal of Visual Impairment & Blindness, 78*, 158-159.

Lowenfeld, B. (1971). Psychological problems of children with impaired vision. In W.M. Cruickshank (Ed.), *Psychology of exceptional children and youth* (3rd ed.) (pp. 211-307). Englewood Cliffs, NJ: Prentice-Hall.

National Society for the Prevention of Blindness (1980). *Vision problems in the U.S.: Data analysis*. New York: NSPB.

Peterson, C.D. (1968). *The educability of dynamic spatial orientation in blind children*. Unpublished master's thesis, UCLA, Dept. of Physical Education.

Rowland, C. (1984). Preverbal communication of blind infants and their mothers. *Journal of Visual Impairment & Blindness, 77,* 297-302.

Sherrill, C., Rainbolt, W., & Erwin, S. (1984). Attitudes of blind persons toward physical education/recreation. *Adapted Physical Activity Quarterly, 1,* 3-11.

Siegel, I.M. (1966). *Posture in the blind.* New York: American Foundation for the Blind.

Sklar, M.J., & Rampulla, J. (1973). Decreasing inappropriate classroom behavior of a multiply handicapped blind student. *Education of the Visually Handicapped, 5,* 71-74.

Sommers, V.S. (1944). *The influence of parental attitudes and social environment on the personality development of the adolescent blind.* New York: American Foundation for the Blind.

Steele, A.L., & Crawford, C. (1982). Music therapy for the visually impaired. *Education of the Visually Handicapped, 14,* 58-61.

Stillman, R. (Ed.). (1978). *Callier-Azusa Scale.* Dallas: University of Texas, Callier Center for Communicable Disorders.

Warren, D.H., & Strelow, E.R. (1985). *Electronic spatial sensing for the blind.* Boston: Martinus Nijhoff.

Weitzman, D.M. (1985). An aerobic walking program to promote physical fitness in older blind adults. *Journal of Visual Impairment & Blindness, 79,* 97-99.

Williams, H.G. (1969). A comparison of selected behaviors of identical twins, one blind from birth. *Journal of Motor Behavior, 1*(4), 259-274.

Wills, D.M. (1979). Profile of young blind children. *Psychoanalytic Study of the Child, 24,* 217-237.

Winnick, J.P. (1985). The performance of visually impaired youngsters in physical education activities: Implications for mainstreaming. *Adapted Physical Activity Quarterly, 2,* 292-299.

Winnick, J.P., & Short, F.X. (1982). *The physical fitness of sensory and orthopedically impaired youth.* Washington, D.C.: U.S. Office of Education, Special Education Programs.

ADDITIONAL REFERENCES

Brooks, K., & Dunn, S. (1952). Dancers in darkness (interview). *Journal of School Health, 44*(3), 147-151.

Cratty, B.J. (1973). *Physical development for children: Selected perceptual-motor activities to enhance movement attributes and sports skills.* Baldwin, NY: Activity Records.

Fletcher, J.J. (1980). Spatial representation in blind children 1: Development compared to sighted children. *Journal of Visual Impairment & Blindness, 74,* 381-385.

Fraiberg, S., Siegel, B., & Gibson, R. (1966). The role of sound in the search behavior of a blind infant. *Psychoanalytic Study of the Child, 21,* 327-357.

Igarashi, N. (1971). Ocular autostimulation of pre-school blind children. *Bulletin of the Tokyo Metropolitan Rehabilitation Center for the Physically and Mentally Handicapped,* pp. 39-45.

Jansson, G. (1983). Tactile guidance of movement. *International Journal of Neuroscience, 19,* 37-46.

Kephart, J., Kephart, C.P., & Schwartz, G.C. (1974). A journey into the world of the blind child. *Exceptional Children, 40,* 421-427.

Laughlin, S. (1975). A walking-jogging program for blind persons. *New Outlook for the Blind, 69,* 312-313.

Lord, F.E. (1969). Development of scales for the measurement of orientation and mobility skills of young blind children. *Exceptional Children, 36*(2), 77-81.

Resnick, R. (1973). Creative movement classes for visually handicapped children in a public school setting. *New Outlook for the Blind, 67,* 442-447.

Scholl, G.T. (1986). *Foundations of education for blind and visually handicapped children and youth: Theory and practice.* New York: American Foundation for the Blind.

Warren, D.H. (1977). *Blindness and early childhood development* (2nd ed.). New York: American Foundation for the Blind.

Warren, D.H., & Strelow, E.R. (1985). *Electronic spatial sensing for the blind.* Boston: Martinus Nijhoff.

QUESTIONS FOR DISCUSSION

1. How are blindness and various degrees of visual impairment defined? What are the practical implications of these definitions?

2. How might a partially sighted youngster differ conceptually from a totally blind youngster when both are mainstreamed into a physical education class of sighted peers?

3. What are the main causes of blindness? In what ways might these causes affect participation in a physical education program?

4. What further studies might be carried out dealing with the effects of sensory-motor training on the total functioning of blind babies? With the attempts of blind adolescents to learn the streets of their town? With newly blinded older individuals?

5. How are activities modified for the blind in physical education?

6. What kinds of tasks might young blind children participate in to find out about their body and its parts? What tasks might help older blind children become more aware of the spatial dimensions of their classroom or the total school in which they must move?

7. What special cues, instructional aids, and the like might help blind children move about and learn more readily?

8. In what ways could jogging and cross-country running be modified so that blind populations might participate in these sports more fully?

STUDENT PROJECTS

1. Visit and interview a teacher of a blind or visually impaired child. Discuss with the teacher any special social and psychological characteristics that might be relevant to physical activity.

2. Visit the home of a blind child and interview the parents relative to special problems the child may have. How did the child learn about being "different," and what do the parents see as a vocational or professional future for their blind youngster?

3. Review additional literature dealing with the physical characteristics of blind children. Formulate an ideal week-long physical activity program with reference to these abilities.

4. What motor tests might be appropriate for administration to blind or partially sighted youngsters? What kinds of tests are likely to produce scores that approximate those of sighted children? What tests might produce different scores when comparing the abilities of the two populations?

5. Interview a physical educator who has one or more blind children in a class. Observe the class. Attempt to ascertain what principles guide the teacher's behavior. What special equipment and facilities, if any, are provided?

6. What special cues, teaching aids, and equipment might facilitate the teaching of physical activities to blind youngsters? Obtain catalogs that contain motor development equipment for normal children, and determine which kinds of equipment are appropriate for blind or partially sighted youngsters. How might other commercial equipment be modified?

7. Interview a young adult who has impaired vision. Try to determine what experiences revolving around physical activity were critical, if any, during the formative years of the person's life.

RESOURCES

American Association for the Blind
1511 K. St., N.W.
Washington, DC 20005

American Blind Bowling Association
150 North Bellaire Ave.
Louisville, KY 40206

American Foundation for the Blind
15 W. 16th St.
New York, NY 10011

Association for the Education of the
  Visually Handicapped
206 N. Washington St.
Alexandra, VA 22314

Braille Sports Foundation
730 Hennepin Ave. S.
Minneapolis, MN 55403

National Society for the Prevention
  of Blindness
79 Madison Ave.
New York, NY 10016

Royal Institute for the Blind
224 Great Portland St.
London, WIN 6AA
England

The Seeing Eye, Inc.
Morristown, NJ 07960

Ski for Light, Inc.
1455 West Lake St.
Minneapolis, MN 55408

U.S. Association for Blind Athletes
55 W. California St.
Beach Haven, NJ 08008

7 Hearing Impairments

Over 300,000 children in the United States are considered deaf or hard of hearing. These youngsters in turn have mild to severe problems in oral communication, which influence their functioning in today's society. Overall, approximately 40% of all children in the U.S. are born deaf, 30% become deaf before age 2, and the remainder of them become deaf at 3-18 years of age (Schein & Delk, 1974). The *age of onset* of deafness is critical relative to acquisition of speech and communicative skills later in life. Those who have become deaf prelingually (have never acquired spoken language) and those who have encountered deafness after acquiring the ability to vocally communicate show sharp and distinct differences in communication skills.

BACKGROUND AND HISTORY

The first schools for the deaf began to appear in the United States in the early part of the last century. Following sporadic attempts to tutor the deaf (usually by the clergy prior to 1800), Thomas H. Gallaudet established the first residential school for the deaf in Hartford, Connecticut, in 1817.[1] Having prepared himself in France, Gallaudet provided the impetus for institutions of a similar nature. Later his son Edward led in establishing the first college for the deaf, Gallaudet University, now in Washington, D.C. Named in honor of his father, it is the only liberal arts college for the deaf in the world.

During the 50 years from 1817 until 1867, schools founded for the deaf were residential institutions. Then, as now, some students who attended them lived at home. Day schools for the deaf were not instituted until after the Civil War, when schools in Pittsburgh and Boston were among the first to be opened. This pattern has been followed to the present, and most medium and large cities in the country have day schools for the deaf and hard of hearing in addition to state schools for the deaf.[2]

Even in the 1800s it was recognized that providing a bland speech environment for the hard of hearing did not serve their best interests. Some progressive educators of the deaf welcomed hearing children into their schools so their noisy chatter at play and work would help their less advantaged peers learn to speak as well as possible.

Today, with the advent of mainstreaming in the middle and late 1970s, several trends are apparent in various educational contexts:

1. Residential schools continue to try to attract hearing children for at least part of their day to enrich the language and speech of the deaf and hard of hearing.

---

1. Originally named the American Asylum for the Education of the Deaf and Dumb, it is now the American School for the Deaf, located in Washington, DC.

2. A well documented history of education of the deaf may be found in *Educating the Deaf: Psychology, Principles and Practices* by D.F. Moores, 1978, Boston: Houghton Mifflin.

2. More and more deaf and moderately hard of hearing children are being included in at least part of the curriculum of regular schools.

3. Increased efforts are being made to detect slight hearing losses in children and ascertain as early as possible in the life of infants those who may have hearing losses.

Of all the handicapped groups, deaf and hard of hearing children and youth may be expected to participate most vigorously in programs of athletics, recreation, and physical education. Interscholastic participation in many sports has long been a vital part of the interactions between schools for the deaf throughout the U.S. Able physical educators should encourage normal to above-average participation in virtually all individual sports and some team sports, with only minor accommodations to the condition.

DETECTION

Measurement of hearing by simple use of the human voice or ticks of watches has become rare in professional circles. The measure most often employed today is the *pure-tone audiometer*, which produces a variety of controlled tones that can be varied in pitch and loudness. Requiring a voluntary response, such as raising a finger to sounds heard, this type of testing is relatively fast and accurate with children over age 4. In younger children a variety of methods may be employed, including *psychogalvanic skin resistance audiometry*, which measures and records changes in skin resistance via hand-held electrodes when tones are presented to the child.

In some cases conditioning to the sound has been used through prior pairing with a mild electric shock. The child anticipates the shock and responds to the tone by a change in skin resistance. This method, as well as others that do not require overt, voluntary responses from children, is applicable also to some physically handicapped, mentally retarded, and multiply handicapped children.

With standard audiometry children respond to a series of sounds ranging from middle C to five octaves above in both ears. Responses are recorded in the form of an audiogram. Children who do not perceive frequencies above 2000 cycles per second (or 2000 Hz)[3] may have problems recognizing words containing the sounds of the letters *s, z, sh, zh,* and *th*, as well as *ch* (as in *chair*) and the letters *p, b, t, d, f, v,* and *h*.

For the most part, children with slight hearing losses may be able to understand low-frequency sounds better than high-frequency sounds. Dance teachers and physical education teachers should plan their music and vocal communication accordingly and should attempt to speak in well modulated, lower tones if possible.

Although pure-tone testing is helpful, it is most important to determine how well children hear human speech. Using tests developed at Bell Telephone Laboratories during the 1920s and 1930s and studies conducted at Harvard during World War II, various adaptations of tests of speech-sound perception have been made available.

In addition, *bone conduction testing* may be carried out. To accomplish this, a vibrator is placed on the mastoid area at the rear of the ear, and children are asked to respond in

---

3. One cycle per second is equal to one hertz (1 Hz).

the way described above. Thus, both air conduction and bone conduction tests are used to evaluate children's sensitivity to loudness via a decibel (db) measure and to various frequencies of sound and pitch.

A sometimes perplexing variable may intrude on one's best efforts to evaluate the hearing of young children and youth. Not always in concordance with the results obtained from traditional audiometric approaches are indications of how children perceive and organize the words and sentences to which they are exposed. Thus, children with apparently similar hearing losses as measured by pure-tone audiometry may vary markedly in their ability to comprehend what is being said to them. This is one of the areas addressed by professionals who deal with learning disabilities.

Even with the detection procedures briefly surveyed, parents are the most important evaluators of children's hearing early in life. Early detection by parents is critical. By the second and third year, about 70% of the children with hearing losses have been identified as being hearing impaired by a parent—usually their mother. This leaves about 30% whose problem may be identified by teachers and others later. Parent education on the signs of hearing loss is carried out by numerous organizations, including the Tracy Clinic in Los Angeles. Too, programs of early education in which parents play a critical role have proliferated in recent years.

DEFINITIONS AND CLASSIFICATIONS

In general, the classification of hearing losses formulated by Streng (1958) is accepted in most special education programs. It consists of categories for mild, marginal, moderate, severe, and profound hearing loss. Often, however, the boundaries between these classifications are vague, and with maturation and exposure to educational programs and increasingly sophisticated tests, children and youth sometimes pass from one classification into another.

1. *Profound hearing loss.* Children with profound hearing loss are essentially deaf. Because they cannot hear words even when amplified, they may respond only reflexively by turning their heads to extremely loud noises close to the ears. These children should be fitted early in life with hearing aids to help them "hear" loud sounds and may only recognize music through the presence or cessation of vibrations. Overall hearing loss in this category is 75 db.

2. *Severe hearing loss.* Children with a severe hearing loss of 60-75 db are considered educationally deaf. Although some residual hearing is present, a great deal of special training is needed for them to learn language. Using hearing aids with strong amplification, these children can distinguish between various loud sounds, horns, and the rhythm of music. Some words may be distinguished if spoken a few inches from the ear.

3. *Moderate hearing loss.* Children with an overall loss of 40-60 db can hear loud conversation within a 3-foot range, but meanings often are garbled. As a result, some children in this category are initially considered retarded. Like the previous category, children with moderate hearing losses must obtain special training in speech.

All children in the first three categories are considered deaf and require extensive special education in both oral and signed communication.

4. *Marginal hearing loss.* Children with an overall 30-40 db loss cannot hear conversation farther than 3 feet away. They may miss at least half of what a teacher says in class, unless they can see the speaker's lips. If the loss is in the higher frequencies, children may exhibit various speech defects. With a hearing aid, however, these youngsters usually hear normally. Thus, within safety constraints, instructors should permit children with this degree of hearing loss to retain the hearing aid in physical education classes.

5. *Mild hearing loss.* Often these children are overlooked, as they generally do not experience learning problems. Preferential seating in a classroom is helpful. Although these children's speech is usually normal, they may require some help with vocabulary development. Pupils in this category have a 20-30 db loss and occasionally are fitted with a hearing aid.

CAUSES OF HEARING DEFECTS

Most hearing losses are caused by some dysfunction of the outer or middle ear that prevents sound vibrations from reaching the inner ear. Figure 7.1 illustrates the ear and its parts. Less frequent are hearing losses resulting from damage to the inner ear, the auditory nerve, or the brain. Damage to the vestibular branch of the auditory nerve, or to the inner ear, can cause concomitant balance problems. Often damage to these areas is caused by meningitis.

Almost two thirds of all hearing losses are considered *congenital* (present at birth), and the other third are *acquired*. Of the hearing losses designated congenital, some are attributable to hereditary causes (ranging from 8% to 26% in various surveys published) and others to the mother's having contracted German measles (rubella) during pregnancy.

Temporary conductive hearing losses at times result from bacterial or fungal inflammations of the outer ear. The resultant swelling, partial closing of the external meatus, and pain, plus a watery discharge, preclude students from participating in swimming. Similarly, any infection that causes blockage of the eustachian tube between the ear and throat may require the insertion of artificial tubes—which also precludes children from swimming while the middle ear heals.

The most prevalent cause of conductive hearing loss is an infection or inflammation of the middle ear called *otitis media*. Chronic inflammation may produce fine tears between the ear drum (tympanic membrane) and the three small bones of the middle ear (the ossicles), which normally transmit sound waves. Infection of this nature in the middle ear is dangerous insofar as it may spread into the air cells of the mastoid process within the temporal bone, causing *mastoiditis*. Chronic otitis media is a potentially dangerous infectious condition that can move into the meninges of the brain, causing meningitis and accompanying hearing loss.

Conductive hearing losses and sensorineural losses have several important differences, which are discussed briefly here.

Conductive Hearing Loss

Conductive hearing losses are usually not as severe as sensorineural losses and may be corrected through amplification (hearing aids). The problems that cause this type of loss

Figure 7.1 Parts of the Ear

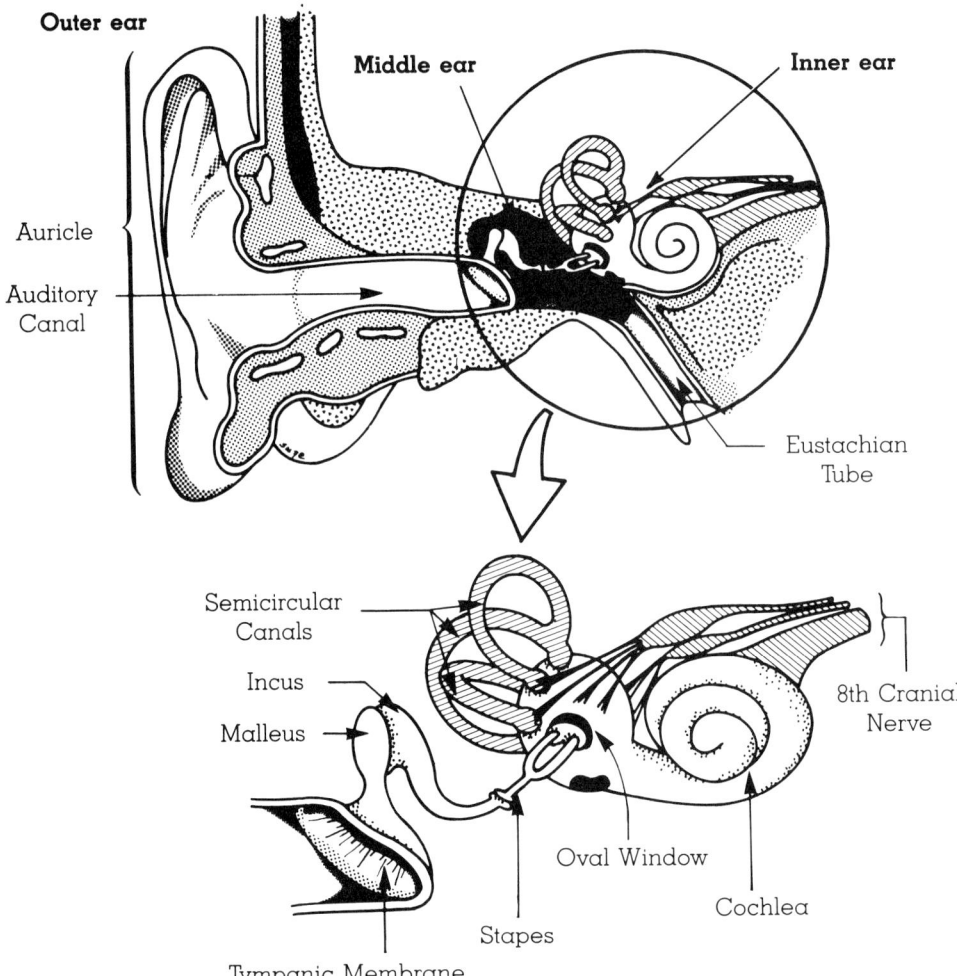

occur in the middle or outer ear—including the tympanic membrane, ossicles, and eustachian tube—manifest in a partial hearing loss usually not exceeding 60 db. Discrimination of sounds is often normal, but amplification is needed. Indeed, a person with this type of loss often can hear well via telephone because of the ability of the facial bones to conduct sound. Speech and language development typically are not seriously impaired.

Sensorineural Loss

In contrast, the individual suffering from a sensorineural loss is often profoundly or severely impaired both in hearing and in language. Noise can be frustrating, and shouting or amplification of other kinds does not help. A person with this type of loss may not discriminate speech sounds well but does better with higher than lower frequency sounds. The individual tends to speak loudly and in ways that are difficult to understand, mispronouncing words frequently.

Even with the most contemporary diagnostic tools available, ascertaining the causes of deafness in children remains a difficult undertaking. The catch-all classification "etiology unknown" is comonplace on graphs listing causes of deafness. The causes for deafness were ascertained in only slightly more than half of the 21,000 students surveyed in a report by Reis (1973). The most common cause of hearing impairments in the past was the rubella form of measles, contracted by pregnant mothers. Vaccinations against rubella have reduced the incidence in newborns in recent years. Other causes stem from hereditary factors, prematurity, meningitis, and Rh blood incompatibility. All of these causes except meningitis are prenatal.

CHARACTERISTICS OF THE DEAF AND HARD OF HEARING

Traditionally, reviewers have painted a rather negative picture of various dimensions of the deaf and hard of hearing. They have been described as socially withdrawn, concrete rather than plastic in their thinking, intellectually inferior to the hearing, and somewhat depressed emotionally. Fortunately, more enlightened contemporary inspections of recent research findings, plus more flexible interpretations, have produced more positive assessments of the attributes of the deaf and the near-deaf.

Social-Emotional Characteristics

Moores (1978) pointed out that deaf children tend to acquire feelings of inferiority, stemming from infancy, when they are received in the family with some alarm and reared under tensions not experienced by normally communicative infants and children.

The deaf or near-deaf understandably feel cut off if placed in a social environment composed primarily of the hearing. It is analogous to an individual in the midst of a group speaking a foreign language.

Most clinical observations now indicate that, among themselves, the deaf often are extremely gregarious and outgoing, constantly communicating with their peers in animated signs, spoken words, and facial expressions. When members of a hearing population make overt attempts via gestures and facial expressions to communicate with a deaf person, the communication often is readily reciprocated with social behavior in the form of gestures and easily understood signs.

Intellectual Characteristics

Intellectual behaviors of the deaf have been variously interpreted by social scientists. In the past the deaf (as the blind) have been described as able to think primarily in concrete rather than abstract terms. Writers, however, have not adequately defined the terms *concrete* and *abstract*, and intelligence tests administered to the deaf often have contained inappropriate items. Results sometimes indicate how well the tester administered the test rather than real intellectual abilities.

Three historical stages may be drawn in assessment of intelligence of the deaf:

1. Reviewing the research, Pinter, Eisenson, and Stanton (1941) concluded that although the results of some investigations were confusing, deaf children appeared to be inferior in intelligence to children with normal hearing.

2. Myklebust (1964), reviewing some of the same studies surveyed by Pinter, concluded that the deaf were not generally quantitatively inferior in intelligence but were *qualitatively* different in the manner in which they thought. Myklebust contended that deaf children did better with more concrete concepts while not functioning as broadly and in as concrete a fashion with the content of intelligence tests.

3. A third phase, reflected in reviews of the literature by Rosenstein (1961) and Vernon (1967), suggested that the terms *concrete* and *abstract* were vague. They argued that deaf and hearing youngsters have no real differences when linguistic factors are within the language experience of deaf subjects. Vernon reviewed 31 studies from 1930 to 1960 and reported that "these language impoverished youths do well in a wide variety of tasks that measure thinking, as do youngsters of normal language development." Vernon also pointed out that deaf populations often contain higher percentages of children with neurological impairment, as well as some from low socioeconomic backgrounds—both factors to consider when comparing results of intelligence test scores obtained from children with and without hearing.

Despite the rather positive flavor of these more recent assumptions concerning intellectual abilities of the deaf, children with extremely poor hearing may have problems with any one of the three types of speech attributed to youngsters: (a) *internalized* speech, which may be a partial parallel support of thought; (b) overt *expressive* language; and (c) *receptive* language—the ability to understand others. The next section discusses how physical activities may contribute to development of each of these types of speech.

As is true in any population, some deaf children are retarded intellectually. But any blanket assumptions about the intellectual make-up of deaf children applied to one or a few children with poor hearing is shortsighted and likely to do a disservice to youngsters to whom various spurious stereotypes may be applied, resulting in inferior services to the children, as teacher expectations may be incongruent with the children's real abilities and attitudes.

Motor Characteristics

Until recently, comprehensive studies of the motor abilities of deaf youngsters were few. Much of the early research was summarized in Myklebust's (1964) text. This early information was superficial at best and incorrect at the worst. Data from early studies, however, did begin to indicate that, as a group, deaf youngsters may possess balance problems. For the most part, when a population of deaf children is compared to hearing youngsters, the primary motor deficit in the former group is likely to be balance (Brunt & Broadhead, 1982) and closely related tasks involving "dynamic coordination" (Wiergersma & Van der Velde, 1983).

Recently a comprehensive study was published contrasting various fitness, motor control, and body composition measures of 1,468 deaf and hard of hearing youngsters to scores in the same tasks posted by normal youth 10-17 years of age (Winnick & Short, 1982). Also included in the investigation were youngsters labeled orthopedically handicapped and those who were blind or visually impaired. In most of the tasks compared, scores of the auditorily impaired were similar to scores posted by hearing youngsters of the same age. When differences did occur, most were about .25 standard deviations. The auditorily impaired, however, did seem to fall behind the hearing youngsters to whom they were compared in a long-distance run (.63 S.D. when girls were contrasted and .72 when boys were compared).

Scores of the youngsters with auditory impairments generally exceeded scores posted by the other handicapped groups contrasted (blind, visually impaired, and orthopedically handicapped). In most tasks the variability of scores posted by those with auditory impairments was not greater than the variability of scores of normal youngsters. But the lack of consistency in scores on the same tasks recorded for the other handicapped groups in this investigation (the visually and orthopedically handicapped) was quite apparent and exceeded the variability of scores posted by the normal subjects.

In recent, carefully conducted studies, sub-populations of deaf youngsters (those evidencing additional signs of neurological impairment) were evaluated (Wiergersma & Van der Velde, 1982). As might be expected, these children evidenced clearly inferior motor abilities. Thus, when programming for deaf youngsters, they should be separated into at least two groups: (a) those showing average to above-average abilities, and (b) those exhibiting coordination problems that need special attention.

With remediation, deaf youngsters are likely to improve in motor abilities, even on tests of balance (Effgen, 1981). This improvement, however, may be attributable to more mature strategies the youngsters apply to balance tasks rather than to any "real" improvement in this neuromotor quality (Brunt, Layne, Cook, & Rowe, 1984). But, except for balance deficits in deaf youngsters possessing vestibular etiology for their hearing impairment, deaf youngsters may be inferior motorically to hearing youngsters only because they lack experience in a given skill or group of skills or they possess some other neuro-motor deficit reflecting, for example, a mild form of cerebral palsy (Schmidt, 1985; Winnick, 1986).

Fine-motor abilities are extremely important in younger deaf populations. The ability to sign—and thus to communicate—relies upon the ability to move the hands and fingers with precision. Thus, the deaf or hard of hearing child with motor problems, including mild forms of cerebral palsy, is often doubly handicapped when using communication skills. Surprisingly, though, young deaf children, even those with deaf parents, acquire the ability to sign and communicate with these "finger-words" earlier than hearing infants begin to communicate vocally! Deaf infants frequently display their first signs by the eighth or ninth month of life, and by the middle of the second year, sign combinations (signed sentences) emerge (Bonvillian, Orlansky, & Novack, 1983). The "finger abilities" used in signing do not necessarily parallel the emergence of locomotor abilities and other larger muscle activities.

Some believe that *thinking* about tasks, including motor tasks, may be impeded in the deaf because of a postulated deficit in internal speech. In studies we have carried out evaluating the motor planning abilities of deaf and hearing youngsters, however, the deaf often perform better (Cratty, Cratty, & Cornell, 1986). The possible reason for this superiority is that the deaf must give close visual attention to others—to their signs as well as their nonverbal communication cues. The deaf bring this same close visual attention to physical skills, facilitating their abilities to replicate complicated movement series.

PROGRAMMING GUIDELINES

Whether they are in charge of a class totally composed of hard of hearing youngsters or a class in which some deaf children have been mainstreamed, uninitiated physical educators have the immediate challenge of communicating with children whose receptive speech may be impaired or totally absent. At first physical educators may experience a feeling akin to panic, but acquiring a few survival signs should help make initial physical education lessons relatively painless for all concerned. Indeed, it has been found in recreation programs containing partially sighted children and deaf children that the former have mastered enough signs to make themselves understood by the latter. Because "survival signs" are so important, some of them are pictured in this section.[4]

One controversy continually appearing in the literature on deafness during the past 150 years concerns whether some kind of oral communication or some kind of signing is best for the hard of hearing. Although the arguments for either will not be dwelt on here, many sensible educators of the deaf advocate *total communication* involving signs and accompanying verbalizations of what is being transmitted through the hands. I agree with this position.

A communication environment in which signs rather than spoken words are being used has many social and psychological dimensions:

1. Although teachers may have one or more years of instruction in signing, it may take them a year or more in a school environment before they are able to tell precisely what two deaf children are communicating to each other in rapid "slurred" conversation.

2. When facing a deaf group, to accompany one's signs with the spoken words, clearly enunciated, is not only helpful but almost mandatory so that the hearing impaired person does not consider the speaker impolite.

3. Hearing impaired individuals in each environment—school, home, and workplace—will develop their own unique signs. Like spoken English, these signs constantly evolve, change, and are added to. A teacher's challenge then, is to decode these subtle and highly individualistic signs.

4. Each child and adult answers to his or her own name sign. The sign may stand for a personality trait of the individual, a physical characteristic, a habit, or an initial. Pointing to an obvious mole on the cheek might be a child's sign, or a gesture meaning "shy" might indicate Shy John. These signs may change as children or youth try to divest themselves of negative self-images. For example, a boy may try to have other children call him something besides Nail-biter.

---

4. These survival signs are in Ameslan. This system and others, their philosophies and uses, have been reviewed in chapter 9 of *Educating the Deaf* by D.F. Moores, 1978, Boston: Houghton Mifflin.

Survival Signs

1. Signs useful for beginning a lesson

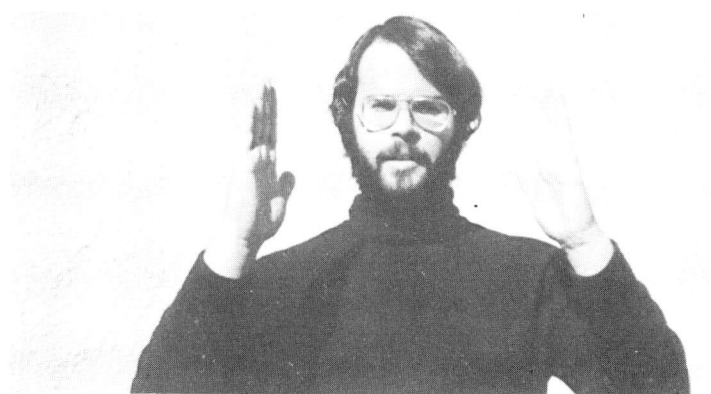

Pay attention!
Short, forward motions of the hands outward; limits field of vision.

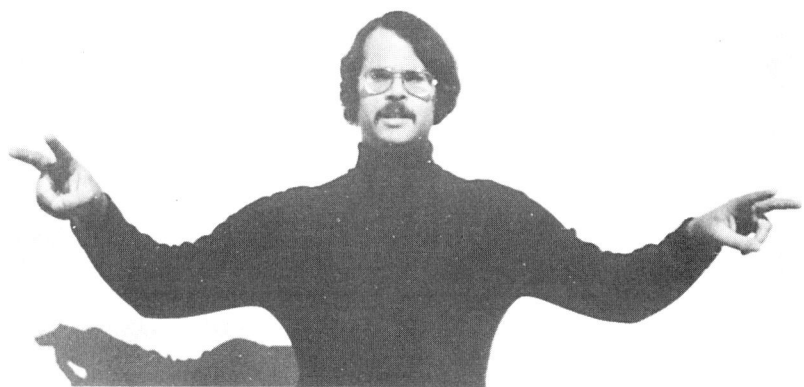

Watch me! *Both hands, fingers apart, move together, from outward motion...*

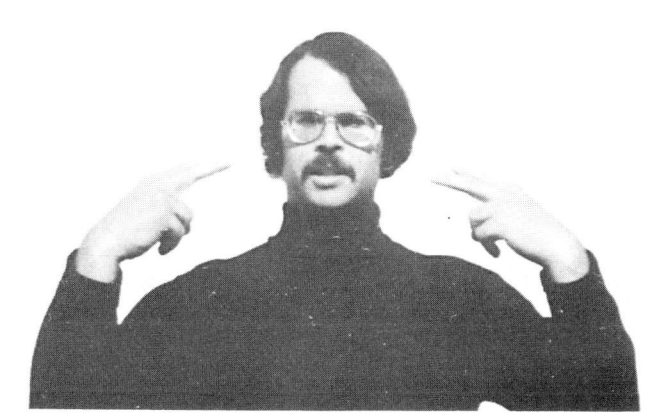

... inward toward eyes.

Start!
First finger
makes twisting
motion (turning
a key) into the
division of the
first and
second fingers
of the second
hand.

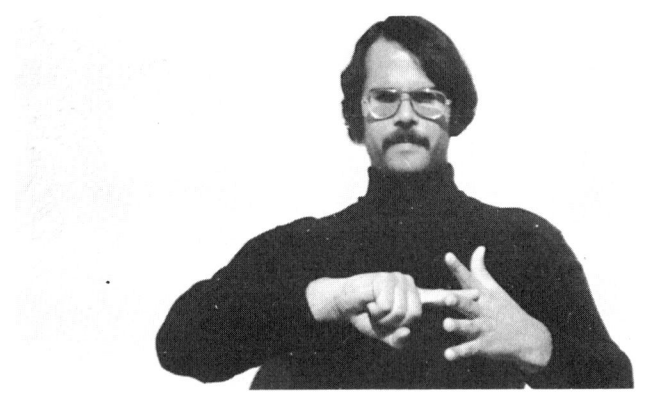

Have fun!
Hands move
inward toward
chest until
fingertips
touch.

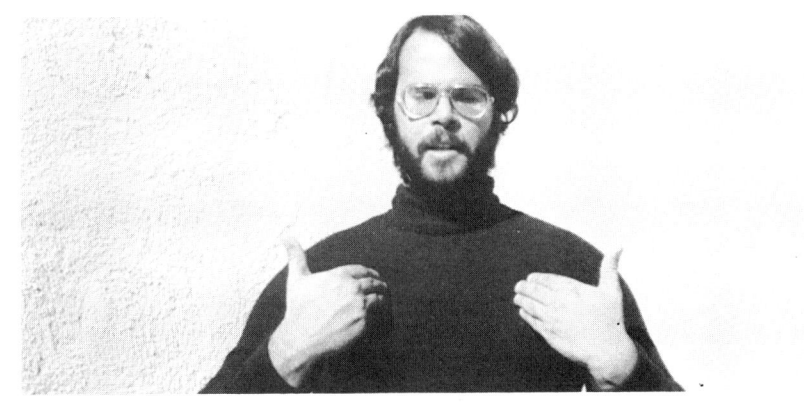

Two fingers
travel together
from nose...

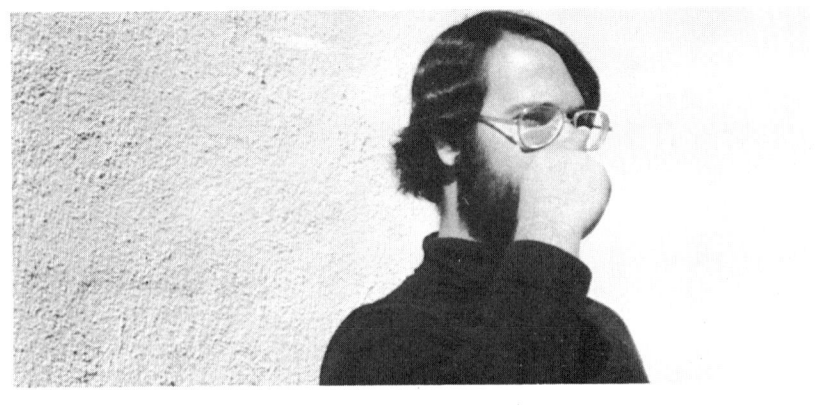

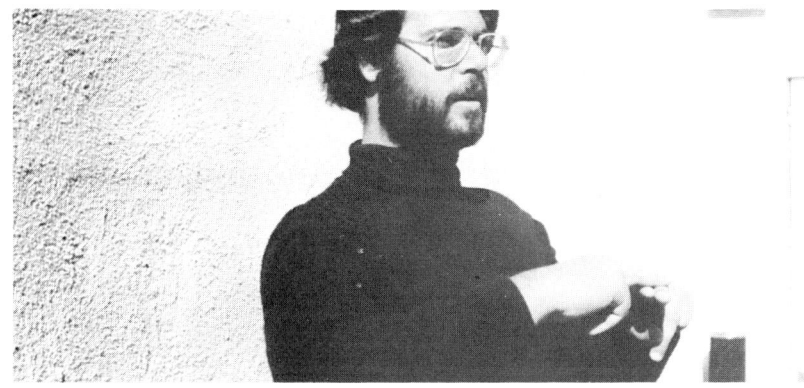

*...to two
fingers of
opposite hand.*

2. *Signs that inform, give commands during a lesson*

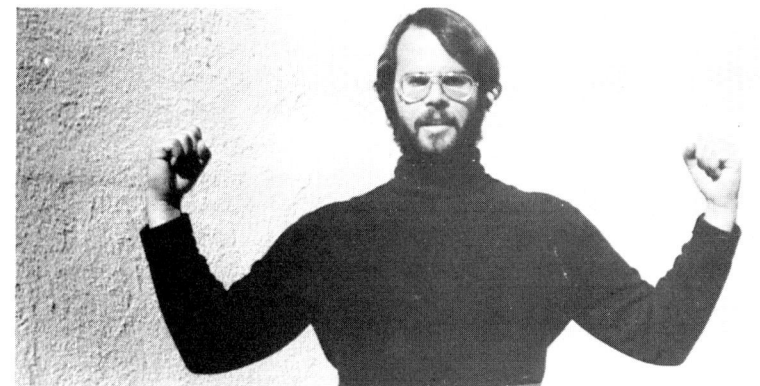

Exercise
*Slight flexion,
extension in
and out at
elbows.*

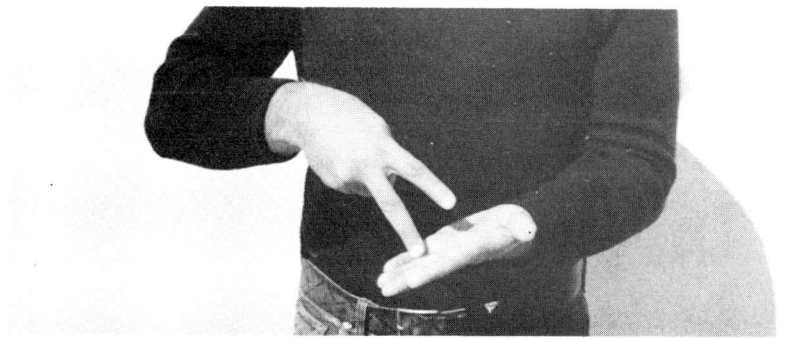

Dance
*Two fingers
twist in dance
on palm of
opposite hand.*

Right!
*Hands come
together once,
with fingers
extended, from
position shown.*

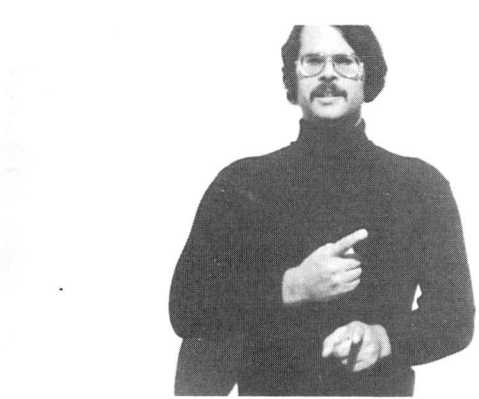

Wrong!
*Hand moves
from a position
away from the
chin to
touching
knuckles to
chin as shown.*

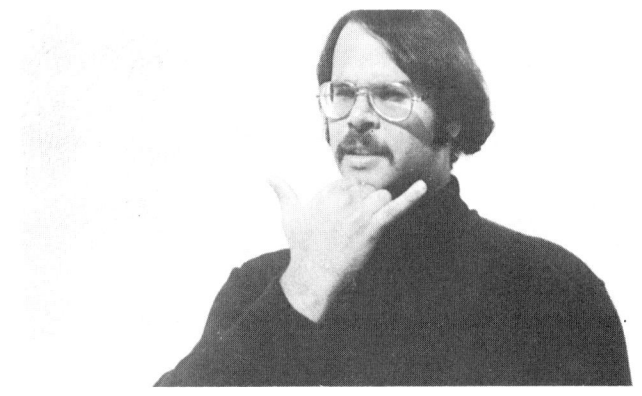

Yes!
*Hand in fist
nods up and
down by
flexions and
extensions at
wrist.*

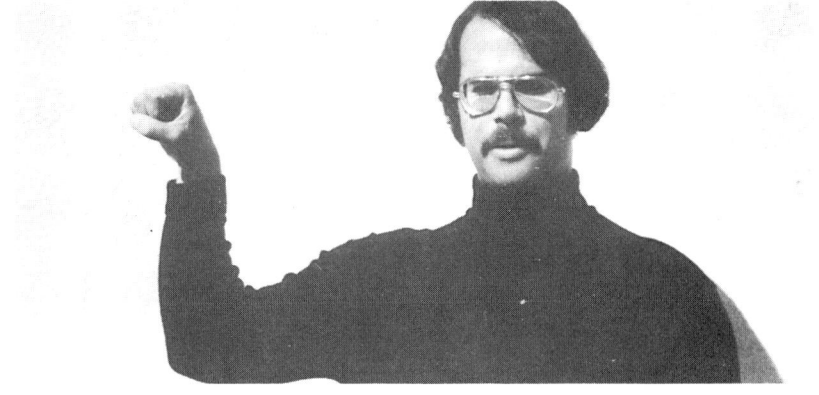

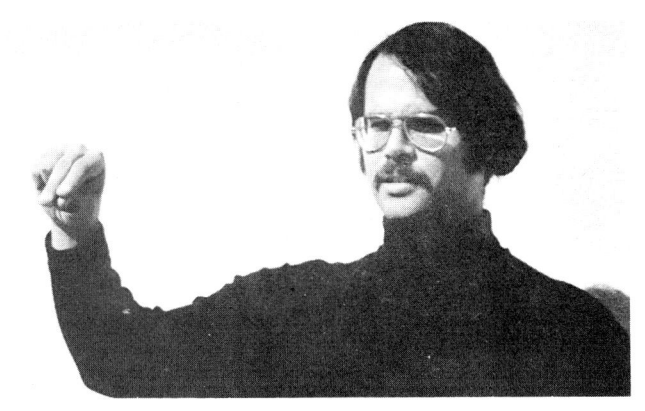

No!
First and
second fingers
move up and
down to thumb
at least twice.

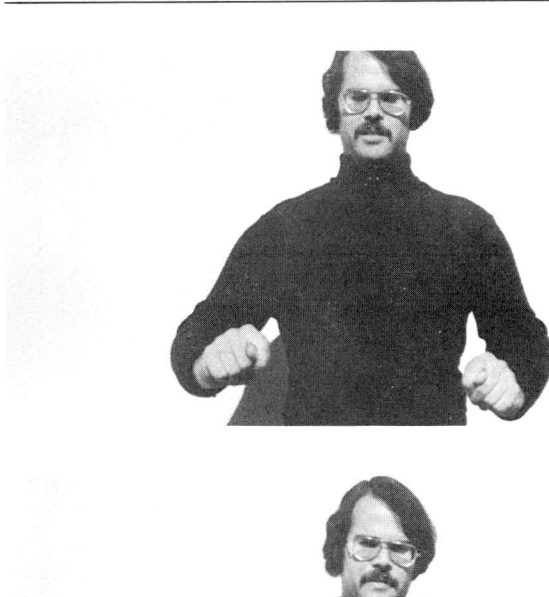

Try again!
Try.
Thumbs are be-
tween first and
second fingers;
hands make
short pushing
away motion
from body,
moving
together.

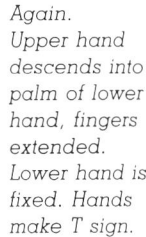

Again.
Upper hand
descends into
palm of lower
hand, fingers
extended.
Lower hand is
fixed. Hands
make T sign.

Slow!
*Top hand,
fingers
extended,
brushes
upward from
wrist...*

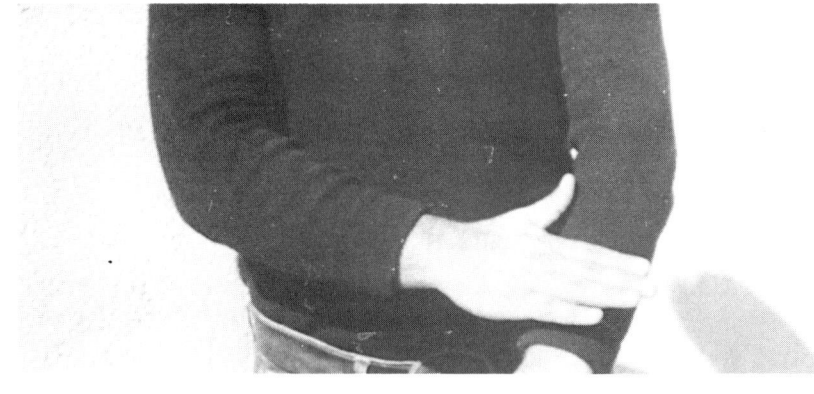

*...to elbow of
other arm.*

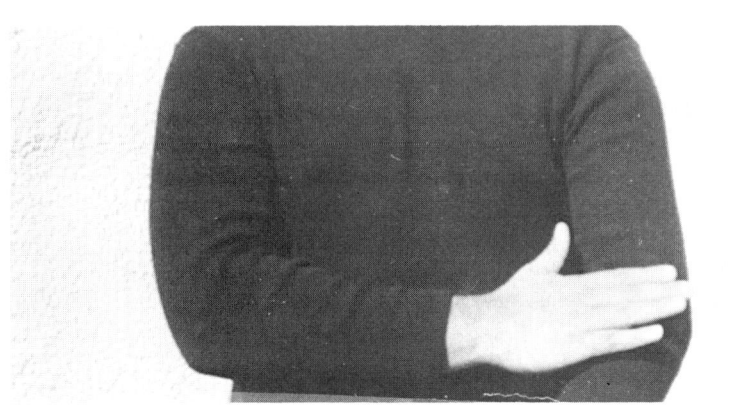

Fast!
*Hands in fists
remain in
place...*

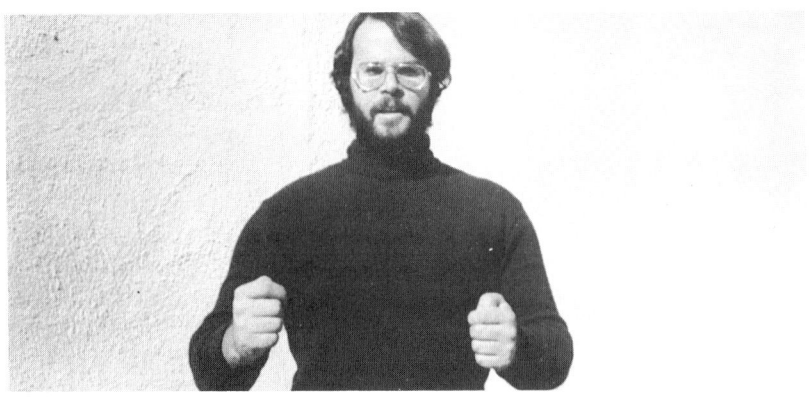

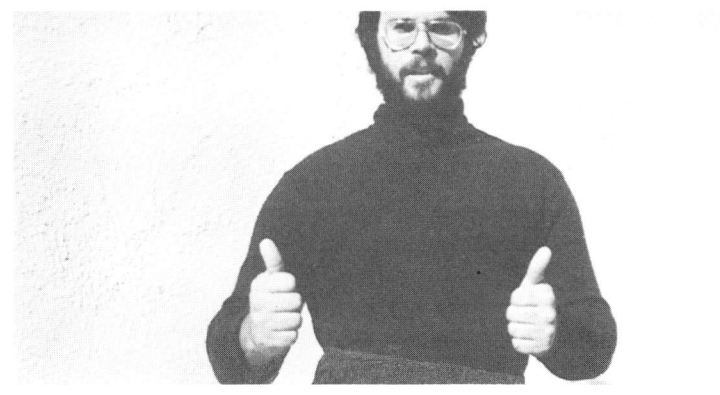

. . .while thumbs flick up and down rapidly.

Run!
First finger of one hand hooks on thumb of lower hand; whole two-hand unit moves rapidly away from body, with both thumbs and first fingers wiggling (flexing and extending last two joints).

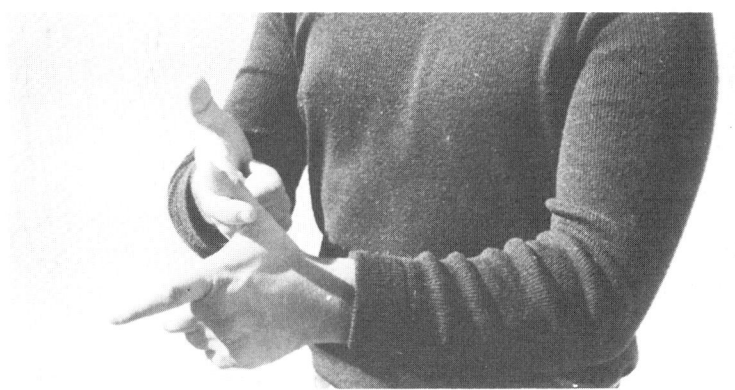

---

3. Questions, during a lesson

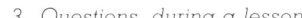

Does it hurt? Where?
Hurt?
Fingers face each other, and twist rapidly in opposite directions.

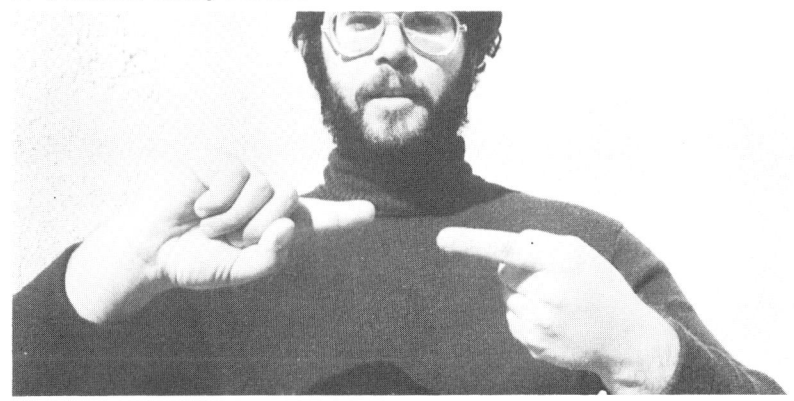

Where?
Finger up, arm moves back and forth at elbow, in windshield wiperlike motion.

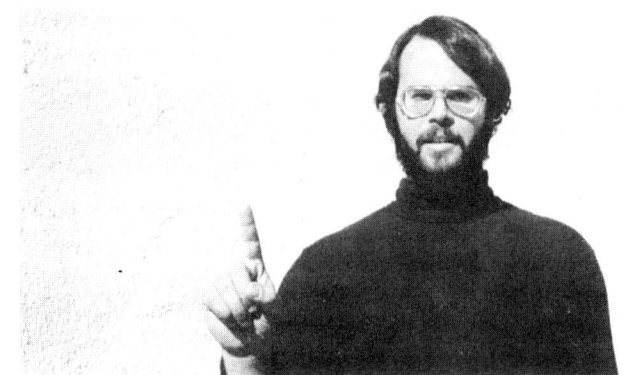

Location of hurt may be a question or response with hurt sign made at various body parts, such as leg...

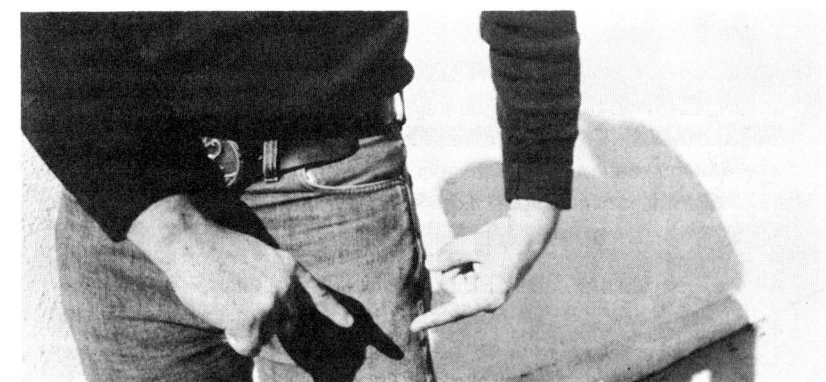

...or shoulder.

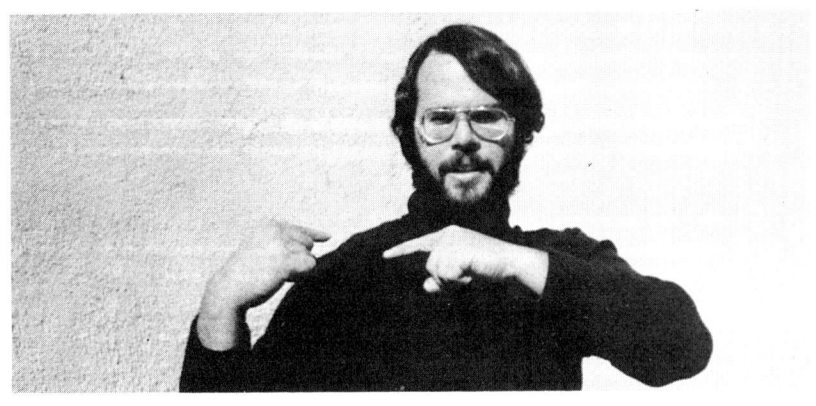

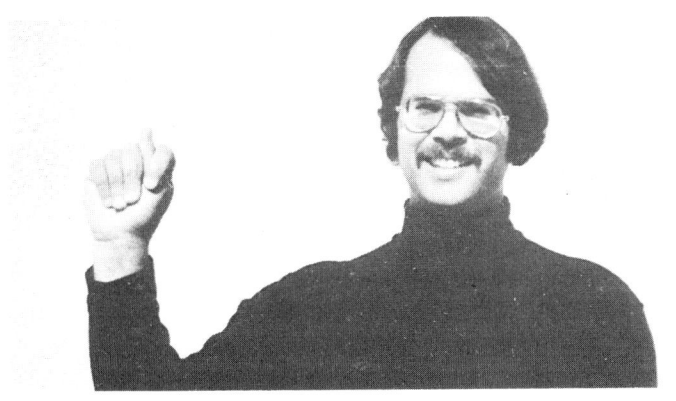

Toilet?
Sign for letter
T, or two R
signs (see sign
for rest),
standing for
restroom.

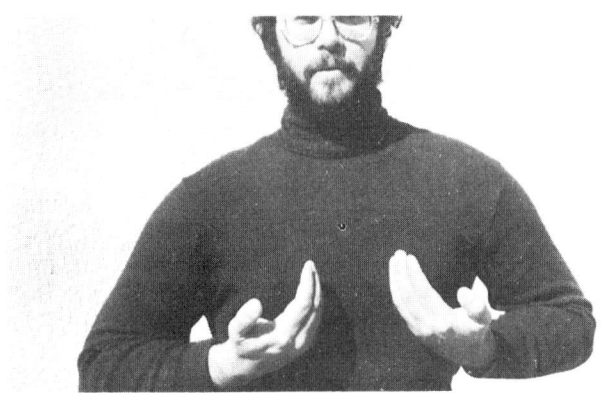

Tired?
Rotation of
cupped hands
together from
outward
position, palms
up, inward
until fingertips
touch chest.

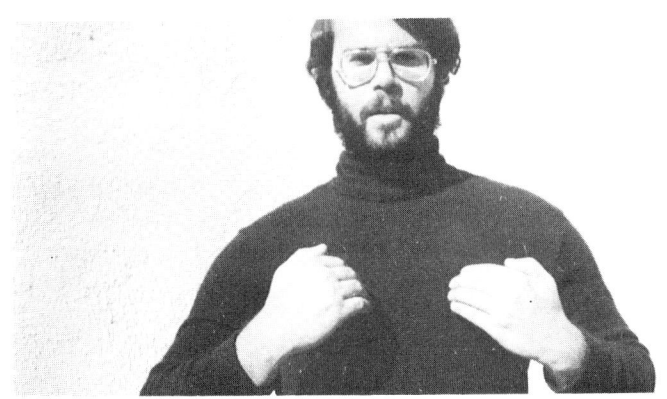

Final position
for tired
accompanied
by tired
expression on
face.

Do you understand?
Fist is held in place; first finger flicks out in quick extensions.

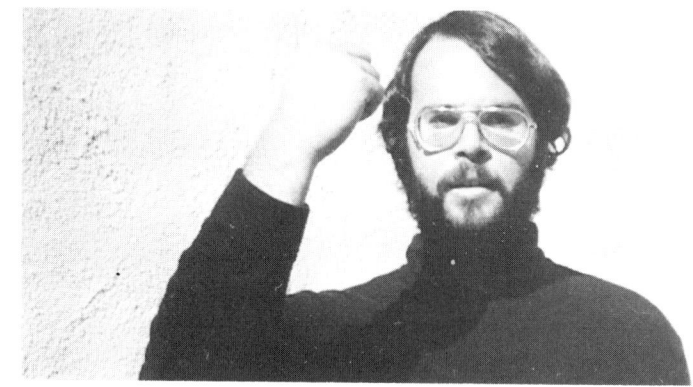

Sign suggests a light bulb going on, for having an idea.

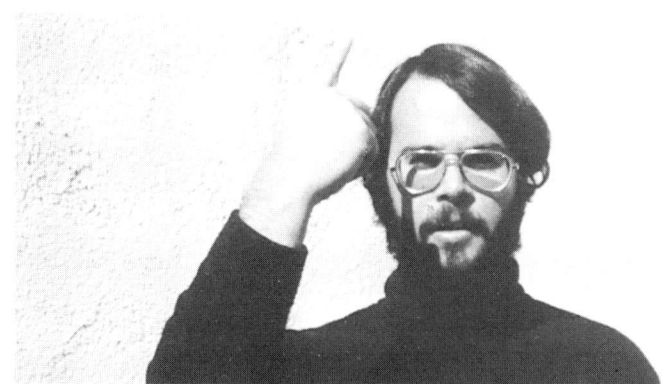

---

4. Signs that reward, give approval

Fantastic!
Hands make small pushes outward.

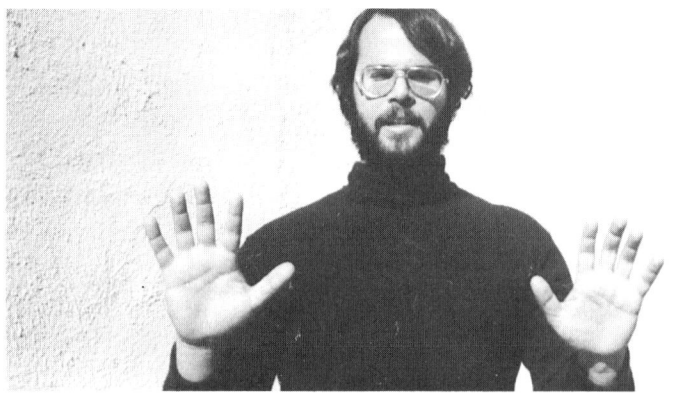

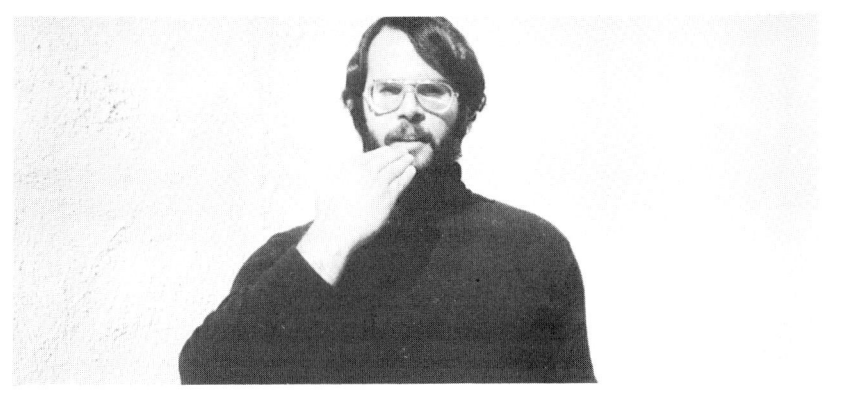

Good! Thank you.
Fingertips travel from mouth...

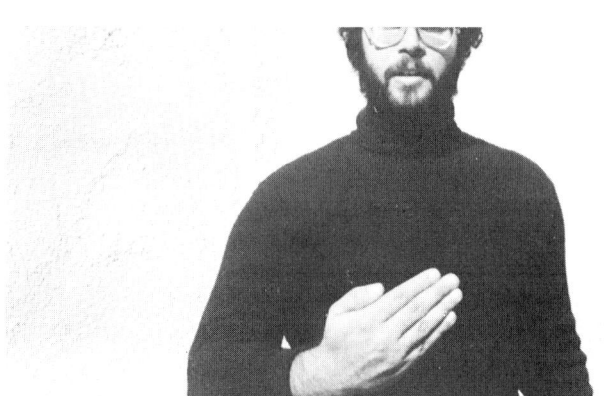

...outward. For emphasis, slap palm of opposite hand with back of moving hand.

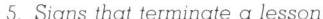

5. *Signs that terminate a lesson*

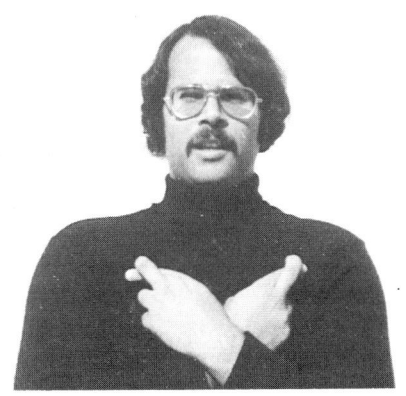

Rest.
Hands, first two fingers crossed, are immobile on chest, making R sign.

Shower.
Fingers held above head flex into fist and extend, simulating showering action.

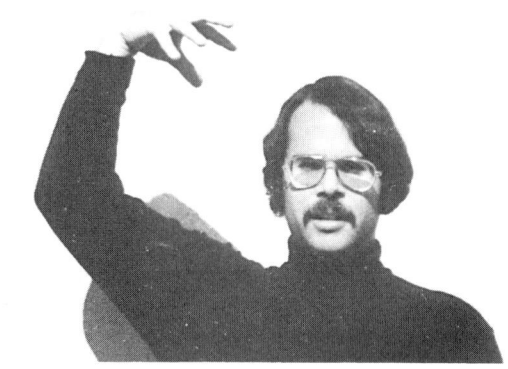

Stop!
Hands start apart...

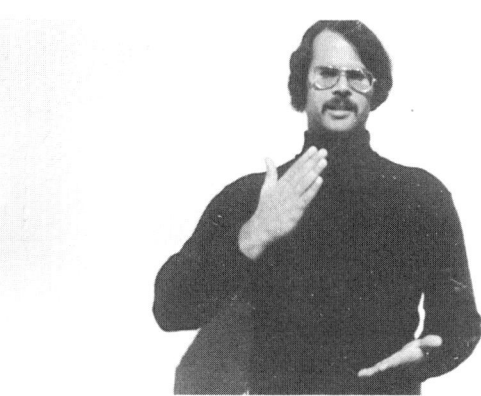

...and upper hand chops downward into palm of opposite hand.

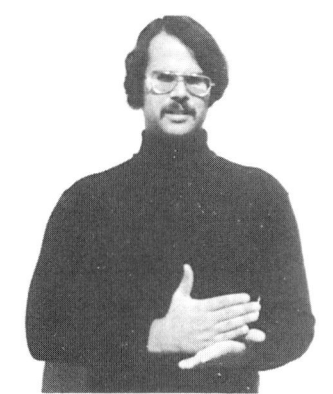

138

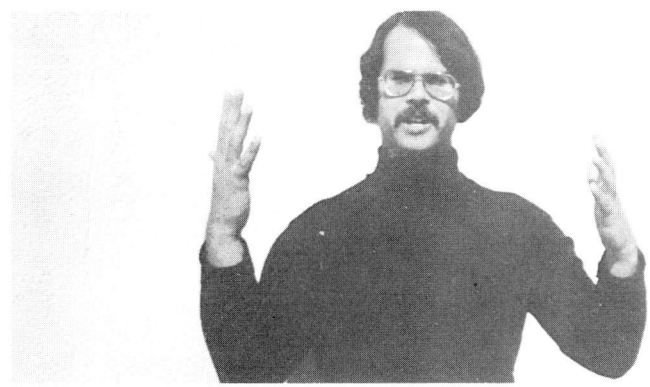

Cut it out!
*Hands start
facing each
other...*

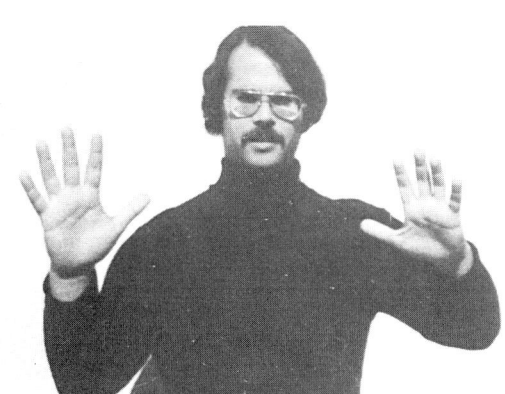

*...and rotate
outward and
with palms
toward listener.*

A new teacher also is given a name sign by the class—maybe even two signs, one that is used to their face and another with somewhat negative connotations used in other contexts!

5. Hearing teachers new to the deaf may not at first realize that a class is not "listening" (i.e., watching them). Apparently attentive silence may in truth be heavily loaded with sign communication, indicating that the children have many other things on their minds besides the instructions for beginning a lesson.

6. Teachers of the deaf, including physical education teachers, have to take care when attempting to elicit language from their charges. Youngsters' language may be depressed when a teacher forces the child to repeat words and phrases excessively or poses frequent questions requiring language responses.

Physical education teachers should be prepared to meet the deaf at least halfway by learning rudimentary signs at first and then acquiring formal instruction if they will have prolonged exposure to the deaf or hard of hearing. Obviously, hearing teachers should be prepared to enter this "foreign country" to a greater degree when working with one or more severely or profoundly deaf students. Failure to do so will doom one's best attempts to convey a physical education program to even the most motivated child with this kind of sensory handicap.

The photographs depict some of the more basic signs needed initially by physical education teachers working with the deaf or hard of hearing. These may be added to, and the students themselves may teach the teacher many more. Teaching physical education through signing is not too difficult, insofar as the ideas often involve actions that are replicated exactly by a sign. For example, holding one hand over the head and alternately spreading and contracting the fingers is the sign for "shower." Throwing and other physical skills also may be simply imitated. Some signs are needed immediately to ensure the health and safety of children and youth in the class.

IMPLICATIONS FOR PHYSICAL EDUCATION

Deaf and near-deaf children grow up in a world in which they tend to feel relatively isolated. No one, at first, is able to penetrate their consciousness, and they may appear withdrawn and be reluctant to participate in childhood games with others to whom they appear strange and uncommunicative.

Some writers have suggested that primary emphasis be given to individual sports in their physical education programs—archery, shooting, and the like—rather than team sports in which interpersonal communication is important. Individuals advocating this approach point out that the deaf, alone in many ways, function best if not forced to participate in team games. An opposite viewpoint seems to be more uplifting and useful: Because the deaf and hard of hearing are in a world separate from the hearing, participation in group games and team sports *is* helpful and educational for them and may enhance their social and communicative skills.

The lack of opportunity to play vigorously in neighborhood games often is reflected in poor development of basic skills, such as throwing, dribbling, and kicking, and lack of understanding of the nature of team sports and tactics (e.g., the necessity for quickly changing from offense to defense). Thus, prior to introducing deaf and hearing impaired students to a team or group sport, teachers should start with lead-up activities:

1. Introduce children to the skills in a developmental manner. Do not introduce too many sub-skills at once.

2. Incorporate activities that engender basic concepts of team play—for example, staying between the person you are guarding and the basket while playing defense in basketball. These concepts may be practiced while the students move slowly through standing positions on the court or field. Concepts of this type may be diagrammed or represented by disks and stick figures on a table before children move to the court or the field.

3. If the team sport mixes deaf and hearing youngsters, stress to the latter that their deaf teammates are not likely to respond to them unless the two make visual contact. Equipping hearing youngsters with some of the basic signs (shown earlier) also would help with communication in fast-moving team sports. For the most part, gestures (e.g., indicating "throw the ball to me") often suffice. If the team is composed entirely of the deaf, referees must substitute flags for whistles, and gestural communication is a must.

My observation, after spending some time in schools for the deaf, is that deaf youngsters often display skills that are less than adequate because of experiential deprivation rather than because of any kind of subtle neurological deficit. Physical education teachers, therefore, should provide physical experiences in sequentially sound and motivating ways for children who are hard of hearing and deaf.

There are signs that exposure to motor development programs will have generally positive effects upon groups of deaf children (Pennella, 1979). Kraft (1981) and others have set forth guidelines for teaching physical education to the deaf. Among these principles are the following:

1. Class size should be under 10 students.
2. Once games are started, they should not be interruped with frequent instructions.
3. Games should be scaled to children's maturity levels, not their chronological ages.
4. Activities should emphasize social interaction opportunities and be taught using visual cues (to signal fouls, etc.).
5. When possible, hearing and deaf students should be treated equally in game and physical activity situations.

Finally, cochlear implants now are being done with some deaf children. A child with this type of implant, however, does not receive full auditory information but, rather, a "buzzing" sound array, and speech is not heard as speech, nor is music heard as music (Schein, 1984).

SUMMARY

The history of education for the deaf and hard of hearing is not dissimilar from that for the blind and visually impaired. Initially, residential schools were established during the last century. Today several models exist, ranging from special schools to mainstream classes within regular school settings.

Deaf children may possess movement characteristics that make them different from their peers who hear normally. Any deficiencies that do exist, however, likely are caused by sparse experiences in movement activities rather than any differences connected with the inability to hear well.

Early literature indicated that the deaf were generally inferior to the hearing in mental abilities. More recent evidence suggests, however, that differences that do exist are superficial and not critical to the construction of their educational program.

Physical educators who work with the deaf and hard of hearing should become familiar with and use survival signs—gestures that help get a lesson going and provide for the children's safety by ensuring communication between teacher and pupils. Signs permit physical educators to move into the exotic world of their charges with facility and increase their effectiveness greatly.

Because of minimal to moderate neurological problems, some deaf youngsters may benefit from special developmental activities such as tumbling and balancing. Most, however, should be introduced to regular physical development activities and recreational sports. Special help and encouragement should be extended for them to take up group games and to enhance their social and communication skills by interacting with hard of hearing peers and hearing youngsters alike.

REFERENCES

Bonvillian, J.D., Orlansky, M.D., & Novack, L.L. (1983). Developmental milestones: Sign language acquisition and motor development. *Child Development, 54,* 1435-1445.

Brunt, D., & Broadhead, G.D. (1982). Motor proficiency traits of deaf children. *Research Quarterly for Exercise & Sport, 53,* 236-238.

Brunt, D., Layne, C.S., Cook, M., & Rowe, L. (1984). Automatic postural responses of deaf children from dynamic and static positions. *Adapted Physical Activity Quarterly, 1,* 247-252.

Cratty, B.J., Cratty, I.J., & Cornell, S. (1986). Motor planning abilities in deaf and hearing children. *American Annals of the Deaf, 131,* 281-287.

Effgen, S.K. (1981). Effect of an exercise program on the static balance of deaf children. *Physical Therapy, 61,* 873-877.

Kraft, R.E. (1981). Movement experiences for children with auditory handicaps. *Physical Education, 38,* 35-38.

Moores, D.F. (1978). *Educating the deaf: Psychology, principles and practices.* Boston: Houghton Mifflin.

Myklebust, H. (1964). *The psychology of deafness* (2nd ed.) (pp. 180-201). New York: Grune & Stratton.

Pennella, L. (1979). Motor ability and the deaf: Research implications. *American Annals of the Deaf, 124,* 366-372.

Pinter, R., Eisenson, J., & Stanton, M. (1941). *The psychology of the physically handicapped.* New York: Appleton-Century-Crofts.

Reis, P. (1973). *Reported causes of hearing loss for hearing impaired students.* Washington, DC: Gallaudet College Office of Demographic Studies.

Rosenstein, J. (1961). Perception, cognition, and language in deaf children. *Exceptional Children, 27,* 276-284.

Schein, J.D. (1984). Cochlear implants and the education of the deaf. *American Annals of the Deaf, 133,* 324-332.

Schein, J., & Delk, M. (1974). *The deaf population of the U.S.* Silver Spring, MD: National Association of the Deaf.

Schmidt, S. (1985). Hearing impaired students in physical education. *Adapted Physical Activity Quarterly, 2,* 300-306.

Streng, A. (1958). *Hearing therapy for children.* New York: Grune & Stratton.

Vernon, M. (1967). Relationship of language to the thinking process. *Archives of Genetic Psychiatry, 16,* 325-333.

Wiegersma, P.H., & Van der Velde, A. (1983). Motor development of deaf children. *Journal of Child Psychology & Psychiatry, 24,* 103-111.

Winnick, J.P. (1986). Physical fitness of adolescents with auditory impairments. *Adapted Physical Activity Quarterly, 3,* 58-66.

Winnick, J.P., & Short, F.X. (1982). *The physical fitness of sensory and orthopedically impaired youth.* Washington, DC: U.S. Office of Education, Special Education Programs, Project Unique.

ADDITIONAL REFERENCES

American Alliance for Health, Physical Education, and Recreation. (1976). *Physical education, recreation and sports for individuals with hearing impairments* (annotated bibliography). Washington, DC: Author.

Bergés, S.A. (1969, March). The deaf student in physical education. *Journal of Health, Physical Education, & Recreation, 40*(3).

Birch, J. (1975). *Hearing impaired children in the mainstream.* Reston, VA: Council for Exceptional Children.

Curtis, S., Donlan, C., & Wagner, S. (1970). *Deaf-blind children: A program for evaluating their multiple handicaps.* New York: American Foundation for the Blind.

Del Rey, P., & Steiner, S. (1947). Pursuit-motor performance of deaf and hearing girls. *Research Quarterly, 47,* 184-187.

Fant, L.J. (1972). *Ameslan: An introduction to American sign language.* Northridge, CA: Joyce Motion Picture Co.

Fant, L.J. (1976). *Signed English dictionary: 2000 of the most used signs for parents and teachers.* Northridge, CA: Joyce Media.

Furth, H. (1966). A comparison of leading test norms for deaf and hearing children. *American Annals of the Deaf, 111,* 461-462.

Gallaudet, E. (1886). History of the education of the deaf in the United States. *American Annals of the Deaf, 31,* 140-147.

Korones, B. (1976, August). Congenital rubella—An encapsulated review. *Teratology, 14,* 111-114.

Lynch, T. (1973, February). The development of language-training programs for postrubella hearing-impaired children. *Journal of Speech & Hearing Disorders, 38,* 15-24.

Myklebust, H. (1946, April). Significance of etiology in motor performance of deaf children with special reference to meningitis. *American Journal of Psychology, 59,* 249-255.

Nesbitt, J., & Howard, G. (1975). *Proceedings of the National Institute on Recreation for Deaf-Blind Children, Youth and Adults.* Iowa City: University of Iowa Press.

Nix, G.W. (1976). *Mainstream education for hearing impaired children and youth.* New York: Grune & Stratton.

Pender, R.H., & Patterson, P.E. (1983). A comparison of selected motor fitness items between congenitally deaf and hearing children. *Journal for Special Educators, 18,* 71-75.

Potter, C.N., & Silverman, L.D. (1984). Characteristics of vestibular function and static balance skills in deaf children. *Physical Therapy, 64,* 1071-1075.

Rubella Group for Deaf-Blind Children. (1961). *Report on Conference on Children with a Combined Visual and Auditory Handicap.* New York: American Foundation for the Blind.

Wisher, P. (1969, March). Dance and the deaf. *Journal of Health, Physical Education, & Recreation, 40*(3).

QUESTIONS FOR DISCUSSION

1. What are the various types of deafness, and which are more likely to be accompanied by movement problems?

2. How might the lack of internal speech impede the learning of motor skills? How might internal speech be enhanced through physical activities?

3. What special movement problems are said to beset deaf youngsters? Is there evidence to substantiate these claims?

4. What special games may be employed to enhance the language of deaf students?

5. What conceptual problems might a deaf youngster of 10 have when playing basketball for the first time with hearing children? How might these problems be overcome?

STUDENT PROJECTS

1. Visit a class for the deaf. What problems, in addition to deafness (if any) do some members exhibit? In what type of physical education program do these students participate?

2. In three pages, prepare an outline with

which a hearing youngster might be aided in helping a new, hard of hearing student enter a physical education class. List pertinent, specific information.

RESOURCES

Alexander Graham Bell Association for the Deaf
3417 Volta Pl., N.W.
Washington, DC 20007

American Athletic Association of the Deaf
c/o Art Kruger, Chairman
2835-F Hilliard Rd.
Richmond, VA 23228

American Instructors of the Deaf
5034 Wisconsin Ave., N.W.
Washington, DC 20016

Council of Organizations Serving the Deaf (COSD)
P.O. Box 894
Columbia, MD 21044

Gallaudet University
800 Florida Ave., N.E.
Washington, DC 20002

National Association of the Deaf
814 Thayer Ave.
Silver Spring, MD 20910

Section III

Behavioral and Learning Disorders

8 Learning Disabilities

During recent decades no other type of child has attracted so much interest as the youngster with learning disabilities. Following the programs instituted by Frostig, Kirk, Dubnoff, and others in the United States following World War II, educators and parents have continued to concentrate a great deal of attention on children who seem intelligent but who somehow are not performing up to their potential in academic programs.

DEFINITIONS

During the 1960s and up to the present, people have been seeking a definition for these children. Because their characteristics are varied, getting a handle on what they are all about seems to have eluded many. Some definitions imply a medical etiology and include labels such as "minimal brain damage," "neurological impairment," and "minimal brain dysfunction." Other definitions reflect a psychological or educational orientation and refer to "learning disability," "distractibility," and the like.

One of the more accepted definitions, formulated by the National Advisory Committee on Handicapped Children (1968), makes these points: (a) a disparity exists between these children's potential and their actual performance; (b) several processes individually or in some combination may be responsible for the learning disorder; and (c) certain handicaps, such as hearing and visual disorders, are excluded. The definition is as follows:

> Children with special learning disabilities exhibit a disorder in one or more of the basic psychological processes involved in understanding or using spoken or written language. These may be manifested in disorders of listening, thinking, talking, reading, writing, spelling, or arithmetic. They include conditions which have been referred to as perceptual handicaps, brain injury, minimal brain dysfunction, dyslexia, developmental aphasia, etc. They do not include learning problems which are due primarily to visual, hearing, or motor handicaps, to mental retardation, emotional disturbances, or to environment disadvantage. (p. 4)

This definition postulates that a variety of problems may be inhibiting children from learning well. At times a single process may be disturbed enough to prevent good learning. In most cases, however, learning disabled (LD) children exhibit problems of several types in attempting to compete with their peers in a regular classroom. For this reason the over 600,000 children in the United States who carry this label often are placed in classes for the whole day or for part of the day to receive special attention. Estimates of the incidence of learning disabled children within the normal population range from 3% to over 20% and depend largely on the criteria used when evaluating a population of school children.

Despite the interest in learning disabled children in more recent years, these children always have been with us. The population, which is made up of 70% to 90% boys, consists of children who seem a little slow in the regular classroom, have trouble sitting still, or act dreamy during lessons. In physical education classes, they historically have been chronically late to class, perhaps have had trouble working their locker combinations, or have had difficulty dressing and undressing quickly. In class they may have had trouble keeping up with the others, particularly in games requiring precise hand-eye coordination. They have been conundrums for physical education teachers for years.

Learning disabled children may pose special problems in integration into regular physical education classes. The regular children are often less accepting of newcomers with apparent problems that somehow seem under their control to prevent. Moreover, several research studies during the 1980s give clear indication that learning disabled children are deficit in basic social skills—an area that makes them irritating to socially more mature youngsters. For example, in an investigation by Gresham and Reschly (1986), teachers, parents, and peers rated LD children as severely deficit in social skills. They were found to lack basic social skills and courtesies including not saying "excuse me" when appropriate, not waiting their turn when playing, and not following basic rules in games and in class.

BACKGROUND AND HISTORY

In his history of thought and practices dealing with learning disabilities, Wiederholt (1974) divided his discussion into three phases: (a) a foundation phase, from the early 1800s to the 1940s; (b) a transition phase, from 1940 to about the middle 1960s, during which various isolated systems and tests emerged; and (c) a contemporary integration phase, recognizing the validity of a *team approach* to the diagnosis and educational remediation of learning disabilities. Wiederholt dated his final period from the founding of the Association for Children with Learning Disabilities in 1963, which arose from a conference organized by Samuel Kirk, sponsored by the Fund for Perceptually Handicapped Children.

Foundation Phase

During the early foundation phase, theoretical positions on learning disabilities were formulated by observing problems of post-stroke patients. Most of the work was clinically based. Controlled research procedures, however, were not employed to objectify the observations that damage to various portions of the adult brain resulted in various perceptual and learning problems at times resembling those of "word-blind" children (Hinschelwood, 1917).

The principle of individual differences in learning problems began to emerge during this early time. For example, post-stroke aphasics (without speech) often could write their thoughts, much as children who had been afflicted with the same symptoms at birth. Thus, even then some researchers were beginning to understand that children and post-stroke adults might be considered intellectually able and yet possess sensory, conceptual, or motor blocks.

By the 1930s neurologists, including Head (1926), Orton (1939, 1943), and others, began to isolate specific symptoms typical of children who evidenced difficulties in adapting to home and school situations. These symptoms included disruption of perceptual-motor functions, problems of attention termed the Strauss syndrome, perseveration, and other reactions. Some realized that so-called learning disabled children may have suffered perinatal insults to the nervous system that were in many ways similar to the problems encountered by middle-aged and aged cerebral stroke victims.

Transition Phase

The transition phase was marked by the emergence of a group of hardy pioneers who in rather isolated situations began to attempt programs for the remediation of learning disabilities and formulate tests that might substantiate their claims for progress. Among these innovators were Marianne Frostig, who concentrated on perceptual problems and contributed a test of visual perception (Frostig, 1961). Kirk (1966) focused upon psycholinguistic abilities and auditory perception. The Illinois Test of Psycholinguistic Abilities (Kirk, McCarthy, & Kirk, 1978) is important and still in use. William Cruickshank's concept of a stimulus-free environment also was an important contribution (see Cruickshank, Bentzen, Ratzeburg, & Tannhauser, 1961). During this same period Kephart and others, perhaps influenced by the text by Strauss and Lehtinen (1955), *Psychopathology and Education of the Brain-Injured Child*, began to formulate perceptual-motor approaches to the remediation of learning disabilities. Kephart's theories and contributions, as well as those of others with a similar orientation, including Getman and Delacato, are reviewed in chapter 5.

Contemporary Phase

Wiederholt termed the final contemporary phase the *integration period*. During this time educators and teachers have taken a more eclectic and comprehensive approach to the remediation of learning problems, incorporating materials and tests from a variety of sources rather than being tied into a single system. This period is marked by a helpful scrutiny of the programs and tests that emerged earlier and the formulation of comprehensive programs to aid children with learning problems, including remediation focusing on the specific symptoms exhibited. Although some people today seem to resist a symptom-specific approach (notably Ayres, 1972), I and others believe that the symptom-specific avenue is and will be the most helpful channel in the years immediately ahead.

Additional information on the past and present historical development of remediation programs, leadership training programs, and theoretical assumptions may be obtained from Myers and Hammill (1976), Schuell et al. (1964), and Hallahan and Cruickshank (1973), as well as earlier works by Head (1926) and Hinschelwood (1917). Hallahan and Cruickshank discuss disorders of perceptual-motor performance, including the Strauss syndrome. A book by Schain (1977) presents a clear look at learning disabilities from a medical viewpoint.

CAUSES OF LEARNING DISABILITIES

One important *possible* cause of learning disability is some kind of brain dysfunction. One could make the case that because all human behavior, intelligent and emotional, has neurological underpinnings, all deviations from the norm are predicated on some disruption of neurological functioning. Many people, however, object to the neurological disruption concept and to terms indicating that some apparent injury or insult to the nervous system is present in all learning disabled children. Clear-cut evidence of such disruption is seldom present, nor is it always easy to ascertain, even with the most thorough neurodiagnostic work-up.

Nevertheless, in a percentage of the learning disabled, insults around the time of birth, including anoxia (deprivation of oxygen shortly after birth) and other conditions caused by physical trauma at birth and chemical imbalances (the Rh factor), probably *do* lead to some neurological insult—subtle, unseen damage that becomes manifest in later symptoms, including delayed motor development, poor speech and language functioning, emotional instability, or conceptual problems associated with the acquisition of written language such as reading.

Children whose learning disabilities are accompanied by mild or severe convulsions are generally assumed to have problems that are organically based rather than problems attributable to other factors such as a deprived environment or emotional instability. Children or youth who exhibit various symptoms resulting in learning disabilities after traumatic injury are assumed to have had disrupted neurological functioning.

Two other possible causes of learning disabilities have been hypothesized: (a) early environmental deprivation, and (b) emotional disturbance. At times, of course, disentangling these causes from one another, as well as from the previously mentioned neurological insult, is impossible. Children with minor neurological problems often begin to exhibit signs of an emotional overlay on finding themselves at a disadvantage in competition with siblings and peers. Early environmental deprivation sometimes is accompanied by nutritional deficits, which affect neurological functioning.

Among the kinds of environmental deprivation that may be seen by physical education teachers who are working with the learning disabled are children whose physical and emotional environments have discouraged manipulative and exploratory behaviors. Sometimes this deprivation has been rather specific. For example, a child may have been left alone to roam the streets, acquiring unusually good sports skills, while being deprived of a closely attending parent who would encourage early scribbling and printing behaviors.

Human development is an extremely complex process. Studies of so-called deprived children in which child-rearing practices discouraged early ambulation (e.g., Dennis, 1940) found that the walking behaviors of the children involved were not significantly blunted. To cite another example, Kagan (1976) studied children who were raised in windowless huts during the first two or three years of life in primitive Guatemalan villages; even this kind of religiously sanctioned restriction failed to prevent them from becoming "gay, alert, active, and attractive" children by age 11.

In programs conducted over the years on children with motor delays, I have tested youth who might be described as "apartment children." They generally exhibit no impairment in basic motor functions (e.g., balance) but do not demonstrate the vigorous sports skills typical of other children their age who have had less restricted home environments. These motor deficiencies may or may not be accompanied by learning disabilities reflected in delayed academic performance.

Failing to find basic physical functions below normal when testing a large population of children labeled learning disabled is not uncommon. Even so, my associates and I have found that many of the children tested indeed do have disabilities. Although not exhibiting obvious skill deficiencies, they sometimes reveal emotional immaturities that prevent them from engaging in games that engender even a minimal amount of frustration, complexity, or stress.

As is true in attempts to untangle the causes of a variety of handicapping conditions, one is faced with a chicken-and-egg dilemma. Children who are frustrated when confronted with school tasks inevitably will have emotional reactions ranging from passive avoidance to moderate avoidance (usually called distractibility) to rages reflecting extreme frustration. Thus, determining whether conceptual, perceptual, and motor deficiencies came first, or whether emotions stemming from frustration tended to distort children's thoughts, coordination, and perceptions of the world is difficult, if not impossible.

CLASSIFICATIONS AND STRATEGIES

The assumption here is that learning disabled children and youth will evidence one or more of a number of symptoms. Further, these symptoms will be evidenced not only in children's home and classroom life but also in physical education classes. Finally, it is assumed that these symptoms, when recognized and dealt with sensitively and intelligently, will facilitate children's progress in physical education; when ignored, misunderstood, or dealt with inappropriately, these symptoms not only will cause students to fail to experience growth in the objectives set for physical education but also may cause real harm to their total personalities and result in trauma that will become apparent at home and in the classroom.

As a precautionary note—a given type of activity or teacher behavior, even if selected and plugged in properly, will not automatically work. Those in the field know that pat solutions to the complexities of learning disabled children's problems do not always occur. The following pages present information that will optimize physical education teacher-student contact based on the *probabilities* that a given strategy will produce a *possible* change in the child.

For purposes of organization, the following learning disabilities have been divided into four areas of difficulty: (a) conceptual, (b) perceptual, (c) attention and activity level, and (d) motor. A given learning disabled child will not necessarily possess any or all of these problems. Each child is unique, exhibiting a mosaic of symptoms, not all of which will appear in a given situation. Thus, teachers of learning disabled children should recognize the general pattern of disorders in a given child, the probability of certain problems appearing in given situations, and, most important, how to cope with the specific problem or set of problems (syndrome) that a child or youth brings to class each day.

Conceptual Problems

Learning disabled children may show rather diffuse patterns of conceptual disorganization or may evidence specific types of intellectual problems. An example of the former is difficulty in integrating pieces of information to form logical conclusions. An example of a more specific problem is one involving short- or long-term memory.

Generally, learning disabled children evidencing conceptual problems do not stick out at first in physical education classes, as do those beset with clumsiness, for example. But, youngsters who have difficulty remembering, drawing conclusions, and the like will have difficulty remembering the rules for a complex game and quickly calling up the correct rule or skill in a fast-moving game. LD children may remember a rule or strategy when it is repeated, evidencing recognition memory, but at the same time be unable to recall or to formulate the correct rule, skill, or strategy when it is called for. Often, memory deficiencies of this type are connected to problems in attention; the children apparently cannot remember because they never attended closely enough to learning in the first place!

Teachers may employ a number of strategies for children who evidence conceptual deficiencies in physical education settings:

1. The complexity of games should gradually be built up from simple sub-skills and lead-up games to the entire sport. Blake and Volp's (1964) excellent book on lead-up games would be of some help here.

2. The logical place of each skill, sub-skill, and strategy in the total game effort should be carefully explained. Learning disabled children might not readily grasp the meanings of drills, rules, and the like for the entire game or recreational situation. Likewise, they may not understand long-term goals for drills and fitness exercises without precise explanation.

3. Some overteaching of rules may be necessary. Learning disabled children with memory problems must overlearn conceptual skills, particularly those that must be recalled under the stress of athletic or sports competition. Moreover, children should be taught in several modalities because these children typically have reading problems. Thus, for best understanding, rules, skills, and tactics should be stated, demonstrated, and explained, and also be available in print.

4. The complexity of the social situation should be reduced for perceptually and motorically involved children alike. Some older (6 and over) learning disabled children may not at first be able to cooperate in games involving just two children. The instructor may be surprised to find that two children standing a few feet apart cannot cooperate in a simple game of catch. If this is true, the activities should be moved back developmentally from a social standpoint. The instructor should start with parallel play (in which both are doing the same thing but not in concert), whatever the age of the children involved. After this stage is successfully mastered, the games and activities should gradually assume increasing complexity, from parallel play, to dual activities, to small-group activities with simple games and rules, and finally to complex games played in a group according to codified rules.

Perceptual Problems

Learning disabled children may exhibit a number of perceptual problems. With the development of motor-free tests of perception, the percentage may not be as high as once thought, but these children and youth sometimes evidence any one or a combination of the following perceptual problems:

1. Tactile perception may be poor. For example, children may not be able to identify which of their own fingers have been touched when their hands are hidden from view. This kind of problem is called *digital agnosia*, but similar agnosias may affect other body parts and surfaces as well. These deficiencies conceivably can interfere with the accuracy of perception, as in the the case of digital agnosia when a ball has reached the hand.

2. Often, learning disabled children are unaware of the positions, movements, and locations of their own body parts in relation to their total body. This kind of problem may not be measurable in the usual tests of verbal identification of body parts (e.g., "Where is your elbow?") but may be seen when children's bodies suddenly become limp or floppy

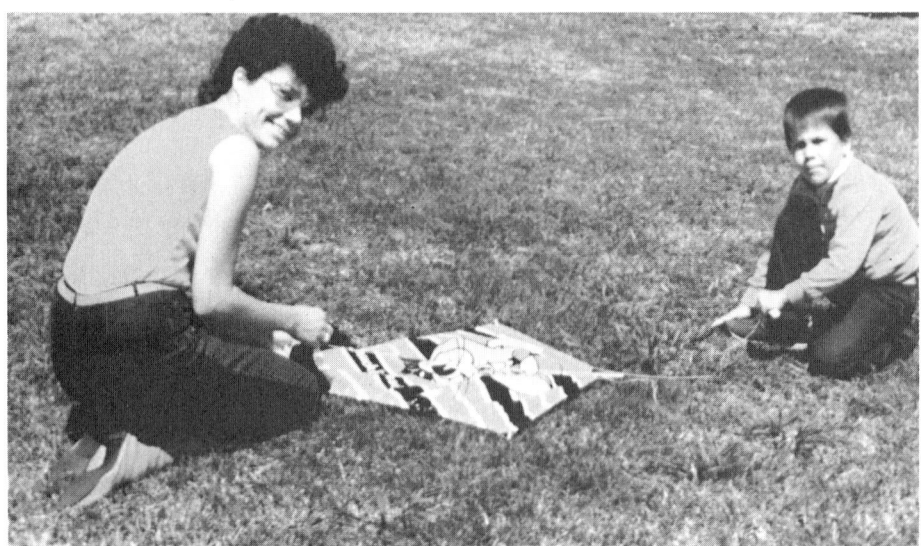

Kite flying may be one appropriate activity for a learning disabled child, as it does not engender stress through competition but does require some motor skills and coordination.

Courtesy, Special Education Branch, Los Angeles City Schools

when they are required to perform a task or when they fail to walk between or crawl under obstacles. If a child does not react correctly when asked to "lie down with your legs toward me" or "stand against the wall with your back to the wall," teachers may interpret the response as disobedience rather than perceptual problems.

3. Children may not be able to pick a figure out of a background. This problem of *figure-ground perception*, often discussed in the literature, may impede performance when balls are thrown at children or when they must select teammates out of a confusing background to whom to pass in a game.

4. Children may not integrate the parts of a situation with a whole. They may not be able to synthesize visual information properly when observing a demonstration of an action to be copied. Tests in which children attempt to imitate gestures, both simple and complex, may help educators objectify this condition. The same kind of problem may have caused children to exhibit some degrees of clumsiness early in their development; they might have failed to "see" the movements of other children in developmentally appropriate activities (running, throwing, and the like), and thus were unable to copy the actions unconsciously during their formative years as children usually do.

5. Auditory perception problems may plague children with learning disabilities—and confuse physical education teachers attempting to offer verbal directions to the youngsters. Often these children are able to hear clearly but cannot properly organize the words in sequence. Thus, children who have an auditory sequencing problem may perceive a direction to "get the balls out of the bag" and "bring them to me" as something entirely different. Again, teachers may interpret children's confusion or incorrect actions as naughtiness and admonish the children instead of repeating the directions more slowly and in simpler terms.

Other auditory confusions may be similar to the figure-ground problem. That is, from among a number of noises or voices, children may be unable to select appropriate directions and words to which to react.

The implications of these subtle perceptual problems for teachers of physical education are numerous. Some implications simply revolve around being more careful and precise relative to the rapidity and amount of information offered children in attempts to instruct them. Others involve formulating special training activities and game modifications that will help children with these perceptual confusions improve or at least not feel as inadequate. Physical education teachers should not be surprised when these subtle perceptual problems manifest themselves in some of the ways described. When children react improperly to sensory information in a game, they should first be given the benefit of the doubt. Most important, if perceptually handicapped, learning disabled children are attempting to interact with a class of normal youngsters—especially in a complex game involving difficult hand-eye coordinations (e.g., interception of balls)—special care should be taken to educate their peers about the nature of these confusions.

Specifically, some principles that may be applied to learning disabled children with perceptual handicaps include:

1. Verbal information concerning a skill, game, strategy, or exercise should be offered slowly, carefully, and in small bits. One should take a multimodal approach to instruction; verbal direction should be accompanied by easy-to-understand demonstrations, preferably by children about the same age and size.

2. Care should be taken not to place a perceptually handicapped child in complex game situations in which too many things (e.g., people and missiles) are moving at once. Rather, the usual games may be scaled down and made simpler, or they may be gradually built up until the whole game sequence is assimilated.

3. Sports that do not have too many perceptual components may be welcomed by perceptually handicapped children. The children are elated to find that sports such as swimming and running do not require them to make complex perceptual judgments involving three-dimensional space. Moreover, one's improvement in these and similar individual sports is highly measurable and apparent to the youngsters who participate. Care must be taken even here, though, as children with *somatoagnosia* (body agnosia) often find the first exposure to water frightening and difficult because the absence of the usual forces of gravity makes their bodies seem to "disappear" at first. Aquatics activities are the subject of chapter 31.

4. Various verbal and tactile body-image games may be introduced with useful outcomes. Games of various degrees of difficulty have been devised for the blind and neurologically impaired relative to verbal identification of body parts. The sequence of body-part identification abilities appears in chapter 30.

5. Perceptually confused children often have difficulty participating in games in which space has to be managed. For example, children with left-right confusion are as likely to run to third base as to first on striking the ball. Prior to placing children in this situation, various lead-up activities should be initiated. The bases should be walked to, given different colors, and in other ways made different from each other to prevent left-right confusions.

Some perceptual handicaps may prevent children with learning disabilities from reading well. They may not be able to select specific words out of a background or identify shapes easily or listen to sentences and then reproduce them verbally. Upon encountering these children, physical education teachers not only should take steps to accommodate and help rectify the children's confusions but also provide a friendly place in which children may succeed in stages rather than an environment fraught with frustrations.

Attention and Activity Level Problems

Perhaps no type of disability is more publicized than *hyperactivity*. The "too-busy" child has been described in clinical terms and has been subjected to many experiments, particularly during the past 20 years. Interventions have included rearrangement of the environment, behavioral modification, medication, muscular relaxation, mental exercises, and changes in diet. Hyperactivity has been ascribed to neurological deficiencies, emotional problems, chemical imbalances, and even variables as elusive as the weather. To many, the concept of hyperactivity is singular and always accompanies motor awkwardness.

Hyperactivity and other attentional disorders are the focus of chapter 26. Here, four practical implications for the physical education teacher are:

1. Attentional disorders may or may not be accompanied by excessive activity, and hyperactive children may or may not have problems reflecting motor incoordination.

2. Most of the time, children described as hyperactive are not excessively active but are usually doing the wrong things. They are engaging in asocial behaviors rather than being excessively active.

3. Hyperactivity receives much attention, while *hypoactivity* often is ignored. Passivity in the classroom does not attract the same concern as the activity of children who seem to "bounce off people and climb the walls." Many of the activities outlined in chapter 26 are useful when applied to hypoactive children.

4. A final attentional disorder has been termed *perseveration*. Unlike hyperactivity, which reflects an inability or disclination of children to pay attention to tasks for prolonged periods, children evidencing perseveration remain fixed overly long on a given stimulus, or they engage in repetitive, inappropriate motor behavior in an almost hypnotic manner. To "unstick" these children from a task is difficult. Perseveration is found not only among learning disabled children, but also among the retarded and the emotionally disturbed.

Motor Problems

Awkward, or uncoordinated, children do not necessarily have learning disabilities, but they probably represent a slightly higher percentage than do normal children (the research is yet unclear) within populations of those labeled learning disabled. Indeed, one specific learning disability, *dysgraphia*—the inability to print with clarity and facility—involves motor abilities.

By the time children are 4 or 5 years old, motor functioning becomes highly specific. Children with problems in balancing may not have difficulties in printing, while children who print letters well may have difficulty buttoning their clothes. General qualities, however, may permeate more than one task. These include: (a) difficulties in motor planning (*praxic* behavior); (b) overflow movements (excess associated movements in noninvolved body parts); (c) problems with integrating body parts, as in shifting the weight from foot to foot when throwing; (d) *asymmetries*, as evidenced by children who always jump with one foot slightly in front of the other or who cannot move well laterally; and (e) degrees of *hypertonia* or *hypotonia*—an excess of muscle tone or increased resistance to stretching, or an insufficiency in muscle tone or lack of resistance to stretching, respectively.

For the most part, although these general qualities are not easily measurable, they are obvious and observable to professionals and peers alike. Their presence at times seems to make the children "look funny" to others. These qualities detract from the mechanics and interfere with the physics of movements children are attempting to execute.

Learning disabled children who have movement difficulties should be attended to. The principles and guidelines contained in chapter 12, dealing with motor problems, should be consulted.

SUMMARY

Ever since the end of World War II, accommodating educational programs to children with learning disabilities has had increased emphasis. Generally, this label is given to children and youth who have difficulties acquiring academic skills but who score reasonably well on standard tests of intelligence. Their problems may stem from one or more sources, including visual perceptual difficulties, motor awkwardness, conceptual immaturity, attentional disorders, or auditory perceptual abnormalities.

Historically, during the last century clinicians noted that some children and youth displayed rather exotic and specific perceptual and conceptual problems similar to disorders exhibited by stroke patients and others incurring cerebral dysfunctions later in life. After a period during which various clinicians in the United States developed tests and training regimes, the general approach now taken toward learning disabilities is rather symptom-specific and includes attention to motor awkwardness, if present. Accommodation to learning disabled children within a physical education setting may take the form of special aids to help them control their own activity level, perceptually easier games and sports, and special developmental activities to enhance sports skills and hand-eye coordination.

Special attention often has to be given not only to LD children's motor problems at play but also to social immaturity under the stress of competitive sports and games. Activities might have to be scaled down in complexity and difficulty to make them manageable for learning disabled children. Perceptual problems may take the form of various kinds of spatial agnosias influencing children's perception of their bodies, as well as visual perceptual problems that create difficulty in handling fast-moving ball games. Thus, special lead-up activities often must be substituted for the more difficult games in which their more able peers participate. Motor and attentional problems and activities are discussed further in chapters 12 and 26, respectively.

REFERENCES

Ayres, A.J. (1972). *Sensory integration and learning disorders.* Los Angeles: Western Psychological Services.

Blake, O.W., & Volp, A.M. (1964). *Lead-up games to team sports.* Englewood Cliffs, NJ: Prentice-Hall.

Cruickshank, W.M., Bentzen, F.A., Ratzeburg, F.H., & Tannhauser, T. (1961). *A teaching method for brain-injured and hyperactive children.* Syracuse, NY: Syracuse University Press.

Dennis, W. (1940). The effect of cradling practices upon the onset of walking in Hopi children. *Journal of Genetic Psychology, 56,* 77-86.

Frostig, M. (1961). *Developmental tests of visual perception.* Palo Alto, CA: Consulting Psychologists Press.

Frostig, M. (1968). Education for children with learning disabilities. In H. Myklebust, *Progress in learning disabilities* (Vol. 1). New York: Grune & Stratton.

Gresham, F.M., & Reschly, D.J. (1986). Social skill deficits and low peer acceptance of mainstreamed learning disabled children. *Learning Disability Quarterly, 9,* 23-32.

Hallahan, D.P., & Cruickshank, W.M. (1973). *Psychoeducational foundations of learning disabilities.* Englewood Cliffs, NJ: Prentice-Hall.

Head, H. (1926). *Aphasia and kindred disorders of speech* (Vols. 1 & 2). London: Cambridge University Press.

Hinschelwood, J. (1917). *Congenital word blindness.* London: Lewis.

Kagan, J. (1976). Resilience and continuity in psychological development. In A.M. Clarke & A.D.B. Clarke (Eds.), *Early experience: Myth and evidence.* New York: Free Press.

Kirk, S.A. (1966). *The diagnosis and remediation of psycholinguistic disabilities.* Urbana: University of Illinois Press.

Kirk, S.A., McCarthy, J., & Kirk, W. (1978). *Illinois test of psycholinguistic abilities* (1968). Baltimore: University Park Press.

Myers, P.I., & Hammill, D.D. (1976). *Methods for learning disorders* (2nd ed.). New York: John Wiley & Sons.

National Advisory Committee on Handicapped Children. (1968, January). *Special education for handicapped children.* Washington, DC: U.S. Dept. of Health, Education, & Welfare.

Orton, S.A. (1939). A neurological explanation of the reading disability. *Educational Record, 20*(12), 58-68.

Orton, S.A. (1943). Visual functions in strephosymbolia. *Archives of Ophthalmology, 30,* 707-713.

Schain, R.J. (1977). *Neurology of childhood learning disorders* (2nd ed.). Baltimore: Williams & Wilkins.

Schuell, R.A., et al. (1964). *Aphasia in adults.* New York: Haeber Medical Division, Harper.

Strauss, A.A., & Lehtinen, L. (1955). *Psychopathology and education of the brain-injured child* (Vol. 1). New York: Grune & Stratton.

Wiederholt, J.L. (1974). Historical perspectives on the education of the learning disabled. In L. Mann & D.A. Sabatino (Eds.)., *The second review of special education.* Philadelphia: JSE Press.

ADDITIONAL REFERENCES

Cratty, B.J. (1975). *Remedial motor activity for children.* Philadelphia: Lea & Febiger.

Dubnoff, B., & Chambers, I. (1966). A multifocal approach to the development of the concept of body image. In Council for Children with Behavioral Disorders, *Yearbook.* Washington, DC: CCBD.

QUESTIONS FOR DISCUSSION

1. Discuss the definition of learning disability presented in this chapter. What specific concepts does it contain? How might it be improved on?
2. Discuss the history of awareness of learning disabilities. In what ways did movement attributes contribute to the history?
3. Might learning disabled children do poorly on a battery of motor tests and yet possess average to above-average motor abilities? Explain.
4. How might physical education teachers, when designing a physical program, accommodate learning disabled children's conceptual disorders, their possible perceptual handicaps, and their attentional deficiencies?
5. In what ways are learning disabled children different from retarded children?

STUDENT PROJECTS

1. Interview a teacher of learning disabled children. Discuss the unique characteristics, and types of possible motor problems.
2. Survey literature and tests purporting to evaluate visual, perceptual, and auditory perceptual attributes of learning disabled children.
3. Discuss the special problems in child rearing that may be encountered with learning disabled children by interviewing the parents of an LD youngster. Discuss accompanying educational diagnoses, remediation, and school placement.
4. Outline a curriculum containing movement activities intended to (a) calm down a hyperactive child with learning disabilities or (b) promote physical vigor and skill.

RESOURCES

Association for Children and Adults
   with Learning Disabilities (ACLD)
4156 Library Rd.
Pittsburgh, PA 15234

California Association for
   Neurologically Handicapped
   Children
P.O. Box 61067
Sacramento, CA 95860

Division for Learning Disabilities
Council for Exceptional Children
1920 Association Dr.
Reston, VA 22091

Marianne Frostig Center for Educational
   Therapy
5981 Venice Blvd.
Los Angeles, CA 90034

Orton Dyslexia Society
724 York Rd.
Baltimore, MD 21204

Quebec Association for Children with
   Learning Disabilities
6338 Victoria Ave.
Montreal
Quebec, Canada

9 *Emotional/Behavioral Disturbances*

Those who come in contact with emotionally disturbed children and youth see various facets of their behavior. Peers are shocked by meaningless aggression in play. Parents are concerned when their child does not want to go to school. Teachers label these children "bad." Sensitive counselors become concerned with children who withdraw into themselves and seem to function as impervious beings in a kind of shell. Psychiatrists may speak of "dissociation" between affect and behavior, or perhaps of paranoid schizophrenia.

DEFINITION AND PREVALENCE

Estimates of the prevalence of emotional disturbance in school populations range from 2% to between 10% and 15%, depending on the severity of the conditions considered. Essentially, *emotionally disturbed children are those whose functioning is at an extreme on various scales.* They are overly active or inactive, or perhaps extremely aggressive or passive.

In addition to comprising a separate classification, emotional disturbance is found within several handicapped groups. Many children with learning disabilities are emotionally disturbed, and the prevalence of emotional disturbance in retarded populations usually is found to be greater than within groups of normal children.

Disturbed children usually have learning difficulties but may possess extremely high intelligence or slightly below average intelligence or a sharp contrast of low and high academic/intellectual abilities in specific areas. Emotionally disturbed children are generally assumed to be performing at less than their optimum level in most academic subjects.

Perhaps in no other part of their school day do emotionally disturbed children and youth confront both problems and sources of potential help as much as when they are engaged in organized or informal physical education and play situations. Not always obvious in a classroom, withdrawn children stand out immediately when teams are selected. Moderately aggressive children become enraged as the heat of competition rises during a closely contested game. The behaviors of perseverating autistic children may become exaggerated when they are confronted with play implements and other children.

Physical education teachers are in a position either to aid or to inadvertently harm children with symptoms reflecting emotional disturbance or mental illness. Insensitivity on the part of a play leader can crush the already downtrodden youth, while succorance can bring out the best in an overly anxious class member. During the 1960s one of the more common folk definitions of a disturbed child was one who could not function socially with normal children. And yet, with the advent of mainstreaming, this same child in the 1980s is often placed in a potentially treacherous social context.

When attempting to deal with emotionally disturbed youngsters, physical education teachers should be knowledgeable in a number of related areas. This knowledge should include (a) information about emotional disturbances themselves—their symptoms and potential educational-therapeutic strategies; (b) the ways in which emotional disturbances are manifested in feelings about the body and how the person performs or fails to perform in a vigorous setting (many psychic disturbances involve symptoms revolving around the body, its performance, and bodily feelings); and (c) useful practical operations to employ in classes when attempting to reduce the disturbed behaviors of children and youth.

Among recent trends in the literature are indications that vigorous physical fitness activities including jogging (Allen, 1980) can have important therapeutic effects upon the emotionally disturbed. In a recent review of the literature, Van Andel and Austin (1984) pointed out that aggressive tendencies, as well as depression and anxiety, can be reduced through appropriate physical activity. Other recent innovations include the use of game-like situations to reduce asocial tendencies and promote positive social contacts, including an increase in vocal communication among the emotionally disturbed. These trends and new interventions are explored further later in the chapter.

CLASSIFICATIONS AND CHARACTERISTICS

Previous attempts by the American Psychiatric Association (APA) to classify mental disturbance employed a three-part breakdown: (a) the more severe *psychoses*, including schizophrenia, (b) less severe *neuroses*, including phobias (e.g., school phobia), obsessions, compulsions, and hysteria, and (c) a number of "everyday" *behavioral disorders*. Among the behaviors placed in the latter group were distractibility, overly aggressive behaviors, excessive shyness, and various delinquent habits seen in large numbers among children who otherwise function reasonably well in school settings.

APA Multiaxial Classification System

More recently the American Psychiatric Association (1980) has developed the "Multiaxial Classification System," set forth in its *Diagnostic and Statistical Manual*. This more contemporary typology includes five dimensions. The first relates to disorders usually first evident in infancy, childhood, or adolescence and includes organic mental disorders, substance abuse problems, anxiety disorders, and others. Among these "somatoform disorders" are:

1. Long-lasting pain with no apparent cause.
2. Hypochondriasis (imaginary illnesses and conditions).
3. Conversion disorders (body parts cannot function because of some psychologically based paralysis).
4. Somatization disorders involving the fear of *getting* symptoms!
5. Vague fears, nausea, weaknesses, and fear of doing anything.
6. An "effort syndrome" that includes breathlessness, without any apparent and real physical exertion connected with the condition.

The second axis within this classification system contains various personality disorders accompanying paranoia, schizophrenia, antisocial tendencies, and aggressive behaviors, as well as specific developmental disorders in reading, arithmetic, language, and even articulation problems. The third axis deals with specific and real physical disorders and symptoms.

The fourth axis refers to the severity of the psychosocial stresses that are likely to bring on the disorder. These range from 1 (none) to 3, which may involve, for example, a mild argument with a neighbor, through 7 on the scale, which involves some catastrophe.

The fifth and final axis within this system addresses the individual's highest level of social-adaptive functioning within the past year. These levels also are arranged on a 7-point scale, from 1, reflecting superior social and occupational functioning, through 4, involving moderate impairment, to 7, reflecting gross impairment in virtually all areas of functioning including maintenance of personal hygiene. Thus, an individual believed to be mentally/emotionally disturbed is classified at various points within each of the axes defined.

Childhood Psychoses

Psychoses, considered the most serious form of mental illness, may be differentiated from neuroses insofar as they severely limit or prevent normal daily functions of the individual afflicted. Three major groups of psychoses have been identified: (a) maladaptive *character disorders,* including alcoholism, drug dependency, and socially aberrant sexual behavior; these symptoms usually are not seen in childhood but manifest themselves in early to late adolescence; (b) *affective disorders*, ranging from extreme depression to elation; behavior is marked by swings of mood between these two extremes—the manic-depressive syndrome; and (c) various forms of *schizophrenia*—by far the most common psychosis, afflicting about one half of those considered psychotic. An additional psychosis that is seen rarely but nevertheless is present in some children participating in physical education classes is *autism*.

Relatively little information is available concerning the fitness levels of emotionally disturbed children. Recently, however, Van Pelt and Kalish (1983) surveyed motor proficiencies in children with diagnosed psychoses. The pre-adolescent boys they surveyed scored low on a wide range of skills involving limb coordination and balance. In general, they were more deficient in gross-motor skills than in fine-motor skills. Hypertonicity (excess tension) was seen in over half of the 21 boys tested.

Schizophrenia   The original criteria for diagnosing childhood schizophrenia, developed in the early 1930s, are:

—withdrawal of interest in the environment.
—unrealistic feelings, thoughts, and actions.
—thought disturbances and decreased speech, including mutism.
—rigidity, distortion, and decrease in emotional behaviors.
—hyperactivity or hypoactivity, including bizarre, repetitive behaviors.

Thus, schizophrenia involves various types and kinds of symptoms indicating personality disorganization. These disturbances may be thought of as splits or cleavages between (a) thoughts and feelings, (b) thoughts and reality, and speech and reality, and (c) the attention given to various objects at the same time. Many children diagnosed as schizophrenic are known to later manifest these symptoms in adulthood. Only 4% of adult schizophrenics, however, manifested symptoms in childhood.

Schizophrenic children and adults alike have symptoms that place them in one of four categories:

1. *Catatonic.* This form is characterized by rigid posture, a stupor-like state that reflects denial of reality or an attempt to "leave the world." The patient may spend hours in one position not communicating with others.

2. *Paranoid.* Paranoid patients believe others are speaking of them negatively and have heightened anxiety and fear of social contact and situations. At times these delusions involve religious symbols or ideas and feelings of grandeur. Schizophrenic children in physical education classes may exhibit a paranoid reaction, for example, when they are not chosen first or are discriminated against in team situations.

3. *Hebephrenic.* Hebephrenia involves a defense mechanism that results in regression into childhood behaviors and fantasies. Childish giggling and speech patterns and nonsensical rhymes inappropriate to the speaker's age level permeate the individual's behaviors.

4. *Undifferentiated.* Individuals in this category exhibit behaviors that cannot be neatly classified under any of the previous three areas. When more than one type of behavior (e.g., paranoia plus catatonic reactions) is present, the individual often is classified as undifferentiated.

Working with the schizophrenic child or youth is an extremely difficult undertaking, even under the most advantageous circumstances. Each child or youth may present a different combination of symptoms. Age of onset and family constellation constitute other important variables. For example, children who are psychotic are likely to remain disturbed to some degree as adults, while psychoses appearing in adolescence or in early or late adulthood apparently are not natural outcomes of earlier disturbed conditions.

For physical educators to try to act as family counselors or to make inferences relative to the influence of the family unit on youths' problems is not helpful. A more positive tack is to take a rather direct approach to children evidencing specific symptoms and attempt to use the vivid situations found in physical education classes to help them.

For the most part it is advised not to enter the fantasy life of a hallucinating child but instead to bring the child into reality (e.g., "Now catch the ball"). If the child indicates that he or she is not "letting go" of some extraneous idea, the teacher might say, "That's not true . . . now pay attention to what we are doing." Physical education situations in which attention is required to avoid slight harm, such as walking balance beams, may be useful in focusing the child's attention on the here and now.

Autism Leon Kanner (1943) made the first attempts to describe the severe and relatively rare type of childhood psychosis called "autistic behavior." His description of the characteristics included: (a) severe withdrawal from other people, (b) an intense need to preserve sameness, (c) an inability to deal with people, (d) unique, rhythmic movement mannerisms, (e) apparently good intellectual potential, as reflected by average or better than average scores on some tasks and by an "intelligent facial expression," and (f) severe disturbance of language functioning.

Autism originates very early in life and, in addition to the factors mentioned above, often is accompanied by rather harsh, self-destructive behaviors. Autistic features may first be brought to the attention of professionals at around age 3 or 4, when children whose speech is minimal or absent are referred to clinicians for treatment.

The movement behaviors of autistic children are a mixture of remarkable skill in some visual motor tasks, such as completing puzzles, and bizarre movement patterns including rhythmic arm flapping, hand twisting, spinning the whole body while seemingly out of contact with reality, facial grimacing, and walking on the toes. When confronted with toys, they may become preoccupied with a single function of the toy (e.g., spinning the wheel of a small car) and engage in it insistently.

Their sensory functioning is likewise a mixture of sensitivity and insensitivity. They often are apparently insensitive to pain and do not cry or complain when physically hurt. At the same time, a slight noise or other unusual but harmless sensory experience, such as the touch of another person, may send them into a prolonged, hysterical tantrum reflecting extreme anxiety.

Self-awareness seems to be a significant problem among autistic children. In general, studies exploring the self-concept and image of autistic children are rare, but the findings that have been forthcoming indicate that autistic children are aware of themselves in general, but not specific, ways (Dawson & McKissick, 1984).

Moreover, they display an abundance of neurological signs that indicate motor impairment and dyspraxia, problems that may cause difficulty in engaging in gestural communication as well as normal motor activities including play and self-care (Jones & Prior, 1985).

Obviously, autistic children do not display the same severity of symptoms; the range is great. Recently Schopler (1986) formulated an evaluation scale with which to evaluate the degree and severity of the condition.

Some have postulated that autism has genetic roots. Although the occurrence of autism in siblings of autistic children is only 2%, this is 50 times greater than would occur by chance (Meryash, Szmanski, & Gerald, 1982). More and more, biochemical factors are being explored as possible triggers of autistic behaviors. An elevated level of serotonin, for example, is one suspect in this search for the etiology of autism (Young, Kavanagh, Anderson, Shaywitz, & Cohen, 1982). Increases in amphetamine levels in animals have resulted in the same type of motor activity seen in autistic children.

Positive results have been seen in clinical studies using epinephrine and norepinephrine. Some neuroleptics, such as dopamine, have been shown to modify autistic behaviors including self-mutilation (Young et al., 1982). Although the possibility of mineral and other nutrient intake of autistic children has been explored as a potential controller of behaviors, the results of these studies have not been promising.

Moderate to mild changes have been elicited in autistic children through various interventions including behavior modification and psychotherapy. Some children seem to "grow out of" the more severe manifestations and appear in middle childhood to be simply frightened children who do not listen to directions. Other children do not improve to any great extent, despite the best efforts of professionals and parents. I do not understand how severely autistic children can be comfortably mainstreamed with a class of normal children, but children who apparently are growing out of the symptoms might be integrated into a regular physical education class with careful handling and reasonable precautions.

Anxiety-producing or frustrating situations should be avoided, and class members should be oriented to the autistic child's condition. In general, these children should be approached in an indirect way (e.g., the teacher might enter the room bouncing a ball), not imposing himself or herself directly on the child. With repeated exposure, children then might pick up another available ball and begin to bounce it.

Two studies illustrate ways in which movement experiences may be structured for autistic children. Black, Freeman, and Montgomery (1975) discovered that autistic children modeled after a normal child peer in an obstacle course. This study verified that a nondirective approach in situations involving a logical transition from one movement to another may attract the attention of autistic children. Miller and Miller (1973) also used an obstacle course requiring movement and attention with 19 mute autistic children (mean age 11 years). The intent was to help them learn simple manual signs for the various movements, transfer the concept of signing to things and concepts other than actions, and finally to transfer the concept of signing to the formation of words. Upon completion of the intervention, these children evidenced remarkable change in their behaviors and conceptual abilities. All of them learned signs and some speech and could generalize the signing concept and produce hand signs for objects and other components of their environment.

Among a number of more recent interventions intended to reduce autistic mannerisms has been *vigorous physical exercise*. Kern, Vogel, and Dunlap (1984), for example, found that vigorous exercise indeed reduced manneristic behaviors in a group of young autistic children. They suggested that exercise resulted in the production and release of natural body tranquilizers (beta-endorphins), resulting in the calming of autistic children.

One of the more important types of intervention that a physical education teacher may employ with autistic youngsters is *music therapy* (Baker, 1982), as music is relatively impersonal—emanating from a neutral source and not from a feared other person. Using music, the child's focus upon internal stimulation reflecting isolation may be shifted to an awareness of external qualities in the world. After this shift has been achieved, self-care skills and social relationships may be developed. Because autistic children tend to relate to rhythmic activities, however, care must be taken so that the music does not simply encourage the child's undesirable repetitive mannerisms.

Relaxation training has been shown to be helpful in reducing unwanted aggressive behaviors in autistic children. Hughes and Davis (1980), for example, used muscular feedback to encourage autistic youngsters to decrease the frequency of both verbally and physically aggressive responses by reinforcing the emission of a competing relaxation response, using EMG feedback. Through this method, unwanted aggression was reduced over 67%.

More and more, *game settings* are being carefully constructed to induce positive outcomes. McGee, Krantz, and McClannahan (1984), for example, have reported improving assertiveness as well as conversational skills among autistic adolescents within a "naturalistic game setting." Careful preparation was carried out before the games; modeling of appropriate behaviors was encouraged; and contingency rewards were given when the adolescents expressed assertiveness and verbal skills in positive ways.

These studies, as well as clinical observations of autistic children, reveal that if one is to work with them, indirect approaches not involving forced social contacts are best. Further, movement situations, while challenging and sequential, should be relatively impersonal at first, and peer models can be used effectively. Children must be lured, rather than forced, into moving in ways that are more in keeping with their rhythmic mannerisms.

Working with these children often is a long, painstaking process, requiring inordinate patience. Regressions can be expected along the way. Longitudinal studies are needed on the possible effects of various interventions, including movement activities, on the social, linguistic, and motor behaviors of these complicated children. Movement experiences may prove to be an important part of their therapy, with potentially good payoffs.

GENERAL STRATEGIES AND GUIDELINES

Physical educators and therapists might observe the three roles outlined by Goodrich and Boomer (1958) when working with emotionally disturbed children: (a) preventive, helping to avoid controls that might threaten the child's personality; (b) supportive, helping the child maintain self-control under stress; and (c) restitutive, aiding the child to regain control after temporary failure. Operationalized, these three types of behavior might appear as follows in physical education classes:

1. *Preventive.* The teacher should look ahead in program planning, seeking to include activities that emotionally disturbed children can clearly master and placing them in situations that are not potentially threatening. Such a child, even in middle childhood, might not be ready to cooperate directly in games with other children. Thus, a program that at first might involve parallel play (a child engaging in an activity similar to that of another child—e.g., ball bouncing versus playing catch) may prove useful.

2. *Supportive.* When stress occurs in a class (e.g., a child is ridiculed by a classmate or is chosen last on a team), the teacher should be ready to take the disturbed child aside, sympathize with the problem, and at times, create unobtrusive social circumventions with the aid of more understanding, mature, and emotionally stable members of the class. For example, the disturbed child could be selected to lead exercises.

3. *Restitutive.* Helping a child regain control after an outburst can be a difficult undertaking. The impact on both the normal class members (if in a mainstreaming situation) and on the emotionally disturbed child must be assessed. In most cases, when the *reason* for the problem is discussed with the youngster, it serves to reduce the problem's seriousness in the mind of that child. The instructor then should offer specific advice as to how to avoid the problem in the future (People do not like balls thrown at their heads!), as well as suggest how the child might calm down at the present time ("Why don't you go over and lie down on a mat until you feel better?"). Various kinds of impulse control and relaxation training can be helpful tools when working with a child after an "incident" has occurred.

Recently, more refined teaching strategies that are effective in teaching physical education activities to the emotionally disturbed have been described in the literature. Loss of free time is often effective as a punishment when working with the emotionally disturbed in a physical activity context. Heltma and Vogler (1985) described how such a contingency program improved on-task behaviors more than did simple peer pressure to conform.

Paul and Epanchin (1982) have suggested that the child's removal with an adult, as well as physical restraint (a "therapeutic hold"), plus soothing talk can improve the behavioral management of emotionally disturbed children in educational settings. Redl and Wineman (1957) presented a whole "laundry list" of methods useful in dealing with the aggressive child, including: (a) nonverbal signals and warnings, (b) caring behavior from the teacher, (c) interpreting situations for the child, (d) direct appeals ("please cooperate"), (e) removal from the group, (f) limiting space and tools, (g) using humor to reduce tension, and (h) engaging the child in interesting conversation.

Programs of relaxation and physical training (fitness) should be carefully tailored to individuals rather than simply applied in a blanket manner to a group of disturbed children, youth, or adults (Van Andel & Austin, 1984). Moreover, exposing the emotionally disturbed to fitness, recreational, and exercise activities will result in gains not only in fitness and various emotional states but also in self-esteem and self-concept.

SUMMARY

The range of emotionally disturbed behaviors is wide, ranging from extreme withdrawal to overt aggression. In any form, the more severe manifestations are the most difficult for teachers to handle. The Multiaxial Classification System of the American Psychiatric Association has largely replaced the older classification system of psychoses, neuroses, and behavioral disorders. The APA system has five dimensions, related to disorders first evident in childhood ("somatoform" disorders), personality disorders, physically related disorders, severity of stresses, and social-adaptive functioning. Among the emotional disorders more commonly seen in school-age children are schizophrenia and autism.

When attempting to work with emotionally disturbed youngsters, physical educators should proceed with a great deal of care. In general, three types of strategies are recommended: (a) preventive, in an attempt to allay stresses and controls that may upset the student, (b) supportive, in which an effort is made to prevent various social situations from "unhinging" the youngster, and (c) restitutive, to help children regain self-control after some behavioral incident.

Abrupt or severe discipline may cause emotionally distant children to withdraw even more. An accepting, warm approach is best, ignoring possible mild behavioral transgressions that do not disrupt the class or the general flow of the lesson. Of course, at the other extreme, physical aggression, whether directed against the teacher or another child, requires action. If aggression against a teacher is mild, overreaction is not as acceptable as a quiet question asking the reason for the flare-up, explaining that the minor assault caused hurt, and asking the child not to do it again. If the aggressive act is more violent, the child must be physically restrained and removed from the setting.

If the structure of the situation and the complexity of the activities are not overly threatening and result in disturbed children achieving some success and pleasure, the chances of emotional outbursts are likely to be reduced greatly. Careful planning is an important beginning in keeping emotionally disturbed children calm during class time. The physical educator has many choices and sometimes must guess how best to proceed when working with emotionally disturbed children. The teacher may have to decide whether to intervene in a child's fantasy life, when and how to exhibit control and discipline, and how to structure the situation socially so that it will be of minimal stress to the emotionally disturbed youngster.

At times specific strategies are helpful when working with emotionally disturbed youngsters. These may consist of games that elicit cooperative rather than competitive behaviors, calming-down activities after the excitement of play, and the gradual introduction of youngsters to social situations of increasing complexity as the children become ready for them.

REFERENCES

Allen, J.I. (1980). Jogging can modify disruptive behaviors. *Teaching Exceptional Children, 12*, 66-70.

American Psychiatric Association. (1980). *Diagnostic and statistical manual of mental disorders.* Washington, DC: APA.

Baker, B.S. (1982). Music therapy as a treatment modality for autism. *Journal of Psychosocial Nursing & Mental Health Services, 20*, 31-34.

Black, M., Freeman, B.J., & Montgomery, J. (1975). Systematic observation of play behavior in autistic children. *Journal of Autism & Childhood Schizophrenia, 5*(4), 363-371.

Dawson, G., & McKissick, F.C. (1984). Self-recognition in autistic children. *Journal of Autism & Developmental Disorders, 14*, 383-394.

Goodrich, D.W., & Boomer, D.A. (1958). Some concepts about therapeutic intervention with hyperaggressive children. *Social Casework, 39*, 207-213, 286-292.

Heltma, K., & Vogler, E.W. (1985). Effects of an individual contingency program on behaviorally disordered students in physical education. *Adapted Physically Activity Quarterly, 2*, 127-135.

Hughes, H., & Davis, R. (1980). Treatment of aggressive behavior: EMG and biofeedback training. *Journal of Autism & Developmental Disorders, 10*, 193-202.

Jones, V., & Prior, M. (1985). Motor imitation abilities and neurological signs in autistic children. *Journal of Autism & Developmental Disorders, 15*, 37-44.

Kanner, L. (1943). Autistic disturbances of affective contact. *Nervous Child, 2*, 217-250.

Kern, L., Vogel, R.L., & Dunlap, G. (1984). The influence of vigorous versus mild exercise on autistic stereotyped behaviors. *Journal of Autism & Developmental Disorders, 14*, 57-67.

McGee, G.G., Krantz, P.J., & McClannahan, L.E. (1984). Conversational skills for autistic adolescents: Teaching assertiveness in naturalistic game settings. *Journal of Autism & Developmental Disorders, 14*, 319-325.

Meryash, D.L., Szmanski, L.S., & Gerald, P.S. (1982). Infantile autism associated with fragile-X syndrome. *Journal of Autism & Developmental Disorders, 12*, 295-299.

Miller, A., & Miller, E.E. (1973). Cognitive-developmental training with elevated boards and sign language. *Journal of Autism & Childhood Schizophrenia, 3*(1), 65-85.

Paul, J.L., & Epanchin, B.C. (1982). *Emotional disturbance in children.* Columbus, OH: Charles E. Merrill.

Redl, F., & Wineman, D. (1957). *The aggressive child.* New York: Free Press.

Schopler, E. (1986). *Childhood autism rating scale* (CARS). New York: Irvington.

Van Andel, G.E., & Austin, D.R. (1984). Physical fitness and mental health. *Adapted Physical Activity Quarterly, 1*, 207-220.

Van Pelt, M.V., & Kalish, R.A. (1983). Motor proficiency in children with psychosis. *Physical Therapy, 63*, 194-199.

Young, G.J., Kavanagh, M.E., Anderson, G.M., Shaywitz, B.A., & Cohen, D.J. (1982). Clinical neurochemistry of autism and associated disorders. *Journal of Autism & Developmental Disorders, 12*, 147-161.

ADDITIONAL REFERENCES

Campbell, A., Scaturro, J., & Lickson, J. (1983). Peer tutors help autistic students enter mainstream. *Teaching Exceptional Children, 15,* 64-69.

Elio, M.R., & Norman, A. (1981). Toward more success in mainstreaming: A peer-teacher approach to physical education. *Teaching Exceptional Children, 13,* 110-114.

Watters, R.G., & Watters, W.E. (1980). Decreasing self-stimulatory behavior with physical exercise in a group of autistic boys. *Journal of Autism & Developmental Disorders, 10,* 379-387.

QUESTIONS FOR DISCUSSION

1. Describe an emotionally disturbed child. Give an example of an incident in a physical education class that might set off such a child. What might the physical educator do when confronted with the situation you construct?

2. What are the characteristics of autistic children? What are their unique movement characteristics? How might these children be approached when attempting to introduce them to physical activity?

3. How might a game (e.g., kickball) gradually be made more and more socially stressful and complex to accommodate the "stress training" of an emotionally disturbed child?

4. When and how often might relaxation training be given to an emotionally disturbed youngster?

5. What principles can you formulate that might be followed before and during the first class in which an emotionally disturbed child of 10 has been placed with normal youngsters of the same age?

6. What kinds of questions would you ask the consulting psychologist who has done a work-up on an emotionally disturbed boy of 12 before he enters your class in physical education composed of normal youngsters of the same age?

7. What special problems might an emotionally disturbed girl of 15 have on being confronted with a social dance class composed of normal adolescents her age of both sexes?

STUDENT PROJECTS

1. Observe a class having one or more emotionally disturbed children without knowing in advance which ones they are. Attempt to ascertain which children have been diagnosed as emotionally disturbed. What behaviors helped you decide who was emotionally disturbed? Were you correct in your identification of the disturbed youngster(s)?

2. If possible, observe, via one-way mirror, the evaluation of an emotionally disturbed child or youth.

3. Discuss the problems of integrating an emotionally disturbed child within a regular classroom with a teacher who has had to do so. Are the problems similar to those that might be encountered by the physical education teacher? If not, why not?

4. Interview a child psychologist or psychiatrist concerning the types of assessment tools employed when evaluating an emotionally disturbed child for the first time. What questions are asked the child? The parents? What objective and projective tests are given? What kinds of follow-up procedures are employed?

5. Devise a physical education program for a week, with classes meeting each day for 45 minutes, in which activities appropriate for psychotic 10-year-olds are planned.

RESOURCES

American Schizophrenia Foundation
Box 160
Ann Arbor, MI 48107

National Society for Autistic Children
Suite 1017
1234 Massachusetts Ave., N.W.
Washington, DC 20005

10 *Mental Retardation*

The label "mental retardation" often is attached to youngsters after they have failed to complete tasks appropriate for their age on standarized tests of mental functioning. Signs of delayed development in infants encourage some observers to designate them spuriously as mentally retarded also. Other infants, particularly victims of various kinds of genetic disturbances including Down syndrome, have identifiable morphological characteristics at birth indicating that they most likely will perform in subnormal ways on intelligence tests administered several years after birth.

The term *mental retardation* is falling out of favor among some professionals and parent organizations. *Mentally handicapped* is preferred by some. And *developmental disability* and *developmentally delayed* are terms achieving more and more recognition as the word *development* includes the broader context of social and adaptive behaviors along with performance on intelligence tests.

Perhaps no handicapped group has been accorded more attention by physical educators since the late 1960s than the mentally retarded. Following the beginning of the Special Olympics in 1968, the public and those working directly with the retarded, including teachers and parents, have become aware of the physical capabilities of these children and youth, as well as the social and emotional benefits they derive from participating in sports contests and physical education programs.

CLASSIFICATIONS, PREVALENCE, AND CAUSES

The United States government and other entities tend to stratify mentally retarded children and adults—usually on four levels. But many children and youth apparently falling within these neat classifications display traits that in reality result in a rather uneven profile of abilities. For example, children with Down syndrome may show a delay in expressive language but are often better at receptive language (understanding); these same children sometimes display social competencies within normal ranges while remaining deficient in school performance. Differences between social intelligence and school functioning have encouraged the use of the term *6-hour retardation*, describing children who are behind in school subjects yet function reasonably well as family members and playmates.

By far the vast majority of the so-called retarded population of over 6 million in the United States are *mildly retarded*. Almost 90% bear this label. Relatively few are considered to be at the lowest level, the *profoundly retarded*. In between are the levels of *moderately retarded* and *severely retarded*.

Several generalizations may be made about these four levels relative to physical capacities and related function.

1. As one descends the intellectual scale in testing the physical abilities of children: (a) the percentage of children and youth with obvious motor dysfunctions rises; (b) the percentage of children with speech and language deficiencies increases; and (c) the number of specific and separate ability traits decreases.

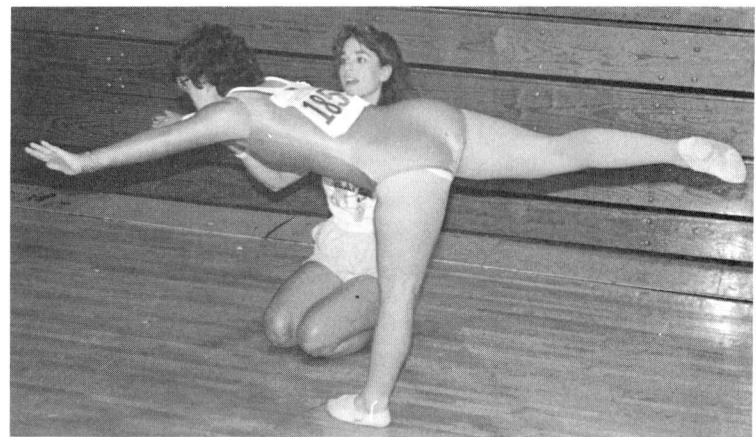

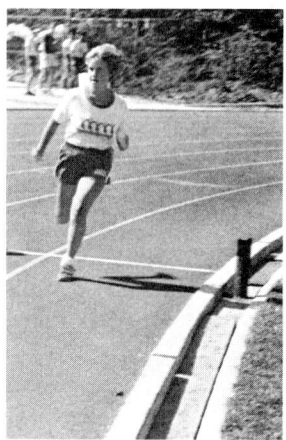

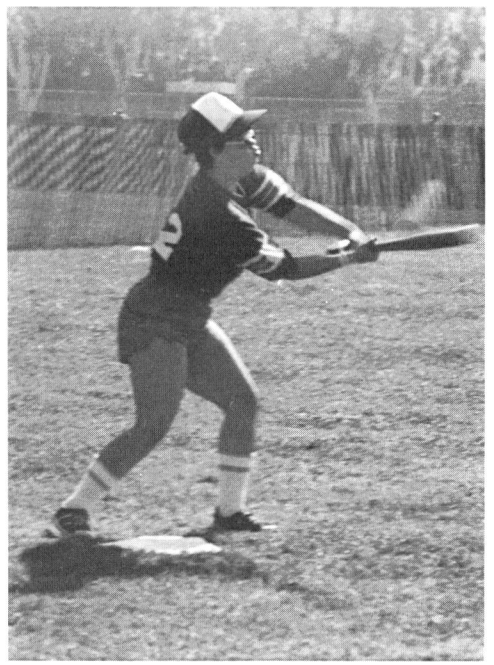

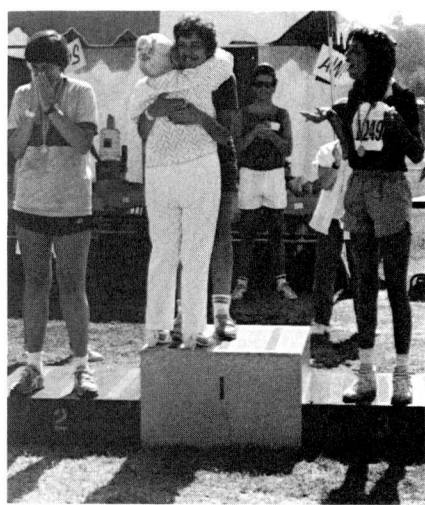

A greatly expanded program of activities is present in the
modern Special Olympics, including gymnastics, running events,
and team sports. All events end with hugs and medals.

Courtesy, California Special Olympics

2. A relatively substantial percentage of mildly retarded children and youth have normal or above-average physical abilities and capacities. Many can compete on interscholastic teams with normal youngsters in a variety of sports.

3. So-called averages of physical abilities computed for children and youth at various levels of intellectual functioning are often less than useful. Compilers of these means usually have failed to differentiate between children with obvious neurological problems reflected in physical awkwardness and children who, although they may be academically retarded, do not show impaired coordination.

4. Averages reflecting physical prowess for various levels of retardation generally suggest that *groups* of retarded youngsters evidence motor abilities comparable to intellectual age. Even general relationships between intellectual age and motor ability, however, are likely to be low when (a) mildly retarded individuals are the subjects, and (b) the motor task scores recorded are relatively simple and direct measures of strength and force rather than complex, sequenced coordination tasks.

5. With careful teaching and prolonged practices, the physical abilities of some mildly and moderately retarded youngsters will approximate or even exceed the skill levels of normal children and youth.

The quality of instruction that can be imparted to a retarded child partly depends on the degree and cause of the retardation. Classification systems used to categorize retarded individuals are of two types: *assessments of adaptive behavior* and *medical classification systems.* Standarized intelligence tests such as the Wechsler Scale and the Stanford-Binet are no longer the sole means whereby a child is classified as retarded. Educators and testing psychologists now look further and deeper into these children's personalities, evaluating social competencies, self-confidence, and ability to maintain themselves independently in society as they mature. From a behavioral standpoint, the following four groups are the usual ones considered.

Classifications Based on Adaptive Behavior

The Mildly Retarded   Generally possessing an IQ of 50 and above, the mildly retarded constitute almost 90% of all retarded children, youth, and adults. During their early years they may show some motor lags and are often late in developing language competencies. They are able to function academically but are about two years behind persons of normal intelligence. They are aware of social expectations. Many become self-sufficient as adults, taking particular care to meet their financial and social obligations in ways often superior to those of normal adults. The mildly retarded at play may become frustrated when confronted with too many rules to learn and assimilate in rapidly changing game situations. Much of the time, however, they are indistinguishable at play from their intellectually average peers. Mildly retarded students can be expected to assimilate academic content up to the sixth-grade level.

The Moderately Retarded   Moderately retarded children require special help as soon as their condition is suspected. The most noticeable early symptom is a delay in language development. This is sometimes, but not always, accompanied by a delay in the acquisition of motor competencies during the early years of life.

By late childhood many moderately retarded youngsters can learn rudimentary reading (at the first- and second-grade level), counting, and making change. They are usually delayed in the onset of language and speech and have speech difficulties. The prognosis for job placement in early adulthood is most often a sheltered workshop situation; moderately retarded persons need supervision and guidance in managing personal affairs and under conditions of stress.

The Severely Retarded   Because these children show delayed motor development, an initial goal is to achieve locomotion in early childhood. Speech is minimal or absent; therefore, other types of communication, such as signing, may be helpful. Basic self-care skills, such as washing and toileting, require extended practice and sequential development, often with the help of behavior modification techniques. After learning some self-care skills such as eating and dressing, children are able to be maintained with decreasing supervision. Training and education consists to a large degree of sensory and sensory-motor activities in efforts to increase the children's general alertness to the environment. About a quarter of a million persons in the United States are within this category.

The Profoundly Retarded   The profoundly retarded usually lack locomotion and always lack speech. They respond to stimulation if exposed to sensory-motor training and need a one-to-one ratio of teacher to learner when attempting to achieve even slight gains. In adulthood the lack of mobility results in constriction of joints and muscular contractures unless these are counteracted by physical therapy services. Some may respond in minimal ways to training in self-care skills. Some 90,000 individuals in the United States are profoundly retarded.

Medical Classifications

Nine medical classifications of retardation account for only about 10% of the retarded population in the United States. The remaining 90% is placed in the tenth category—retardation caused by "other conditions and environmental influences." This category is composed of children and youth for whom there is no evidence of a physical cause, structural defect, or evidence of familial subnormal functioning or of psychosocial causes that may contribute to retardation.

The first nine medical classifications, based on cause, are:

1. *Environmental influences.* Mental defects are caused by severe environmental trauma, including neglect, sensory deprivation (e.g., closeting the child), and other forms of emotional deprivation.

2. *Chromosomal abnormalities.* A number of genetically related conditions have been identified, of which the most common is Down syndrome (to be discussed later).

3. *Unknown prenatal influences.* These include malformations of the brain, including the absence of a portion of the brain (anencephaly), microcephaly (a small head), spina bifida and other disorders involving faulty closure of the neural tube, as well as rare syndromes (Cornelia de Lange's syndrome, Apert's syndrome, Laurence-Moon-Biedl syndrome, etc.).

4. *Problems involving metabolism or nutrition.* Various metabolic, endocrine, or growth dysfunctions, such as phenylketonuria (PKU), hypothyroidism (cretinism), and galactosemia fall in this category.

5. *Rare postnatal diseases of the brain.* One of these conditions, von Recklinghausen's disease, is characterized by tan spots on the skin (café-au-lait spots), also termed neurofibromatosis. Other conditions include Sturge-Weber-Dimitri disease, one of whose symptoms is port-wine stains on the face and scalp, and tuberous sclerosis, a condition characterized by nodules throughout the central nervous system and tumors on various organs.

6. *Postpsychiatric disorders.* This category refers to retardation following psychiatric disturbances, with no obvious organic base.

7. *Gestational disorders.* Retardation stems from perinatal problems, including low birth weight, premature birth, or postmature birth.

8. *Trauma or retardation caused by physical agents.* Injuries to the brain before, during, or after birth include the battered-child syndrome and injury caused by insufficient oxygen as the result of shock, poisoning, convulsions, or severe anemia.

9. *Infections and intoxication.* Retardation may be caused by prenatal and maternal infectious conditions such as rubella (German measles) and syphilis.

The causes of about 90% of the retardation in children and youth are unknown. Moreover, only a relative small percentage of the retarded have any overt physical or facial anomalies that mark them as retarded. The vast majority of retarded people not only resemble normal people but also, if given the opportunity to progress at a reasonable pace, sometimes acquire physical attributes approximating those of normal children and youth. Children and youth at the lower levels—moderately, severely, and profoundly retarded—need special help to attain a variety of sensory and sensory-motor abilities.

CHARACTERISTICS

The Mildly Retarded

Mildly retarded children are the ones most often found in regular physical education classes and are most likely to be mainstreamed now and in the years ahead. Their primary characteristic in the physical education setting is that they may not quickly comprehend directions from a teacher or their peers when exposed to complicated game situations or skills to be acquired.

Many, if not most, are socially competent and, if not made to feel inferior, will strive hard to keep up with and at times surpass the intellectually more able in physical education classes. They are more likely to excel in activities that require simple efforts reflecting strength or endurance (e.g., distance running) than they are at intricate team sports. Even when exposed to team sports, however, they will make a valuable contribution to the team and in the process expand their self-concept and feelings of personal worth if given enough practice.

In one extensive study by Rarick and his colleagues, involving the testing of 4,000 mildly retarded students (Rarick, Dobbins, & Broadhead, 1976):

1. The averages of the mildly retarded were inferior 85% of the time to the scores achieved by normal students. In the 300-yard run, for example, the former posted scores 4 yards behind those posted by the latter. Similar inferiority was seen in scores obtained from the broad jump, softball throw, and 50-yard dash.

2. Sex differences similar to those seen in studies of normal children were found in the data on retarded children.

3. Age trends were similar in the normal and retarded populations. For example, the retarded girls' scores plateaued in the 50-yard dash at about age 12, as is true in normal girls.

This study, as well as others, does not clarify whether inferiority in the scores is attributable to the failure to place retarded children in vigorous physical education programs (or when in such programs, their feelings of reluctance and inferiority, which prevent them from participating fully) or the presence of children with minimal to moderate neurological impairment, which tends to depress mean scores of large groups. And many neurologically intact but intellectually inferior children and youth may be in the groups as well.

For example, Maloney and Ward (1970) found significant differences in the perceptual-motor performance of retarded children diagnosed as having "organicity" versus those whose retardation was "functional" (social-environmental) in nature. Until norms for the mildly and moderately retarded reflect attention to these differences in various subpopulations, the average scores attained are not very useful when planning programs.

Most studies indicate that retarded children and youth react more slowly to stimuli than do normal children and that reaction time tends to increase when the task to be performed or the stimulus to be reacted to is made more complex. These findings hold important implications for teaching skills to the mildly retarded, relative to pacing the presentation of verbal and visual demonstrations and material. The rapidity with which information is presented must be compatible with their ability to assimilate, process, and act on the information. The channel capacities of mildly retarded youngsters can be easily overloaded, particularly when they are exposed to potentially stressful and competitive physical education activities.

In a detailed task analysis of mildly retarded youngsters and adolescents (Cratty, 1967), I found that:

1. Not until after age 12 could mildly retarded students correctly (better than by chance) locate their left and right body parts (arms, hands, etc.).

2. Not until after age 13 could the mildly retarded accurately hop and jump in a series of six $1' \times 1'$ squares.

3. Catching a ball (8″ diameter) bounced to them was difficult for the majority until late childhood.

4. Few could posture on one foot with eyes closed from 4 to 6 seconds.

5. Jumping backward with any accuracy was impossible for all except 10% of the children and youth tested.

The Moderately Retarded

Moderately retarded children and youth are significantly inferior to mildly retarded youngsters in measures of balance and coordination, as well as fitness (Cratty, 1967; Hayden,

1966). The sub-scores most predictive of average scores attained in a six-item motor ability test battery were reflected in verbal responses to a body image test (Cratty, 1967). Subsequent analyses found that this sub-test is primarily an assessment of children's verbal-cognitive abilities rather than that of a motor ability trait. Thus, when purportedly evaluating the motor abilities of the moderately retarded, it is difficult to ascertain the extent to which comprehension of the verbal instructions or the visual demonstration has influenced the scores achieved and, thus, whether the final outcomes are valid indices of motor abilities.

Down Syndrome Within populations of moderately retarded youngsters, a highly recognizable type of retarded child is the youngster with Down syndrome. This syndrome originally was identified in 1886 by Langdon Down, a London physician, whose clinical description has endured almost intact over the years. His explanation that the condition probably had its roots in some kind of emergent genes from the Mongol race (hence the formerly used term "mongolism") was wrong, though.

By the first half of this century, over 40 explanations had been set forth as the source or cause of Down syndrome. Work by Lejune, Gauthier, and Turpin (1959) involving the analysis of cells from tissues collected from nine "mongoloid" children was a breakthrough in that it indicated that the cells contained 47 rather than 46 chromosomes.

The most common type of Down syndrome is *trisomy 21* constituting about 96% of Down syndrome individuals. During meiosis (chromosome dysjunction) a chromosomal pair (the 21st) fails to separate, resulting in 24 instead of 23 chromosomes. The fertilization of this cell, which has three #21 chromosomes instead of only a pair, with a normal gamete, results in a zygote with 47 rather than 46 chromosomes (Scarbrough, 1982). The overall incidence of trisomy 21 is about 1 per 800 live births. The risk of having a trisomy 21 child increases in mothers from age 35 (1 in 365 live births) to mothers of 45 (1 in 32 live births) (Kovar, 1981).

In 1966 a girl who had 46 chromosomes and apparently was a Down syndrome child was discovered. This *translocation type* (typical of only about 4% of all Down syndrome cases) occurs when an extra 21st chromosome is transferred to the 15th chromosome. The total count is 46 instead of 47, but extra material is present. In general, this type may have higher intelligence than trisomics, and the condition may be inherited. I am unaware of any studies indicating motor ability differences between the translocation and trisomy types.

A third, rare type of Down syndrome is *mosaicism*. It also occurs from nondysjunction during meiotic division of early embryonic cells. The child's body contains both normal and abnormal cells, and the appearance (phenotype) varies from characteristics that obviously are identified with Down syndrome to almost normal appearance.

According to Hook (1981), the rate of Down syndrome has dropped recently. The reasons postulated include the decline of older child-bearing mothers and the increased use of birth control. Further hope for correcting or preventing the condition may come from the laboratories of genetic engineers (Smith, 1985). Some have predicted that the complete linkage of chromosome 21 will soon be achieved.

The majority of children with Down syndrome possess characteristics, both internal and external, that set them apart from other retarded children. Differences in their internal functioning, including abnormalities in cardiovascular and endocrine functions and visual abilities, as well as other physiological and neurological processes, mark them as "unfin-

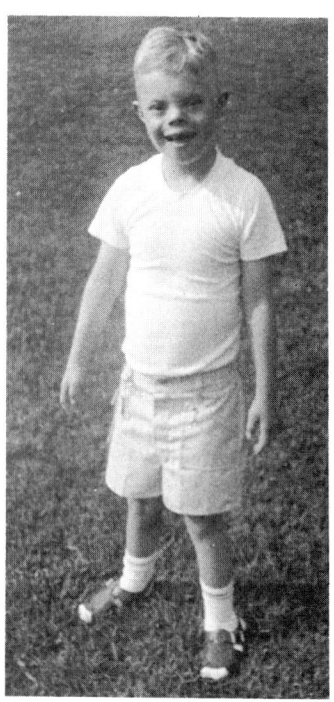

This Down syndrome boy has the characteristic features, but to a lesser extent than some.

ished children." Most of their organs and many of their larger, more observable structures never fully mature.

In trisomy 21 the characteristic signs include short, broad hands with atypical fingerprints; almond-shaped, slanting eyes; flat bridge of the nose; and a protruding tongue. The latter leads to dryness of the tongue and mouth, which often results in a parched, split appearance of the tongue. The hair is straight and coarse. The skin is often dry. The child walks with a wide gait. In fact, walking seems to create balance problems most of their life. The teeth usually are maloccluded; dentition is immature; and dental caries (cavities) are excessive.

The joints seem loose, and the children sometimes seem to "fold in half," touching their knees with their chin while in a seated position. Muscle tone is poor, which has led to the term "floppy children." All tests of muscle tone and of the vigor of various reflexes in Down syndrome youngsters attest to the presence of hypotonicity (Morris, Vaughn, & Vaccaro, 1982). This reduced muscle tone is accompanied by slow reaction time and poor kinesthetic awareness. Weight also has been problematic, although this is better controlled now than in the past, through diet and reasonably vigorous exercises.

A serious physical disorder known as *atlantoaxial instability* involves greater than normal mobility of the upper two cervical vertebrae at the top of the neck, so an afflicted child may squeeze or even sever the spinal cord if the neck is vigorously or forcibly flexed. Symptoms of this disorder are deterioration in walking, changes in bowel or bladder control, weakness in the body extremities, and limited range of motion in the neck (Cooke,

1984). For this reason, undue pressure on the neck region (as might be experienced in a tumbling program) should be avoided.

Internally, various organ systems do not function well. The frontal lobes of the brain are usually not completely myelinated. Because the optic nerve has not developed normally, whatever visual input these children receive may be distorted, contributing to their obvious balance problems and difficulties in locating balls rolled to them. Congenital heart disorders (commonly a leakage in the septum) are prevalent. The aorta and other arteries within the circulatory system may remain small and narrow, and the children are often diagnosed as having a systolic heart murmur. Thus, the exercise load placed on these children should be carefully monitored and reduced whenever the children show symptoms such as breathlessness or blue lips. Because of the deficient immune system, Down syndrome youngsters tend to have a vast number of respiratory and other infections and diseases. Recent experiments with dietary supplements (i.e., zinc), however, have shown that the immune system can be improved.

Research on Early Stimulation   Although Down syndrome youngsters are said to be more deficient in motor skills than in cognitive skills (Harris, 1981), extreme language delays occur in the Down syndrome population. It has been estimated that these youngsters require about twice as much time (46 months) to form a correct three-word sentence as the normally expected sentence formation time (24 months). Research cited by Barnard (1975) indicates that early stimulation, in the form of linguistic interactions from the mother and

When their weight is held in check, children with Down syndrome sometimes show surprising physical skill.

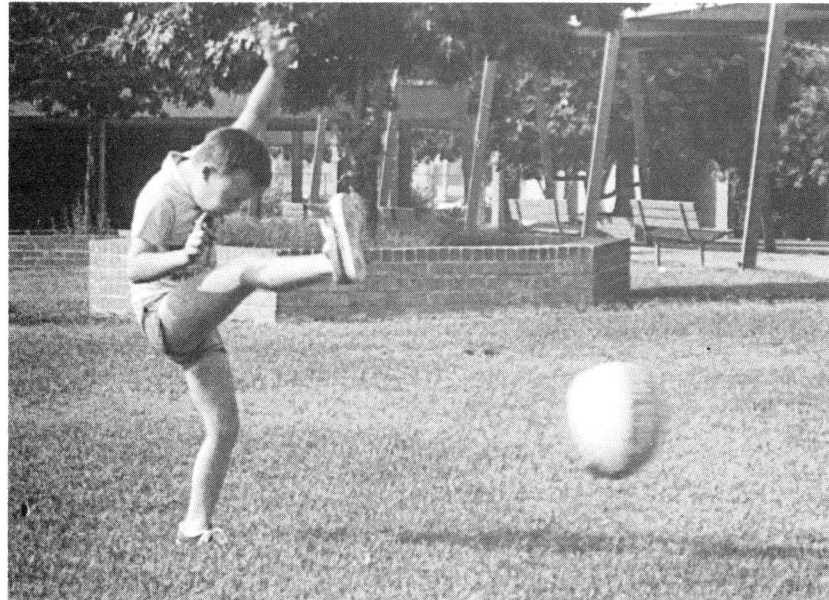

Courtesy, Fontana, California Public Schools

of passive exercises, exerts positive influences on both verbal and motor abilities, as reflected in measures obtained on the Bayley Scales of Infant Development (Bayley, 1984) and the Gesell Infant Scale (Gesell & Amatruda, 1947). Most important, these studies of the early stimulation of Down syndrome infants indicate that this kind of enrichment during the first 4 to 6 months of life is critical in eliciting improvement. Early motor manipulation does not seem to accelerate the development of normal infants, but early stimulation of premature, neurologically impaired, and Down syndrome neonates seems critical during the first days and weeks of life. Stimulation of this kind often offsets the drop in development that occurs in many Down syndrome infants at about the 8th month. Chapter 25 is devoted to a thorough discussion of infant stimulation techniques, with a brief introduction here.

In the 1980s early stimulation programs have been applied to Down infants with positive results (Harris, 1981). One program, called "developmental coaching" (Esenther, 1984), involves the parents helping to stimulate tasks in five areas (gross-motor, fine-motor, daily living skills, socialization, and language). This program resulted in positive changes in the onset of locomotion. The Read Project (Piper, 1980) is another recent program aimed at early stimulation and improvement of Down sydrome youngsters (Esenther, 1984; Piper, 1980).

Connolly, Morgan, Russell, and Richardson (1980) have reported that Down syndrome children from birth to age 5 who were stimulated evidenced improvement in scores reflecting intellectual, motor, and social growth. A recently published longitudinal study in Australia found that 39 Down syndrome children ranging from birth to 5 years of age evidenced increased intellectual status. The researchers attributed this trend to the presence of more and more programs aimed at early stimulation of this population (Berry, Gunn, & Andrews, 1984).

As Down syndrome children are more and more exposed to social-vocal interactions with normal children via mainstreaming efforts, their development should continue to improve. Language usage, for example, is likely to be greater when they are exposed to children who are normally endowed with linguistic abilities (Knox, 1983). Increased parent education also is likely to result in improved attention spans and social interactions on the part of these children (McInerney, McLaughlin, & Truhlicka, 1982).

The Severely and Profoundly Retarded

Severely and profoundly retarded children and youth pose special problems for those wishing to improve their functions. Changes, if forthcoming, often are slight, but even minimal improvements in self-care skills (self-feeding, toileting, and the like) produce marked differences in the number of custodial personnel (and thus monies) needed to maintain them.

The categories labeled severely and profoundly retarded are often vague and ill-defined. Thus, studies carried out with these lower two levels of retarded people are difficult to interpret (Switzky, Haywood, & Rotatori, 1982).

In any case, a primary effort usually is directed at eliciting locomotion. Locomotion is acquired in gradual stages, similar to the sequence of normal children (see chapter 28), with the help of patient educators, therapists, physical educators, and volunteers. After becoming mobile, these children, like all toddlers, have little judgment concerning their comings and goings. They are either extremely explosive in their jaunts or need to be prodded out of lethargy to maintain locomotor behaviors. The first steps resemble the first steps of any child. They are awkward, with feet wide apart, and often are terminated by stiff-legged sits, unaccompanied by appropriate parachute reactions (knee-bend, with hands reaching out to catch their fall).

In work with the severely and profoundly retarded, several principles seem worth considering:

1. There is no substitute in one's educational armament for a thorough and detailed knowledge of normal child development—particularly the sensory and sensory-motor stages seen in the normal child from birth to the 2nd or 3rd year, because severely and profoundly retarded children function like children of this age. Their developmental quotients may drop below 20, so a child of 10 or 12 may be functioning like an infant less than 2 years of age.

2. First goals may be simply to elicit reactions to various kinds of sensory stimulation. Thus, educators should be equipped to engage in tactile, auditory, visual, and temperature (heat-cold) stimulation to elicit simple responses.

3. The educator should gain a thorough knowledge of behavior modification techniques. The most profoundly retarded children might not be able to associate reward with behavioral change, but they may gain self-care skills if the skills are carefully reinforced and presented to them in sequenced sub-stages. The act of putting on a shirt, for example, may be divided into 10 to 20 sub-stages, ranging from simply looking at the shirt and then touching it to the completed act of getting the shirt over the head and both arms through the proper holes. Toilet training likewise may be divided into sub-stages (at one conference the number of sub-stages was set at 76!).

4. Profoundly and severely retarded children and youth are generally at the extremes of hypotonicity or hypertonicity. Either they are virtually rigid and must be given a great deal of help to relieve spasticity and contractures that prevent movement, or they are so hypotonic and floppy that they cannot even support the trunk in ways that permit them to engage in manipulative or locomotor activities. The hypotonic child must be given a program of assisted movements simulating simple, voluntary movements seen in babies. The hypertonic, spastic-type child must be exposed to heat hydrotherapy in addition to general stretching, to create *some* range of motion necessary for the child to begin to move in minimal ways.

5. When locomotion and simple manipulative activities have been mastered, carefully designed sequences of activities may combine the two. These can include simply holding an object for increased periods of time during locomotion, to later picking up an object, carrying it to another point, and releasing it into a box. The several stages and sub-stages of these complex hand-eye-locomotor behaviors must be carefully introduced, reinforced, and molded by patient educators—a process that may last from months to several years.

6. Reluctant administrators might be convinced of the worth of sensory-motor training—a necessary precursor to self-care skills—if the therapist or special educator carefully ascertains how much of the budget will be saved if, for example, children learn to feed themselves, as contrasted to the costs of sensory-motor therapy necessary to achieve this type of skill. Toilet training also can be shown to represent not only a humanitarian step forward but an economic saving as well.

7. Lower functioning children work best when they are emotionally satisfied and soothed.

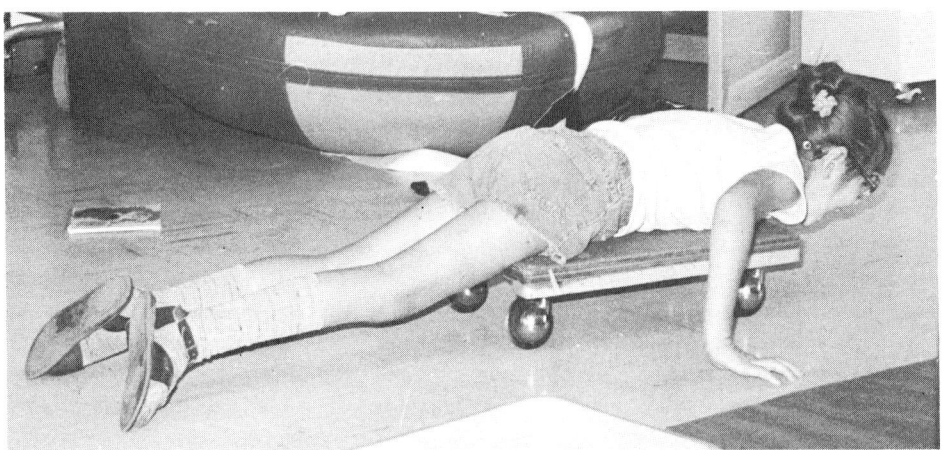

A scooterboard can help severely handicapped children easily change position in space.

Courtesy, Fontana, California Public Schools

Accompanying sensory-motor training with music, in an environment painted in soft colors and softly lighted, can optimize therapeutic efforts.

8. Profoundly and severely retarded children must be placed in situations that require their attention, some adjustment by them, and movement of some kind. Exposing them to a "crowded box" filled with other children against whom they might move is one helpful experience. Placing them in a situation that requires them to act (e.g., to move a box to get food or to enter a tunnel while not being permitted to move backward on an obstacle course, or to mount stairs—perhaps with assistance—with no other alternatives available) is a forced therapeutic strategy.

9. Any activity that requires increasing periods of attention is likely to be helpful and to transfer to other situations that require attention. Walking a line or a wide balance beam for increased periods of time or rolling a ball "just one more time" are examples of useful, easily modified activities.

10. Attempts to improve cardiovascular functions among profoundly retarded clients have met with success (Mulholland & McNeill, 1985). The activities used in this study consisted of simple assisted rolling, lying on and bouncing with assistance on the trampoline, and other assisted exercises.

Therapeutic Strategies   Strategies useful for the profoundly and severely retarded generally emphasize some kind of sensory stimulation. Attempts are made to make individuals more responsive and movement-responsive. At first children are assisted by the therapist or physical educator. Types of sensory stimulation are:

1. *Visual stimulation:* Moving a light placed over the youngster's eyes while the child is in a supine position. The bright light hopefully will attract the attention of the child or youth and visual following responses will begin to occur for increased periods of time.

2. *Auditory stimulation:* Making a noise (clapping two blocks of wood together) to the side of the supine youngster in the hope that it will attract attention and that the child's head will turn toward the direction of the sound. At first, the therapist may move the head manually at the time of the sound. Later, when prehension is acquired, the child may be shown how to make sounds by banging blocks against the floor.

3. *Heat-cold.* Placing two pans of water, one with cold water, the other with water slightly warmer than warm, by the seated child. Alternately, the child's hands are placed in each pan in an attempt to make the child feel the temperatures, the changes and differences, and to elicit some reaction.

4. *Tactile stimulation:* Stroking the back or other body parts in an effort to (a) calm the agitated child before engaging in other therapy, or to (b) help the child become aware of body parts and surfaces of the trunk of which he or she may be unaware. Tactile stroking may be accompanied, or immediately followed, by assistive movements of the limbs or body parts stroked. Verbal input is helpful at this time: "There we are, rubbing your arm. . . . Now we are moving your arm. . . . Look at it move."

5. *Olfactory stimulation:* Having the child smell extreme odors—spices, ammonia, and so on—in efforts to elicit avoidance or responses indicating pleasure. Perfumes can be paired with aversive smells, for example.

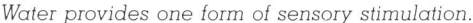

Water provides one form of sensory stimulation.

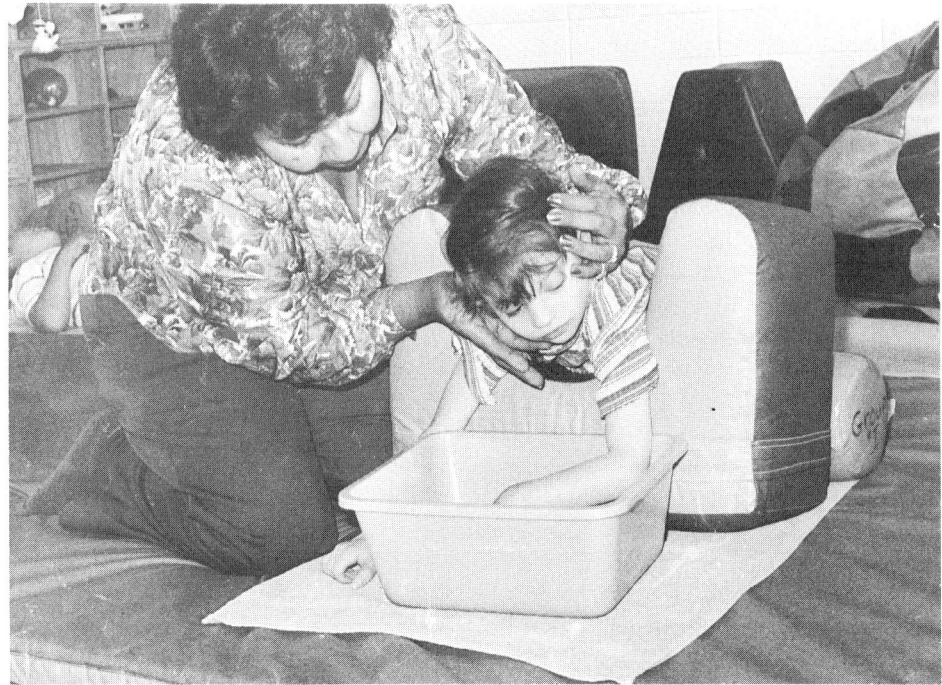

Courtesy, Fontana, California Public Schools

6. *Taste.* Touching bits of stimulating substances (alum, salt, sweets, and the like) to the child's tongue in an effort to elicit either pleasurable or avoidance reactions. This type of stimulation may be successfully worked into a reinforcement schedule when the child clearly recognizes and seeks a given type of taste (e.g., sugar).

7. *Kinesthetic stimulation.* Molding movements of various kinds to trigger patterns that will eventually lead toward at least rudimentary voluntary movements. For example, the child's head may be turned while in a supine position, and then the child's hips aided to follow the head in a roll-over from the back to the front. Assisted sit-ups may be attempted, in which the child is pulled gently by the hands from a supine to a seated position in an effort to get the head to accompany the body's sit-up action and, finally, to get the head to anticipate the pull to a seated position.

Innumerable complex movements may be sought using assisted movements together with various kinds of sensory stimulation. For example:

- With the child in a prone position, place the arms so that they support the child (elbows straight), and then move a visual stimulus across the child's field of vision. As the child's head turns to watch (or is turned by the therapist), help the child's body turn over (by assistance at the hips) to a supine position (on the back).
- Elicit reaching behavior by making objects more vivid—making noises with them, using shiny objects, and so on—in an effort to have the child reach for things with more frequency while in a supported prone position or a supported seated position; or when the child is on all fours, to encourage the first crawling reactions.
- When the child is ready, encourage the first standing reactions by showing stimuli just out of reach overhead. Objects should be attractive, noisy, shiny, or even pleasant to taste (if the child has previously associated the object (e.g., a sugar cube) with a pleasant taste.
- Reduce unwanted reflex positions via tactile and verbal stimulation. For example, in helping a child roll over, the asymmetrical and impeding tonic neck reflex may be reduced by rubbing the arm, which automatically extends when the head is turned toward it (thus impeding the rolling action), and then gently bending it at the elbow and placing it at the child's side so that a rolling movement may be made in the direction toward which the head is turned without the extended arm braking the movement.

These suggestions are just a few examples of many strategies that may be employed. They are based on sound principles of behavior modification, awareness of the nature of normal perceptual and motor development, and knowledge of the way in which infant reflexes can impede or facilitate the onset of rudimentary voluntary movements. Examples of movement strategies are given in chapter 25.

When working with profoundly and severely retarded youngsters, thorough evaluative methods are important for two primary reasons: (a) knowledge of progress is imperative in planning future strategies; and (b) the mental health of therapists, physical educators, and others working with "slow-to-improve" individuals is greatly enhanced if *some* evidence of improvement is forthcoming on a regular basis.

Testing severely and profoundly retarded adults is difficult. Often, special preparations must be made—familiarizing them with the testers and test situation in order to obtain valid information. One attempt to achieve this has been to use partners, with the more able guiding the less able through a testing situation. This type of modeling was moderately successful, but even these efforts did not prepare all the clients for testing (Tomporowsky & Ellis, 1984).

Because the developmental patterns of the severely and profoundly retarded are generally those of early childhood, a number of scales intended for use with normal infants are helpful. These include the Bayley scale (Bayley, 1984), as well as the Gesell scale (Gesell & Amatruda, 1947). Also used are scales specifically formulated for these youngsters, including the Adapted Behavior Scales (Nihara, Foster, Shellhaas, & Leland, 1969), as well as the Webb (1969) index (evaluating awareness, manipulation, and posture). Some portions of the Vineland Social Maturity Scale (Doll, 1985) are useful when working with these children. A classification system by Hasazi, Streifel, and Edgar (1971) presents eight levels at which the social competencies of severely retarded children and youth may be classified via observational ratings: autistic behavior, unoccupied behavior, independent play, observational behavior, attempted interaction, parallel play, associative play, and co-operative play. This classification system is useful when evaluating general alertness and social levels of the severely and profoundly retarded, as well as moderately retarded individuals in early and middle childhood.

PKU One condition commonly associated with the severely retarded is phenylketonuria (PKU). This and many other genetic and metabolic disorders can be accompanied by retardation. PKU is caused by a build-up of phenolic compounds that leads to brain damage in infants and young children. Although PKU is a lifetime condition, almost all of the damage is done during the first few years of life (Lyman, 1963).

PKU was discovered in the 1930s by a Norwegian doctor, Asbjorn Folling. In addition to reduced intellectual development, PKU children may be violent and destructive and have unpredictable rages. Seizures are common, as are serious motor impairments including extremes of either hypotonus or hypertonus. The presence of phenylacetic acid may give the child a musty or "mousy" odor.

Although the effects of PKU cannot be reversed, some improvement can be seen if the condition is treated before the end of brain growth. Detection of PKU is inexpensive; the most widely used test is carried out by adding ferric chloride to a urine sample. Further, the amount of phenylalanine in the body can be reduced through a special diet containing amino acids. The diet often can be stopped after the brain growth years, when its discontinuance does not result in noticeable drops in intelligence or changes in temperament. Almost all states in the U.S., as well as many foreign countries, now test for PKU. Success in preventing the unwanted effects of PKU depend on its early detection (Seakins, Saunders, & Toothill, 1973; Winick, 1979).

EVALUATION INSTRUMENTS FOR PHYSICAL ABILITY TESTING

A number of observational rating forms and physical ability test batteries have been specifically designed for use with retarded populations. As has been pointed out, individual scores, when contrasted to the available norms, should be interpreted with discretion because of the variations within retarded populations relative to inherent motor capacities.

The AAHPER-Kennedy Foundation Fitness Test is among the most widely used of these instruments. Norms on this test have been established on moderately retarded children and youth ages 8-18. Achievement of prescribed standards for both sexes, by age, results in awards (American Association for Health, Physical Education and Recreation, 1971).

The Fait (1972) Physical Fitness Battery consists of six items, evaluating cardiorespiratory endurance, static muscular endurance of the arm and shoulder girdle, static balance, dynamic endurance of the leg flexors and abdominals, agility, and sprinting ability. Averages are established for boys and girls in three age groups: 9-13, 13-16, and 17-20. Criteria for low, average, and high are reflected in the scoring table.

Various versions of the Oseretsky Tests of Motor Proficiency have been employed to evaluate the retarded, including racial comparisons carried out by Alley and Snider (1970) with mildly retarded children ages 7-12. Kershner and Dusewicz (1970) developed a modification of the Oseretsky , also for use with retarded children, in which they advanced techniques for group administration.

The shortened Purdue Perceptual-Motor Survey has been employed by Neeman and Phillips (1970) and others to screen mildly and moderately retarded children and youth. Both the Minnesota Rate of Manipulation Test and the Purdue Pegboard Test have been used by Hirsch (1965) and others to evaluate the manual abilities of retarded populations.

Drawing tests used with retarded children include the hand-eye portion of the Frostig (Frostig, Maslow, Lefever, & Whittlesey, 1964), as well as the Bender-Gestalt (Bender, 1938). Maloney and Ward (1970), for example, purportedly were able to differentiate between what they termed "functional" and "organic" retarded individuals using this instrument. Reaction time and movement speed tests are plentiful—and many of these have been employed with retarded populations. A review is found in the chapter by Malpass (1963) in Ellis's *Handbook on Mental Deficiency*.

A number of self-concept scales may be applied to retarded populations. One of these (Gallagher, 1959) is an observational rating scale useful for classifying the self-concept or emotional development of both mildly and moderately retarded children and youth. Children are rated on eight dimensions: isolation, dependency, omnipotence, adult imitation, adult identification, peer imitation, peer identification, and self-determination.

STRATEGIES AND TRENDS WITH THE RETARDED

When working with the retarded, feedback from the teacher should be positively attuned to the possibility that with effort they can improve. Often, feedback has consisted of statements indicating that retarded children possess poor basic abilities and are not likely to change, even by working hard (Raber & Weisz, 1981). The physical education teacher should emphasize the positive role of effort through statements such as "If you try harder, you will get it."

Often, even mothers of the retarded react differently in social and vocal ways to their handicapped offspring. They tend to dominate or overprotect the retarded child; as a consequence the child is less likely to initiate social interactions with other children. Physical education teachers, too, should be supportive and encouraging rather than dominating in interactions with retarded youngsters.

Motor learning studies and research have become more focused upon skill acquisition. For example, transfer between tasks has been found to be more likely if the variations of an initial task have been practiced. A specific skill in ball throwing is more likely to improve if the child has been exposed to a variety of ball throwing tasks rather than to a single specific one (Portella, 1982).

Also, increased emphasis is being placed upon the cognitive aspects of motor learning and training retarded children to carefully plan how to do a motor task before executing it. In this way, improvement in planning behaviors will likely transfer to the performance of other tasks, including those that are more perceptual and academic than motor (Hoover & Wade, 1985). Moreover, the precise use of reinforcers, including social reinforcement, has been studied as influencing basic actions of the severely and profoundly retarded. One case study indicated that basic walking behavior may be positively influenced with well applied social reinforcement (Hester, 1981).

Obesity frequently is found among the mentally retarded. Kelly, Rimmer, and Ness (1985), for example, found that approximately 50% of the retarded they evaluated were markedly obese. The increased incidence of illness and death among retarded adults may be partially attributable to obesity (Larson, Bjorntorp, & Tibblin, 1981). Parental training about correct nutrition may be needed before positive results will take place (Jackson & Thornbecke, 1982). Exercise, combined with nutritional advice and control, is helpful in weight reduction (Beasley, 1982). Obesity is covered in more detail in chapter 17.

Jogging programs with retarded adults have produced positive outcomes (Beasley, 1982). Improvement may be expected not only in cardiovascular efficiency but also in measures of self-confidence and self-control. And Edmondson and Han (1983) described the positive effects of "socialization games" on the aggressive behaviors of mentally retarded women.

SUMMARY

Retarded individuals are classified according to severity levels—mildly retarded, moderately retarded, severely retarded, or profoundly retarded. This placement, however, is not necessarily a precise reflection of a variety of social, intellectual, emotional, and physical qualities.

In descending this classification scale, the incidence of individuals with obvious motor problems increases. Mildly retarded children or youth may or may not evidence some kind of motor ineptitude, but severely and profoundly retarded youngsters usually cannot adequately engage in self-care skills. They exhibit marked difficulties in managing the larger muscle groups and have obvious problems with locomotion.

Formulating valid norms on physical attributes for retarded youngsters is a difficult undertaking because of wide individual differences and the presence in some retarded populations of neurological impairment as part of the syndrome. Among the moderately retarded are children exhibiting Down syndrome, a constellation of symptoms including perceptual and motor difficulties more marked than those of other moderately retarded populations.

When evaluating the motor abilities of the retarded and when formulating program content for their improvement, a number of factors should be kept in mind:

1. What level of "testability" do the youngsters exhibit?

2. What degree of social control and emotional stability is possessed by individuals and groups of retarded youngsters for whom one wishes to develop programs?

3. What percentage of a mildly retarded population can participate in regular physical education with only slight, or no, special modifications? What percentage needs special help in skill development?

4. What tools are available to measure the often slight changes in groups of profoundly and severely retarded when exposed to sensory-motor and sensory education?

5. How can conditions, facilities, and equipment be arranged to ensure optimum attention and participation by often distractible youngsters within a physical education or physical development program?

REFERENCES

Alley, G.R., & Snider, B. (1970). Comparative perceptual-motor performance of Negro and white young mental retardates. *Developmental Psychology, 2,* 110-114.

American Association for Health, Physical Education and Recreation (1971). *The best of challenge* (Vol. 1). Washington, DC: AAHPER.

Barnard, K.E. (1975). Infant stimulation. In R. Koch & F. de la Cruz (Eds.), *Down syndrome (Mongolism): Research, prevention and management.* New York: Brunner-Mazel.

Bayley, N. (1984). *Bayley scales of infant development.* New York: Psychological Corp.

Beasley, C.R. (1982). Effects of jogging program on cardiovascular fitness and work performance of mentally retarded adults. *American Journal of Mental Deficiency, 86,* 607-612.

Bender, L. (1938). *A visual motor Gestalt test and its clinical use.* New York: American Orthopsychiatric Association.

Berry, P., Gunn, V.P., & Andrews, R.J. (1984). Development of Down syndrome children from birth to five years. *Perspectives & Progress in Mental Retardation, 1,* 167-177.

Connolly, B., Morgan, S., Russell, F.F., & Richardson, B. (1980). Early intervention with Down's syndrome. *Physical Therapy, 60,* 1405-1408.

Cooke, R. (1984). Atlantoaxial instability in individuals with Down's syndrome. *Mental Retardation, 22,* 193-194.

Cratty, B.J. (1967). *The perceptual-motor attributes of mentally retarded children and youth.* Unpublished monograph, County Mental Retardation Services Board, Los Angeles.

Doll, E.A. (1985). *Vineland social maturity scale.* Circle Pines, MN: American Guidance Service.

Edmondson, B., & Han, S.S. (1983). Effects of socialization games on proximity and prosocial behavior of aggressive mentally retarded institutionalized women. *American Journal of Mental Deficiency, 87,* 435-440.

Esenther, S.E. (1984). Developmental coaching of the Down's syndrome infant. *American Journal of Occupational Therapy, 38,* 440-445.

Fait, H. (1972). *Special physical education.* Philadelphia: W.B. Saunders.

Frostig, M., Maslow, P., Lefever, D.W., & Whittlesey, J.R. (1964). *Marianne Frostig Developmental Test of Visual Perception.* Palo Alto, CA: Consulting Psychologists Press.

Gallagher, J.J. (1959). Measurement of personality development in pre-adolescent mentally retarded children. *American Journal of Mental Deficiency, 64,* 296-384.

Gesell, A., & Amatruda, K. (1947). *Developmental diagnosis.* New York: Harper & Row.

Harris, S.R. (1981). Physical therapy and infants with Down's syndrome: Effects of early intervention. *Rehabilitation Literature, 42,* 339-343.

Hasazi, J., Streifel, J., & Edgar, C.L. (1971). Promotion of positive social interaction in severely retarded young children. *American Journal of Mental Deficiency, 75,* 519-524.

Hayden, F. (1966). *The nature of physical performance in the trainable retardate.* Paper presented at the Joseph P. Kennedy Foundation Third International Scientific Symposium on Mental Retardation, Boston.

Hester, S.B. (1981). Effects of behavioral modification on the standing and walking deficiencies of the profoundly retarded child. *Physical Therapy, 61,* 907-911.

Hirsch, W. (1965). *Motor skills transfer by trainable mentally retarded and normal children.* Doctoral dissertation, University of California, Los Angeles.

Hook, E.B. (1981). Down's syndrome: Its frequency in human populations and some factors pertinent to variation in rates—Trisomy 21 (Down's syndrome). *Research Perspectives, 2,* 3-15.

Hoover, J.H., & Wade, M.G. (1985). Motor learning theory and mentally retarded individuals. *Adapted Physical Activity Quarterly, 2,* 228-252.

Jackson, H.J., & Thornbecke, P.J. (1982). Treating obesity of mentally retarded adolescents and adults. *American Journal of Mental Deficiency, 87,* 302-308.

Kelly, L.E., Rimmer, J.H., & Ness, R.A. (1985). Obesity levels in institutionalized mentally retarded adults. *Adapted Physical Activity Quarterly, 2,* 167-176.

Kershner, K.M., & Dusewicz, R.S. (1970). KDK-Oseretsky tests of motor development. *Perceptual & Motor Skills, 30,* 2020.

Knox, M. (1983). Changes in the frequency of language use by Down's syndrome children interacting with non-retarded peers. *Education & Training of the Mentally Retarded, 14,* 185-190.

Kovar, R. (1981). Pregnancy and increased maternal age. *Nebraska Medical Journal, 66,* 7-12.

Larson, B., Bjorntorp, P., & Tibblin, G. (1981). The health consequences of obesity. *International Journal of Obesity, 5,* 97-116.

Lejune, J., Gauthier, M., & Turpin, R. (1959). Etude des chromosomes somatiques de neuf enfants mongoliens. *Academy of Science, 248,* 1721-1722.

Lyman, L. (Ed.). (1963). *Phenylketonuria.* Springfield, IL: Charles C Thomas.

Maloney, M.P., & Ward, M.P. (1970). Bender-Gestalt test performance of "organic" and "functional" mentally retarded subjects. *Perceptual & Motor Skills, 31,* 860.

Malpass, L.F. (1963). Motor skills in mental deficiency. In N.R. Ellis (Ed.), *Handbook of mental deficiency.* New York: McGraw-Hill.

McInerney, M.F., McLaughlin, T.F., & Truhlicka, M. (1982). Increasing eye-contact and instruction following behavior with a three-year-old Down's syndrome child with parents as therapists. *Journal of Special Education, 18,* 71-80.

Morris, A.F., Vaughn, S.E., & Vaccaro, P. (1982). Measurements of neuromuscular tone and strength in Down's syndrome children. *Journal of Mental Deficiency Research, 26,* 41-46.

Mulholland, J.R., & McNeill, A.W. (1985). Cardio-vascular responses of three profoundly retarded multiply-handicapped children during selected motor activities. *Adapted Physical Activity Quarterly, 2,* 151-160.

Neeman, R., & Phillips, H.E. (1970). *Perceptual-motor evaluation of mental retardates in a sheltered workshop*

(Studies in Mental Retardation Monograph). Buffalo: State University of New York, School of Health Related Professions.

Nihara, K., Foster, R., Shellhaas, M., & Leland, H. (1969). *Adapted behavior scales.* Washington, DC: American Association on Mental Deficiency.

Piper, M.C. (1980). Effects of home environment on the mental development of Down syndrome infants. *American Journal of Mental Deficiency, 84,* 111-116.

Portella, D. (1982). Motor schema formation by EMR boys. *American Journal of Mental Deficiency, 87,* 164-177.

Raber, S.M., & Weisz, J. (1981). Teacher feedback to mentally retarded and non-retarded children. *American Journal of Mental Deficiency, 86,* 148-156.

Rarick, G.L., Dobbins, D.A., & Broadhead, G.D. (1976). *The motor domain and its correlates in educationally handicapped children.* Englewood Cliffs, NJ: Prentice-Hall.

Scarbrough, P.R. (1982). A review of trisomies 21, 18, 11. *Alabama Journal of Medical Sciences, 19,* 167-169.

Seakins, J.W.T., Saunders, R.A., & Toothill, C. (1973). *Treatment of inborn errors of metabolism.* London: Churchill Livingston.

Smith, G. (1985). *Molecular structure of the no. 21 chromosome and Down's syndrome.* New York: New York Academy of Science. (Monograph)

Switzky, H.N., Haywood, H.C., & Rotatori, A.F. (1982). Who are the severely and profoundly mentally retarded? *Education & Training of the Mentally Retarded, 13,* 268-277.

Tomporowsky, P.D., & Ellis, N.R. (1984). Preparing severely and profoundly mentally retarded adults for tests of motor fitness. *Adapted Physical Activity Quarterly, 1,* 158-163.

Webb, R.C. (1969). *AMP Index* (7th ed.). Glenwood, IA: Glenwood State Hospital.

Winick, M. (1979). *Nutritional management of genetic disorders.* New York: John Wiley & Sons.

ADDITIONAL REFERENCES

Berry, P., & Gunn, V.P. (1984). Development of Down's syndrome children from birth to five years. *Perspectives & Progress in Mental Retardation, 1,* 167-177.

Brinker, R.P. (1985). Interactions between severely mentally retarded students and other students in integrated and segregated public school settings. *American Journal of Mental Deficiency, 89,* 587-594.

Cleland, C.C. (1979). *The profoundly mentally retarded.* Englewood Cliffs, NJ: Prentice-Hall.

Crain, L. (1984). Application of a multiple measurement approach to investigating the effects of a dance program on the educable mentally retarded. *Research Quarterly of Exercise & Sport, 55,* 231-236.

Pueschel, S.M. (1984). *The young child with Down's syndrome.* New York: Human Sciences Press.

Rarick, G.L., & Dobbins, D.A. (1972). *Basic components in the motor performance of mentally retarded children: Implications for curriculum development* (Monograph). Washington, DC: U.S. Office of Education, Bureau of Education for the Handicapped.

QUESTIONS FOR DISCUSSION

1. What considerations, both academic and operational, should one keep in mind when testing retarded youngsters?

2. What sports might be played by both mildly and moderately retarded youngsters 14 years old? What characteristics of traditional games and sports make some more amenable to a program of physical education than others?

3. What motivational problems might you encounter when working with mildly retarded children within a physical education class of normal youngsters? How might you circumvent or overcome these problems?

4. What are the unique characteristics of youngsters with Down syndrome? How do these characteristics influence program planning and content?

5. What scales are available with which to evaluate motor competencies of the moderately retarded? What criteria should be used when selecting the instrument and the subtests that might make up a test battery you choose to administer?

6. When working with a group of severe-ly retarded 10-year-olds, what might a daily program of sensory and sensory-motor stimulation consist of? What developmental level might this group exhibit relative to social, psychological, and motor abilities?

7. What differences might you build into a program for retarded children whose make-up is attributable to organic problems?

8. What sources can you locate that contain program contents appropriate for moderately retarded children?

9. What components of the family constellation (e.g., birth order, other siblings) might contribute to positive versus negative environment, influencing a productive home program for motor development?

STUDENT PROJECTS

1. Observe a classroom in which one or more retarded youngsters are participating. What behaviors do you note that suggest how the children might function in a physical education class into which they might be mainstreamed?

2. What agencies in your community serve retarded populations? Interview a representative of one or more of them. What components of the program, if any, deal with physical attributes, motor skills, and recreational skills?

3. Discuss with a parent of a retarded youngster the order and time of appearance of various developmental signposts (e.g., crawling, walking, throwing). Compare the answers to the time of life these behaviors are expected in normal youngsters.

4. Observe the motor evaluation of a retarded youngster. What problems, if any, did you note? How might these problems be overcome? What was the make-up of the test battery? How might the test battery be improved? What were the implications for programming the child you saw tested?

5. Obtain motor tests for retarded youngsters. Test a child labeled "retarded," and compare the results with those obtained on the tests by a normal child of the same chronological age. Attempt to ascertain what differences, if any, were a result of cognitive versus motor problems.

6. Take part as a helper in a Special Olympics competition for retarded youngsters. Write up your observations.

RESOURCES

American Association on Mental
  Deficiency
5101 Wisconsin Ave., N.W.
Washington, DC 20016
  Publications:
  Mental Retardation
  *American Journal of Mental
    Deficiency*

Association for the Severely
  Handicapped
1660 W. Armory Way
Seattle, WA 98119

Canadian Association for
  Retarded Children
149 Alcorn Ave.
Toronto 7
Ontario, Canada

Division on Mental Retardation
Council for Exceptional Children
1920 Association Dr.
Reston, VA 22091
  Publication:
  *Education and Training of the
    Mentally Retarded*

Joseph P. Kennedy Jr. Foundation
1701 K St., N.W.
Suite 205
Washington, DC 20006

President's Committee on Mental
  Retardation
Washington, DC 20201

11 *Speech and Language Impairments*

Youngsters may have difficulties in the manner in which they pronounce sounds, words, and phrases. These are called *speech problems.* Or they may have problems formulating sentences, selecting correct words, or developing vocabulary. These are *language problems.* If the problems are marked enough, children may be placed in special sessions with a speech pathologist one or more times a week. If the problems are obvious, they may pose difficulties for the children at play and in work with peers in physical activities.

At times these impairments have anatomical bases. A cleft palate, for example, causes difficulties in managing the flow of air within the mouth, which results in different sounds. More subtle neurological problems may prevent speech altogether. The *aphasic* child may be partially or totally unable to utter words because of impairment in the auditory-coding centers of the parietal area of the brain or of other components of the cortex that mediate speech.

The emerging expressive language in normal children has an interesting relationship to the development of voluntary motor functions. Initially, young children speak in advance the actions they are about to take, in the third person ("Johnny is going to pick up the ball"). At the same age they also are likely to accompany actions with speech ("Look at Johnny pick up the ball"). Later, children verbally program in advance but carry out actions without speech. With further maturation the actions are preprogrammed silently, before the actions are undertaken. By middle childhood many actions, particularly those often practiced, are carried out without any silent speech.

Knowledge of the manner in which language and motor development interact can be used to help children who are having language delays. A type of play therapy may take place in which children are encouraged to say what they are about to do, talk while they are doing it, and say what actions they have just completed. A theoretical argument among those interested in speech and language is whether language instigates thought or simply reflects it. In either case, it is a vital part of most of our lives.

NORMAL LANGUAGE DEVELOPMENT

Developmental linguists have identified a number of important pre-speech behaviors occurring during the first year of life (Bellugi & Brown, 1971; Schiefelbusch & Lloyd, 1976). The infant at birth emits a cry, which affords the first clue to the vigor of the child's vocal apparatus. By the end of the second month, the infant begins to vary the nature of the crying sound. The sensitive mother can recognize cries that indicate hunger (usually shriller) in contrast to those that indicate lesser needs.

By the 12th week the infant begins to sustain vowel-like cooing sounds. At this point young children in all cultures emit relatively similar sounds. A month or two later the infant begins to search visually for various sound makers (including other humans) and begins to make definite cooing responses to those individuals and objects.

Table 11.1 Language Development

Age in months	Comprehension and Response to Sounds	Vocabulary	Articulation	Expressive Language
1	May respond with different bodily gestures to different voices.		Makes vowel sounds.	Differentiates crying according to need (e.g., hunger, pain, need for attention).
2-4	Responds to voices with smile and may stop making sounds when adult enters room.			Begins babbling. Laughs and coos when comfortable.
5-6	Often responds to babbling of parents. Can distinguish between pleasant and angry tone of voice and responds with either smile or cry.		Produces about one-half of all consonants.	Imitates own sounds. Begins to tune up speech mechanism. Begins to use intonational patterns and directs speech to objects and people.
7-8	Attends to many different sounds in environment.			Repeats sound sequences. Tries intonational patterns.
9-10	Understands and responds to name, "no-no," and "hot." Responds with appropriate gestures to "patty-cake" and "down."	Word-like syllables (e.g., "ma-ma-ma," "da-da-da").		Imitates melody patterns but does not produce sounds in correct order. Child is trying to imitate others.
11-12	Understands action words such as "up," "fast," "down."	First meaningful words.		Copies melody patterns more accurately, but speech is still largely unintelligible. May imitate animal sounds.
12-24	Understands simple commands such as, "Go get the ball."	From 5 to 200 words. About half are nouns.	Typically omits final consonants in words.	May use one name for several unrelated things. Speech may be 50% intelligible to unfamiliar listener.

Note. From *Speech and Language Problems in Children* by J.S. Curran and B.J. Cratty, 1978, Denver: Love Publishing, pp. 17-19.

By the fourth month rudimentary but reciprocal communication between adults and infants begins to occur. Different sounds may be used to instigate various events, such as feeding. Halfway through the first year infants' babbling begins to take on more and more of the sounds exclusive to the unique language environment in which they are born. By the end of the first year they begin to echo real speech—at first simple echoes of repetitive sounds such as "bye-bye."

Table 11.1   Continued

Age in months	Comprehension and Response to Sounds	Vocabulary	Articulation	Expressive Language
24-36	Will listen to simple stories. Begins to comprehend prepositions (e.g., "under," "up," "on").	200 to 900 words, mostly nouns and verbs.	Has unstable pronunciation.	Begins to put two words together. Names objects. Overall intelligibility may increase to 75%. Talks about self to others (egocentric speech). Frequently asks questions. May lack fluency.
36-48	Recognizes plurals and adjectives. Can comprehend compound and complex sentences.	900 to 1,500 words.	Still mispronounces some sounds. Masters *t, d, k, g, f,* and *v.* Omission of final consonants decreases.	Increases intelligibility of speech in context to 100%. Sentence structure still not accurate. Speech becomes more useful—mostly simple sentences. Uses pronouns, some adjectives, adverbs, and prepositions. Can recite poems and songs and relate experiences.
48-60	Carries out longer commands with two to three actions involved.		Can pronounce multisyllable words. Infantile articulation disappears.	Fluency improves. Speech is intelligible even though some sounds are faulty. Uses articles ("the," "a") and plurals. Uses self-made rules of grammar.
60-72	Responds correctly to complex sentences but still may become confused at some involved sentences.		Masters *r, l,* and *th* but still may have difficulty with *s* and blends such as *gr, thr, sk,* and *st.*	Uses grammar correctly almost all of the time. More multisyllabic words are present. Uses 5- to 6-word simple, compound, and complex sentences.

A complete picture of the development of speech and language is presented in Table 11.1. As can be seen, by the beginning of the second year, children begin to emit words that can be understood by nonfamily members. By the end of the second year the speaking vocabulary may reach 200 words, with an understanding of 100 or 200 more.

From the middle of the third year, children begin to show individuality in speech—favorite words and phrases. In some 4-year-olds enunciation becomes almost adult-like with articulation errors occurring less and less frequently. The easier sounds heard within the third year (*m, n, b, p, w*) are augmented with the more explosive consonant sounds (*t, f, k, g*) by the fourth year. The typical 4-year-old can master the more difficult sounds of *sh, s, ch, z, zh, v, l, th,* and *r.*

The table represents approximations rather than absolute milestones. Within so-called normal ranges children may not evidence some behaviors at the precise times indicated. The material in the table has been divided into four categories: (a) comprehension and response to sounds—listening behaviors during the early months of life; (b) vocabulary—the quantity of words expected during various periods in a child's life; (c) articulation—the clarity with which a child produces sounds; and (d) expressive language—the ways in which messages are sent and their clarity.

During the acquisition of these complex components of behavior, children may evidence what to some may appear to be speech problems. These so-called problems include:

—difficulties with the abstruse nature of English language pronunciations (e.g., *ph* and *f* both have an *f* sound, as in *fun*).
—difficulties with English as a second language.
—difficulties in enunciating certain sounds during first attempts, such as the blends in *mists (sts)* and *asked (skt).*
—reversing sounds, as some children of 4 and 5 do, saying *spaghetti* as *pasketti* or *Michigan* as *Mikishan.*
—baby talk, which is normal for 3- and 4-year-olds, although it usually is phased out by age 7—omitting, slurring, or changing sounds (*rabbit* becomes *wabbit, baby* may be *bay,* and *cat* is *tat*).
—controlling and modulating pitch and loudness, using an overly loud voice as an attention-getter at times.
—normal stuttering, which occurs in virtually all children between ages 3 and 4 (they seem to be trying to develop normal speech rhythms and to pair the speed of their thoughts with the speed of speech transmission).

Normal stuttering is an important phase to be aware of, insofar as an overreaction to this normality may prolong the stuttering and transform it into a real problem. When working with younger children or those whose developmental level may parallel that of normal children attempting to acquire adequate speech rhythm (and who evidence periodic stuttering), teachers of physical education should not overcorrect or call children's attention to the problem unduly by saying, "Take a big breath and start over" or "Stop and think before you talk."

LANGUAGE DELAY

In contrast to their peers, some children are delayed in the acquisition of language. Their vocabulary may not be as rich as other children's. The manner in which they express themselves may be less than adequate. They may resort to gestural language or withdraw emotionally in social contexts (Berry, 1969). At times a language delay may be an early sign of possible retardation; other times it may arise for a number of reasons, including the following:

1. The general home environment may not be conducive to the acquisition of language at a normal rate because of (a) the lack of a rich spoken language environment, or (b) the presence of adults or older siblings who are too anxious to meet the child's every whim without making him or her ask for services and objects. Overpressured parents may be too busy to explain things, or siblings and parents may interrupt a child so often that the youngster literally gives up attempting to start, much less complete, a thought verbally.

2. Emotional causes for language deficiencies are found in autistic children and those with childhood schizophrenia, as well as less obvious emotional disorders.

3. Structural and physical problems may cause language delays. These include functional problems with the hearing apparatus (outlined in chapter 7) as well as central nervous system disorders (e.g., cerebral palsy), abnormalities of the oral cavity (e.g., cleft palate), and malformations of the teeth, lips, jaw, and gums. Some genetic disturbances, such as Down syndrome, are accompanied by language delay.

SPEECH PROBLEMS

Traditionally, speech impairments have been divided into three main categories: (a) *articulation* (pronunciation) difficulties; (b) *stuttering*, or *dysfluency*—deficits of rhythm; and (c) *voice* quality problems.

Articulation Disorders

Of the over 3 million children needing speech therapy in the United States, about 70% have problems when attempting to pronounce certain sounds. In working with children who have gross motor coordination problems, physical educators are likely to find a larger percentage with articulation problems than are found in populations free of neuromotor problems.

Failure to speak clearly has obvious social and emotional implications (Winitz, 1969). Articulation problems, if caught early, stand a reasonable chance of remediation. The four basic types of articulation errors are *omissions, substitutions, distortions,* and *additions* of sounds. The checklist provided in Table 11.2 sometimes is used to determine whether children can pronounce 17 major speech sounds at the beginning, middle, and end of the words indicated. When using such a checklist, children should be given a chance to organize their thoughts and lip-mouth-breath actions.

Remedial activities should be guided by a professional speech pathologist but also can be aided with useful outcomes by parents, teachers, and even physical education teachers, if the pathologist recommends this. Physical education teachers should not unilaterally attempt to correct the problem. Nor should they permit other members of the class to ridicule children with articulation problems. Physical educators also should provide a personal model of good articulation, enunciating clearly to the class and to individual class members.

Many games may be played to help the speech pathologist improve children's articulation. Games might include practice in front of a mirror and breath control games similar to those recommended for asthmatic and cerebral palsied individuals to develop the power necessary to undergird and sustain good speech. Balloon blowing and moving ping-pong balls with the breath may also be useful. One of these games is illustrated in Figure 11.1.

Table 11.2 Articulation Checklist

Sound	Beginning	Middle	End
p	pig	popper	rip
b	boy	rubber	rub
t	toy	letter	what
d	dog	ladder	red
k	cup	donkey	look
g	go	Peggy	leg
f	fine	telephone	life
v	value	heavy	love
l	leave	balloon	fall
sh	shake	flashlight	bush
ch	chair	watches	church
j	jacks	cages	page
s	sun	pencil	mouse
z	zoo	wizard	choose
th	three	toothbrush	booth
w	wagon	power	wow
y	yellow		

Stuttering (Dysfluency)

Stuttering is one of the most vivid speech problems. The hapless stutterer long has been the brunt of jokes by nightclub comics and those imitating sounds made by a drunk. It appears in many forms. An individual may hesitate, repeat, or prolong only certain sounds while speaking others with fluency. The hesitations of many stutterers occur only in situations that are perceived as stressful. Thus, physical educators may be able to determine when situations or activities are emotionally harmful to stuttering youngsters by observing the occurrence of arrhythmic speech.

Dysfluency usually appears in early childhood, but in most children it disappears by the fourth year. If it continues, most experts agree that the problem is caused by emotional trauma, such as pressures exerted by perfectionist parents or other anxiety-producing persons and situations in the children's environment. No single identifiable structural or neurological abnormality has been found to be associated with stuttering.

Stuttering may appear in one of four forms. Children may pass through these, in order, into adulthood. Or the problem may be arrested in childhood by attention to emotional or social health conditions and instigation of specific remedial activities designed to reduce and eliminate stuttering (Sheehan, 1970).

Stage One: Insipient Stuttering   In early childhood, stuttering may come and go. Children do not think of themselves as stutterers and do not fear speaking. During this stage children stutter when they are fatigued, under stress, or as they try to tell a long story. This stage is usually associated with pre-school children.

Figure 11.1 Articulation Game Using Ping-Pong Balls

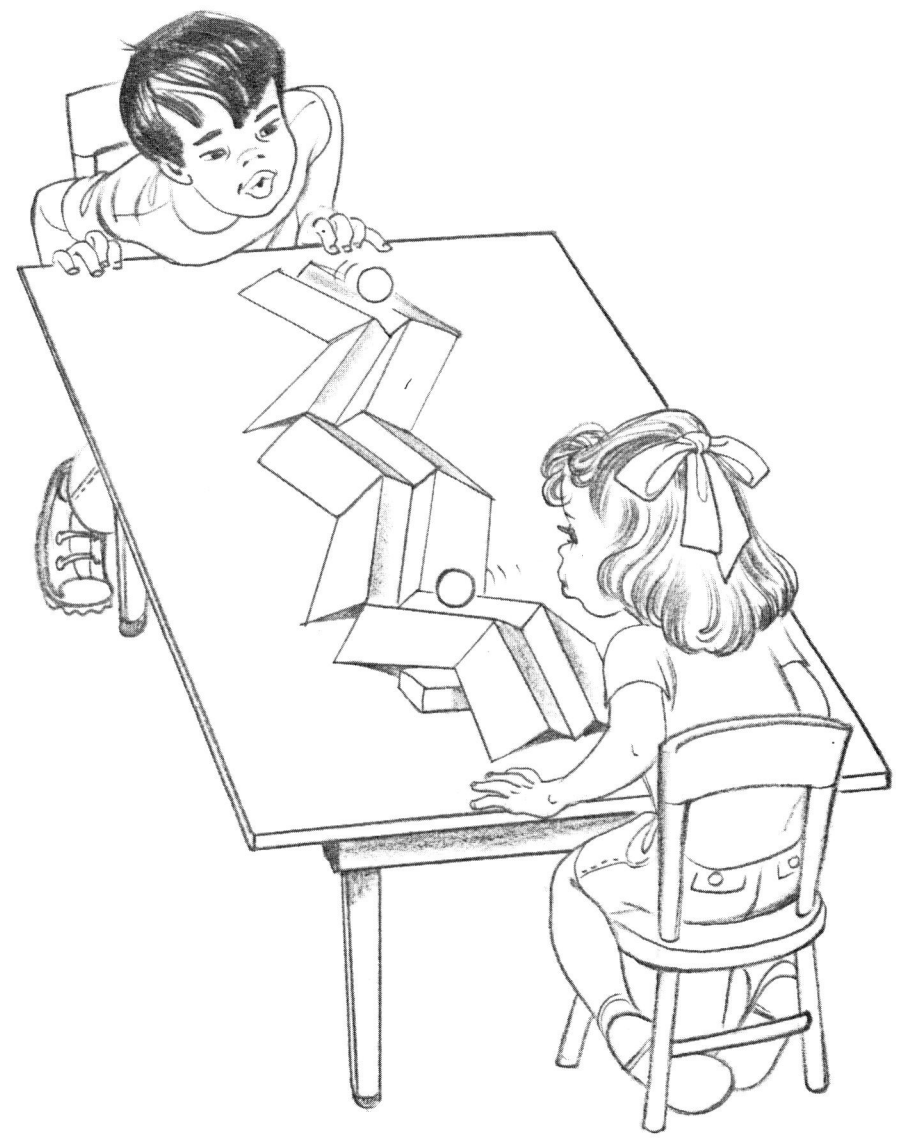

Note. From *Speech and Language Problems in Children* by J.S. Curran and B.J. Cratty, 1978, Denver: Love Publishing, p. 112.

Stage Two: Transitional Stuttering   At stage two, children identify themselves as stutterers. Although they experience situations during which stuttering does not occur, they stutter more than do children in stage one. This stage is aligned with ages 5 through 12.

Stage Three: Confirmed Stuttering   As stuttering children enter junior high school, they become acutely aware of situations that trigger the problem and seek to avoid them. Youngsters may begin to have feelings of marked inferiority and discontinue efforts to talk frequently and freely with teachers, peers, and family members.

Stage Four: Ingrained Stuttering   Generally evidenced in youth of high school age and older, the fourth stage is marked by stuttering accompanied by gesticulations and tensions in the face, limbs, or trunk, and emotional reactions. This stage often is marked by refusal to speak at all. The problem is extremely difficult to remediate if it goes this far.

Behaviors that teachers and parents might engage in with stutterers are not as clear-cut as remedial activities to use with children who have articulation problems. Stress is a highly variable condition, and what may be stressful for one stutterer may not be for another.

Children with problems in rhythm of speech are perceived negatively by children who are free of speech problems. For example, an investigation by Geis-Zaboroski and Silverman (1986) found that "regular" children perceived stuttering children as "frightened, nervous, tense, and unlovable." Therefore, children with this kind of problem may have to overcome negative social evaluations as the result of their speech deficit.

Physical education teachers may find some of the following ideas helpful:

1. Permit the stutterer to act out language roles in private before appearing in front of a class to give directions or to discuss rules of a game.

2. Keep a log on the incidence of and situations that trigger children's stuttering.

3. Deal with derisive or otherwise unacceptable behaviors of peers toward stutterers in private discussions, clearly communicating that this will not be tolerated.

4. When stutterers start to try to reduce or eliminate stuttering in stress situations with the help of the speech pathologist, devise stress situations that are compatible with the goals for that student.

5. Initiate role-play situations, with the speech pathologist's concurrence, as stutterers usually are less likely to stutter when pretending to be someone else.

Voice Problems

A final type of speech problem involves anomalies in a person's voice. Children or youth may speak at an *inappropriate pitch* (too high or too low) or at an *irritating intensity*. They may speak *too loudly* when excited. Various other undesirable voice qualities may include *hypernasality* (talking through the nose), a *metallic* (Mickey Mouse) *voice* (sometimes heard in children with right hemisphere lesions), or a rough or *gravelly voice*.

Speech pathologists often use tape recordings to demonstrate the nature of these problems. Electronic aids such as a vocal intensity meter also are used. Placed around the neck, the meter indicates with a beeping sound when the voice exceeds a predetermined decibel level. At times a wrist counter is used to record how often behaviors that are likely to injure the voice (e.g., yelling too loud when playing games) occur. Use of a counter in a physical education class may be a novelty that attracts positive attention from other children and helps reduce the exaggeration of a potential voice problem.

SPEECH AND LANGUAGE EXPERTS

A complete understanding of normal and abnormal patterns and abilities is within the purview of experts in psychology, medicine, education, linguistics, and speech pathology. These experts should be consulted before physical education teachers take it upon themselves to offer any kind of special attention or teaching behaviors intended to help children who "talk funny." Amateur speech pathology from classroom teachers, interested friends, or ill-advised physical education teachers may not only fail to help a speech or language problem but also may exacerbate the problem. This may be especially true in the emotionally charged environment of competitive sports activities.

Speech Pathologists

Also known as speech clinicians, speech pathologists are the specialists who are most directly concerned with speech and language problems. They work in public schools, in private and public clinics, in hospitals, and sometimes in private practice with medical colleagues.

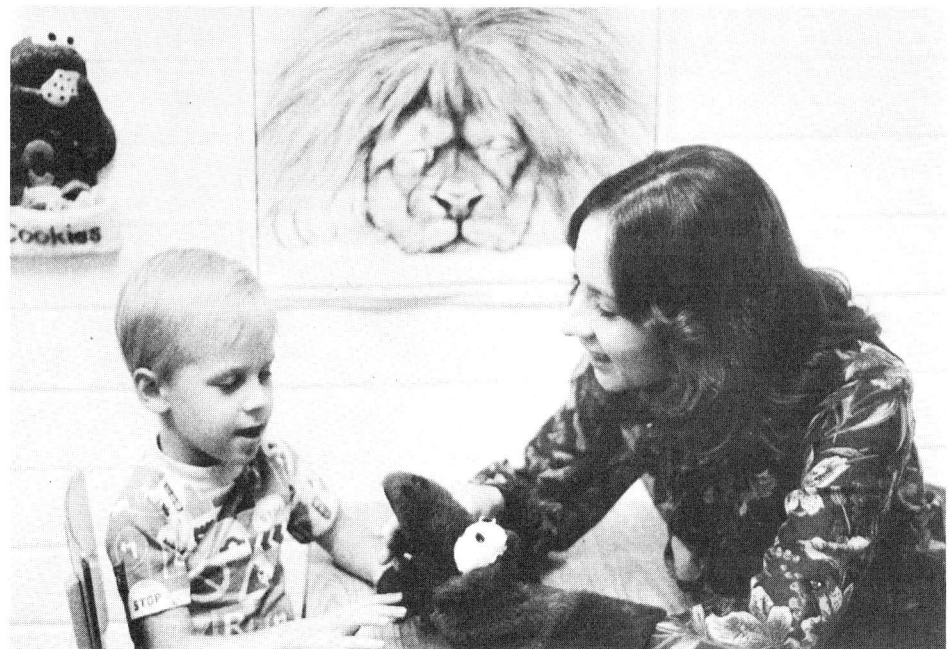

Watching the movement of a puppet's tongue helps a child pronounce difficult sounds.
Courtesy, Special Children's Center, Las Vegas, Nevada

In most states a master's degree is required, followed by a year of clinical experience and an examination formulated by the American Speech-Language-Hearing Association. If successful, speech pathologists are awarded a certificate of clinical competency. Their role is to evaluate the speech and language abilities of suspect children, to counsel parents concerning their findings, and to formulate and to carry out remedial sessions with the child directly.

Audiologists

Using a soundproof booth, the audiologist evaluates the hearing of children to determine not only hearing loss but also the degree to which children may perceive certain sounds. (As discussed in chapter 7, hearing loss has an impact on speech and language development.)

Medical Specialists

Several types of medical specialists focus on children with speech and language difficulties. The plastic surgeon operates on children born with cleft palates, and the oral surgeon corrects structural abnormalities of the jaw and teeth. The pediatrician may be the first to refer children whose language is not developing properly to others for evaluation and help. The pediatric neurologist may be called upon if a neurological problem is believed to contribute to a language or speech delay. The psychiatrist may aid in reducing possible emotional problems that may be the cause or a result of youngsters' inability to communicate with family and peers.

Dental Professionals

The general practitioner in dentistry may refer children with structural problems to a colleague who specializes in dentistry for children. An orthodontist may fit a child with appliances (braces) to help straighten children's teeth to facilitate proper articulation.

Other Professionals

Speech and language are not discrete, isolated human abilities but, rather, should be considered vital components of children's emotional and social life. Thus, social workers, child psychologists, and developmental experts often perform important services in evaluating the total psychosocial context in which children with language or speech problems may be attempting to function. Children's self-concept, interactions with peers, and relationships within their families often hinge to a large extent on their ability to communicate. These other professionals have important roles in assessing the social/emotional/psychological impact of parents, peers, or teachers who may be less sensitive to implications of the child's language problem.

IMPLICATIONS FOR PHYSICAL EDUCATION

Overall, the types of speech and language problems discussed have important implications for physical education teachers. The physical education context is an emotionally stressful one that is likely to trigger stuttering or cause children to abuse their voices by yelling too much. Moreover, physical activities may prove to be a helpful "laboratory" in which to expand the capacities of children whose language may be blunted in various ways.

Most of the implications for physical educators reflect common sense. Nevertheless, strategies should not be applied without the advice and guidance of speech professionals, including the speech pathologist.

1. Physical educators should not call undue attention to youngsters with speech or language problems. At the same time, obviously avoiding them by preventing them from speaking when appropriate may have a worse effect than permitting them to exhibit inadequate speech and language behaviors while alleviating threats and pressures to them.

2. Physical educators should (a) talk to aphasic children and not reduce language input to those who lack expressive language, and (b) listen to the stutterers and children with language deficiencies. Patience reflected in speech ("We have plenty of time to talk") and in facial expressions can have a salutary effect on many speech and language problems.

3. Physical educators should cooperate with the speech pathologist, when indicated, designing specific lessons to enrich children's language output. Storytelling that leads to games, describing games, and discussing rules are examples of ways in which vocabulary may be enriched and facile use of language may be encouraged in children. Figure 11.2 illustrates one activity that encourages language games.

4. Physical educators should be aware of the presence of structural devices that may become dislodged or broken during play and cause choking or other problems.

5. Physical educators should be particularly sensitive to the emotional intensity of games played in class and of the social interactions engendered when dealing with children or youth who stutter. When an increase in stuttering is noted, immediate consultation with the speech pathologist is recommended.

SUMMARY

A large percentage of various handicapped groups have speech/language problems. An additional 10% to 15% of all children exhibit speech or language problems. Speech and language problems interfere with children's ability to express themselves socially, and thus their play behavior often is affected adversely by their inability to communicate well. Conversely, the use of various games, when employed effectively, has been found to facilitate language.

Language difficulties refer to the inability to formulate sentences, to select appropriate words, or to exhibit an adequate vocabulary. Speech problems including *stuttering* and *articulation* (difficulty in sounding letters and letter combinations) problems, as well as various *voice* problems, including inappropriate pitch, hypernasality, metallic voice, and rough, gravelly voice. Generally, children are considered to have speech problems when their speech is noticeably different from that of peers, parents, and experts.

Language delay may be caused by a bland language environment at home or by various emotional and psychosocial deficiencies in a child's make-up or environment. With the help of a speech pathologist and other professionals, children may be encouraged to speak more and more appropriately when engaging in various games.

Because stress is often inherent in a physical education class, physical educators must be sensitive to the presence of possible speech and language problems in the population with whom they are dealing and optimize the emotional tone of the environment so that

Figure 11.2 A Play House to Stimulate Language

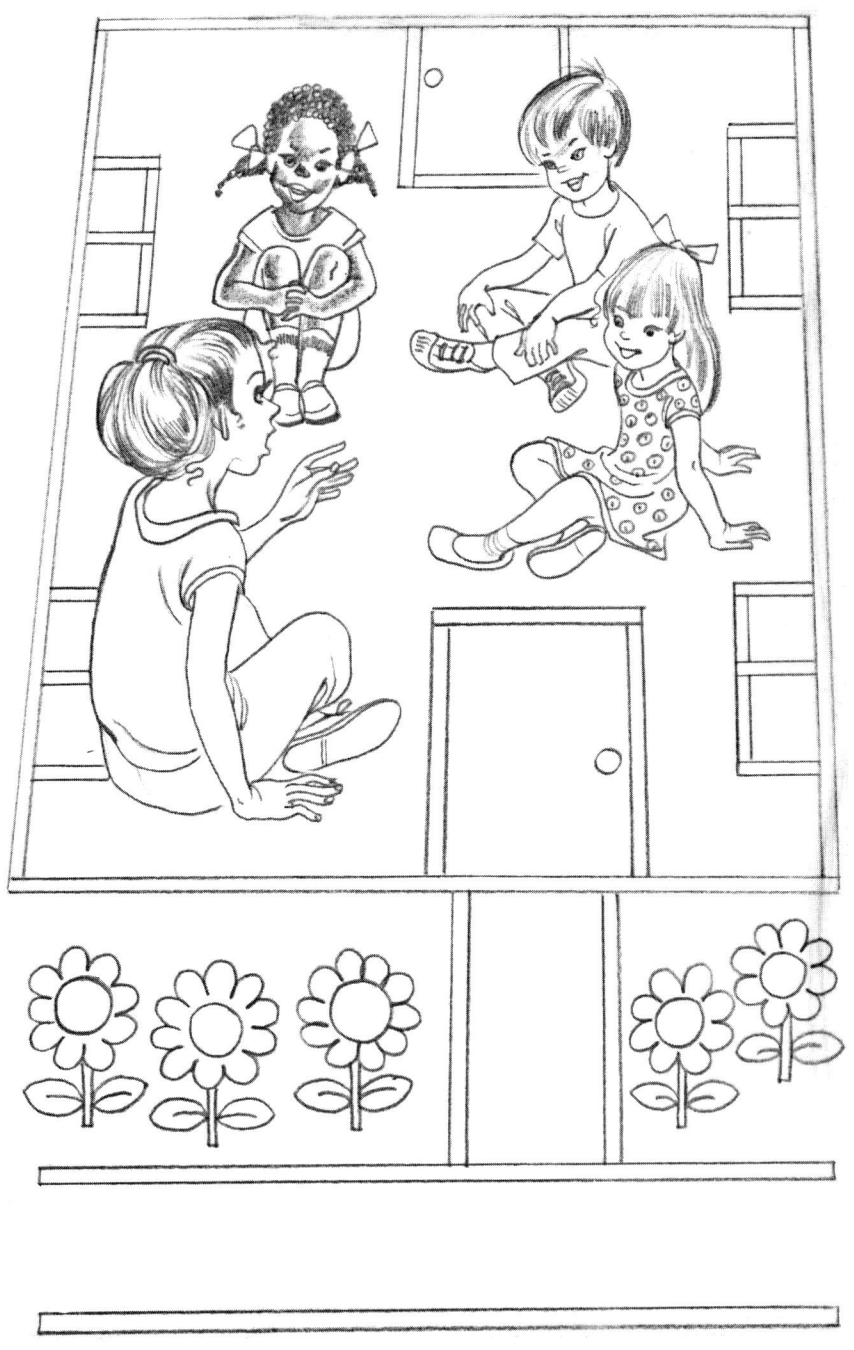

Note. From *Speech and Language Problems in Children* by J.S. Curran and B.J. Cratty, 1978, Denver: Love Publishing, p. 76.

it does not heighten the existing speech and language problems. Physical educators should exercise patience and clarity when speaking to the class and cooperate with the speech pathologist in designing meaningful ways for children and youth to express themselves in appropriate ways prior to, during, and after games or exercise.

REFERENCES

Bellugi, R., & Brown, R. (1971). *The acquisition of language.* Chicago: University of Chicago Press.

Berry, M.F. (1969). *Language disorders of children, the bases and diagnosis.* Englewood Cliffs, NJ: Prentice-Hall.

Geis-Zaboroski, J., & Silverman, F.H. (1986). Documenting the impact of mild dysarthria on peer perception. *Language, Speech & Hearing Services in Schools, 17,* 143.

Schiefelbusch, R., & Lloyd, L.L. (Eds.). (1976). *Language perspectives, acquisition, retardation and intervention.* Baltimore: University Park Press.

Sheehan, J.G. (1970). *Stuttering: Research and therapy.* New York: Harper & Row.

Winitz, H. (1969). *Articulation, acquisition, and behavior.* Englewood Cliffs, NJ: Prentice-Hall.

ADDITIONAL REFERENCES

Luria, A.R. (1960). *The role of speech in the regulation of normal and abnormal behavior.* London: Pergamon Press.

Van Riper, C. (1972). *Speech correction* (6th ed.). Englewood Cliffs, NJ: Prentice-Hall.

Weiss, C., & Lillywhite, H.S. (1976). *Communicative disorders: A handbook for prevention and early intervention.* Baltimore: University Park Press.

Yardley, A. (1971). *Exploration and language.* New York: Citation Press.

QUESTIONS FOR DISCUSSION

1. How much language is a 3-year-old expected to exhibit? How does language at this age interact with the performance of a motor skill?

2. What are some specific problems of articulation? Give examples.

3. When does normal stuttering occur in the life of a child? What dysfluencies are expected at that age?

4. What are the four stages in stuttering? At what age might individuals exhibit speech in the various stages? What might physical educators do to aid stutterers?

5. What might be the social effects of a voice that is too high pitched on a boy of 16?

6. What kinds of games could be played to enrich children's language at age 6?

STUDENT PROJECTS

1. Observe a speech pathologist at work with children evidencing speech problems in articulation or stuttering. What kinds of things are done? What does the therapy have in common with teaching a motor skill on the playground?

2. Discuss stuttering with the stutterer. What brings on stuttering? How does the individual deal with it?

3. Devise two games that normal 5- and 6-year-olds might play to enhance their language skills.

4. Discuss language and speech problems with a physical education teacher.
Find out what percentage of the children
and youth in class have these problems.
How does the teacher accommodate or
deal with these problems?

RESOURCES

American Cleft Palate Educational
  Foundation
331 Salk Hall
University of Pittsburgh
Pittsburgh, PA 15261

American Speech-Language-Hearing
  Association
10801 Rockville Pike
Rockville, MD 20852

National Association for Hearing and
  Speech Action
10801 Rockville Pike
Rockville, MD 20852

Section IV

Central Nervous System and Neuromotor Problems

12 *Awkwardness*

Physically inept children traditionally have not been assigned to special programs for the obviously handicapped. At the same time, however, their visibility to the general public and to educators has gradually come into focus after World War II. In their early text, *Psychopathology and Education of the Brain Injured Child*, Strauss and Lehtinen (1947) described a syndrome of conditions including physical awkwardness, hyperactivity, perceptual problems, and learning disabilities.

HISTORY AND INTERPRETATION

In the decades following publication of the Strauss and Lehtinen book, many clinicians, observers, and writers have focused their attention on poor coordination in children. The primary intent of these theoreticians was to substantiate general theses that physical ineptitude always accompanies learning disabilities and attempts to rectify learning disabilities must invariably include (or consist entirely of) attempts to change motor coordination.

As the result of the writings of Kephart (1962), Delacato (1963), Getman (1962), Barsch (1965), and others, a plethora of perceptual-motor, sensory-motor, sensory-integration, and motor-sensory programs emerged. Their purposes invariably included the heightening of academic and conceptual abilities by placing children in programs consisting primarily of movement activities.

Evaluation of the programs of the multitude of well meaning "perceptual-motor zealots" passed through three major phases during these same decades. Some skeptics initially pointed out that given the knowledge of both motor functions and intellectual-academic abilities at that time, together with information about transfer of training, balance beam walking probably would not help anything other than the dynamic balance qualities inherent in the task (Cratty, 1969).

A second evaluation phase involved literally hundreds of studies whose results, while often pointing to the educational efficacy of motor training, were frequently poorly conceived, lacked adequate controls, and were beset with methodological and statistical problems. Upon examining the results of these studies, Hammill, Goodman, and Wiederholt (1974) and Hirsch and Anderson (1976), among others, attested to their inadequacies. A third, most recent effort to evaluate the outcomes of perceptual-motor programs has consisted of *meta-analyses*—collecting the data from numerous studies of this kind to determine whether any positive outcomes resulted from the application of motor programs with children who had motor difficulties associated with learning disabilities (or to populations containing only children with learning disabilities).

The outcome of one of the most ambitious of these meta-analyses has important implications for educational practices focused upon awkward children, as well as those who continue to believe that application of motor tasks will heighten academic proficiencies (Kavale & Mattson, 1983). The data from this survey, based upon 180 studies (containing 13,000 subjects!), indicated that perceptual-motor training programs of various types resulted in insignificant changes in reading and were far inferior to changes expected if a traditional program of reading had been applied. A second finding was of critical importance for physical educators as well as classroom teachers confronting physically awkward children: The programs of perceptual-motor training had no significant effect upon the motor competencies of the children to whom they were applied!

At my university I conducted programs focused on awkward children. The continual finding was that with carefully designed individualized programs directed at motor ineptitude itself, change was often difficult to come by. Change did occur, however, if individual programs were carefully planned and we reached youngsters in early childhood.

In the years during which we conducted this program, the children themselves, as well as their parents, constantly informed us that being an awkward child was socially and emotionally devastating. Our own efforts and observations led to the firm conclusion that the reduction and remediation of physical skill problems provided adequate justification for the program of motor training.[1] One need not allude to the possible changes in academic or reading ability that might transpire. Transfer of simply applied motor-task training to academic skills is a myth. But, clearly, physical awkwardness in and of itself is important to identify and remediate. Physical awkwardness often renders youngsters unable to play well with peers, prevents them from expressing their intelligence adequately, and makes them ineffectual in job-related tasks.

Unfortunately, changes in physical coordination and performance are extremely difficult to instill. Only carefully conceived and applied programs are likely to make inroads into the physical coordination improvement of awkward children.

PREVALENCE

Physical incoordination is seen within various atypical groups, including the developmentally delayed. At the same time, awkwardness can appear in youngsters who have no diagnosed educational or medical problems. The prevalence of awkwardness in youngsters has been estimated at 10%-15% of children who have been assigned to a regular elementary school setting and who have not been found to have sensory, motor, emotional or learning problems. Awkwardness, however, is greater within groups of children said to be learning disabled, as well as within populations of the retarded and those evidencing visual and hearing problems.

CAUSES

The causes of physical awkwardness are often difficult to ascertain. Physical incoordination can stem from subtle inherited qualities, from undiagnosed, mild types of cerebral palsy (covered in chapter 13), from endocrine abnormalities, or from an environment that prevents a child from developing normally. Additionally, a measurable deficiency in motor coordination at a given point in a child's life may be a sign of a degenerative condition

---

1. "Lisa says that during her dreams at night she hears the voices of children teasing her at play." "Alex refuses to go to school on Friday for physical education; he gets sick and barricades himself in his room in the morning so he doesn't have to go to school." These are two representative statements by parents of awkward children after we evaluated their youngsters.

of the type discussed in chapter 14. Normal maturational processes within the first three or four years of life can mask an exotic or rare condition that may begin to make its overt appearance during the late pre-school years or during the first years of school. Muscular dystrophy is only one of many possible examples (see chapter 16). For this reason, physical educators who are adroit at administering a battery of useful motor tests to a group of children should not assume that they are the "last word" when discovering some problem. Rather, they should suggest or even encourage a more thorough medical work-up if the youngster has not already had one.

To cite only one example of misdiagnosis or superficial assessment that might occur: A physical educator may observe that a child is unable to intercept a ball well and conclude that more practice with balls—catching them, hitting them, attempting to bat them on swinging strings—will constitute an adequate answer to the problem. In truth, the child may not see balls coming from various angles because of restriction in the visual field, which may be caused by a growing tumor within the visual-ocular apparatus! If the child is not examined thoroughly by appropriate medical-ophthalmological personnel, a serious condition might be permitted to persist.

Perinatal Conditions

The various conditions discussed in chapter 13 surrounding cerebral palsy also may contribute to mild or moderate awkwardness. Lack of adequate oxygen around the time of birth—*birth anoxia*—is believed to be responsible for some later problems in coordination. Other traumas during this critical period include breech birth and prolonged labor.

Nutritional Conditions

Under the broad label "nutritional conditions" one can include problems traced to abusive substances in the mother's system. These include nicotine, alcohol, and cocaine. Descriptions of infants with *fetal alcohol syndrome*, for example, bring up problems in coordinating the larger and smaller muscle groups. Moreover, children who are poorly nourished after birth or whose mothers reside in a nutritionally impoverished environment can develop later problems such as hyperactivity and awkwardness.

A malnourished fetus with low weight at birth, whether born at full term or prematurely, is more likely to have later motor problems than is an infant whose size is normal (whether premature, or full term). Although these children may catch up, their need for extra help in achieving motor milestones of development is often apparent.

Trauma

At times physical awkwardness can result from trauma. A fall from a bike, an injury from or within a car involving a blow to the head may cause bilateral or unilateral (if one side or the other is affected) distortions of motor coordination. Because parents may not recognize the effects of an infant's fall from a crib or chair early in life, the cause of later motor problems may remain a mystery. Or, tragically, motor inadequacies can result from physically abusive actions toward children.

Deprivation of Experience

Some children live in environments that prevent them from gaining normal motor development. A number of apartment-reared children we have tested have not had the opportunity to play actively but instead spend their time complacently seated in front of the television set. One child we evaluated—a 5-year-old whose student-parents were from a foreign country—had not been permitted to leave the home, even to play in the back yard! His lack of motor experience was apparent during the assessment period.

Often one is unable to pinpoint the cause of a child's motor coordination problem. And caution is advisable in pointing a finger at the child's home environment, because of parental guilt-taking and inter-parent blaming that may ensue. But all of these children should be considered as having an educational problem that requires the proper attention. Many also should be considered for additional diagnostic help.

CHARACTERISTICS AND CLASSIFICATIONS

Each awkward child has a subtle mixture of elusive motor irregularities. Moreover, each has developed an often elaborate (depending upon age and sophistication) manner of dealing with the social/emotional demands of the environment that his or her muscles cannot meet. Each needs thorough assessment using the appropriate evaluation tools (discussed later) as well as subjective but careful observations of how the child compensates motorically and socially in school, home, and neighborhood settings.

Movement Characteristics

Body-Part Integration   Awkward children do not integrate parts of their body well. They do not shift the appropriate foot forward when throwing a ball. They may lift the arms when jumping, but they do so too late—or earlier than when the leg extends at the knee. Biomechanical analyses of their efforts reveal that forces are not summated correctly when they try to apply force; forces are dissipated rather than being channeled in the directions and with the power seen in the efforts of their peers.

The result of this lack of integration is the inability to transfer a pattern from one side of the body to another, as when trying to alternately hop from one foot to the other or when doing jumping jacks. Likewise, the upper part of the body is not well integrated with the lower part in throwing, catching, jumping, and similar actions in which the arms and legs must work in concert.

Motor Planning (Praxic Behavior)   Awkward children have difficulty replicating a complex movement either demonstrated to them or that they have been asked to do verbally. They often are described as *apraxic* (literally, without action). Gubbay (1978) has used the term *developmental apraxia* to describe awkward children in general.

In a series of tests we have researched over the years, many children cannot observe one or two consecutive movements of the hands or limbs (presented one per second) and

This 7-year-old girl can integrate her arms and legs well in a jumping jack—a task difficult for a 5- or 6-year old.

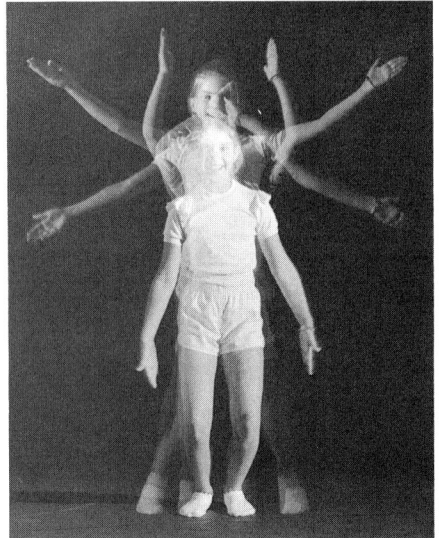

The integration of arms and legs is better in this 9-year-old boy than in the 7-year-old girl when both are asked to jump up.

Reprinted from *Perceptual and Motor Development in Infants and Children* (3rd ed.) by B.J. Cratty, with permission of the publisher, Prentice-Hall

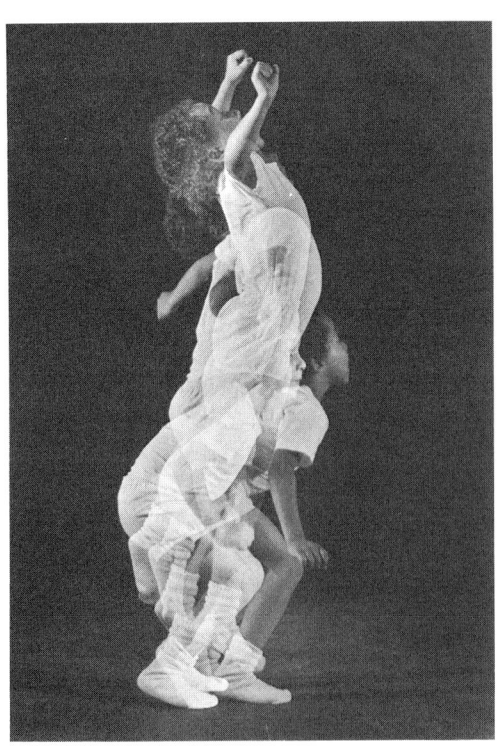

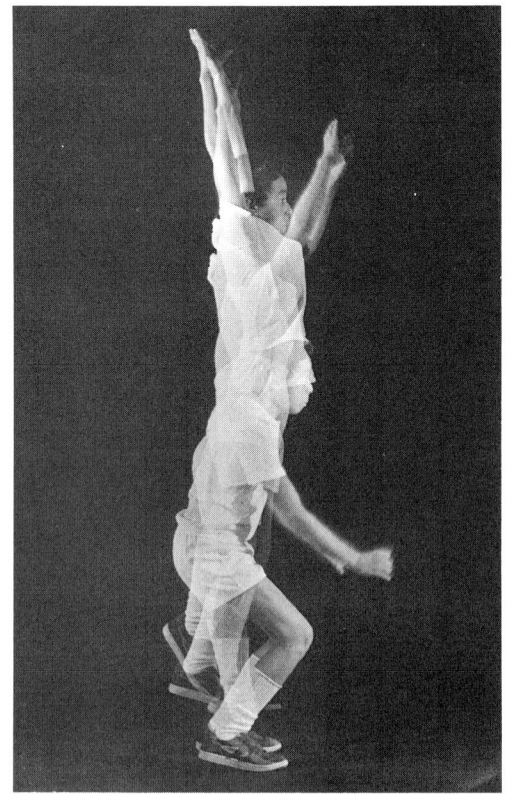

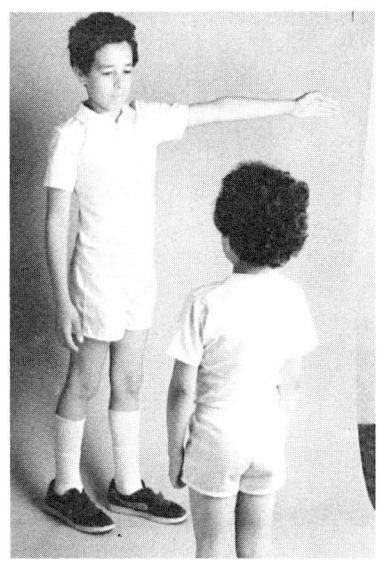

The ability to replicate a series of arm positions, hand positions, or positions of the total body can indicate motor planning abilities.

Reprinted from *Perceptual and Motor Development in Infants and Children* (3rd ed.) by B.J. Cratty, with permission of the publisher, Prentice-Hall

then successfully replicate them. Normally, youngsters by the age of 5 can replicate three or more such positionings, and by age 7, up to five or six action-positions of this nature (Cratty & Samoy, 1984).

Apraxia (more accurately, *dyspraxia*) may be relatively specific to the task involved. For example, in our work we have found relatively low correlations between motor planning tasks involving the replication of hand movements, limb positions, strokes to make a drawing, and positions of the total body first demonstrated and then replicated. A child with a minor right hemisphere problem involving spatial-motor functioning may have difficulty duplicating bodily positions, but the same child may be more successful in another complex movement task to which a verbal formula (involving the left hemisphere) can be applied.

A 17-year-old we evaluated recently had severe dyspraxia. His intelligence was permitting him to enter college, but he had been fired from a part-time job in a fast-foot restaurant because he could not construct hamburgers! He was dropped from the basketball team in high school because he could not remember and execute the plays. His social life was a shambles because he could not dance.

Apraxic children require extremely patient teaching. They must be presented with parts of whole-complex movements permitting them to gradually evolve larger and larger parts out of more minute components of tasks (the additive method of teaching skills).[2]

Four motor planning tests have been developed over a 12-year period at the UCLA Perceptual-Motor Learning Laboratory. They are intended to assess short-term motor memory for visually presented stimuli. They represent separate and discrete measures of

---

2. Recent attempts to evaluate this quality are appearing with frequency in the literature (e.g., Cornish, 1980).

these capacities and have been found to be reliable on a test, retest basis and on inter-observer measures. The tasks within each sub-test are designed to be free of "culturally loaded" and biased movements.

The tests are administered individually in distraction-free settings. The tester presents each movement in the series in an additive manner (i.e., the first one is shown and the child is permitted to respond, a second is added, etc.) until the child shows within two consecutive turns that he or she is unable to produce the series of movements given accurately and in order.

Test #1—Limb Praxis: The tester demonstrates the action(s) standing 10' to the front and 3' to the right (if subject is right-handed) of the subject. As with all tests, the movements are given one per second, followed by a period of 10 seconds to allow the subject to respond. Figure 12.1 illustrates the positions in limb praxis.

Figure 12.1 Test for Limb Praxis

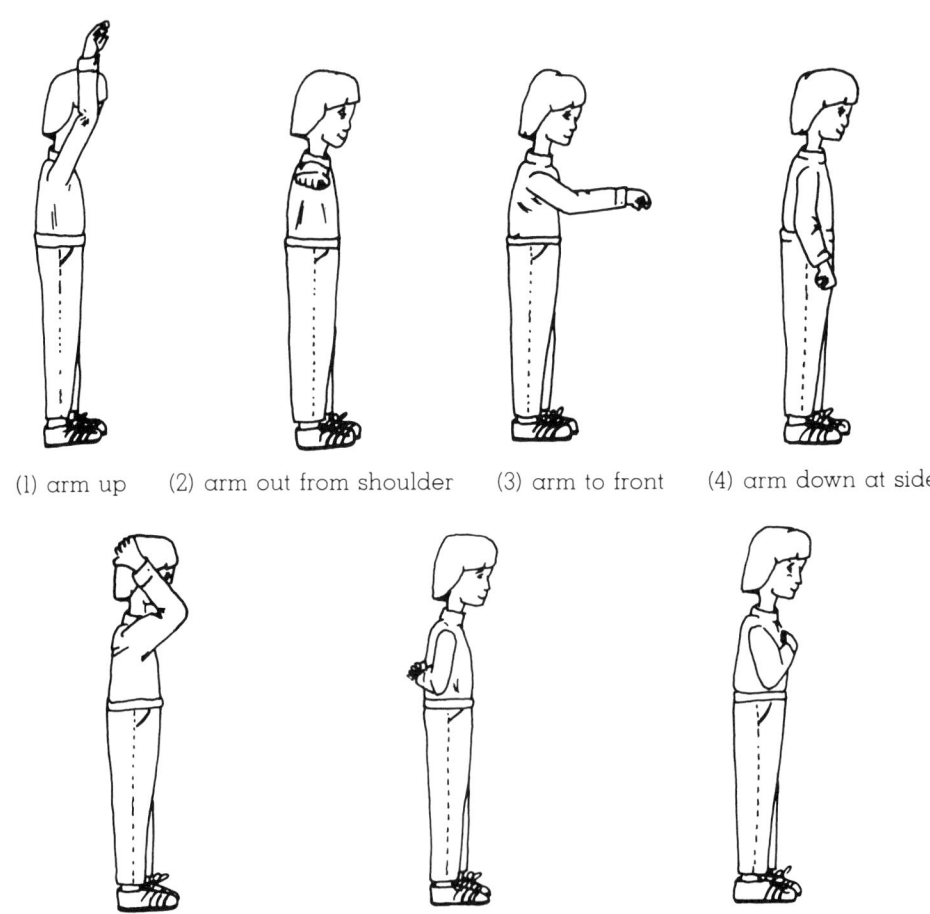

(1) arm up   (2) arm out from shoulder   (3) arm to front   (4) arm down at side

(5) hand behind head   (6) hand behind waist   (7) hand across chest

Test #2—Hand Praxis: The tester sits to the side of the preferred hand of the subject (based upon printing preference). The movements are presented in order until the child fails to reproduce the previous series presented in order. The demonstrator's hand lifts about 12″ in the air between each movement. Scoring is similar to that used for limb praxis, above. This test is illustrated in Figure 12.2.

Test #3—Trunkle Praxis: The mat is marked as shown in Figure 12.3 (but numbers shown are omitted). The tester jumps in the square marked 1, and the child is asked to duplicate the position (simply walking there if jumping capacities are absent). Squares are jumped into until the child either fails in two consecutive turns to complete a series correctly or the entire series is replicated correctly. The tester remains in each square approximately 1 second.

Test #4—Drawing Praxis: In this test the child is shown and then asked to replicate a series of strokes that together make a completed figure. Each sub-test (stroke or stroke combination) is first demonstrated, and then the drawing (model) is removed while the child tries to replicate the stroke(s) previously demonstrated. The test remains an assessment of short-term motor memory, as is true of the previous three tests. The tester sits to the side of the subject's preferred hand. The subject is not permitted to see previous renditions as he or she attempts subsequent parts of the test. Figure 12.4 contains 7 stroke patterns.

Figure 12.2   Test for Hand Praxis

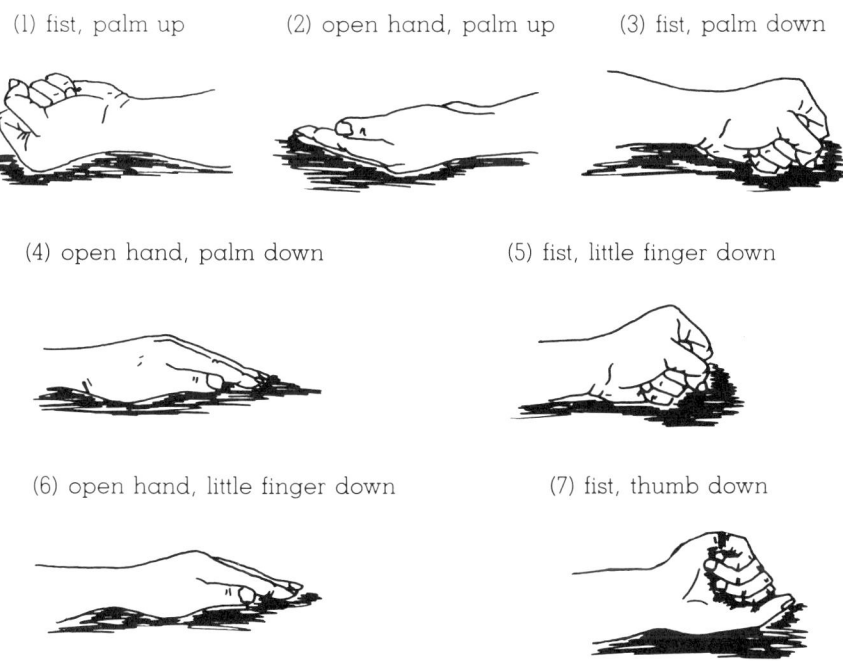

(1) fist, palm up   (2) open hand, palm up   (3) fist, palm down

(4) open hand, palm down   (5) fist, little finger down

(6) open hand, little finger down   (7) fist, thumb down

Figure 12.3   Test for Trunkle Praxis

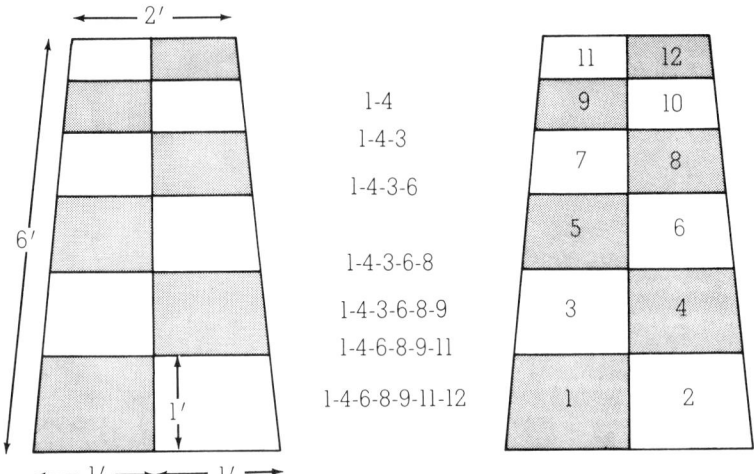

Figure 12.4   Test for Drawing Praxis

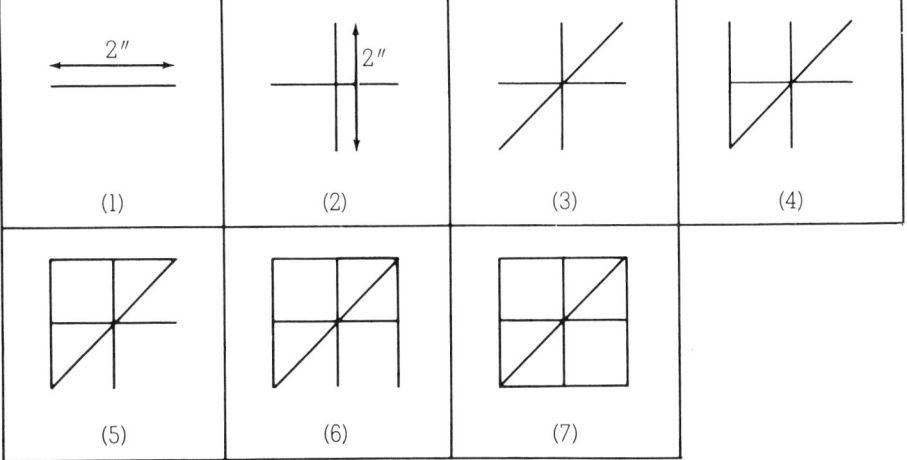

Asymmetries   A child may be asymmetrically awkward. Perhaps evidencing a mild form of hemiplegia (see chapter 13), the youngster might be able to move laterally to the right better than to the left. One hand may be significantly better than the other at manipulative tasks. Often the difference is not great; it may be very subtle. Even a small difference, however, may cause the child to run on the bias—moving ahead with the left side and shoulder, for example, and pushing the weaker left side of the body with the stronger right side and leg.

At times asymmetry is seen in children with speech problems whose left side is involved—producing right-sided weakness in the larger muscle groups. Aphasic children, for example, may evidence this type of problem.

Among the tasks that might uncover this kind of asymmetry are: (a) finger opposition (touching the fingers of each hand, in order, to the thumb of the same hand); (b) lateral movement of the total body both ways (the child will move best away from the side of the "good" leg, indicating a weakness of some kind); and (c) marked differences in the ability to hop on one foot or to balance on one foot at a time.

Overflow (Associated Movements)   Since the 1960s, researchers have taken increased interest in the phenomenon of overflow movements, first defined early in this century as "motor irradiations that are outside the subject's awareness and accompany, but are not necessary for, the performance of an intended movement" (Noica, 1912). These extraneous, unnecessary motions are believed to be caused by immaturities in the nervous system. They usually diminish by ages 6-8 and disappear altogether by age 9 or 10 in children who are otherwise free of signs of neuromotor immaturity or damage.

Excess overflow presents two problems to children: (a) They look "funny" (unaesthetic) to others and thus may attract social derision, and (b) they are likely to be biomechanically

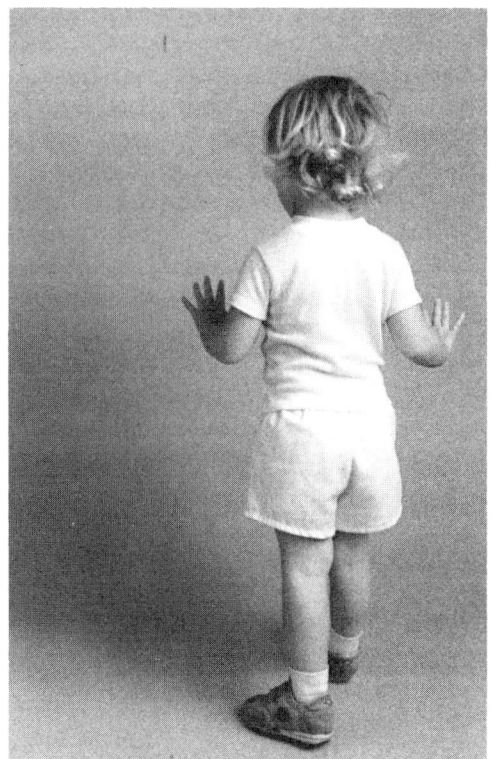

Overflow is normal in this 2-year-old. When asked to walk on his heels, the arms and wrists flex.

Photos on pages 215-218 reprinted from *Perceptual and Motor Development in Infants and Children* (3rd ed.) by B.J. Cratty, with permission of the publisher, Prentice-Hall.

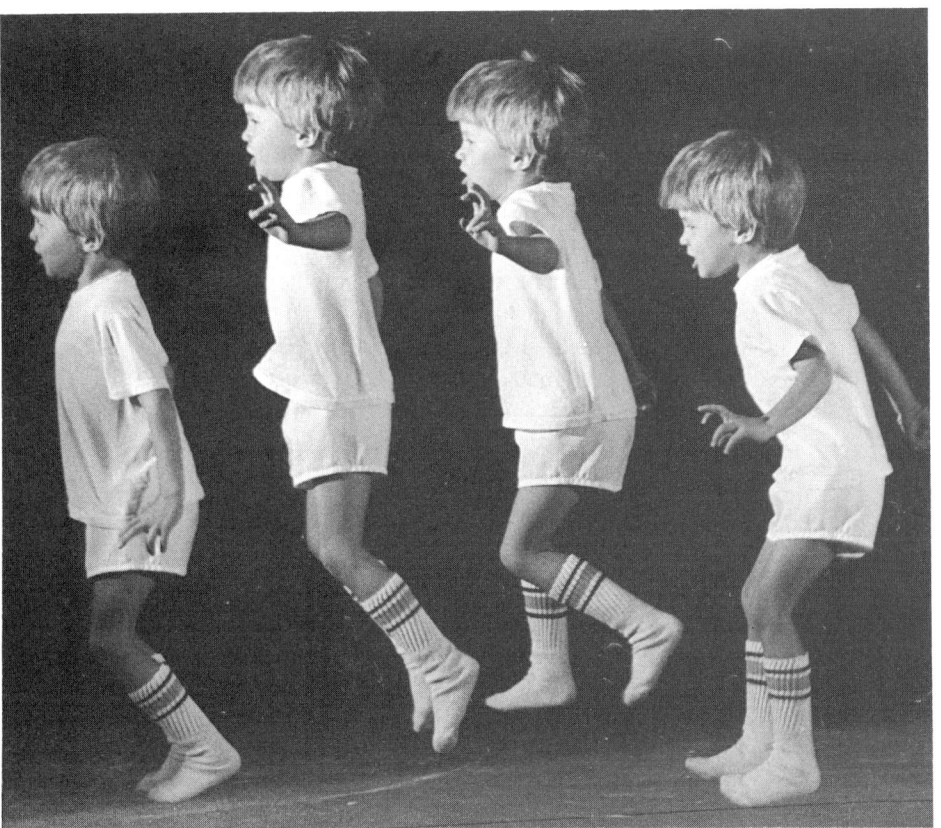

When asked to jump, this 4-year-old reveals overflow in the upper limbs.

less efficient (for example, the arms and hands are too tense and do not move appropriately in conjunction with the legs when running). Children who rated high in this unwanted quality in a recent investigation also were judged as having poor task-attentional qualities and were otherwise judged as immature (Waber, Mann, & Merola, 1985). In general, boys evidence more of this later in life than do girls, who tend to mature earlier neurologically.

Overflow is evaluated in a number of ways, usually based on a three-part rating system (1 = absent, 2 = slight, and 3 = marked). The tasks may include (a) finger opposition, (b) alternate toe or hand tappings, and (c) alternate pronated and supinated hand touches to the thigh while in a seated position. Another task involves *stress gaits*, which requires the child to walk on tiptoes, on the inside and outside of the feet, and also on the heels. Overflow emanating from gait stress is revealed in flexions, pronations, and extensions of the elbows and wrists.

A specific type of overflow is called *mirror movements*. These are elicited by asking the person to spread his or her fingers and lift a finger. Mirror movements are evidenced by unintended (and unaware?) movements made in the same way with the opposite hand (Cohen, Lawrence, Mahadeviah, & Birch, 1967; Wolff, Gunnoe, & Cohen, 1982).

In all cases, observations of movements, twitchings, and so forth are noted in body parts that are not directly instructed to move. Often, in finger spreading, for example, the mouth moves excessively.

Investigations have revealed an excess of overflow in various atypical populations including the retarded (Connolly & Stratton, 1968) and brain damaged (Fog & Fog, 1963; Abercrombie, Linden, & Tyson, 1964). The precise neurological meaning of these movements remains controversial. The findings indicate, for example, that various kinds of associated movements seem to appear and then diminish at various chronological ages. Moreover, different types of pathways (and their relative maturation) probably contribute to and detract from the presence of these actions. Associated movements from stressed gaits, for example, probably reflect the maturity of ipsilateral neural pathways, while the so-called mirror movements, or overflow from one side of the body to the other, are probably transmitted by motor pathways that cross (Zulch, 1942; Hopft, Schlegel, & Lowitzsch, 1974).

Findings by Wolff and his colleagues (1983) indicate that each type of associated movement may have a specific maturational meaning at a specific age. Combining the results of several associated movement signs may obliterate important neurodevelopmental information. At the same time, these intriguing actions probably provide (if they are carefully interpreted) important indices of neuromotor maturation uncontaminated by the effects of

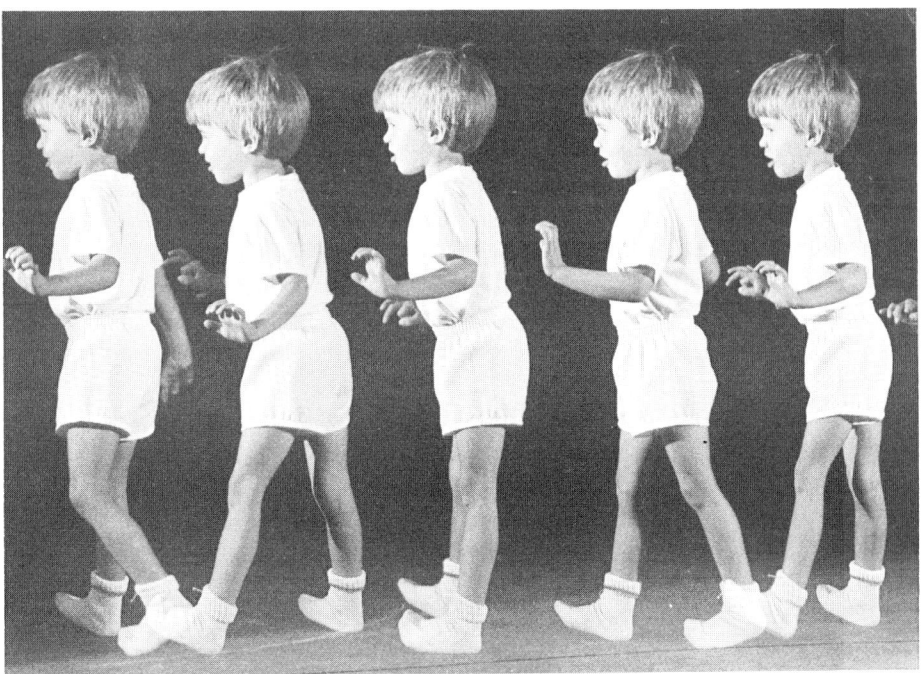

The 4-year-old reveals overflow in the upper limbs when asked to heel-walk . . .

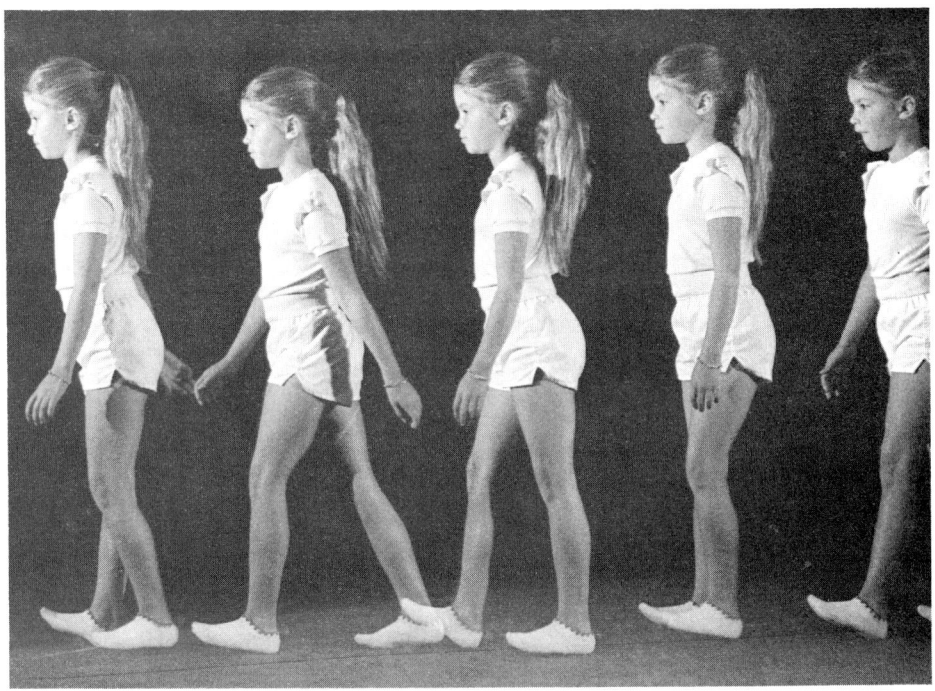

. . . while the 7-year-old shows no upper limb overflow or tension in the heel-walk.

learning, size, strength, or other cultural variables. Moreover, children with neuromotor immaturities seem less able to consciously restrain the presence of these actions than is true of children who are free of other neurological soft signs.

In short, the presence of overflow movements may provide important information when giving an overall neurological examination (Cohen et al., 1967). Their presence indicates that inhibitory processes may not yet be mature. Their absence in late childhood is a reflection of the adequate maturation of inhibitory processes and structures.

Reducing overflow may be difficult and can involve the use of mirrors (watch how you move your mouth when writing), relaxation training, and so forth. This quality should be carefully taken into consideration when assessing awkward children and when designing programs for them.

Perseveration   Undue persistence in a behavior is a pervasive characteristic of many emotionally disturbed children. Awkward children also may evidence this kind of problem in motor behaviors. It can be described as an inflexibility in the ability to transfer or change from task to task when change is appropriate and called for in a given situation.

Clinically the quality might be assessed by asking a child to draw a series of capital S's and then to draw reverse S's. If the child continues to draw correct S's, he or she can be said to have problems with persistence and perseveration. In general play this characteristic may become apparent when the skills or strategies of a previous game intrude into a subsequent one.

Impersistence   In some ways impersistence is in opposition to perseveration. Impersistence refers to a child's inability to maintain a required position for a reasonable time. Speech pathologists are concerned, for example, when a child cannot persist in a "tongue thrust" (holding the tongue out rigidly from the mouth); impersistence is revealed as the tongue begins to slowly curl inward. Impersistence also may be spotted by asking a child to hold both hands out in front of the body, at right angles to the body, with eyes closed; a further request to quickly open and close the fists may result in one arm slowly being dropped to the side.

Impersistence may be a sign of poor kinesthetic perception. In any case, its presence may be determined within an evaluation program for awkward children, accompanied by other tests of kinesthetic awareness (e.g., limb positioning at targets without vision).

Tonus Problems

Hypertonicity   Children who perform poorly in physical tasks may have problems with tonus, reflected in how much or how little residual, resting muscle tone they display. The child may be *hypertonic*—overly tense, with extraneous twitchings and tremor. This child further might have a mild to moderate form of spastic cerebral palsy (see chapter 13). A mild spastic condition in children who are participating in normal, often competitive classroom settings can cause excess emotional stress, which can lead to increased muscle tone. The hypotonic child will be seen to grip a pencil too hard and exhibit writing and printing movements that require great force to restrain. The knuckles and fingers appear white while gripping the pencil. On the playground this youngster may have problems in varying the force of thrown balls, for example, throwing too hard at a teacher or peers while not meaning to do so.

Relaxation training may help a hypertonic child. This can be incorporated into physical education lessons or applied before and afterward. Special strategies may have to be adopted when teaching a child with this problem to function more adroitly in play situations.

Hypotonicity   An equally serious problem is presented by the child whose muscle tone is poor. The *hypotonic* younger child may have difficulty holding a writing instrument or a ball. The eyelids may droop, as poor muscle tone is present even here. At times a hypotonic condition in the pre-school years is a precursor to athetoid cerebral palsy (see chapter 13), so suspect youngsters must be carefully evaluated.

In the later school years these youngsters often are considered "fat and lazy." Thus, moral judgments are made about their character when in fact the problem is neurological. They are unable to apply force well, and they run slowly and poorly. In later years they cannot even support their weight off the ground when asked to do so on a high-bar in preparation for pull-ups, which are equally impossible for them.

This condition may be caused by a brain stem malfunction—a failure to adequately supply a steady stream of impulses necessary to maintain adequate muscle tone. Attention to and consideration of hypotonicity should be a part of programs dealing with awkward children.

Imbalance, Unsteadiness, and Tremor

A number of problems revolving around unsteadiness and balance may beset children who do not perform physical skills well. These problems may be confined to the upper or to the lower parts of the body (the hands versus the legs and feet, for example), or all parts of the body in some cases.

This constellation of movement symptoms may reflect moderate problems in the part of the brain—the cerebellum—that makes movement precise and promotes kinesthetic awareness. A mild form of cerebellar ataxia (see chapter 13) may be present in the make-up of a youngster with these characteristics.

One specific symptom may be a somewhat unsteady gait, with a short extension at the knee just after the foot strikes the ground when walking. In printing, each line drawn may have small, regular fluctuations. This kind of printing problem sometimes can be aided by helping the child to anchor the elbow when forming letters and shapes.

Balance problems involving the motor apparatus may accompany this kind of unsteadiness. One-foot stands may be impossible for the child (an average child may posture on one foot by about age 7). This lack of balance may prevent adequate sports performance. For example, in throwing behaviors, lateral movements either way may be difficult. Controlled, relaxed landings after a jump also may be troublesome for the youngster who displays the pattern of unsteady traits just described.

Dysgraphia

Another frequently encountered problem within populations of awkward children is reflected in scrawly, immature attempts to draw or to print and write letters and words. This usually becomes obvious when children enter school, and it has been classified as a specific learning disability (also see chapter 8). Dysgraphic problems are not entirely of a motor nature. A child who is unable to develop good "internal speech" in trying to write or print will fail not only at the motor part of that communicative effort but also in observing and replicating the complicated steps in executing a capital G or a written capital H, for example.

When trying to transcribe their thoughts to paper, dysgraphic children may have a number of difficulties, including: (a) tensely executed words and letters, resulting in efforts that leave them fatigued and discouraged by long written lessons; (b) a tremor in their printing that may be caused by a minor cerebellar ataxis, or a rambling look to letters that may result from a minor athetosis; (c) letters that are not aligned properly or are not separated well or combined well, because of their spatial-motor deficiencies.

These problems may be present without the presence of motor coordination problems in the larger muscle groups. Nevertheless, dysgraphic children as a group are over-represented in populations classified as awkward.

If begun early enough in the child's life, remedial efforts may be successful. These efforts should be made upon first discovering that the child cannot print and draw well. Corrective therapy may be hastened by carefully sequenced, well thought-out lessons (Cratty, 1984).

Sensory Problems

A number of sensory problems, including visual, auditory, or perceptual impairments and agnosias, may interact with some of the movement characteristics described previously. A case can be made for the fact that blind children who are awkward have not been able to adequately perceive appropriate movements of their peers to copy. Without appropriate models, they need to be taught in special ways how to move with power and accuracy.

Body Awareness Sensory problems may involve children's awareness of their bodies, limbs, fingers and hands, and their total positions in space. These conditions have been described by clinical neurologists as *agnosias* (literally, without awareness). *Digital agnosia* means a lack of awareness of sensations impinging on the fingers. *Somatatoagnosia* refers to the child's lack of awareness of the body or its parts. The symptoms of *spatial agnosia* are reflected in a child's seeming to be totally "lost in space" when trying to get from one place to another.

Many awkward children have good body vocabularies. Thus, evaluating how aware they are of their bodies by asking them to name body parts can be deceiving. They can name their body parts and make judgments (e.g., "touch your left hand to your right shoulder"). What they lack is the kinesthetic or tactile awareness of their body surfaces and the positions of limbs when vision is obstructed.

Evidence of agnosias can come in many ways when these children are engaging in physical activities. As two examples: (a) when they throw, they may have to keep the throwing arm and hand in sight and therefore do not pull back the arm behind the shoulder because that would restrict their vision of the motion of the throw; thus, long, powerful throwing efforts are not possible; and (b) when asked to execute a standard front roll in tumbling, a child may lose awareness of where the arms and hands are when the head is tucked through the arms at the beginning of the movement; thus, undue pressure will be placed on the head and neck as the arms do not position themselves correctly or fail to exert force against the ground, preventing the head from coming through properly.

Spatial agnosias may be indicated if a youngster has difficulty responding correctly to directions such as "lie down with your feet toward me" during the course of a lesson. Complex directions concerning retrieval of equipment and the like may seem to go unheeded or may be performed incorrectly. A superficial interpretation of such poor response may be that the child is stupid or bad, while in truth the child may have difficulty locating his or her body in space or performing a series of actions when going from one place to the other.

Body agnosia (somatatoagnosias) may be signified when an awkward youngster has difficulty putting on or taking off clothing in a physical education class. This sometimes is called "dressing agnosia," denoting the difficulty a child has in executing movements of this kind using clothing and body parts.

In digital agnosia, children simply are not aware of the location of, and cannot feel, delicately applied touches to their fingers. They may fumble frequently when trying to execute manual skills. Clinically this condition is assessed by asking a child to close his or her eyes. Then the child's fingers are gently stroked, one at a time, with the instruction, "Move the finger I touch." Children who do poorly in manual dexterity tasks often have finger or digital agnosia. Digital agnosia may be accompanied by *acalculia*, the inability to perform mathematics well. Children may not begin to count well because the "tools" initially used for counting—their fingers—are relatively insensitive.

Visual-Auditory Perceptual Problems   Marked, or even moderate, auditory or visual perceptual problems tend to result in awkwardness. Some of these awkward children have problems at play while classroom tasks involving these same abilities remain intact (or have been overlearned successfully). Other times, the play environment poses auditory or visual perceptual stresses not found in other parts of the child's life—hence, a breakdown in performance. One situation may be when a youngster is confronted with fast-moving games in which balls and people move rapidly.

Multifaceted visual-spatial problems, coupled with movements, become even more difficult when these children must remember and call up rules when appropriate. Whereas most boys and girls in mid-childhood can accommodate the visual/auditory and cognitive complexities of more advanced games, awkward children often fail. They make many compensations, including: (a) pretending to play (following the flow in a soccer game, for example, but not getting too near the ball or coming in contact with it); (b) staying out of such games at all costs; or (c) even cowering on the sidelines in fear.

Corrective lenses do not necessarily change the movement problems of children who have visual perceptual impairments. Visual-spatial abilities of a dynamic nature are not altered simply by helping the child see more clearly by introducing lenses. Careful build-up to the complexities of games is necessary to reverse the "failure syndrome."

Social-Emotional Characteristics and Compensations

Awkward children and youth, as is true for all of us, simply cannot tolerate constant social pressure, derision, and censure when attempting to interact and play with others. Awkward children *must* compensate in various ways in physical education, sports, and recreation. The following list of compensations probably could be lengthened by any perceptive teacher who carefully observes children at recess and during physical education. Awkward children may be first identified by watching for these compensations within a school population with as much accuracy as individually assessing motor competencies in them!

The Aggressor   Rather than engage in socially approved, cooperative game behaviors, the awkward child may run after others (smaller than he or she) and even strike others. This kind of behavior is well known among those who identify "problem children" in school. The aggression can be seen during a game or as a sidelight to the game itself. Some case study evidence suggests that sociopathic behaviors occurring later in life stem from physical awkwardness and an inability to engage in socially approved sports and games during early development, particularly in boys.

The Teacher's Helper   Elementary teachers and physical educators should be suspicious of children who want to help too much. These children often substitute teacher-helping for recess or even physical education, if permitted to do so. Overly cooperative behaviors can constitute a cover for their unwillingness to engage in vigorous activity and should be cause for concern rather than pleasure on the teacher's part.

The Infant   Perhaps the most common type of compensation, often supported during the pre-school years by the mother, is infantilization and learned helplessness. Before entering school the child has become aware of the parental concerns for his or her ineptitude and late development. These children use this means to elicit overly supportive behaviors from parents and other caregivers. They constantly request help for even the simplest tasks, and when help is given, their capacities are further blunted.

Upon entering school this type of behavior becomes even more pronounced if further overly permissive behaviors are forthcoming from teachers. Moreover, the child plays in immature ways, preferring solitary play to the more mature group play of other children. The "infant" also may pair off with an equally immature (or awkward) peer and avoid the more socially and physically complex games usually seen by the second and third grades.

The Scientist-Scholar   Perhaps one of the more reasonable and useful social compensations is a marked effort to be smart! Hours spent at a computer or with school books can adequately shield a student from exposing himself or herself to the mockery of others in games and sports. This compensation, while more approvable than the others covered here, may result in an overly tense child, one whose body does not develop as it should because of the lack of physical activity during the important development and growth years. An accurate picture of the awkward child's real intellectual capacities is helpful so that this kind of compensation may be correctly guided and the proper academic loads placed on the eager young scholar.

The Joker   Because awkward children, like all of us, abhor being ignored, they sometimes try to gain attention through jokes and humor. For these youngsters, play periods are a time to entertain others. Teachers who permit themselves to be deceived by this type of behavior may fail to notice that the "funny" youngster does not engage in the game being satirized! A child exhibiting this kind of behavior, as is true with the other compensations discussed, should be gently guided into achievable physical situations when possible.

The Psuedo Player   The most ingenious, interesting compensation may be false-playing. Unless the child is closely scrutinized, he or she will successfully blend into a game without exerting any physical effort or skills! This youngster may line up, cheer while moving to the head of a line (ready to bat or to play handball), and then when his or her turn comes to participate, subtly fade away and resume a position at the end of the line again, without having to expose any physical skills.

Overall compensations of the type discussed are evidence that awkward youngsters are aware of their skill deficiencies and are seeking socially acceptable, or even unacceptable, ways to avoid participation. This avoidance results in further loss of capacities and further ineptitude. A circle of failure is started and reinforced during the elementary school years. Avoidance of activity may become extreme, possibly resulting in school phobic reactions of an exaggerated nature.

DIAGNOSIS AND PROGNOSIS

Diagnosis-Evaluation

Careful assessment of youngsters suspected of having motor problems is essential. The assessment, using some of the tools described in chapter 3, should be designed so that specific areas of ineptitude are described. Not all awkward children have similar patterns of abilities and disabilities. Screening tests such as the Stott are useful in this respect (Stott, Moyes, & Henderson, 1984). Screenings of large groups may be followed up with more thorough work-ups for children identified as well below the norm (Sugden, 1985).

Additionally, the evaluation can concentrate upon various movement qualities discussed earlier, as well as the product of the child's movement (e.g., how far he or she can throw). Figure 12.5 illuminates three dimensions that may be considered in evaluating awkward children: (a) the mechanics of execution, (b) the task as executed, and (c) general qualities. This matrix also lists some of the motor tasks that might be evaluated.

Figure 12.5   Dimensions of Motor Problems in Children

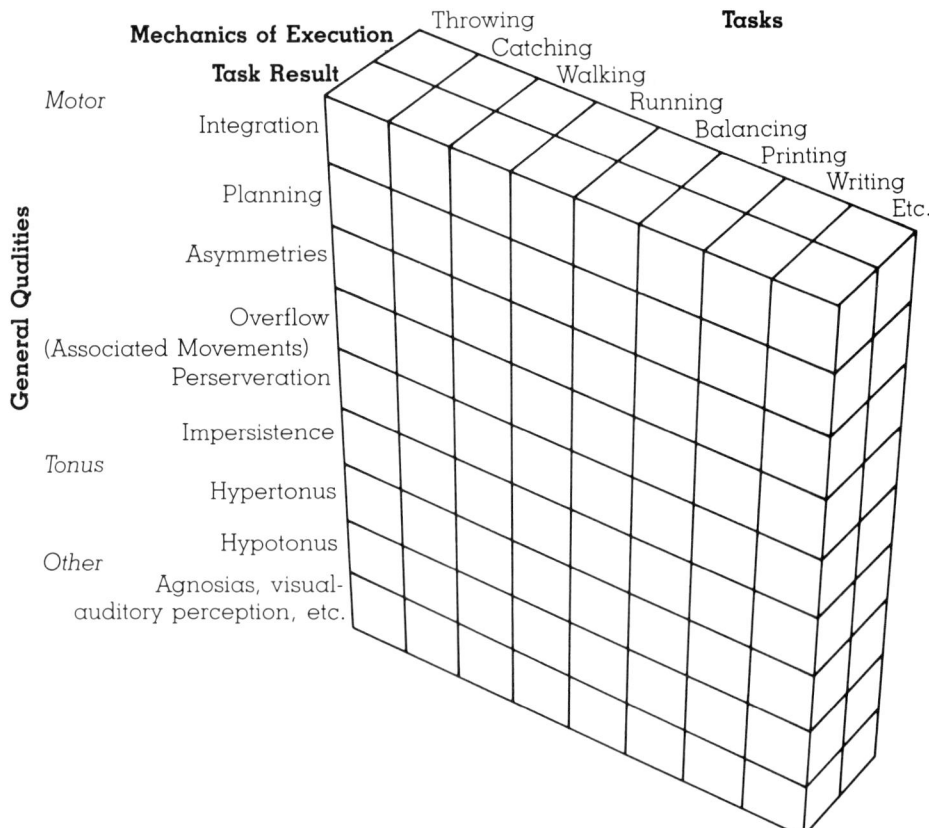

The decisions that physical education teachers should make based on the concepts and qualities in Figure 12.5 and the results of tests administered to children relate to the following questions:

1. Given the chronological ages of the children and youth in my charge, what activities are appropriate, and what developmental activities should be administered to improve their skills, relative to the performance of others of a similar age?

2. How can I correct the general problems that appear in more than one motor task?

3. How many sports skills versus basic developmental activities (e.g., balance beam walking) can I teach children of a given age and social sophistication?

4. How might I introduce developmental activities, such as agility drills, into a game that has a high degree of social value in the eyes of the children and youth with whom I am dealing?

5. How many types of activities should I introduce within a given, often limited time period?

Some of these decisions might be made after you have expanded the matrix in Figure 12.5 to a checklist, such as that shown in Table 12.1.

Table 12.1   Dimensions of Throwing: A Checklist

General Qualities	Behavior
Integration of body parts	Forward step with leg/foot opposite to throwing arm/hand. Note weight shift during release.
Motor Planning (Praxic behavior)	Body segments brought into use in proper order—foot, through leg, hip, waist, to shoulder/arm in spiral-shaped pattern.
Asymmetries	In two-handed push or throw, one hand may push too much.
Overflow (Associated movements)	Extraneous tensions in face; flopping of arms after release.
Perseveration	Unable to easily adapt to different throwing task demands for speed, distance, accuracy, etc.
Impersistence	Cannot maintain a constant, reliable effort when task demands remain the same or similar.
Hypotonia	Difficulty throwing hard, or far; difficulty in expressing effort.
Hypertonia	Bursts of effort result in ball being thrown too hard relative to demands; cannot vary force; cannot throw softly.
Mechanics of Execution	Appropriate weight shift as ball is released. Rotation of body and at shoulders, relaxed, well timed release from hand.
Task Result	Throwing accuracy and/or distance appropriate for age group.

After identifying specific areas of difficulty, the evaluation should translate into program guidelines. The specific areas should be dealt with individually, as transfer from one skill area to another cannot be expected. We have found that transfer will not occur, for example, between fine- and gross-motor skills. If a child has printing deficiencies and throwing difficulties, these must be worked on separately. Work on larger muscle groups will not aid manipulation or fine-motor skills. And transfer between many gross motor skills may not occur. We have found that intercepting balls swinging on a string does not correlate with intercepting balls bounced to children. Although more transfer may occur with younger or less able children, practice in specific skills is usually more productive.

Periodic reassessment is needed both in culturally desirable activities such as throwing and catching balls and in more basic qualities such as balance. This kind of reassessment, mandated by law in the U.S., should occur at approximately 6-month intervals.

Prognosis

Remarkably little research has been done to determine if changes can be elicited in motor coordination and control through training efforts. What work that has taken place indicates, first, that training effects should be highly individualistic. Some children improve rapidly, and others seem resistant to change. A student of mine recently tried to change the throwing patterns of 5-year-old girls. Some changed, and some did not. In research I have conducted over the years, younger children have been found to change more markedly than older ones when exposed to a program of remedial motor education (Cratty, Ikeda, Martin, Jennett, & Morris, 1970).

Second, children with subtle and slight problems change more than those who have obvious signs of central nervous system involvement reflecting some type of mild or moderate cerebral palsy. Third, the emotional-social climate in which the child lives, as well as the emotional environment within the remedial program, is critical. In the programs we have administered, children sometimes have been suddenly removed from a program when their parents saw progress! The parent or caregiver should be carefully informed and counseled regarding the program's aims and objectives. Family counseling by emotional health specialists may be necessary when subtle parental needs to overprotect the child come in conflict with program efforts to elicit change (and thus to promote more independent behaviors by an overprotected youngster).

The social environment may have to be readjusted to provide more positive feedback. I have often recommended that a child change schools, if possible, after he or she has improved in some obvious aspect. In this way the child can leave behind his or her reputation for being clumsy. The child's original school environment and peers tend to perpetuate that image, which makes the improvement more difficult to maintain and continue.

Most important, parents must be made acutely aware of any improvement so that they will modify their expectations and social judgments accordingly. A child who improves but whose parents, family, and peers remain negatively judgmental, is almost doomed to further failure. These attitudes should never be underestimated in planning for a child's improvement.

SUMMARY

After World War II, interest in awkward children heightened, primarily because many believed that remedying physical awkwardness would improve deficient academic ability and performance. By the 1980s, however, clear-headed educators, heeding the evidence focusing upon perceptual-motor training programs, began to perceive that (a) physical awkwardness was not necessarily associated with academic deficiencies and that helping a child to move better would not invariably provide an easy way to improve reading skills, (b) physical awkwardness was an important deficit to focus upon in and of itself, and (c) physically awkward children often display a number of other qualities such as dysgraphia (the inability to write or print well) and emotional effects including lower self-concept.

These kinds of observations have led to two helpful outcomes. Penetrating looks are directed at the qualities surrounding physical awkwardness, including emotional overcomes (Wall, McClements, Bouffard, Findlay, & Taylor, 1985). A further and most helpful trend has been the development of more and more useful instruments to evaluate physical awkwardness at younger and younger ages (Harris, Halty, Tada, & Swanson, 1984; Noller & Ingrisano, 1984), as well as instruments to assess possible clumsiness in children within the middle childhood years (Hughes & Riley, 1981; Stott et al., 1984).

The causes of awkwardness are many and often are difficult to determine, as they may be interrelated. Physical ineptitude can stem from a mild type of cerebral palsy, from an endocrine abnormality, or from malnutrition or an environment that simply does not allow for normal physical movement. It can be related to a visual defect or to a neurological abnormality. It can be part of a syndrome. It has been associated with learning disabilities. For this reason, a battery of carefully selected assessment and evaluation instruments is needed, along with possible input from a physician, to know how best to proceed.

An awkward child not only displays obvious signs of ineptitude, including the inability to apply proper biomechanics and to produce the proper performance outcomes (e.g., throwing with accuracy and for distance) but also evidences a range of subtle movement problems including:

—*problems in integration of body parts* (left and right, upper and lower, etc.)
—*apraxia, or motor planning problems* (the inability to replicate a series of movements)
—*asymmetries* (subtle differences in the efficiency with which each side of the body and limbs are employed)
—*overflow, or associated movements* (tension carryover from a part of the body used in a task to another part that is not used)
—*perseveration* (inflexibility in transferring from one task to another)
—*impersistence* (inability to maintain a position of a limb or other body part)
—*hypotonicity* and *hypertonicity* (inappropriate tension levels, either too low or too high)
—*tremor, unsteadiness,* and *imbalance* (reflecting possible neurological conditions such as that found in cerebral palsy)

—*dysgraphia* (a disorder in writing/printing skills that is also cognitive in nature and has been identified as a specific learning disability)

—*sensory problems* or *agnosias* (manifested in an inability to locate the body or any of its parts in space or in relation to other things)

—*perceptual problems*, visual or auditory (caused by a defect in one of the bodily senses that relates to movement and physical skills).

Motorically unskilled, awkward youngsters often have gaps in their emotional-social development attributable to their physical deficiencies. Not only may they not get along with others at play, but they may even devise a number of compensations to avoid negative attention from peers and others.

Physical educators and other motor development specialists have an obligation to provide a motor learning environment that promotes both physical and social-emotional success in awkward children. In addition, they should seek to gain the support of parents and families in an effort to reduce negative reactions toward clumsy children. The sensory aspects should be addressed along with the motor aspects, although getting a child corrective lenses or other aids cannot be expected to produce a magical transformation. And evaluation instruments should be carefully selected in assessing and programming for individualized activities that will promote specific skills.

Finally, as recent writers have pointed out, awkward children may lack adequate knowledge of how to move and about the nature of action in general (Wall et al., 1985). Thus, a comprehensive approach to the remediation of movement difficulties should include straightforward efforts to change movement results and qualities, help with parallel feelings of inadequacy and other emotional overtones stemming from a failure to do well in culturally important tasks, and attention to the meta-cognitive aspects of movement experiences. Helping awkward children to think about how to perform better may be as useful as trying to teach them in traditional ways to perform more efficiently (David, 1985).

REFERENCES

Abercrombie, M.L.J., Linden, R.L., & Tyson, M.G. (1964). Associated movements in physically handicapped children. *Developmental Medicine & Child Neurology, 6*, 573-579.

Barsch, R. (1965). *Achieving perceptual-motor efficiency* (Vol. 1). Seattle: Special Child Publications.

Cohen, H.J., Lawrence, T.T., Mahadeviah, M.S., & Birch, H.G. (1967). Developmental changes in overflow in normal and aberrantly functioning children. *Journal of Pediatrics, 71*, 39-47.

Connolly, K., & Stratton, P. (1968). Developmental changes in associated movements. *Developmental Medicine & Child Neurology, 10*, 49-56.

Cornish, S.V. (1980). Development of a test of motor planning ability. *Physical Therapy, 60*, 1129-1132.

Cratty, B.J. (1969). *Perceptual-motor behavior and educational processes.* Springfield, IL: Charles C Thomas.

Cratty, B.J. (1984). *From scribbling to printing: Guidelines for beginning handwriting skills.* Los Angeles: IMED Publications.

Cratty, B.J. (1986). Qualitative changes in movement behaviors. Ch. 9 in B.J. Cratty, *Perceptual and motor development in infants and children* (3rd ed.). Englewood Cliffs, NJ: Prentice-Hall.

Cratty, B.J., Ikeda, N., Martin, M.M., Jennett, C., & Morris, M. (1970). *Movement activities, motor ability and the education of children.* Springfield, IL: Charles C Thomas.

Cratty, B.J., & Samoy, L. (1984). Ein vergleich praxischer verhaltensweisen bei bjahrigen kindern [A comparison of praxic behaviors in young children]. *Motorik, 7*, 52-58.

David, I.S. (1985). Motor sequencing strategies in school-age children. *Physical Therapy, 65*, 883-889.

Delacato, C.H. (1963). *Neurological organization and reading.* Springfield, IL: Charles C Thomas.

Fog, E., & Fog, M. (1963). Cerebral inhibition examined by associated movements in minimal cerebral dysfunction. *Clinics in Developmental Medicine* (No. 10). London: Spastics Society.

Getman, G. (1962). *How to develop your child's intelligence.* Luverne, MN: Research Publications.

Gubbay, S.S. (1978). The management of developmental apraxia. *Developmental Medicine & Child Neurology, 20*, 643-646.

Hammill, D.D., Goodman, L., & Wiederholt, J.L. (1974). Visual-motor processes: Can we train them? *Reading Teacher, 27*, 469-478.

Harris, S.R., Halty, S.M., Tada, W.L., & Swanson, M.W. (1984). Reliability of observational measures of the movement assessment of infants. *Physical Therapy, 64*, 471-475.

Hirsch, S.M., & Anderson, R.P. (1976). The effects of perceptual motor training on reading achievement. In R.P. Anderson & C.G. Halcomb (Eds.), *Learning disability/minimal brain dysfunction syndrome.* Springfield, IL: Charles C Thomas.

Hopft, H.C., Schlegal, H.J., & Lowitzsch, K. (1974). Irridiation of voluntary activity to the contra-lateral side in movements of normal subjects and patients with central motor disturbances. *European Neurology, 12*, 142-147.

Hughes, J.E., & Riley, A. (1981). Basic gross motor assessment: Tool for use with children having minor motor dysfunction. *Physical Therapy, 61*, 503-511.

Kavale, K., & Mattson, P. (1983). One jumped off the balance beam: Meta-analysis of perceptual-motor training. *Journal of Learning Disabilities, 16*, 166-173.

Kephart, N.C. (1962). *The slow learner in the classroom.* Columbus, OH: Charles E. Merrill.

Noica, A. (1912). Etude sur les mouvements associes. *Encephale, 7*, 201-221.

Noller, K., & Ingrisano, D. (1984). Cross-sectional study of gross and fine motor development. *Physical Therapy, 64*, 308-313.

Stott, D.H., Moyes, F.A., & Henderson, S.E. (1984). *Test of motor impairment: Henderson revision.* Guelph, Ontario: Brook Educational Publications.

Strauss, A.A., & Lehtinen, C.E. (1947). *Psychopathology and education of the brain injured child.* New York: Grune & Stratton.

Sugden, D. (1985). Review of the Test of Motor Impairment: Henderson Revision. *Adapted Physical Activity Quarterly, 2*, 167-169.

Waber, D.P., Mann, M.B., & Merola, J. (1985). Motor overflow and attentional processes in normal school-age children. *Developmental Medicine & Child Neurology, 27*, 491-497.

Wall, A.E., McClements, J., Bouffard, M., Findlay, H., & Taylor, M.J. (1985). A knowledge-based approach to motor development: Implications for the physically awkward. *Adapted Physical Activity Quarterly, 2*, 21-42.

Wolff, P.H., Gunnoe, C.E., & Cohen, C. (1983). Associated movements as a measure of developmental age. *Developmental Medicine & Child Neurology, 25*, 417-425.

Zulch, K.L. (1942). *Die mitbewegungen bei hirneverletzten zentralblatt fur neurochirurgie, 7*, 160-186.

ADDITIONAL REFERENCES

Arnheim, D., & Sinclair, W. (1979). The clumsy child. St. Louis: C.V. Mosby.

Cratty, B.J. (1975). *Remedial motor activity for children*. Philadelphia: Lea & Febiger.

Dare, M.T., & Gordon, N. (1970). Clumsy children: A disorder of perception and motor organization. *Developmental Medicine & Child Neurology, 12,* 178-185.

Gubbay, S.S. (1975). *The clumsy child: A study of developmental praxia and agnostic ataxia.* Philadelphia: W.B. Saunders.

QUESTIONS FOR DISCUSSION

1. What does *apraxia* mean? How might it be evaluated? What might be done to improve the condition?

2. What does *agnosia* mean? What are some types of *agnosias*? How do they specifically affect performance in a physical education class?

3. What kinds of assessment principles and instruments might you use when instigating a movement remediation program for the awkward children within an elementary school? How many awkward children might populate a program in a school whose total enrollment is 1,000?

4. What kinds of social compensations do awkward children seem to use when confronted with play/recreation situations requiring physical skill? Which of these, if any, may be more socially acceptable than others?

5. What kinds of *qualitative* changes in movement skills may be necessary to help a child improve in motor performance and look better when performing? How might these qualities be improved?

6. Might a child labeled "clumsy" function well within one family and be subjected to derision and ridicule within another? Could the same child be subjected to different kinds of social demands and stresses in different elementary schools? Why?

STUDENT PROJECTS

1. Visit an elementary school playground and observe children who seem to be "fringers"—avoiding vigorous play. How are they acting and what kinds of social compensations are they using? Check with their teachers relative to popularity, self-confidence, and their participation in formal physical education lessons.

2. Ask an elementary school teacher to single out two or three children who are most uncoordinated. Observe these children at play. If possible, expose them to several age-appropriate physical tasks to see if their throwing, balance, and similar skills are what is to be expected for children their age.

3. Using a book on perceptual-motor development (the one by Cratty (1986) comes to mind!), formulate a checklist similar to the one in this chapter. Use it in a convenient elementary school, surveying a class of your choice. Try to identify children with movement problems and who might benefit from extra help in motor abilities. (Be sure to obtain parental and school permission for your project.)

4. Interview the parent(s) of a child who has been identified as clumsy or awkward. Discuss any difficulties the child seems to be having with peers and in other aspects of his or her life. How have family members, including brothers and sisters, reacted to the problem? Is the problem specific to large muscle groups, or do handwriting and fine-motor control seem to be part of the picture? How does the child seem to deal with it?

13 *Brain Injuries and Cerebral Palsy*

Injuries to the central nervous system may involve either the brain or the spinal cord, or both. Unlike the degenerative diseases discussed in the next chapter, the conditions discussed in this chapter are a result of a trauma or insult to the central nervous system in which the effects may be permanent but do not worsen except in relation to secondary complications resulting from restricted movements and so forth. The manifestations are related to the point of trauma, its severity, age at occurrence, and many other variables. Thus, the range of potential repercussions is wide, and the prognosis is variable, although individuals with this type of condition are generally considered good candidates for physical therapy. In fact, it often is mandatory in a program of intervention.

DEFINITIONS OF BRAIN INJURIES

Accidents, and sometimes intentional acts, can result in trauma to the brain. If the injury results in relatively stable symptoms of motor dysfunction, the diagnosis may include reference to cerebral palsy (discussed later in the chapter). Head injuries may be classified into two major groups: (a) *open-brain injuries*, involving some penetration of the skull and brain, and (b) *closed-brain injuries*, in which the skull is not penetrated but the blow to the head results in various intellectual, sensory, or motor dysfunctions. Penetrating head injuries often result from injuries incurred in wartime (Sweeney & Smutok, 1983) or as the result of a crime.

Both open and closed brain injuries fall under a broader category called *acquired brain injuries* (ABI), which also include cerebral vascular accidents (strokes), brain tumors, hypoxia, infections of the brain, and the results of intake of toxic substances (Consortium, 1987). In general, acquired brain injuries are triggered by *external events* or *internal events*.

Injuries from either penetration or a jolting of the brain result in damage at the point of penetration or contact, as well as damage across from the site of the impact. These secondary injuries and complications can include hemorrhages (hematomas or bleeds), edema (swelling in the white matter at the site of the lesion), diffuse brain swelling, ischemia (insufficient blood flow), or raised intracranial pressure. The point of contact is termed *coup*, and the point opposite to the point of contact (or penetration) is referred to as *contra coup*, as shown in Figure 13.1.

In closed-brain injuries rotational forces act upon the tissue causing a tearing, shearing, and sometimes a stretching of the axons that integrate all or most of the brain's functions. This phenomenon is called *diffuse axonal injury*, and its results include a wide variety of perceptual, cognitive, emotional, and motor disorders.

CHARACTERISTICS OF BRAIN INJURY

Head injury cases often present rather unique groups of social-emotional and physical symptoms. Adult victims often respond in emotionless, mechanical ways to their environments,

231

Figure 13.1   Physical Results of Brain Injury

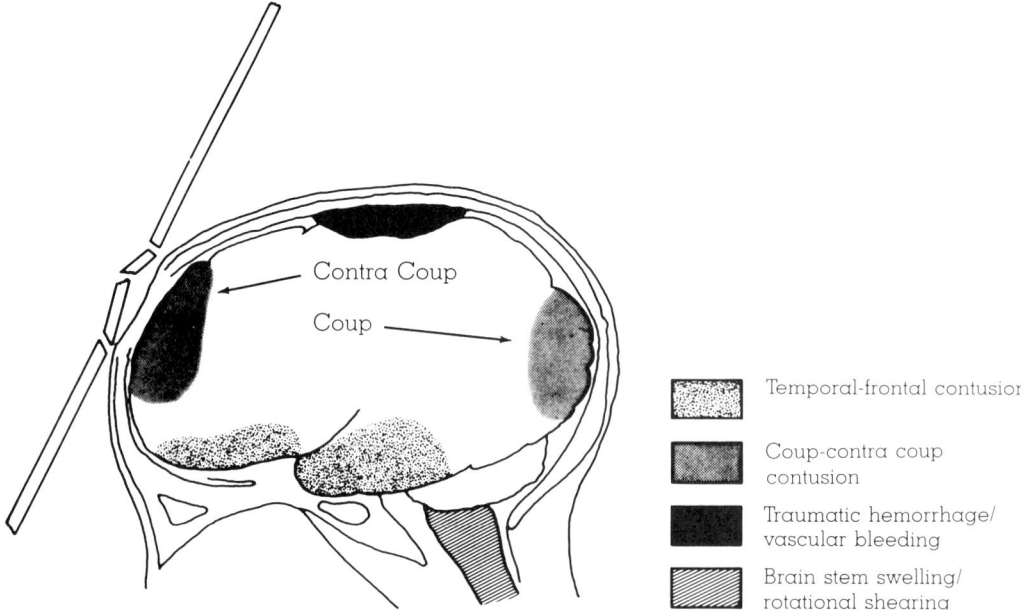

displaying a "robot syndrome," with symptoms that include depression, boredom, fears of attempting motor tasks that they once accomplished, and inactivity accompanied by overeating and weight gain (Mercer & Boch, 1983). The physical and sensory accompaniments to head trauma, as would be expected, depend upon the severity of the injury and its location. Symptoms might include hyperactivity and distractibility, as well as speech and language dysfunctions.

ASSESSMENT OF BRAIN INJURY

The severity of the injury shortly after the trauma, as well as the degree of recovery, are often assessed using the Glasgow Coma Scale (Jones, 1979), which evaluates the depth and severity of the initial coma, The scale, shown in Table 13.1, results in a score ranging from 3 ("none" in all categories—eye opening, motor response, and verbal response) to 15.

In addition, standard motor assessments are used. There is a moderate relationship between the depth of the coma and the eventual outcome, but age is the most critical factor in predicting recovery of functions. In several studies (for example, Heiden, Small, Caton, Weiss, & Kurze, 1983; Talmadge & Collins, 1983) recovery of functions, with the help of intense and useful therapy, has been far better in those under 20 years of age than if the injury had occurred after that time. For example, in the Heiden study 61% of the subjects 19 years and under evidenced either moderate disabilities or "good recovery" 1 year after the injury, whereas only 13% percent of those between 40 and 49 posted similar

Table 13.1   Glasgow Coma Scale

Assessment	Response	Score[*]
Eye opening (A score)	Spontaneous	4
	Speech	3
	Pain	2
	None	1
Motor response (B score)	Obey	6
	Localize	5
	Withdrawal	4
	Abnormal flexion	3
	Extension	2
	None	1
Verbal response	Oriented	5
	Confused conversation	4
	Inappropriate	3
	Incomprehensible	2
	None	1

[*]Responsiveness or coma sum = 3 to 15 points.

Note. From "Glasgow Coma Scale," by C. Jones, 1979, *American Journal of Nursing, 79,* pp. 1551-1553.

Table 13.2   Five-Category Glasgow Outcome Scale

1. Death	
2. Vegetative state	Not obeying commands or vocalizing, spontaneous eye movements, sucking and chewing reflexes, occasional visual tracking, and stereotyped motor responses.
3. Severe disability	Awake and dependent, assisted for activities of daily living, major cognitive or physical problems or both.
4. Moderate disability	Independent but disabled, independent in activities of daily living and some independence in home and community skills, vocational goals limited to lower level of responsibility, and residual problems such as cognitive changes, impaired communication skills, motor skills, or balance problems persist.
5. Good recovery	Able to pursue normal occupational and social activities with minor physical deficits or complaints.

recovery rates. All of the 26 subjects over 60 were either dead or remained in a coma ("persistent vegetative state") a year later. Of those in the age 20-39 category, slightly over 40% had a good or moderate recovery, based on the Glasgow Outcome Scale (Jones, 1979), shown in Table 13.2.

A study of head-injured patients by Talmadge and Collins (1983) also found that age 20 seemed to be the "positive limit for complete recovery" and age 40 seemed to be the positive limit for survival alone. Other factors influencing recovery included the individual's level of functioning before the accident, cardiovascular measures and the amount of blood loss, and other trauma incurred at the time of the injury (Talmadge & Collins, 1983).

In recent years hospitals, as well as independent medical-therapy units, have become better equipped to deal with the results of head trauma, including the socio-emotional overtones and vocational retraining needs of victims. Physical therapy efforts often have to begin with simple sensory stimulation, together with assistance in the simple actions of infants— turning, sitting, kneeling, and finally walking. Moreover, visual processes may have been lost, and maybe language and speech as well. Indeed many of the suggestions found in chapter 25 (Infant Stimulation) are useful for application to individuals with head injuries.

DEFINITION AND INCIDENCE OF CEREBRAL PALSY

The term *cerebral palsy*—coined in the 1930s by Dr. Winthrop Phelps, an orthopedic surgeon in Baltimore—literally means "brain paralysis." Although the public is aware of the condition, confusion often surrounds it. Cerebral palsy (CP) can be defined as a nonprogressive disorder of movement or posture, or both, resulting from one or more insults (injuries) to the central nervous system. Estimates of the incidence of cerebral palsy range from 1.7 to approximately 2.0 per 1,000 births—a figure difficult to formulate because of the difficulty of diagnosing mild forms of the condition as well as the lack of necessity to report cerebral palsy (unlike the necessity to report various communicable diseases and other infant and adult disorders). About 85% of the people afflicted with the various forms of cerebral palsy have had the condition since birth (an estimated 5,000 new cases each year), and a smaller percentage has similar symptoms because of accidents or damage caused by tumors later in life. Overall, about 700,000 U.S. residents have cerebral palsy.

CHARACTERISTICS OF CEREBRAL PALSY

Cerebral palsy is not a single dysfunction but, rather, a group of movement and posture disorders. These may be characterized by the locations of the body in which they are found, the specific types of dysfunction that occur, and the level of severity. Unlike some other crippling disorders that are manifested only in peripheral dysfunction, the central nature of cerebral palsy often brings with it associated problems of visual perception and learning, as well as auditory perception. Speech and language defects are present in about half of the children with cerebral palsy. These may be attributable to partial paralysis or incoordination of the speech apparatus itself or to the child's inability to organize and choose words correctly when speaking. Overall, about 30% of all cerebral palsied persons are likely to be mentally retarded, and 70% are classifiable as normal or above normal in intelligence.

Other problems accompanying the various types of cerebral palsy include personality disorders, with sometimes high levels of anxiety; drooling (because of a defective swallowing reflex); dental problems, including tooth malformations and cavities; sensory deficiencies, including those of touch; and poor body awareness.

A study by Winnick and Short (1982) produced results that contrasted the fitness and body composition of children with cerebral palsy with normal youngsters. The subjects consisted of 396 youngsters 10-17 years of age with cerebral palsy. Approximately 40% were confined to wheelchairs, and the others were ambulatory. Overall, the cerebral palsied children were not overly obese, based upon skin-fold measures comparing them with normal youngsters. When various measures of muscular strength were contrasted, however, the children with cerebral palsy were considerably inferior. Their fitness measures were 1-2 standard deviations below those of normal youngsters to whom they were contrasted. But test scores recorded by the cerebral palsied population in this study were highly variable—more variation than was seen in the scores of normal youngsters performing the same tests and tasks.

Some cerebral palsied children are susceptible to seizures, ranging from petit mal to grand mal in nature. Estimates of the percentage of these children subject to seizures range from about 15% to 60%. (Seizure disorders are discussed in chapter 15.)

Thus, cerebral palsy encompasses a wide array of symptoms and disorders that may be present in a given child. The physical educator or movement specialist should be prepared to deal with possible emotional, personality, and other affective components, as well as linguistic, sensory, and physical limitations when confronted with children and youth with this type of disorder.

CAUSES OF CEREBRAL PALSY

Cerebral palsy usually arises prior to and during birth, stemming from a variety of insults to the growing fetus and emerging neonate. In a few cases, cerebral palsy may even be inherited. Among the major causes, however, are various infections (usually German measles) occurring in the mother during the first 3 months of pregnancy. Sometimes a lack of sufficient oxygen at birth (because of knotting of the umbilical cord, shock resulting from blood loss by the mother, or trauma to the placenta) is a factor. Or Rh incompatibility (in which the mother's defenses manufacture antibodies that destroy the infant's red blood corpuscles, producing anemia, and the products of the blood cell destruction, when combined with the lack of oxygen, damage the brain) can be the cause of cerebral palsy.

Premature birth or a birth weight of 5 pounds or less constitute one of the main causes of cerebral palsy, accounting for 30% to 60% of the cases recorded in surveys carried out in the 1950s and 1960s. Prematurity can result in spastic diplegia, manifested neuroanatomically by damage to either side of the ventricles of the brain. Metabolic disorders in the mother (primarily diabetes) also may cause cerebral palsy in the infant. Finally, about 30% of all prenatal cerebral palsy is of unknown etiology, reflected in cerebral anomalies emerging during the first 12 weeks of pregnancy when fetal brain development is most rapid.

Cerebral palsy also can occur from trauma during and immediately after birth. Among the main causes during delivery are birth anoxia (lack of oxygen resulting from lung collapse or pneumonia), too much sedation, or physical trauma to the skull during delivery. The latter may be caused by the baby's being very large or born feet first or by a difficult or prolonged delivery. Birth anoxia can result in various types of spasticity, including quadriplegia (involvement of all four limbs) because of damage to the surface cells within the motor cortex of the brain.

Factors that may contribute to the various types of cerebral palsy after birth include head injuries from accidents or parental battering and brain infections and toxic conditions (e.g., encephalopathies, meningitis, lead poisoning). These conditions account for approximately 60% of postnatal cerebral palsy. Brain hemorrhages or clots after birth can cause cerebral palsy manifested on one side of the body (hemiplegia). Carbon monoxide poisoning, near drowning, stopping of the heart (cardiac arrest), and electric shock are other examples of traumatic conditions that may cause movement disorders of this type. Damage after a brain tumor has been removed also may result in cerebral palsy.

To compare the causes of cerebral palsy by age of onset:

—about 60% of all cases are perinatal (during birth) in origin.
—approximately 30% result from prenatal (before birth) factors.
—the remaining 10% can be attributed to postnatal factors.

CLASSIFICATIONS OF CEREBRAL PALSY

Classification by Body Parts Affected

Individuals having cerebral palsy are classified according to the bodily areas affected or predominantly involved, as depicted in Figure 13.2. At the same time, however, a pure monoplegic (or other type) is not likely, as the entire body usually is afflicted to some extent by the disorder. Therefore, the five definitions below refer to the primary characteristic of the cerebral palsied person.

Paraplegia involves the lower extremities only. Sometimes in children with mild signs of cerebral palsy, the lower limbs are relatively hypotonic, while the upper limbs may function better.

In *hemiplegia* involvement is on one side of the body, affecting both upper and lower limbs. Most often the right side is affected. Studies have indicated that the hemiplegic may be more employable later in life than individuals whose condition involves more than two limbs.

Triplegia refers to the involvement of three limbs—usually both legs and one arm.
Monoplegia means involvement of one limb only—a relatively rare occurrence.
Quadriplegia refers to involvement of all four extremities.

Figure 13.2   Cerebral Palsy as Defined by Body Part(s) Affected

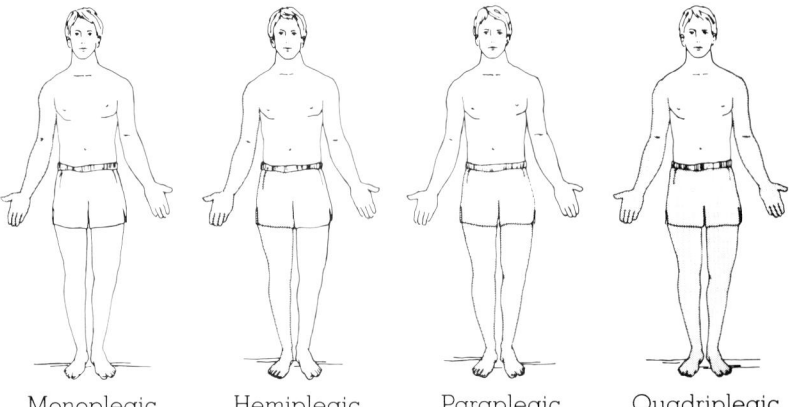

Monoplegic   Hemiplegic   Paraplegic   Quadriplegic

Neuromotor Classifications

Cerebral palsy has been classified by the nature of the atypical movements and postures exhibited. Six neuromotor classifications are recognized by the American Academy for Cerebral Palsy: (a) spasticity, (b) athetosis, (c) ataxia, (d) tremor, (e) rigidity, and (f) mixed. Approximately two thirds of all those with cerebral palsy are spastic; 20%-30% evidence some degree of athetosis; those with ataxia and rigidity account for only 8% and 4%, respectively. For the most part, those classified as mixed do not show a predominant type of movement. Most children with cerebral palsy show signs of more than one type, with spasticity and athetosis being the most prevalent combination.

Spasticity   The spastic person moves in a jerky manner. Movement seems to be characterized by an excess of muscular tension (hypertonia). When the prime movers of the joint (e.g., the biceps in the elbow flexion) are activated, the antagonistic muscles (in this case, the triceps) do not reflex and elongate normally, permitting movement to occur. The antagonistic muscles seem to recoil explosively, in what is termed a *clonus* phenomenon. When an arm reaches upward, for example, it suddenly jerks back involuntarily.

Other movements and postures typical of the spastic individual include an arm that is almost locked in a pronated position, a fist clasped in an unwanted ball, a leg that is chronically flexed (a condition that may have to be surgically modified). Contractures of the lower limbs, accompanied by inward rotation of the leg at the hip joint, result in a *scissoring gait*. This may prevent a child from ever walking because of the tendency of the large head of the femur to dislocate (subluxate) from the hip.

Chronic tension is manifested in generalized ways throughout the body and may be triggered by a noise, a touch, or a condition that results in emotional excitement. Thus, a calm, gentle approach in a teaching situation is more likely to be productive, as are reasonable goals and requests to "go slowly" or "relax," than are instructions to "do your best" or "move fast." The latter directions probably will exaggerate the already excessively hypertonic condition rather than reduce hypertonus to a point that encourages voluntary movements and postures.

From a neuroanatomical standpoint, the spastic child usually has damage to the cells on the surface of the cerebral cortex, which controls voluntary movements of the limbs. Damage to these cells and the nerve fibers within the motor cortex results in *spastic paralysis*.

Among spastic types, spastic diplegia is the most common (Taft, 1985). As might be expected, spastic diplegics have a difficult time in the beginning stages of locomotion. They can move through space only by the end of the first year if their condition is not too grave (Largo & Molinari, 1985). Recently, spastic diplegics have been using elastic braces made of flexible webbing. These assistive devices, less bulky than previous ones, are helpful adjuncts to more moderate therapeutic techniques now being employed (Nuzzo, 1980).

Spastic quadriplegia is caused by degeneration of the surface cells of the cortex. Spastic hemiplegia results from an enlarged cavity or cyst in the brain (porencephaly).

As might be expected, spastic children are limited physically, and at times emotionally. They are frequently fearful, and this fear further reduces their capacities to move (Scrutton, 1984). Often this fear prevents them from leaving the security of others, including their parents, and participating actively with peers. Some observers have noted that spastic persons tend to be rather compulsive in nature and become annoyed at deviations from

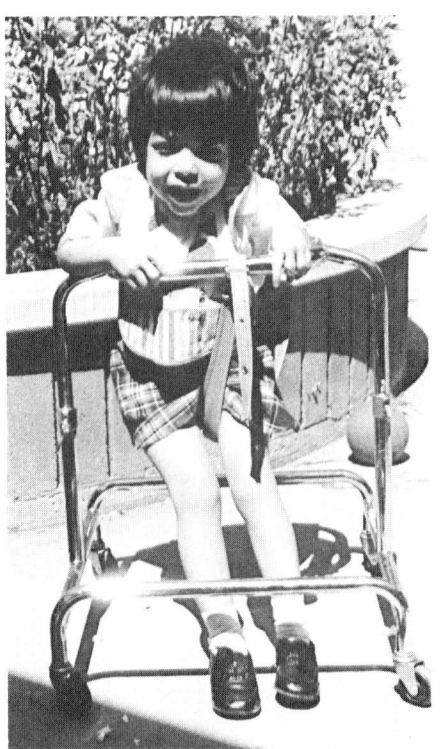

Walkers help cerebral palsied children who are otherwise nonambulatory to achieve upright independence.

Courtesy, Special Education Branch, Los Angeles City Schools

a fixed routine. Intellectually, 20%-25% of spastic students can be expected to possess intelligence above the average for normal children (Katz, 1968). Therefore, educators should not assume inferior learning capabilities based upon physical manifestations of cerebral palsy.

Athetosis   The athetoid person seems like an out-of-tune orchestra—each instrument (muscle) playing its own melody relatively independent of the others. Movements are random, apparently purposeless, often slow, and snake-like. Many younger individuals with athetosis have difficulty even holding their heads up, much less walking. Those who acquire locomotion later must mentally pre-program even the simplest movement prior to attempting its execution. A turn of the head may result in an arm suddenly extending—evidence of failure to suppress the asymmetrical tonic neck reflex. Conversely, in attempting a reaching movement, the head may be jerked away from the outstretched arm. As would be expected, eye movements are not well coordinated.

Frustration accompanies even the simplest activities of life. Some athetoid children have been noted to have obsessive-compulsive traits. Sometimes they have trouble adapting to new situations. They may at times exhibit explosive behavior, as well as other signs of emotional instability. It can be argued that emotional problems in the athetoid (as well as in other types) are caused by the negative feedback they receive from their own movement efforts, as well as from the social context in which they attempt to function. Some also suggest that the psychic instability may stem from concomitant damage to the emotional center of the brain (hypothalamus).

Specifically, three kinds of movements are seen to various degrees in an athetoid child—who, for the most part, tends to be affected in all four limbs:

1. *Intermittent muscular spasms* occur in a predictable pattern and are triggered by changes of head position due to the influence of tonic labyrinthine reflexes. These patterns may end with the child in a fixed position—usually extreme flexion or extension.

2. In *moving spasms* the limbs may alternate in pronation and supination, causing "pawing" of the ground with one foot or uncontrollable stepping (the "athetoid dance"); these movements are often rhythmic in nature.

3. *Brief, localized contractions* can appear in all muscle groups and, if strong enough, can produce exaggerated, bizarre grimaces of the face, as well as unusual movements of the arms and hands. If these localized movements are limited in scope and weaker, they may appear as minor twitches.

These types of involuntary activities make certain voluntary movements difficult or even impossible.

Ataxia   A more subtle type of cerebral palsy, ataxia often does not make itself known until the child begins to walk. The gait is unsteady, and the child's first efforts at drawing reveal a rhythmic periodicity—a "printout" almost like that obtained from an electrocardiogram. Shaky, unsteady movements may appear in the lower limbs, in the upper limbs (when the child is printing), or in both upper and lower parts of the body. Mild forms of ataxia often are undiagnosed in children within a normal school population.

The finite coordination mediated by the cerebellum, when disrupted, is assumed to result in ataxic behaviors. The child may have both kinesthetic and vestibular inadequacies and thus may tend to fall when running, run into things (and other children) in the classroom, and otherwise evidence typical behaviors of an awkward or clumsy child (discussed in chapter 12).

Ataxic movements often appear in a young child who at first may seem only to be lacking good muscle tone (hypotonic). Often, marked improvement in motor performance (e.g., printing) of the mildly ataxic child may be elicited by helping the child to adopt strategies such as anchoring the arm and wrist, that provide a more stable base from which to execute movements. Pure ataxics are relatively rare (about 8% of all those with cerebral palsy), although in a mild form ataxic motor behavior may be more prevalent than current literature suggests.

Figure 13.3 shows the locations within the brain associated with the first three types of cerebral palsy—spasticity, athetosis, and ataxia. It also gives examples of how a child with each of these three types of cerebral palsy might draw a line from one point to another.

Tremor   The limbs of all normal humans vibrate in usually undetectable oscillations. The limbs of the cerebral palsied child diagnosed as "tremor type," however, shake in an ob-

Figure 13.3   Neuromotor Classifications of Cerebral Palsy

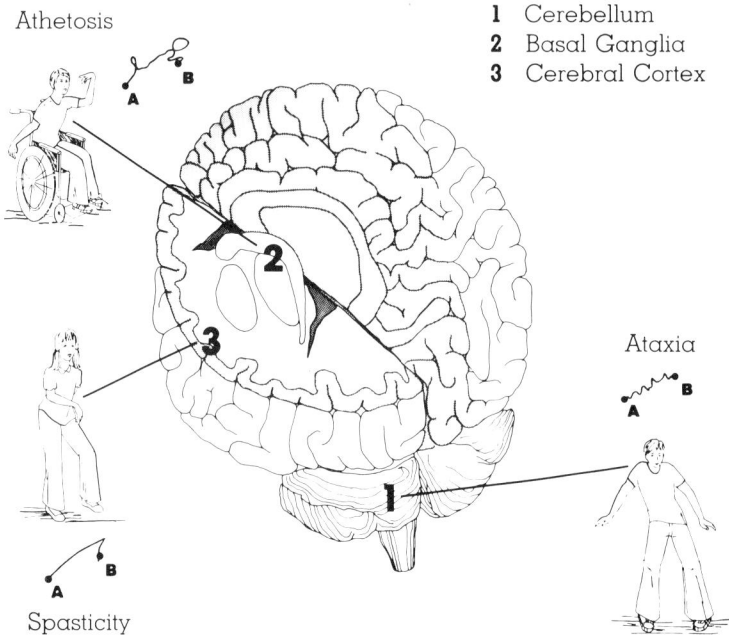

1   Cerebellum
2   Basal Ganglia
3   Cerebral Cortex

Note. Next to each illustration is the type of line each might draw from point A to point B.

vious manner. In more severe forms these tremors may produce either abnormally heightened or greatly reduced muscle tone (dystonia). Like other forms of cerebral palsy, these tremors may produce parallel postural conditions involving heightened curves of the lower back (lordosis) or a C- or S-shaped curve in the spinal column (scoliosis).

Rigidity   Rigid muscular behavior is not only a classification of cerebral palsy but also may be a form of Parkinson's disease. A rigid type of cerebral palsy is always associated with severe mental retardation. The child may be fixed in positions so rigid that the joints cannot be moved manually (lead-pipe rigidity) or in positions that do permit some movement if the child is assisted manually by a therapist (the cogwheel phenomenon). Generally, a physical education teacher will not deal with rigidity, which is seen in only a few of the cerebral palsied.

Mixed Type   Many children diagnosed as cerebral palsied do not exhibit pure types of pathological movements. When no one kind predominates, the condition is classified as mixed. This category has been used less in recent years. Many children in the mixed group are among the multiply handicapped or severely retarded.

Classification by Severity

Minear (1956) suggested a classification system based on the severity of cerebral palsy. The physical educator might consider this system when developing appropriate activities.

The four classifications are:

1. Individuals with a practical limitation of activities. These people have slight symptoms that result in subtle signs of awkwardness; they may be found within so-called normal populations. At times these children do not have a formal label of cerebral palsy attached to them.

2. Individuals with slight to moderate limitation of activity. These children and youth may be exposed to many regular physical education activities with only slight modifications.

3. Individuals with moderate to great limitations of activity. Many children and youth within this population are confined to wheelchairs and require considerable modification in activities. Most of the activities in this chapter are for persons within this category.

4. Individuals unable to carry out any useful activity. For the most part, these people need the careful and constant efforts of well trained therapists and assistants to help them carry out basic functions such as eating and elimination. Physical education teachers usually are not involved in their care or training.

PHYSICAL EDUCATION PROGRAMMING

General Principles and Guidelines

When working with brain-injured or cerebral palsied children, one must keep in mind the total complex of their potential emotional, social, intellectual, perceptual, and sensory disabilities and abilities. Physical education teachers should, in all cases, complement the aims of the physical therapist and other professionals treating the child. They should be conversant with the general principles and main techniques underlying some of the more popular theories of muscle reeducation. The theories of Bobath, Kabat, Gillette, Dreves, and Fay-Doman are among those most employed. Many times these techniques are combined in an eclectic manner.

Physical education teachers should avoid activities that muscularly or emotionally work against the child's best interests. Activities that are too highly arousing should be avoided, as additional excitation is likely to thwart the attempts of athetoid and spastic children to control their movements and direct their efforts toward useful skills. Most important, P.E. teachers should avoid activities that call for movements and efforts opposite to those that are useful to the children. For example, activities adding tension to the musculature that rotates inward and abducts the femur should be avoided. Tasks such as rope climbing (in which the rope is squeezed between the legs) and the elementary backstroke (in which the legs are squeezed inward during the kick) or walking narrow beams or lines (to help balance) also should be avoided, as they involve a feet-together gait and may cause dislocation of the femur at the hip. Figure 13.4 illustrates this concept.

Physical education teachers should select approaches and activities that contribute to the psychological, as well as the physical, well-being of their students. Thus, initial attempts to introduce an activity should be motivating and could include taking an instant picture of the individuals practicing a new activity or beside a piece of apparatus. When looking at the picture, they may identify with the game or sport. The sports and activities should, if possible, resemble those of individuals with normal movement capacities. Most

Figure 13.4   Dislocation of Femur at Hip Caused by Scissoring Gait

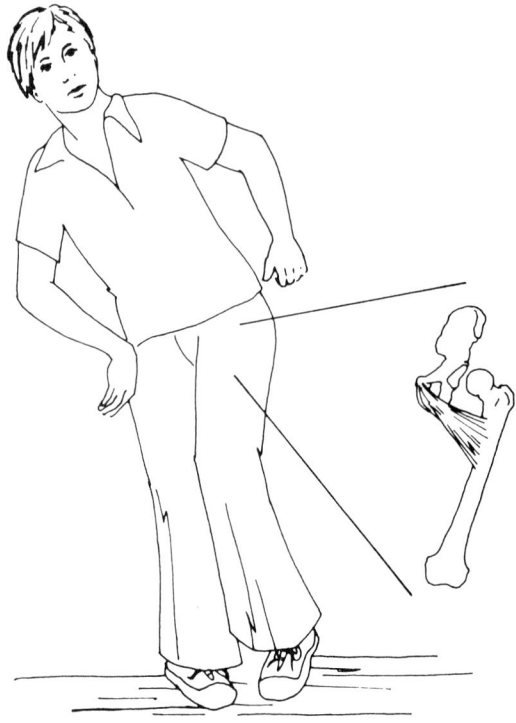

important, students who are able to do so should be encouraged to participate to the limit of their capacity and not be relegated to scorekeeping or watching.

Advancements

New teaching techniques and therapeutic technologies that have been employed to help children move better include the careful use of *behavioral modification* (Hill, 1985). Moreover, *biofeedback* in the form of auditory cues has been used with positive results when attempting to change the asymmetrical gait of the hemiplegic child to one that can be maintained after the training has been completed (Seeger, Caudrey, & Scholes, 1981).

Perhaps the most innovative—as well as a most pleasurable—form of therapy involves horses. Not only do the children have fun, but they also acquire vestibular and neuromotor stimulation, and the horse itself can be considered a "moving therapy platform." In the latter case the child is placed in various positions on the horse's back, and as the animal walks, various kinds of exercise and movements are attempted (Haskins, Bream, & Erdman, 1982).

Treatment models are becoming more eclectic, drawing from several of the traditional theories of rehabilitation (Levitt, 1982). Individual differences in the kinesthetic abilities and emotional characteristics of children with various types of central nervous system damage are resulting in modifications of therapeutic approaches that may have much relevance and validity (Opila-Lehman & Short, 1985). New and useful surgical techniques, as well as improved and innovative orthotic devices for stabilizing and aiding ankle and foot movements while walking, are aiding therapists in their work (Ireland & Hoffer, 1985; Barto, 1984).

One new surgical technique, called *selective posterior rhizotomy*, involves selecting and severing the appropriate sensory nerves in the lower spinal cord to reduce spasticity. Figure 13.5 illustrates this procedure, refined by Dr. Warrick Peacock of UCLA. For decades surgery has been performed to relieve excess muscular tension in spastics, but the objective was usually to lengthen hamstrings and heel tendons to facilitate walking. Therefore, this new operation is a major advance in managing spasticity and, with further refinements, even more relief from spasticity is foreseen.

The technique has been performed with stroke patients, those with spinal cord injuries, and some persons with degenerative neural conditions, but the most success seems to derive from the procedure when it is used with spastic cerebral palsied children who are relatively free of other debilitating conditions. Those most likely to be helped are ones who have not had previous surgery for their disorder, whose emotional stability is good, and whose motivation and intelligence are average to good.

Figure 13.5   Selective Posterior Rhizotomy

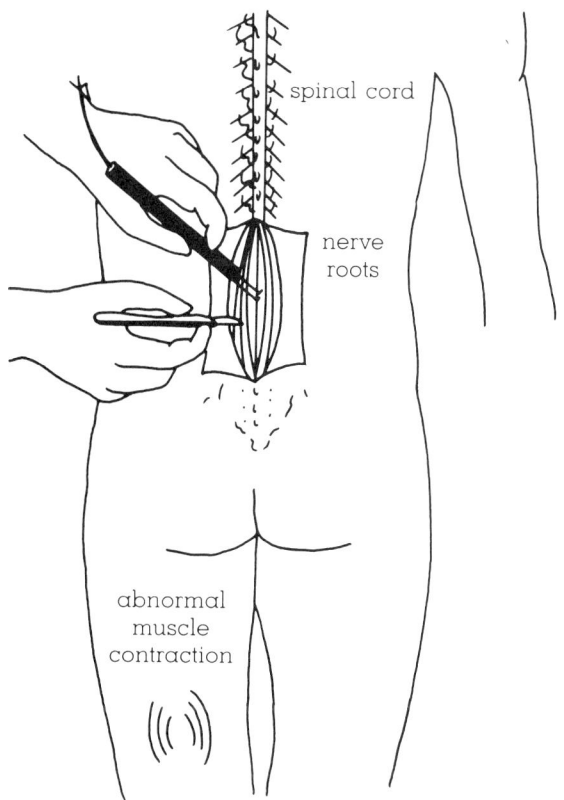

The reduction of spasticity assists therapists in producing desired pre-locomotion tasks and, in some cases, locomotion itself. It reduces therapists' need to manually inhibit abnormal muscle tone, allowing therapy to focus on helping learned behaviors. The facilitation of normal movement patterns is begun shortly after surgery is completed, under a strict protocol. Therapists have begun to describe which therapeutic strategies are most useful in post-operation habilitation (Irwin-Carruthers, 1985; Elk, 1984). The therapy emphasizes correct kinesthetic input.

Specific Activities

A number of specific physical activities are potentially helpful and can be implemented in a physical education class. All of the activities suggested here should not necessarily be imposed on all children with brain damage or cerebral palsy, because manifestations are so widely varied. The specialist ministering to the child and the physician who has jurisdiction over the case should be consulted when planning and implementing any activity program.

Body-Image Games   Many authorities, including the Bobaths, believe that children with cerebral palsy in particular lack an adequate awareness of exactly what movements their bodies are making or are capable of making, as well as the locations and names of various body parts and body movements. The concepts and body perceptions that may be worked on directly or indirectly include the following:

1. "Name Your Body Parts." The child may be asked to touch (or to name as the physical education teacher touches) the various parts of the body. The parts of the face, the hands, feet, and limbs are easiest to locate. The more difficult parts are the elbows, shoulders, knees, and specific fingers. The body planes are good to work on also. The child may be asked to point to them, or to say which part is touching the surface of the floor or may be touching the wall as the child assumes a standing position. Again, the body planes that can be clearly seen, such as the stomach, are easiest. Next in order of difficulty is the back. The sides are the most difficult.

2. "Lefts and Rights." Differentiation of the sides of the body in exact left-right terms is not seen in 75% of normal children until about age 7. Thus, any child whose mental age is below 6 or 7 may have difficulty responding correctly to questions about left and right. Children with a mental age of 5 should be able to make consistent judgments about left and right although they might be consistently backward (e.g., consistent in placing the left arm over the left leg). To name left and right body parts when asked to touch them is easiest. Next in order of difficulty is to place an object to the right or left. Relocating the body relative to left-right directions (e.g., "Lie on your left side," "Place your right side toward the wall") is the type of task most difficult to accomplish.

3. "A Body Can Move." All children must learn a movement vocabulary. For example, children should understand what straightening or bending an arm or leg means. More obvious directions and proper responses are also appropriate. "Stand up," "Get down," "Roll over," "Lie on your back" are examples. An entire list of movement vocabulary terms of this nature should be compiled and the child's reactions tested.

Games of this nature can be administered either by themselves or in conjunction with other developmental activities. For example, the child playing a ball game could be asked, "Which hand are you using to throw the ball?" The child may need nonverbal input in addition to verbal requests to move or touch a given body part. Thus, tactile stimulation may also be used—e.g., a washcloth gently rubbed on a child's limb as the child is asked to bend it or is asked which arm is being touched. Body-parts games also may be effective if the child, particularly the child who is mildly or moderately spastic, is encouraged via relaxation training to isolate and to move specific body parts (e.g., one arm only). (See chapter 28.)

Verbal Programming   Brain-injured or cerebral palsied children may lack adequate sub-vocal guides to movement. Normal youngsters formulate obvious (those that can be heard) or subtle (subvocal) verbal directions to themselves before or during movements. In the nursery school yard the normal child can be heard saying, "Johnny is going to dig a hole" or "See Johnny dig the hole" (as Johnny is doing it), and finally, "I finished digging the hole." If word articulation is a problem, this kind of vocal accompaniment may be lacking.

Thus, children with movement problems resulting from some kind of central nervous system injury may be encouraged to (a) state in one word or simple sentence what they are about to do; (b) if the movement is not too rapid, say outloud what they are doing as they do it; (c) tell the physical educator just what they have done after the action is completed.

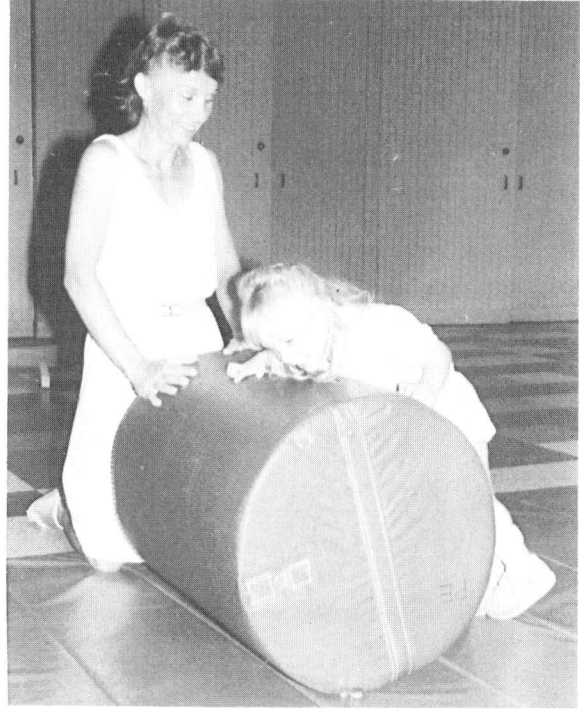

Planning a way to get over this obstacle is a difficult but useful task for a child with cerebral palsy.

Care should be taken not to overpressure the children who have speech problems. Tensions could block a child from carrying out the program at all. Initially the child may be encouraged to represent an action by a single word (e.g., "ball" or perhaps "throw" when throwing the ball). Later, a child who is comfortable with this may be asked to use a subject (e.g., "John throws!"). Still later a more elaborate sentence may be used.

Imagery One interesting method recently has been researched (Opila-Lehman & Short, 1985). This method involves first asking the child to imagine a movement—to retrieve a memory trace from its storage somewhere in the central nervous system. Although proponents of the method report success, one wonders how well a child can recall and mentally rehearse a movement that he or she has never performed.

Speech Games Children with central nervous system disorders frequently lack sufficient power in the diaphragm and intercostal muscles to support speech. Thus, the physical education teacher may encourage games that will help the child and reinforce the speech pathologist's efforts to build up the needed force or wind, which then may be translated into speech sounds by the various parts of the mouth—tongue, teeth, and lips.

Blowing games of all kinds, such as blowing ping-pong balls from side to side on a table, are helpful. Figure 13.6 illustrates this. Precision and variation in lung power are also possible in such games, as the child may be asked to blow a ball with precision at a target, or to blow "half that hard" or as "gently as possible."

Figure 13.6 Blowing Game to Develop Muscles That Support Speech

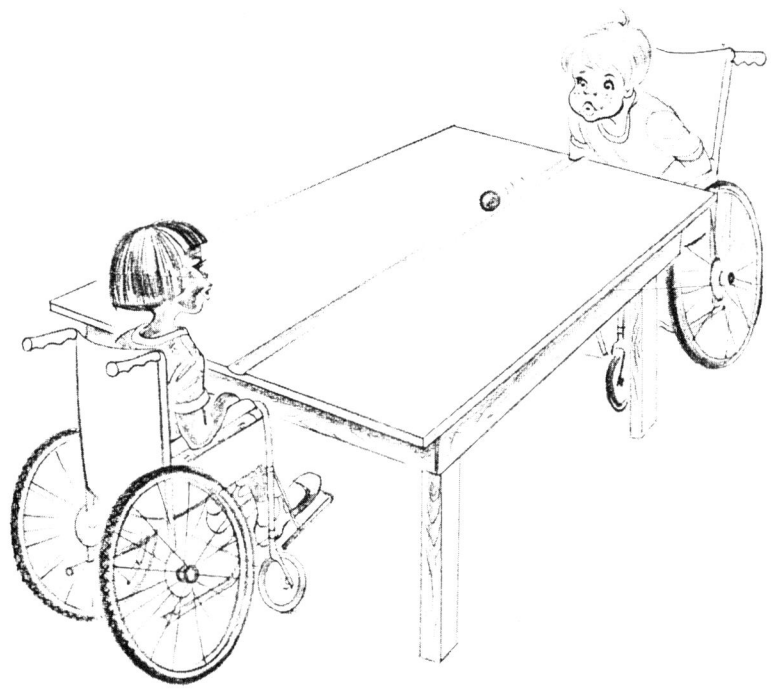

Movement Activities A child may be anxious in situations that require direct motor performance of some kind. Therefore, the physical educator must find strategies to introduce him or her gradually to a new activity in ways that are as nonthreatening as possible. The child may first be introduced to a relatively simple component of a skill—perhaps merely holding a ball and then handing it to another child—before attempting the more difficult task of barely releasing the ball in an upward direction with both hands and then catching it again. Early success in new activities is essential.

The child may be first asked to practice new activities while alone, then with another child present, and finally with two or three more children present. After the tasks have been overlearned at each of these successive levels of social stress, more social stress may be applied, such as an audience of one or more children who may exhort the child to do well or to offer verbal direction as the child tries to perform a motor skill. When competition is desired, the child should be given a chance to win or be successful at least half the time.

Like many handicapped people, children suffering from severe motor impairment may feel ineffectual. These children may have gone through much of their lives feeling that things—people, sharp corners of furniture, balls, animals—may do something to *them* while they have difficulty doing something to things. Thus, games and situations in which these children are made to feel effectual are important. A large skittle-ball game, for example, in which a ball is simply released from the lap of a nonambulatory child and allowed to

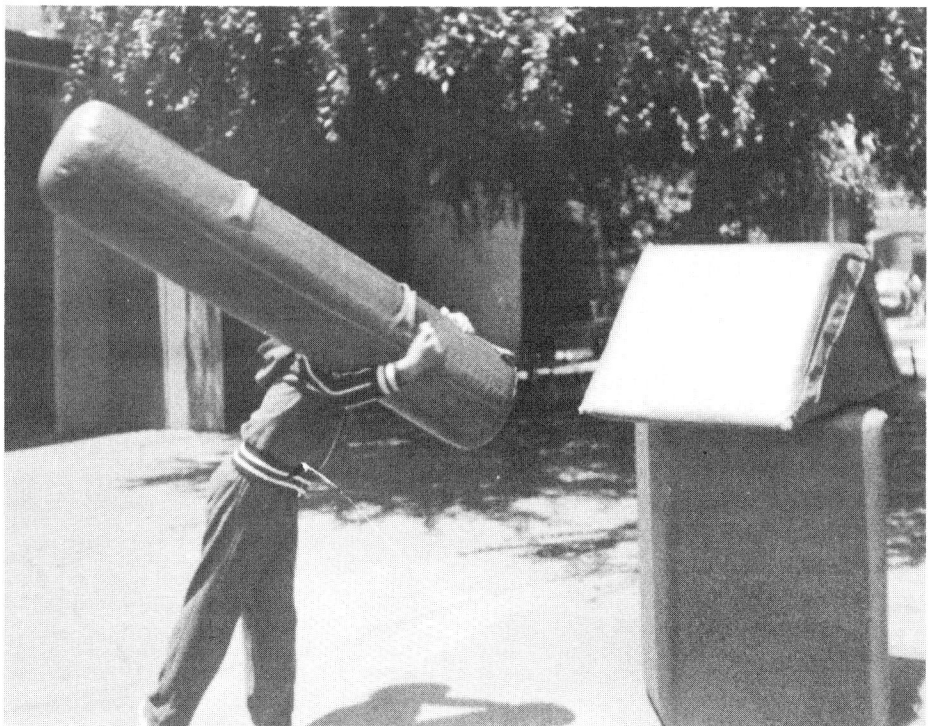

Having an effect on things can be rewarding for children with motor impairment.

swing, hitting three or more bowling pins, may be highly satisfying. Large foam-filled objects, when piled high and knocked down with a gentle push, provide another means whereby the child or youth may be permitted to feel that he or she can have an effect on something else.

Various scooterboard activities are good in this regard. Children who lack the movement capacities to make dramatic changes in their position in space may be able to effect satisfying changes in spatial location when placed on a board mounted on small wheels. A slippery floor may accomplish the same purpose.

Tactile Activities   Instructions to parents should include admonishments to give the child touching experiences via cuddling and the like and to make changes in the child's positions in space by picking up the child and slowly changing his or her position from the vertical to the horizontal in space. Physical education teachers should heed the same advice. A rewarding pat on the head and other tactile experiences are helpful as well as satisfying to the recipient. These types of experiences should be gentle rather than abrupt or rough. Moving the child slowly from a wheelchair to an exercise position is more rewarding than doing this in a rush.

Nonambulatory children or youth are not always placed in positions that permit their hands freedom to explore and manipulate. If braced in upright positions or placed on their stomachs over bolsters, these children may experience tactile sensations and use what capacities their hands possess.

Children who have hemiplegia (who are involved on only one side) may be encouraged to try most hard things with the "good" hand (e.g., throwing, reaching, holding, catching), or perhaps to try doing some things with the more involved side to gain more use of it. Or they might be able to use the hands in a helpful tandem—to hold work or to stabilize themselves or the task with the more involved side while exerting the main effort or precision act with the "good" side.

Righting Activities   Adequate righting reactions are often deficient in children with central nervous system damage. When, through their own efforts or circumstances beyond their control, they are placed off balance, they are unable to come quickly to grips with gravity and have difficulty gaining control or righting themselves. This difficulty in righting themselves may become apparent if they are placed or go off balance in a kneeling, sitting, or standing position.

A number of activities may improve these reactions, from those involving simple adjustments of posture to gravity while seated to the more complicated righting reactions needed when standing and walking. For example:

- With the child in a seated position, the physical educator may, by holding one of the child's shoulders with each hand, gently and slowly tilt the child from side to side while encouraging the child to reach out with the appropriate hand to keep from falling to either side.
- If the child is able to stand, he or she might benefit from gentle assistance in descending to a seated position, together with encouragement and assistance to reach out with one or both hands. Manual assistance may be offered in bending the knees during the descent.

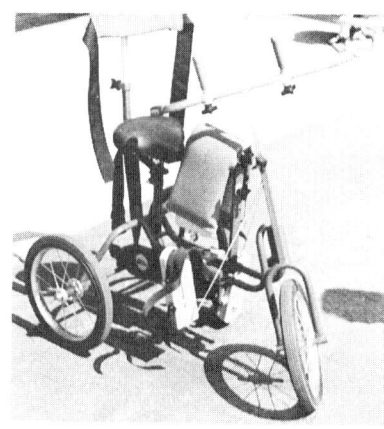

This special bicycle helps reduce scissoring when a child with cerebral palsy is riding it, because of the leg separator shown.

Courtesy, Special Education Branch, Los Angeles City Schools

- Various pieces of equipment may be used to improve righting reactions. Low stools that tilt easily may help trigger the appropriate reactions of hands and head (tilt to the opposite direction of the tilting stool). For those who can stand, a low, unstable "standing board" may be used to help children lean and tilt their heads in a direction opposite to the direction the platform makes them tilt. This apparatus may be used in a side-to-side direction or in a front-to-back direction.

Care must be taken not to overactivate these children and thus heighten tensions and spasticity. Under moderately motivating conditions, however, their reaction times and movement speed may be improved without harmful results (Horgan, 1980).

Finally, the stress of concentration needed for manual activities results in excess drooling in some of these children. This socially unacceptable effect (which is usually apparent to the children) may make them withdraw from tasks that require trying hard. The instructor might want to give the child a washcloth to blot the flow of saliva when engaged in tasks that require physical effort.

SUMMARY

Injuries to the central nervous system may result from physical trauma either before or after birth. Brain injuries are either penetrating or non-penetrating and include strokes, tumors, hypoxia, infections, and the result of intake of toxic substances. Manifestations and prognosis depend upon the severity of the damage and its location, but the major factor in how well a person responds is age; those under 20 years have much more resiliency. Tools to aid in determining severity include the Glasgow Coma Scale and the Glasgow Outcome Scale.

Physical therapy is a vital part of any treatment program for brain-injured individuals. Depending upon the severity, the therapist may have to go back to movement methods used with infants, but individualization is the key, because symptoms and areas of functioning are so widely varied.

The most common type of insult to the central nervous system is cerebral palsy, which encompasses a broad spectrum of conditions, all of which are characterized by nonprogressive dysfunctions reflected in motor and other overt abnormalities. The type of predominant movement, the limbs involved, and the severity of the condition all determine the nature of tasks to which a cerebral palsied child should be exposed in a physical education program.

Spastic cerebral palsy is marked by an excess of muscle tone. In *athetosis* the limbs make meaningless and distracting motions. *Ataxia* is characterized by problems with fine-motor coordination. The limbs and hands of the *tremor*-type individual constantly oscillate. Cerebral palsied persons with *rigidity* have "locked limbs" and sometimes are unable to move at all; this type of cerebral palsy is accompanied by severe mental retardation. Other cerebral palsied children are labeled *mixed* because they have more than one of the forms and no one form predominates. Although a "pure" type is rare, most cerebral palsied individuals manifest one primary movement characteristic among the types mentioned. In classifying cerebral palsy by the limbs affected, *paraplegia* involves the lower extremities only; *hemiplegia* refers to involvement of only one side of the body; *triplegia* means that three of the limbs are affected; *monoplegia* involves one limb only; and *quadriplegia* refers to involvement of all four extremities.

Some children and youth within normal school populations are thought to be clumsy or awkward when in reality they have mild forms of cerebral palsy. The physical educator may be called on to serve the needs of these children, as well as those who have more extensive involvement and may be confined to wheelchairs. The most severely affected cerebral palsied children are found at home or in institutions; their condition is accompanied by severe retardation, and they may not be able to take care of even minimal needs.

Certain personality distortions are found within sub-groups of cerebral palsied children. And cerebral palsied children as a group tend to be mildly to moderately retarded (although many have above-average IQs). Problems in visual function, as well as speech and hearing difficulties, may be present. Tactile sensitivity also may be deficient.

Physical educators should develop activities that contribute to children's feelings of competence in recreational and self-care skills, as well as activities enhancing children's total therapy program. P.E. teachers should avoid activities that overexcite the children or magnify their motor problems, as well as tasks that may be too taxing physically or emotionally for them. Activities from which these children may profit include those intended to enhance body image, those that improve righting reactions and help children balance when kneeling, sitting, and standing, those that encourage imagery, speech, and verbal programming, and those that utilize tactile experiences, as well as movement activities to maintain and strengthen physical abilities or recreational skills.

A promising development in recent years is the availability of several drugs that have been used with positive effects to treat muscle spasms. Liorseal and others have been employed in this context. There are also new surgical techniques and innovative orthotic devices that hold much promise in their application.

REFERENCES

Barto, P. (1984). Dynamic EMG findings in various hindfoot deformity and spastic cerebral palsy. *Developmental Medicine & Child Neurology, 26,* 88-93.

Consortium for the Study of Programs for Brain Injured in California Community Colleges. (1987). *The ABI (acquired brain injuries) handbook.* 1000 Oaks, CA: Author.

Elk, B. (1984). Pre-operative assessment and post-surgical occupational therapy for children who have undergone a selective posterior rhizotomy. *South African Journal of Occupational Therapy, 10,* 212-217.

Haskins, M., Bream, J.A., & Erdman, W.J. (1982). The Pennsylvania horseback riding program for cerebral palsy. *American Journal of Physical Medicine, 61,* 141-144.

Heiden, J.S., Small, R., Caton, W., Weiss, M., & Kurze, T. (1983). Severe head injury: Clinical assessment and outcome. *Physical Therapy, 63,* 1946-1951.

Hill, L.D. (1985). Contributions of behavioral modification to cerebral palsy habilitation. *Archives of Physical Medicine & Rehabilitation, 65,* 341-344.

Horgan, J. (1980). Reaction time and movement times of children with cerebral palsy. *American Journal of Physical Medicine, 59,* 20-29.

Ireland, M.L., & Hoffer, M. (1985). Triple artherodesis for children with spastic cerebral palsy. *Developmental Medicine & Child Neurology, 27,* 623-627.

Irwin-Carruthers, S.H. (1985). Early physiotherapy in selected posterior rhizotomy. *South African Journal of Occupational Therapy, 10,* 212-217.

Jones, C. (1979). Glasgow coma scale. *American Journal of Nursing, 79,* 1551-1553.

Katz, E. (1968). Intelligence test performance of athetoid and spastic children with cerebral palsy. *Cerebral Palsy Review, 16,* 17-19.

Largo, R.H., & Molinari, L. (1985). Development of locomotion: Significance of prematurity, cerebral palsy and sex. *Developmental Medicine & Child Neurology, 27,* 183-191.

Levitt, S. (1982). *Treatment of cerebral palsy and motor delay.* Boston: Blackwell Scientific Publications.

Mercer, L., & Boch, M. (1983). Residual sensorimotor deficits in the adult head-injured patient. *Physical Therapy, 63,* 1988-1991.

Minear, W.L. (1956). A classification system of cerebral palsy. *Pediatrics, 18,* 841-845.

Nuzzo, R. (1980). Dynamic bracing: Elastics for patients with cerebral palsy, muscular dystrophy and myelodysplasia. *Clinical Orthopedics, 148,* 263-273.

Opila-Lehman, J., & Short, M. (1985). Kinesthetic recall of children with athetoid and spastic cerebral palsy and of non-handicapped children. *Developmental Medicine & Child Neurology, 27,* 223-230.

Scrutton, D. (1984). *Management of the motor disorders of children with cerebral palsy* (Clinics in Developmental Medicine No. 90). London: Spastics International Medical Publications.

Seeger, B.R., Caudrey, D.J., & Scholes, J.R. (1981). Biofeedback therapy to achieve symmetrical gait in hemiplegic cerebral palsied children. *Archives of Physical Medicine & Rehabilitation, 62,* 364-368.

Sweeney, J.K., & Smutok, M.A. (1983). Vietnam head injury study: Preliminary analysis of the functional and anatomical sequelae of penetrating head trauma. *Physical Therapy, 63,* 1946-1951.

Taft, L. (1985). Cerebral palsy. *Pediatric Annals, 14,* 789-799.

Talmadge, E.W., & Collins, G.A. (1983). Physical abilities after head injury: A retrospective study. *Physical Therapy, 63,* 2010-2017.

Winnick, J.P., & Short, F.X. (1982). *The physical fitness of sensory and orthopedically impaired youth* (Project Unique). Washington, DC: U.S. Office of Education, Special Education Programs.

ADDITIONAL REFERENCES

Bleck, E.E. (1975). Cerebral palsy. In E.E. Bleck & D.A. Nagel, *Physically handicapped children: A medical atlas for teachers.* New York: Grune & Stratton.

Bobath, K. (1980). A neurophysiological basis for the treatment of cerebral palsy (2nd ed.) (Clinics in Developmental Medicine No. 23). London: Spastics International Medical Publications.

Finnie, N.R. (1970). *Handling the young cerebral palsied child at home.* New York: Dutton.

Kudrjavcev, T., & Schoenberg, B. (1985). Cerebral palsy: Survival rates, associated handicaps and distribution by sub-type. *Neurology, 35,* 1031-1038.

Manley, M., & Gurtowski, J. (1985). The vertical wheeler, a device for ambulation in cerebral palsy. *Archives of Physical Medicine & Rehabilitation, 115,* 717-720.

Neilson, H.H. (1971). Psychological appraisal of children with cerebral palsy: A survey of 128 re-assessed cases. *Developmental Medicine & Child Neurology, 13,* 707-720.

O'Reilly, D.E. (1971). The future of the cerebral palsy child. *Developmental Medicine & Child Neurology, 13,* 635-640.

Rinehart, M.A. (1983). Considerations for functional training in adults after head injury. *Physical Therapy, 63,* 1975-1982.

Robinault, I., & Connor, F.P. (1968). *Realistic educational planning for children with cerebral palsy, pre-school level.* New York: United Cerebral Palsy Association.

Smoot, G.D. (1958). *I'm handicapped for life: The story of an 18-year-old's fight against cerebral palsy.* New York: Vantage Press.

QUESTIONS FOR DISCUSSION

1. What are the two basic types of brain injury, and what are some of the causes?

2. How might a child with central nervous system damage best be introduced to a new physical activity? What cautions should be kept in mind? What feelings and emotions should be taken into consideration?

3. What are the motor and other characteristics of the athetoid, the spastic, and the ataxic person?

4. What are some of the ways of positioning a child with central nervous system damage? What activities and positions might be avoided?

5. What games and activities may be employed to enhance the body image?

6. How might language and speech be aided via physical activities? Be specific.

7. What questions are important for the physical education teacher to ask in a meeting attended by a psychologist, physician, and physical therapist to discuss the total program for a brain-injured child?

8. What special equipment might be needed when working with a group of children who have various forms of cerebral palsy?

9. What are righting reactions? How might these be enhanced through activities within a physical education program?

STUDENT PROJECTS

1. Observe a child with cerebral palsy or brain injury in a physical education class. What special methods are used in remediation?

2. Write a case study of a brain-injured or cerebral palsied child. Describe the family setting and make-up, the child's skills, personality, and learning traits, and social competencies in relation to physical activity. What kind of program is the child in, and how might it be improved? Outline a motor program for the child.

3. Read in the research literature (see the Additional References for this chapter) an article dealing with qualities (other than movement) within populations of cerebral palsied children (intellectual, perceptual, emotional, social, etc.). Discuss the implications when working with a cerebral palsied child in a physical education class.

4. Discuss with a physical therapist the various scales and assessment instruments used to evaluate the motor abilities of persons with a head injury. Are any of these of potential value to the physical educator?

5. Observe a physical education teacher or therapist working with older cerebral palsied or brain-injured students (high school age). To what tasks are these youth exposed? Which seem most appropriate for them?

6. Devise an ideal physical education program for a real (or imagined) cerebral palsied child. Describe the child in detail; categorize the activities; list any special equipment or materials needed; suggest an approximate weekly schedule giving types and duration of activities.

RESOURCES

American Academy for Cerebral Palsy
University Hospital School
Iowa City, IA 52240

American Academy for Cerebal Palsy
    and Developmental Medicine
P.O. Box 11083
2405 Westwood Ave.
Richmond, VA 23230

Head Injury Foundation
1629 Columbia Rd.
Washington, DC 20009

National Association of Sports for
    Cerebral Palsy
66 East 34th St.
New York, NY 10016

National Committee for Multi-
    Handicapped Children
339-14th St.
Niagara Falls, NY 14304

National Society for Crippled Children
    and Adults
2033 W. Ogden Ave.
Chicago, IL 60612

United Cerebral Palsy Association
50 West 57th St.
New York, NY 10019

14 *Degenerative Diseases of the Nervous System*

Innumerable relatively rare, and usually inherited, diseases affect various portions and functions of the nervous system. These conditions, though progressive in nature, often show a mixed clinical pattern. The symptoms of some of them reach a plateau and stabilize for many years, while other conditions cause death in early childhood or before school age.

Most of these diseases are difficult to diagnose, and the symptoms often resemble those of muscular dystrophy or some form of cerebral palsy. Usually the conditions are accompanied by muscular atrophy and contractures, which inevitably lead to changes in posture and bony conformations and thus result in postural abnormalities. The main symptoms are first mild, and then increasingly apparent, muscular incoordination.

These children require immediate referral to expert diagnosticians when the first signs of muscular incoordination are noted by teachers, physical educators, parents, or others who are in a position to observe. Following diagnosis, treatment should be accompanied by careful concern for the type and difficulty of motor tasks to which these children are exposed, together with intelligently applied exercise to maintain or prolong their neuromotor functions. Teachers also should consider activity modifications and employ special devices so that the children can circumvent coordination problems.

Two of these degenerative conditions—Friedreich's ataxia and childhood spinal muscular atrophy—are briefly reviewed in this chapter. These are representative of progressive degenerative diseases of the nervous system. Other diseases affecting the nervous system along with the muscles (e.g., multiple sclerosis) are discussed in chapter 16.

FRIEDREICH'S ATAXIA

Friedreich's ataxia is an inherited disease usually seen within the first two decades of life. Its symptoms may be present in infancy. The signs include poor agility, clumsiness, and impairment of fine-motor control, reflected in handwriting and self-feeding. As the condition progresses, muscular atrophy occurs, together with skeletal malformations, including spinal curvatures (kyphosis and scoliosis), and deformations of the feet. The disease is caused by a progressive degeneration of the sensory cells in the dorsal ganglia and the peripheral nerves to the limbs and trunk. Figure 14.1 gives the signs and symptoms of the disease.

Heart abnormalities are common and may surface at any age. The heartbeat may be irregular, murmurs may be detected, and the heart may become enlarged (Ruschhaupt, Thilenius, & Cassels, 1972). Atrophy of the optic nerve, together with loss of normal eye movements and visual acuity, may occur as the condition progresses. Seizures, mental retardation, and emotional depression are other possible manifestations of the disease. Some of those afflicted may be confined to wheelchairs in their late teens or early 20s, later becoming bedridden, with death occurring in the middle 20s. When afflicted with a minimally

Figure 14.1   Signs and Symptoms of Friedreich's Ataxia

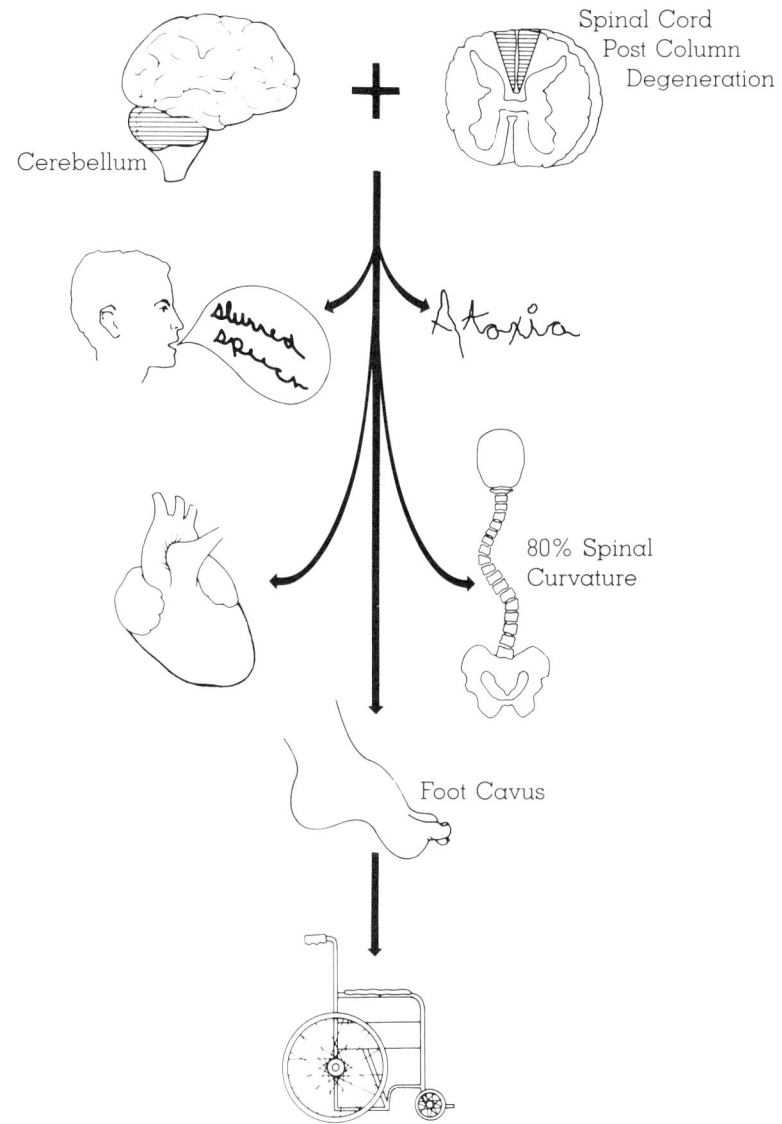

Spinal Cord
Post Column
Degeneration

Cerebellum

Ataxia

80% Spinal
Curvature

Foot Cavus

Note. From *Physically Handicapped Children* by E. Bleck and D. Nagel, 1975, New York: Grune & Stratton, p. 140. Used by permission of the author and the publisher.

progressive form of the disease or with an atypical or incomplete variation, some may live longer.

Needless to say, with the variety of symptoms present, a team approach is necessary to reduce progressive signs of the disease. Carefully planned exercise and recreational activities should be employed, avoiding those that require precise hand-eye coordination. Anti-seizure medicants and cardiac drugs are used. And psychological counseling may be needed both for the youngster and the family.

The child should be kept in a regular classroom as long as possible and receive a specially designed physical education program based on the physician's recommendations. Special devices may be needed if grasping a pencil becomes impossible. Often a special typewriter may be substituted so the child can communicate in writing. Braces enable ambulation, and games can be modified to allow participation. (Chapter 13 presents some games that may be applicable to children with this condition, as the symptoms are often similar to those of cerebral palsy.) When working with children and youth who have this and other degenerative disorders, a great deal of encouragement is needed both to counteract the present effects of the disability and to help the child and family deal with the symptoms, which advance in uncertain ways.

SPINAL MUSCULAR ATROPHY OF CHILDHOOD

This inherited condition is caused by progressive degeneration of the nerve cells of the motor (anterior) portion of the spinal cord and of the motor nuclei of the cranial nerves in the brain stem. The specific cause for this condition is unknown. It has been divided into two forms: (a) a more severe type, characterized by a rapidly progressive course in the young infant (Byers & Banker, 1961), usually ending in death before school age (Werdnig-Hoffman disease), and (b) a less severe type that has a more benign course, begins at a later age, and is sometimes compatible with a long life (Kugelberg-Welander disease). The line between these two subdivisions of the condition may be blurred when attempting to diagnose the often mixed symptoms in a patient.

Symptoms include progressive weaknesses and atrophy of proximal muscles, which may lead to signs resembling those of other muscular diseases. In the young child, weakness in the hip musculature may delay walking or sitting. These same conditions cause the child to fall as he or she attempts to walk or climb stairs. Self-care skills are blunted because of weakness in the shoulders and upper body.

Muscular involvement is reflected in postural problems of the spine, shoulders, and feet. Chest muscle weakness and diaphragmatic problems may result in respiratory insufficiency. Involvement of the lower cranial nerves can cause difficulties when swallowing, a poor coughing reflex, and slurred speech. Atrophy of the muscles often results in joint contractures, and disuse of the muscles leads to brittle bones that are easily broken.

As when working with most children who evidence progressive degenerative diseases of this type, a team approach is needed. Cooperation among neurologists, pediatricians, and rehabilitation specialists is required. Daily exercises combining mild resistance with exercises intended to maintain and extend range of motion are desirable. Lightweight braces to support the knee, ankle, or spine may be needed as the disease progresses. Long-handled spoons to aid in self-feeding and other special implements are helpful.

Daily exercise is imperative despite the apparent downhill nature of this and similar conditions. At times the child may be maintained through exercises until the disease's symptoms stabilize—which may last as long as 2 years. Slight improvement has even been noted in some who are afflicted with this condition. Vigorous therapy also aids in the hardiness needed when the child must combat respiratory infections, the aspiration of secretions, and pulmonary diseases that accompany progressive degenerative diseases of the nervous system.

These children have normal intellectual capacities. They usually require intensive special education and should be prepared to become self-supporting in occupations not calling for muscular coordination.

SUMMARY

The two conditions reviewed in this chapter—Friedreich's ataxia and spinal muscular atrophy—are representative of many progressive degenerative diseases of the nervous system, which are usually inherited and quite rare. The symptoms are often similar to those of cerebral palsy, but the latter is not degenerative.

In any case, the presence of various symptoms of motor incoordination should prompt an immediate and thorough medical work-up, including a neurological exam. Prescribed exercises and physical activity often can maintain or prolong functions that might more rapidly deteriorate without exposure to carefully applied motor activity.

Friedreich's ataxia is characterized by impairment of motor control, muscular atrophy, and skeletal malformations. Death can occur in the middle 20s if the disease is of the more severe type, while those afflicted with a less severe form may live to older ages.

Spinal muscular atrophy in childhood is an inherited condition identified by progressive degeneration of the nerve cells of the anterior portion of the spinal cord and of the motor nuclei of the cranial nerves in the brain stem. It, too, has a more severe and a milder form. Symptoms include atrophy of the muscles, particularly in the hip musculature. Incoordination may be evidenced in poor self-care skills because of weaknesses in the shoulder-girdle region.

In the presence of these and of other progressive diseases of the nervous system, a thorough understanding of the causes and symptoms is necessary. Exercise programs carefully graded in intensity and selective in content should be administered on an individual basis. Frequent consultations with a physician are imperative. Most of the time, physical educators working with these problems perform services in conjunction with occupational and physical therapists.

REFERENCES

Bleck, E.E., & Nagel, D.A. (1975). *Physically handicapped children: A medical atlas for teachers.* New York: Grune & Stratton.

Byers, R.K., & Banker, B.Q. (1961). Infant muscular atrophy. *Archives of Neurology, 5,* 140-164.

Ruschhaupt, D.G., Thilenius, O.G., & Cassels, D.E. (1972). Friedreich's ataxia associated with idiopathic hypertonic subaortic stenosis. *American Heart Journal, 84,* 95-102.

ADDITIONAL REFERENCES

Brown, J.R. (1971). Diseases of the cerebellum. In A.B. Baker & L.H. Baker (Eds.), *Clinical neurology* (Vol. 1). New York: Harper & Row.

Greenfield, J.G. (1954). *The spino-cerebellar degenerations.* Oxford: Blackwell Scientific Publications/Vincent Baxter Press.

Tizard, J.P.M. (1970). *Neuromotor diseases of infancy and childhood.* Springfield, IL: Charles C Thomas.

Van Wijngaarden, G.K., & Bethlem, J. (1973). Benign infantile spinal muscular atrophy. *Brain, 96,* 163-170.

QUESTIONS FOR DISCUSSION

1. What are the symptoms of Friedreich's ataxia? How do they resemble and how are they different from those of cerebral palsy?

2. What are the symptoms of spinal muscular atrophy of childhood?

3. What kinds of questions should a physical educator ask of a physician prior to working with a child who has a degenerative disease of the nervous system?

4. How might a physical educator serve on a committee composed of other professionals, including members of the medical profession, when formulating an exercise and educational program for youngsters with progressive degenerative diseases of the nervous system? How might a physical educator help the parents in planning a home exercise program?

STUDENT PROJECTS

1. From a review of the literature (see Additional References), identify one or more kinds of degenerative neurological diseases not discussed in this chapter. What are their symptoms, and what are the possible implications for a physical education program for these youngsters?

2. Outline an ideal week-long program of developmental activities and recreational opportunities for a child suffering from a type of degenerative neurological disease

you select.

3. Observe a child afflicted with the type of condition under consideration, for an hour, a day, or a week. Keep a careful diary of the child's moods, activities, and social interactions. What problems can you identify with which a physical educator might deal? What kinds of problems might be reflected in the child's social interactions?

15 *Epilepsy and Convulsive Disorders*

$\mathbf{Y}$oungsters with neurological disorders, including cerebral palsy (particularly, spastic), mental retardation, and learning disabilities, are generally more likely to have seizures than are groups of children who do not have these problems. Many afflicted with epilepsy, however, have no other discernible problems, and their epilepsy may be unknown to all but their closest family members and friends, thanks to the use of medicants that can completely control seizures.

CATEGORIES

Seizure disorders fall into two broad categories: (a) genetic, idiopathic, or endogenous, and (b) acquired. In 80% of cases the causes are unknown. Whether epilepsy is inherited is a controversial subject. Even if one or both parents are epileptic, their chances of giving birth to an epileptic child are no more than 1 in 40. Acquired epilepsy is believed to be caused by birth traumas (including those causing anoxia), lead poisoning, cerebral tumors and abscesses, and traumatic injuries to the brain involving penetration.

About 20% of all epileptics have their first seizure before age 10. Another substantial percentage of first seizures occurs in the second decade of life, not infrequently during or just following stressful physical activities in junior high school. Thus, physical educators should be well versed in the nature of seizure disorders, factors that are likely to bring about seizures, and steps to be taken when a seizure occurs (discussed later in the chapter).

TYPES OF SEIZURES

Partial epilepsies are more common than generalized seizures. About two thirds of all adult epileptics incur partial seizures, and about 40% of all epileptic children have partial rather than generalized seizures (Delgado-Escueta, 1983). In general, seven types of seizures account for the majority of those seen in children and youth: petit mal, grand mal, Jacksonian, psychomotor, infantile, autonomic, and mixed.

Petit Mal

These "small" seizures are of three different types:

1. A short suspension of activity accompanied by staring and, at times, eye fluttering. This is the typical variety.

2. The *myoclonic* attack, an atypical variant characterized by a brief contraction of a part or group of muscles, usually sudden neck flexion or extension, accompanied by trunk flexion at times, as well as extension of the arms upward at the shoulders.

3. The *akinetic* attack, known also as *astatic* or *inhibition* epilepsy. This type consists of a sudden drop to the ground, quickly arrested by the individuals, who seem to catch themselves and stop the attack shortly after it occurs.

Seizures of the first kind probably occur more often than they are recorded. According to the literature (e.g., Boshes & Gibbs, 1972), however, they account for under 10% of all seizures occurring in children. They are not seen often in the preschool child, and in many children they disappear at puberty. Their occurrence may be dangerous in physical education class if the child is on a trampoline, climbing, about to catch a ball, or engaged in some other activity that requires close attention. The child's attention should not be called unduly to the occurrence of these seizures, but the child's physician should be notified immediately. Petit mal is uncommon in groups of children who are labeled awkward or who have learning disabilities. Petit mal seizures are not accompanied by obvious limb and trunk movements, as is true with grand mal seizures.

Grand Mal

The grand mal seizure is the most dramatic and easily recognizable type of seizure. During its occurrence the individual loses consciousness and for a brief time (usually under 1 minute) expels air forcibly from the lungs while contracting muscles of the trunk and limbs. Generally the seizure passes through four phases:

1. A warning *aura*, consistent in each person but differing from individual to individual. These warning sensations can consist of smells, visual stimuli (lights), or feelings of fear or elation. Of those who are about to have a grand mal seizure, about half first have an aura.

2. The second, *tonic*, phase, marked by expelling air. The person sometimes utters a cry, and oxygen becomes short. This phase lasts a few seconds, and if the individual is elevated above a surface (such as a diving board) or in deep water, the potential for peril is present.

3. The third, *clonic*, phase, persisting for a few seconds to a few minutes. Because the tongue may be bitten, a soft object should be placed in the mouth at this point. The anal sphincter muscles and those in the urinary tract relax, which may cause spontaneous urination and defecation.

4. The final phase, a sleep or *coma*, lasting from one to several hours before consciousness is regained. After awakening, the person usually has no recollection of the seizure.

Jacksonian

The Jacksonian-type seizure resembles the grand mal type but lacks the aura and tonic phases. The contractions usually begin in one part of the body, a hand or limb, and spread up the limb until all the muscles of the limb are alternately relaxing and contracting. The grand mal and Jacksonian type together account for slightly over half of all seizure types.

Psychomotor

Psychomotor attacks are brief changes in behavior of which the individual is unaware. The behavior takes the form of temper tantrums, aggression against another person, sleepwalking, or hysterics at night. An episode of incoherent chattering may occur. Teachers and parents may misunderstand these attacks and punish children for asocial behavior of which they are unaware. Only 5% of seizure disorders are of this rare type.

Infantile

This convulsive disorder is seen only during the first few years of life and is related to the immaturity of brain development. Various disease states, including tuberous sclerosis, phenylketonuria, and hypoglycemia, are assumed to be associated with these spasms. In about 75% of cases, the spasms occur before the first birthday. Initially the attacks may be focal, but with time a more generalized attack occurs, involving trunk and arm flexion in apparent rhythmic actions. The spells usually occur in series, with a cry uttered between each of the attacks. The infant may flex the trunk, which may lead to incorrect diagnosis of some kind of intestinal problem. At the beginning of a spasm, the infant may become less aware of the environment.

Autonomic

This rare type involves spasms of various functions controlled by the autonomic nervous system. The attack may include abdominal cramping (abdominal epilepsy), headaches, flushing of the skin, dilation of the pupils of the eye, or olfactory sensations. This condition must be subjected to careful diagnosis, as the symptoms may be mistaken for those of other pathological conditions.

Mixed

Mixed convulsive disorders are not uncommon. They usually combine petit and grand mal seizures. From 35% to 40% of all epileptics are in this category.

FACTORS THAT TRIGGER ATTACKS

A number of factors lower a known epileptic's threshold and make a seizure more likely:

1. Edema and other biochemical changes in tissues occurring around the time of menstruation.

2. Stressful conditions that may trigger undue emotions such as anger or fright.

3. Hyperventilation or holding the breath, as in preparation for an endurance event—sometimes seen in competitive swimmers before a race. Dizziness or feelings of faintness experienced by an epileptic while swimming, running, blowing a wind instrument, and the like are warning signs that should be heeded.

4. Chronic head trauma, such as that experienced in contact sports.

5. Excessive intake of alcoholic beverages.

6. Changes in the alkaline/acid balance of the blood, even though minute. These may be caused by changes in the diet. Some diets consist of high-acid foods that are believed to reduce susceptibility to attacks. Accumulation of acid products (such as lactic acid) in the blood as a result of exercise is believed to help prevent seizures.

PSYCHOLOGICAL/SOCIAL FACTORS

Epileptic children may be impaired socially (Kurokawa, 1983). The degree of emotional stability in a child is related to the degree to which seizures have been placed under control. Not only may the condition lead to emotional disturbance, but the brain lesion itself may cause various kinds of psychotic behaviors because of damage to the limbic parts of the temporal lobe (Frasher, 1981).

Parents can have important negative or positive effects upon the mental health of a child afflicted with epilepsy. A dominating, controlling parent may contribute to lowered self-esteem in a youngster (Hoare, 1984). Parental rejection can lead to several social/psychological problems and behaviors.

Epileptics may tend to shun social relationships later in life. In a sampling of Australians, 50% of the epileptics polled had remained single, and an even larger percent believed that their social life had been restricted by the condition. The inability to drive a car is one factor that can limit the social frontiers of an epileptic (Frasher, 1981).

TECHNIQUES AND TRENDS

When a seizure occurs, the child should be kept on his or her side so that mucous and saliva will flow more freely from the mouth. During a seizure the individual's movements should not be restrained. No effort should be made to stop muscular contractions by force. Contrary to popular belief, objects should not be inserted into the child's mouth, as the teeth are typically clenched in a seizure (Laidlaw & Laidlaw, 1984). If there is danger of swallowing or biting the tongue, a piece of gauze should be used. It is also important to reassure and comfort the person so as not to increase the severity of the seizure.

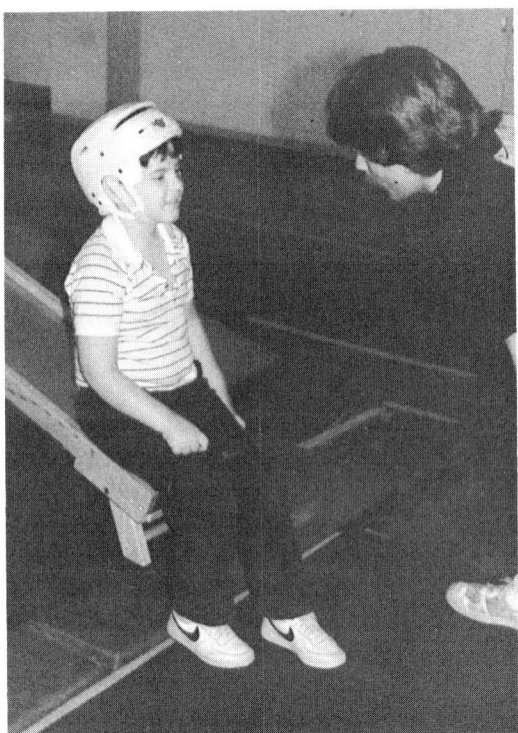

The young child with epilepsy often wears a special helmet to prevent injury if a seizure occurs.

Courtesy, Special Education Branch, Los Angeles City Schools

Among the trends in treating seizure disorders, behavior modification techniques have been used to make the epileptic person more aware of the seizures and to use this awareness to control the seizures. Davis, Armstrong, and Donovan (1984) conducted a study in which cognitive behavior intervention was used to decrease the level of depression in patients with epilepsy. This was done by talking with the patients about their experiences, increasing the cognition of pleasant events, increasing the patients' physical activity, and promoting their assertiveness.

Kraft and Poling (1982) used operant and respondent conditioning in managing seizures. They employed systematic desensitization procedures in which hierarchies of anxiety-producing situations associated with the occurrence of seizures were established and then presented under relaxation conditions designed to be incompatible with anxiety. They also used deep muscle relaxation and a conditioned stimulus (CS) for the relaxation response. The CS was presented by the subject contingent upon an aura or an anxiety-evoking stimulus in order to prevent the seizure. These techniques proved to decrease the number of seizures. Other uses of operant conditioning include reinforcing non-seizure activities and teaching the client self-initiated activities to cope with the seizure. Group therapy also is being used with positive results.

Although behaviorally oriented methods have been shown to help individuals who are prone to seizures, none replaces drug/chemical therapy. Chemical management is continuing to improve the lot of individuals who are subject to seizures. Previously used phenobarbitol treatment has been complemented by new drugs including sodium diphenyl hydantoinate (SDH). Using this new medication, over half of subjects in a study were completely relieved of seizure symptoms, even though previous efforts had been unsuccessful; the remaining subjects also evidenced a decrease in seizure incidents (Merritt & Putman, 1984). Other medications are continually under investigation. It should be pointed out that there are possible side effects when anticonvulsants are used to control seizures (Maddox, 1984). These may include hyperactivity, behavioral problems, and lowering of intellectual vigor.

Sufficient length of sleep is encouraged in patients with epilepsy. Poor sleep may be followed by attacks shortly after the child awakens (Neidermeyer, 1983). Livingston (1972) suggested a ketogenic diet because ketones seem to play a crucial role as an anticonvulsive agent. Alcoholic beverages and caffeine should be avoided as much as possible. Physicians tend to believe that caffeine stimulates the abnormal firing patterns. Biofeedback training, based upon recognition and control of the signs of an impending seizure, constitutes another method of control (Neidermeyer, 1983). Acupuncture also has been attempted with apparent success (Chen, 1983).

IMPLICATIONS FOR PHYSICAL EDUCATION

In terms of physical fitness and exercise for the epileptic child, opinions vary among neurosurgeons. Some believe that epileptic youngsters should be treated like anybody else and all activities, including swimming, contact sports, and gymnastics, should be encouraged. In the past, epileptic children were excluded from underwater and diving events because air is expelled during a grand mal seizure and if the seizure were to occur underwater, the person would sink rapidly. Today, most physicians agree that swimming is a good form of exercise but only under the constant supervision of an adult. Some prominent authorities believe that sports do not trigger seizures but, rather, the excitement or emotional let-downs associated with the games trigger the seizures.

Activities in which seizures could cause a dangerous fall (e.g., parallel bars, high diving, rope climbing, jumping on the trampoline) should be avoided (Committee on Children with Handicaps, 1983). Tennis is a good physical activity that provides exercise and a competitive outlet. Dancing in discotheques is discouraged because children who are photosensitive may be stricken with a seizure as a result of the bright, flashing strobe lights.

Because of the differences in opinion among physicians as to what level of activity the child should be engaging in, physical education teachers in the schools should follow guidelines proposed by the child's acting physician. To summarize, the physical educator should:

1. Treat an epileptic child in ways similar to the way normal children are treated in a physical education class.

2. Encourage vigorous activity and social interaction.

3. Provide special supervision for swimming activities. Avoid contact sports as well as sports in which falling may be a hazard (diving, gymnastics, trampolining).

4. If seizures are not well controlled, encourage the older epileptic child to inform the teacher of a pre-seizure aura occurring.

5. Be well aware of first-aid methods employed during grand mal or other types of seizure that carry risks of injury.

6. Be aware of the signs of petit mal seizures and if these seizures have not been noted previously by parents, teachers, and others, notify parents and the child's physician of their occurrence.

SUMMARY

Seizure disorders may be either inherited or acquired and for the most part are not easy to identify. Most epileptics have their first seizure during the first two decades of life. Seizures usually are controllable with medication. Seizures may be of various types. In *petit mal*, the individual is out of contact with the environment for a short time with no accompanying muscular collapse or writhings. *Grand mal* seizures are marked by the expelling of air and a clonic phase with muscular contractions. This type of seizure resembles the *Jacksonian* type, but the latter is not preceded by a warning aura as is true with a grand mal seizure. A *psychomotor attack*, another variation, consists of brief changes in behavior of which the youngster is unaware, including tantrums and aggressive behavior. Other more rare types also are discussed.

Physical educators should be aware of factors that trigger a seizure in a given child and make attempts to avoid these conditions, including unusual physical or emotional stress. Educators also should be aware of how to proceed during and after an attack. Special supervision for aquatic activities should be provided when working with these youngsters, and, in general, contact sports or those in which falling can occur should be avoided.

REFERENCES

Boshes, L.D., & Gibbs, F.A. (1972). *Epilepsy handbook* (2nd ed.). Springfield, IL: Charles C Thomas.

Chen, K. (1983). Observation of the effects of acupuncture on EEG in epileptic patients. *Journal of Traditional Chinese Medicine, 3,* 121-144.

Committee on Children with Handicaps. (1983). Sports and children with epilepsy. *Pediatrics, 72,* 884-885.

Davis, G.R., Armstrong, H.E., & Donovan, D.M. (1984). Cognitive behavioral treatment of depressed affect among epileptics. *Journal of Clinical Psychology, 40,* 930-935.

Delagado-Escueta, A.A. (1983). Treatable epilepsy. *New England Journal of Medicine, 308,* 1576-1578.

Frasher, R. (1981). Epilepsy. *Annual Review of Rehabilitation, 2,* 147-172.

Hoare, P. (1984). Does illness foster dependency? A study of epileptic and diabetic children. *Developmental Medicine & Child Neurology, 26,* 20-24.

Kraft, K.M., & Poling, A.D. (1982). Behavioral treatments of epileptics. *Applied Research of Mental Retardation, 3,* 151-162.

Kurokawa, T. (1983). Behavioral disorders in Japanese epileptic children. *Folia Psychiatrica et Neurologica Japonica, 37,* 15-19.

Laidlaw, M.V., & Laidlaw, J. (1984). *People with epilepsy.* Livingston, NY: Churchill Press.

Livingston, S. (1972). *Comprehensive management of epilepsy in infancy.* Springfield, IL: Charles C Thomas.

Maddox, D. (1984). Epilepsy: Current therapeutics. *American Pharmacy, 24,* 119-123.

Merritt, H., & Putnam, T. (1984). Sodium diphenyl hydantoinate in the treatment of convulsive disorders. *American Medical Association Journal, 168,* 186-192.

Neidermeyer, E. (1983). *Epilepsy guide.* Baltimore: Urban & Schwarzenberg.

ADDITIONAL REFERENCES

Bagley, C.H. (1971). *The social psychology of the epileptic child.* Coral Gables, FL: University of Miami Press.

Baird, H.W. (1972). *The child with convulsions.* New York: Grune & Stratton.

Epilepsy Foundation of America. *Explaining your brain* [Computer Program]. Landover, MD: Author.

Leppik, I. (1984). Seizures and epilepsy: Understanding the mechanism, and achieving control. *Postgraduate Medicine, 75,* 229-234.

O'Donohoe, N. (1985). *Epilepsies of childhood.* London: Butterworth & Co.

Ososkie, J.N. (1984). Epilepsy: Implications for rehabilitation. *Journal of Applied Rehabilitation Counseling, 15,* 115-124.

Reynolds, E. (1984). *Paediatric perspectives on epilepsy.* London: John Wiley & Sons.

Ward, A.A., Frasher, R.T., & Troupin, A.S. (1981). Epilepsy. In W.C. Stolov & M.R. Clowers (Eds.), *Handbook of severe disability.* Washington, DC: U.S. Office of Education.

QUESTIONS FOR DISCUSSION

1. What are the symptoms of the various kinds of seizures discussed?

2. What physical and psychological/verbal behaviors on the part of the physi-

cal educator are appropriate for dealing with the various types of seizures described?
3. What activities in a physical education class might tend to trigger a seizure? What types of activities should be avoided?
4. What kinds of handicapped populations are more likely to evidence seizures?

STUDENT PROJECTS

1. Talk with a teacher or other person who has administered first-aid procedures to a person with a grand mal seizure, and learn how to administer these procedures yourself.
2. Keep a weekly diary on a child who is subject to seizures (either petit mal or grand mal). Note the incidence of the seizures, conditions that trigger them, their duration, and other variables that seem associated with them.

RESOURCES

Epilepsia
Scientific Publishing Co.
P.O. Box 330
Amsterdam C
The Netherlands

National Spokesman
Epilepsy Foundation of America
1012-14th St., N.W.
Washington, DC 20036

*First Aid for Major Epileptic
    Seizures and Teacher's Tips*
Michigan Epilepsy Association
10 Peterboro St.
Detroit, MI 48201

Horizon Spokesman
National Epilepsy League
116 S. Michigan Ave.
Chicago, IL 60603

16 *Muscular Dystrophy and Other Muscular Disorders*

Muscular weakness or incoordination in a youngster can have a number of causes. Because physical educators may first notice this problem, they should be able to recognize the symptoms of conditions such as various types of muscular dystrophy, anomalies resulting in the atrophy of muscles, inflammatory diseases (including poliomyelitis and polymyositis) influencing movement capacities, disorders of the nervous system involving demyelination or abnormal changes in metabolism, and a group of syndromes reflected in slowness and rigidity of movement (various forms of Parkinson's disease).

THE MUSCULAR DYSTROPHIES

The muscular dystrophies consist of a number of inherited conditions reflected in progressive muscular weakness resulting from changes in the biochemistry and electrical make-up of the muscles. They are x-linked recessive disorders. Thus, most victims are boys. Because of the genetic component, one half of the male offspring of the mother/carrier will manifest the illness, and one half of the girls will be carriers. Most female carriers have minimal non-progressive weakness. About one third of cases are attributable to spontaneous genetic mutation.

Prevalence

Most of those afflicted with the Duchenne and juvenile types of muscular dystrophy are between nursery school and junior high school age. Almost all will die before reaching maturity. Boys are more often afflicted than girls, at a ratio of about 5:1.

Approximately 250,000 persons have muscular dystrophy, with about one fifth confined to wheelchairs. One in 500 children attending public schools has, or will have, some form of muscular dystrophy (Millar, 1971).

Characteristics

The condition itself is not fatal, but the child or youth succumbs to respiratory or cardiovascular problems caused by the weakening of musculature needed to support these functions and may die of heart disease or a simple respiratory infection. A team decision arrived at by the physical educator, parents, and physician must be reached as to how much exercise the child should have in efforts to maintain fitness without making undue demands on a generally weakened system.

Some data indicate that children and youth with muscular dystrophy show a decline in intelligence through the years, but this might well come about because of the emotional overtones connected with the condition. One recent study, however, indicated that up to 30% have IQ's under 75 (Galdi, 1984).

Adler (1973) has identified three main psychological/emotional stages through which the child afflicted with muscular dystrophy may pass: (a) fantasizing normalcy, (b) denial—rejecting the existence of the disorder, and (c) restriction of desires, to be as little trouble as possible. Often as the child tries to cope with the condition, he or she loses initiative, becomes depressed, and has feelings of futility as well as estrangement from the parents.

The dystrophic child, then, also psychologically and socially influences all those around him or her—parents, siblings, teachers, and others. Parents of these children, especially, undergo severe emotional crises and traumas during the course of their child's condition. They often feel guilty and frustrated because they perceive their child's inadequacies as their fault (Carlson & Brumback, 1983). Because the disease apparently is genetically based, parental guilt is often magnified (Charash, 1983). Often they are not given precise information concerning the child's life expectancy, which is important to them (Madorsky, Radford, & Neumann, 1984). Siblings may come to think of themselves as unworthy as a result of the inordinate amount of attention paid to the dystrophied child.

At this time more and more programs of family and child counseling are becoming available within 240 clinics sponsored by the Muscular Dystrophy Association in the United States. Although these efforts are being made, more psychosocial counseling and related services are needed.

Types

The most common types of muscular dystrophy are the Duchenne type, the facioscapulo-humeral types, and juvenile muscular dystrophy.

Duchenne Type   Duchenne, the most prevalent form of muscular dystrophy, is the most severe and may be first seen by the physical educator as general clumsiness in a young child. The infant appears normal until about age 2. At that time the child walks with the heels slightly raised off the ground and is unable to keep pace with peers (Galdi, 1984). Falls are common, and the child may have difficulty arising from them. This is called *Gower's sign,* the action of arising from a lying down position by first "walking" toward the feet, using the hands, and then (while keeping the knees straight) "walking" up the legs with the hands to a standing position. This is illustrated in Figure 16.1.

A waddling gait is seen at ages 3 to 4, and obviously, the child has problems in vigorous activities such as running or tricycle riding. Balance deteriorates with age in children and youth who have Duchenne muscular dystrophy, in contrast to normal children, in whom balance improves with age (Kelly & Redford, 1979). Biochemically, the protein enzyme creatine kinase is elevated in the blood (Ebashi & Ozawa, 1983).

The child begins to assume general bodily characteristics including lordosis (swayback), enlarged calves, and sometimes enlargement of the deltoids and lateral quadriceps. This kind of hypertrophy (termed *pseudohypertrophy*) occurs when fat and connective tissues begin to replace degenerating muscle fibers as the latter become smaller, fragment, and then disappear. At times, hypertrophy gives the impression that the child's musculature is adequate to superior when actually the reverse is true.

Weakness of the anterior tibialis results in a foot drop when walking, which may cause the child to trip. Contractures in the heel tendons begin to appear after the symptoms have

Figure 16.1 Gower's sign

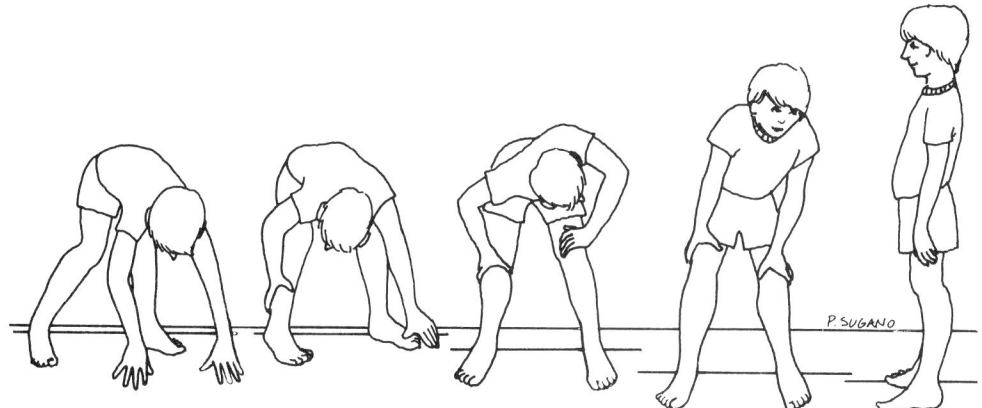

been present for some years, limiting range of motion, increasing the chances of falling, and causing afflicted children to walk on the toes. By late childhood and early adolescence, the youth must spend more time in bed or in a wheelchair. This further exaggerates contractures and postural conditions, including distortions of the chest wall and spinal column (kyphosis and scoliosis).

The Muscular Dystrophy Association of America lists eight stages in the disease:

1. The child walks with a mild waddling gait and lordosis, climbs stairs and curbs without assistance.

2. The child walks with a moderate waddling gait and lordosis, needs help at times to mount stairs and curbs.

3. The child walks with a moderately severe waddling gait and lordosis, cannot get up curbs or stairs, but can rise to an erect posture from a chair of standard height.

4. The child walks with a severe waddling gait and lordosis and cannot rise from a chair of standard height. *This stage is critical. Care should be taken not to place the child or youth in a wheelchair too soon or to permit an unusual amount of bed rest. Instead, the child should be helped and encouraged to walk, to stretch, and to engage in deep-breathing activities, to stimulate what capacities are still present.*

5. The child is relatively independent in a wheelchair and is able to perform activities of daily living from the chair.

6. The child moves in a wheelchair but needs help in some bed and wheelchair activities.

7. The child uses a wheelchair with back support, and the child can roll the chair only a short distance.

8. The child is now a bed patient who needs maximum assistance for all activities of daily living.

As children or youth move toward stage 8, they probably can attend regular school for only part of the day. During the early stages (1 through 5 or 6), however, they should be encouraged to participate in whatever form of physical education and recreation brings them the most pleasure. They should not be excluded from some role in physical activity—if only as scorekeepers. The most helpful activities are recreational games in which they may participate passively, such as shuffleboard, and stretching and deep-breathing exercises of various kinds.

Facioscapulohumeral Type   A less frequently occurring form, facioscapulohumeral muscular dystrophy usually begins in adolescence. It is not as severe as Duchenne's type, and the individual may live to a normal age.

Symptoms include progressive weakness of the shoulder muscles (trapezius, deltoids, and biceps) together with the muscles of the face. This last symptom causes drooping cheeks, "pouting" eyes, and the inability to close the eyes completely. The lower limbs are less likely to be involved. When they are, the waddling gait is seen.

Juvenile Muscular Dystrophy   The juvenile, or limb-girdle, type usually can be seen after the 10th year. Unlike Duchenne's type, which generally involves boys, this type affects both sexes equally.

Initial weaknesses are seen in either the shoulder or hip region. As the disease progresses, both upper and lower extremities are involved. As in Duchenne's type, life expectancy is lowered. Death comes from complications of the respiratory or cardiac systems or is a consequence of other secondary problems stemming from years of inactivity in a bed or wheelchair.

MUSCULAR ATROPHY

Several diseases[1] result in muscular degeneration of the lower motor neuron cell bodies, which in turn results in a failure to transmit impulses through motor nerve fibers that innervate muscles. These conditions produce the following symptoms: (a) partial or complete paralysis, the extent of which depends on the number of cell bodies destroyed, (b) obvious fine or coarse twitchings of parts of muscles (fasciculations), (c) more minute, not directly observable, twitchings or fibrillations, recordable only via electromyographic instruments, (d) loss of strength of reflexes, and (e) impairment of sensory functions.

Muscular atrophy may or may not be fatal. It is extremely rare. Any exercise or physical education program for these children should be prescribed by the attending physician.

INFLAMMATORY AND DEMYELINATING DISEASES

Poliomyelitis (polio) involves inflammation of the motor cells in the spinal cord, which in turn results in muscular weakness. *Polymyositis*, on the other hand, involves an inflammation in the muscle tissue itself.

Widespread availability of the Salk vaccine beginning in the late 1950s has virtually eradicated polio in the U.S. When it was prevalent, therapeutic exercises including swim-

---

1. Werdnig-Hoffman disease, Oppenheim's disease, Thomsen's disease, and Charcot-Marie-Tooth disease, among others, are examples of conditions leading to muscular atrophy.

ming were used with victims. Hydrotherapy in a Hubbard tank, with water temperature approximating that of the body, as well as various flexion and extension movements of the limbs and trunk, also have been employed. Gait training has been moderately successful with polio patients, enabling them to become partially ambulatory, aided by canes or a walker.

Multiple sclerosis (MS) is a progressive disorder involving disintegration of the myelin sheath (the thick, white, fatty covering of nerve fibers). Scar tissue replaces the disintegrating myelin, resulting in lesions throughout the brain and spinal cord. This process ultimately leads to total immobility and death. The cause of MS is unknown.

Recently a study looked at the effects of a 10-week exercise program carried out in water upon the strength and endurance of patients with multiple sclerosis (Gehlsen, Grisby, & Winant, 1984). Although the results were mixed, they were generally positive.

Amyotrophic lateral sclerosis is commonly known as Lou Gehrig's disease. It is reflected in a disintegration of the myelin sheath. A relatively rare condition, it is generally not seen in children or by physical education teachers.

Although experts vary on the utility of exercise for those afflicted with these diseases, physical therapy and related exercise (particularly hydrotherapy) tend to be looked upon as *maintenance* rather than improvement programs. These activities maintain function and delay degeneration as long as possible. Teachers of physical education in elementary and secondary schools seldom encounter individuals with these diagnoses, but when they do, they generally function in a support role to the treatment program prescribed by a physician.

PARKINSON'S DISEASE

Once considered a single condition, Parkinson's disease (parkinsonism) is now fragmented into several varieties.[2] In general, the characteristics of these subdivisions are similar and include muscular rigidity, gait abnormalities, and tremors. During the early stages, the tremor often begins with movement in a single finger and then gradually progresses, first to one and then to the other side of the body. Emotional stress, pain, and illness can increase the tremor rate.

As the condition advances, a flexor posture, accompanied by a mask-like facial expression, is seen. Steps are shuffling, and a patient who falls is seldom able to arise without help, because of muscular stiffness. When individuals with parkinsonism try to stand still, they frequently stagger because of balance difficulties.

Administration of a drug called L-dopa has had a positive effect in increasing mobility and decreasing tremor and stiffness. Side-effects of the drug in some users include restlessness and incoordination, as well as impulsive and aggressive behavior.

The usual therapies applied to individuals with parkinsonism include hydrotherapy and massage to reduce rigidity, passive exercise, and swimming, as well as rhythmic activities carried out progressively. Slow stretching (as done in yoga movements) may help. Motivation for seeking physical activities will vary from patient to patient. Making the program as attractive and individualized as possible may motivate individuals with this affliction.

---

2. Idiopathic paralysis agitans (Parkinson's disease), postencephalitic parkinsonism, and arteriosclerotic parkinsonism.

IMPLICATIONS FOR PHYSICAL EDUCATION

Using animals in experiments, Fowler and Taylor (1982) found that exercise in younger animals did not hasten degeneration of muscles. Translated to progressive muscular disorders, these same researchers have suggested that physical exercise with diagnosed children should begin early in their lives and that these programs should be moderate rather than intense in vigor.

Generally, short therapy sessions or exercise programs each day are helpful for children with muscle disorders. These may consist of activities that moderately tax the breathing and heart systems (possibly only deep breathing during the final stages of a disease), fairly rigorous sports while children are in early stages of a progressive disorder and able to participate at that level, and attention to social overtones by involving classmates in supportive roles.

During the early stages of a progressive disorder, these children should be permitted to perform as vigorously as they wish and as recommended by their physician. If they are withdrawn from an activity because of fatigue, the withdrawal should be carried out unobtrusively. Swimming is helpful and brings into play the larger muscles of the trunk and limbs, as well as exercising the cardiorespiratory capacities without placing undue stress on weakening calf muscles.

Recreational activities of all kinds—nature study, arts and crafts, rock and leaf collections, and so on—should be encouraged, to make the life of the child as pleasant as possible. These types of hobbies can make an afflicted child more interesting and able to relate to normal peers, thus encouraging social contact.

Not unexpectedly, youth with muscular diseases usually are aware of the nature of their condition and go through various kinds of emotional problems and compensations. They may withdraw from achievement-laden situations and from a general interest in their environment. They tend to be emotionally immature at times and to act in asocial ways, knowing that no punishment by the school or physical education teacher can equal the symptoms they are experiencing. Lethargy may be accompanied by a noncaring attitude about personal appearance, dating, dieting, and studying. These negativisms are difficult to counteract but may be overcome at least temporarily by the physical educator's positive approach toward recreational and physical education experiences as satisfying hobbies.

SUMMARY

Progressive muscular disorders are manifested in muscular weaknesses, tremor, slowness, and rigidity of movement. Among those discussed in this chapter are muscular dystrophy, Parkinson's disease, multiple sclerosis, and muscular diseases caused by viral infection. The physical educator or teacher may be the first to notice signs of onset of the condition.

The muscular dystrophies consist of a number of inherited conditions reflected in progressive muscular weaknesses resulting from changes in the biochemistry and electrical make-up of the muscles. Most of those afflicted between nursery school age and early adolescence will die before reaching maturity.

Sensible physical exercise not only serves to maintain functions but also provides a recreational outlet and recognition for youngsters with this kind of condition. Swimming is often helpful, bringing into play larger muscle groups without causing stress to the usually weak muscles of the lower limbs.

Like muscular dystrophy, Parkinson's disease, once considered a single entity, now is categorized into several types of conditions. They all have similar symptoms, including muscular rigidity, gait abnormalities, and tremors. As the condition usually is seen only in adulthood, physical educators are not likely to come into contact with individuals who have this condition.

Other less frequently encountered conditions causing various muscular problems include (a) those in which a degeneration of the lower motor neuron cell bodies results in muscle degeneration, (b) inflammatory diseases, including poliomyelitis, and (c) demyelinating diseases, including multiple sclerosis and amyotrophic lateral sclerosis. For the most part, therapy programs applied to individuals with these problems involve hydrotherapy and other techniques intended to maintain functions.

REFERENCES

Adler, S. (1973). The stigma of handicap and its unlearning: A social perspective of children with muscle disease and their families. *Dissertation Abstracts International, 34.* (University Microfilms No. 73-18, 543.)

Carlson, K., & Brumback, R. (1983). Psychological processes associated with premature death in Duchenne muscular dystrophy. *Psychological Reports, 52*, 165-166.

Charash, L. (Ed.). (1983). *Psychosocial aspects of muscular dystrophy and allied diseases.* Springfield, IL: Charles C Thomas.

Ebashi, S., & Ozawa, E. (Eds.). (1983). *Muscular dystrophy—Biomedical aspects.* Tokyo: Japan Scientific Societies Press.

Fowler, W.M., & Taylor, M. (1982). Rehabilitation of muscular dystrophy and related disorders: I. The role of exercise. *Archives of Physical Medicine & Rehabilitation, 63*, 319-321.

Galdi, A. (1984). *Diagnosis and management of muscular disease.* New York: Spectrum Publications.

Gehlsen, G.M., Grisby, S.A., & Winant, D.W. (1984). Effects of an aquatic fitness program on the muscular strength and endurance of patients with multiple sclerosis. *Physical Therapy, 64*, 653-657.

Kelly, C.R., & Redford, J.B. (1979). *Balance in children with muscular dystrophy.* Unpublished monongraph, University of Kansas, Dept. of Rehabilitation, Kansas City.

Madorsky, J.G., Radford, L.M., & Neumann, E.M. (1984). Psychosocial aspects of death and dying in Duchenne muscular dystrophy. *Archives of Physical Medicine & Rehabilitation, 65*, 79-82.

Millar, J.H.D. (1971). *Multiple sclerosis, a disease acquired in childhood.* Springfield, IL: Charles C Thomas.

ADDITIONAL REFERENCES

Muscular Dystrophy Group of Great Britain. (1968). *Muscular dystrophy—A guide to parents.* London: Author.

Neville, J. (1962). *So briefly my son.* London: Hutchinson.

Swaiman, K., & Wright, F. (1970). *Neuromuscular diseases of infancy and childhood.* Springfield, IL: Charles C Thomas.

QUESTIONS FOR DISCUSSION

1. What are the broad categories of muscular disorders? What is the relative frequency of their incidence in children and youth?

2. What are the various kinds of muscular dystrophy? What type is most likely to be encountered in a school-age child? What are the initial signs a physical educator might see that indicate the onset of muscular dystrophy?

3. What kinds of activities are best for a child with muscular dystrophy? What would be an ideal program for a child in stage 2 of this disease?

4. What psychosocial and emotional problems are likely to be encountered when working with a youngster in late childhood who has a progressive muscular disorder? What kind of counseling might be given to this youngster's normal peers?

STUDENT PROJECTS

1. From a review of of the literature (see References), describe a muscular disorder other than those covered in the chapter.

2. Interview a physical education teacher who has had some experience working with children with muscular dystrophy. What special problems were encountered? How did an exercise program seem to contribute to the child's physical and emotional state?

3. Interview an individual with Parkinson's disease to determine what kinds of therapy and recreational activities are most acceptable and pleasant.

RESOURCES

Muscular Dystrophy Association
  of America, Inc.
810 Seventh Ave.
New York, NY 10019

National Multiple Sclerosis
  Society
205 E. 42nd St.
New York, NY 10017

Section V
Fitness and Structural Problems

17 *Obesity and Fitness*

Obesity and other signs of unfitness are pervasive within populations in the "developed" countries of the world. While members of underdeveloped nations starve, their more affluent neighbors on planet earth eat too much and retain too much of what they eat because of a lack of inclination to move.

Too many fat cells begin to accumulate in infants even before birth and continue to grow in both size and number throughout childhood and adolescence. An estimated 50 million males and 60 million females in the United States are overweight and need to reduce excess fat (Abraham & Johnson, 1980). A recent study found that during the past 20 years the proportion of obese children has risen 50% (Gortmaker & Dietz, in press). This survey, involving over 21,000 children, has produced data indicating an "epidemic" of childhood obesity in the United States and suggesting that adult obesity likewise will rise in the years ahead.

Excess weight, no matter what its cause, constitutes a serious functional problem to growing youngsters. Both handicapped and nonhandicapped overweight children suffer psychosocial punishment at the hands of their playmates, have problems in endurance and skills in games, and lack the flexibility to move well.

Obesity sometimes is classified as an orthopedic handicap, and at other times it is viewed as a medical disturbance in endocrine function. Fat children often are viewed as products of environments that are too nurturing and "soft." Additionally, genetic factors and family eating habits prevent youngsters from achieving and maintaining normal body weights.

Obesity in handicapped populations is likely to be higher than is true among individuals with average sensory, motor, emotional, and intellectual capacities. Recent studies, for example, place about half of mildly and severely retarded people within the "obese" category (Kelly, Rimmer, & Ness, 1985). Moreover, obesity itself can lead to handicapping conditions such as cardiovascular problems and diabetes. Other conditions associated with obesity include hypertension, pulmonary disease, degenerative bone conditions including osteoarthritis, and several types of cancer (McArdle, Katch, & Katch, 1986; Larsson, Bjorntorp, & Tibblin, 1981).

In this chapter the mechanisms of obesity are covered first, followed by the role of exercise and diet in controlling obesity. The chapter concludes with descriptions of exercise programs for various atypical populations and the results of their application, together with a model fitness program and exercises intended to improve endurance, strength, and flexibility.

Several trends are apparent in the current research and clinical literature. More vigorous programs of physical activity and exercise are being applied with success to a diverse group of handicapped individuals, including severely, moderately, and mildly retarded children, adolescents, and adults (Beasley, 1984; Jackson & Thornbecke, 1982), as well as wheelchair-bound people (Glaser & Sawka, 1984), persons afflicted with multiple sclerosis (Gehlsen,

Grisby, & Winant, 1984), the blind (Di Natale, Lee, & Ward, 1985) and the multiply handicapped (Mulholland & McNeil, 1985). Moreover, an increasing range of modalities is being used to impart exercise and fitness programs, including the trampoline (DeVries, Wiswell, Bulsulian, & Moritani, 1984), jogging (Beasley, 1984), and exercises conducted in water (Gehlsen et al., 1984).

OBESITY: CAUSES, MECHANISMS, AND IMPLICATIONS

Obesity may be defined as having an inordinate number of fat cells, as well as enlargement of fat cells already present. Usually an obese person suffers both from an overabundance (hyperplasia) of cells and an enlargement of the cells already present (hypertrophy). The fat cells of fat children, youth, and adults are 30%-40% larger than the same cells in leaner individuals, and obese persons may possess 3 to 4 times as many fat cells as thinner, fit people do (La Vau, 1977).

Infants and children begin to add fat cells during the final months before birth, during the first year or more, and again at adolescence. At the same time, with dietary conditions amenable to the accumulation of fat, the number and size of fat cells may increase throughout childhood.

For the most part, fat children simply eat more than they use in energy in everyday activities. Significant numbers (10% or more), however, suffer from glandular conditions including:

—overstimulation of the adrenal cortex; this may be accompanied by the early development of secondary sexual characteristics.
—malfunction of the thyroid (including cretinism, juvenile hypothyroidism, and myxedema) causing tissues to swell and give the appearance of obesity.
—problems with the pituitary gland, which may be accompanied by excess hair growth (hirsutism), menstrual irregularities, and deposits of fatty tissue around the breasts, abdomen, and rear of the neck (a "buffalo hump").
—cerebral hypothalamic disorders including Laurence-Moon-Biedl syndrome, Fröhlich's syndrome, and pseudo-Fröhlich's syndrome, all of which involve undeveloped genitalia and weight concentrated around the breasts, hips, and abdomen.

In addition, long-term administration of cortisone or other adrenocortical steroids, for the control of asthma, arthritis, allergies, nephrosis, or leukemia, can cause iatrogenic obesity, which may be accompanied at times by growth retardation and hypertension.

The available data indicate that the control of dietary intake and the application of exercise should be undertaken early in life. By adulthood, a fixed number of adipose cells is present, and the only hope for weight loss is to reduce the size of each fat cell rather than to reduce the number of cells. Fat cell size in newborn infants and children up to age 1 year is about one fifth the size of an adult fat cell. Fat cell size triples during the first 6 years of life, with little further increase until age 13. A further expansion of fat cell size seems to occur around the time of adolescence, although the data are fragmentary on this point (Brook & Lloyd, 1973). Figure 17.1 compares cell size and number of a normal and an obese individual.

Figure 17.1   Comparison of Fat Cells of Thin and Obese Individuals

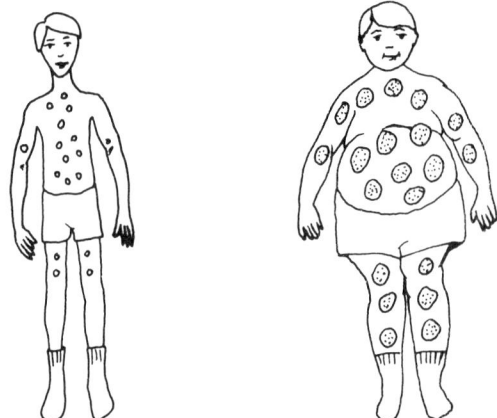

Thus, control in infancy seems imperative. Breast feeding, which limits food consumption, seems to be more helpful in reducing the early onset of obesity than weaning the infant too soon and subjecting him or her to adult ideas of amounts and types of food to consume.

Overall obesity in adolescent males and adults can be expressed in percent of body fat and usually is about 20%-25%. In females the "permitted limits" are somewhat higher—30%-35%. In general, the location of adipose tissue is important, with fat in the abdominal regions posing a greater health risk than fat deposits on the thighs and hips. But trying to "spot-reduce" deposits of fat by exercising specific body parts or areas does not work. Exercising the abdominal area, for example, will not "burn off" fat from the stomach. Weight loss in general reduces fatty deposits, whose location is largely genetically determined.

Training-Sensitive Zone

In cardiovascular conditioning an individual must work hard enough to produce a heart rate within what has been termed a "training-sensitive zone." This zone assumes that the individual's heart/lung system is normal and that the individual is free from coronary heart disease or other debilitating conditions that would be contraindicative of maximum work. Maximum heart rate varies but generally is established as 220 minus the person's age. This, however, is only a convenient rule-of-thumb. For example, normal 40-year-olds will have maximum heart rates of 160-200 beats a minute. (This maximum may be determined after about 2-4 minutes of all-out exercise.)

To train for cardiovascular improvement, a normal individual should select a training heart rate equal to about 70% of the age-predicted heart rate (220 minus age) and then by trial and error (using light and then moderate exercise loads) arrive at a load that produces the desired heart rate during training. Figure 17.2 illustrates the training-sensitive zone and age-predicted maximum heart rates. Increases in training heart rates within the training-sensitive zones indicated should be made with caution and medical supervision when dealing with special populations such as those discussed within this book.

Figure 17.2 Maximal Heart Rates and Training-Sensitive Zones for Various Ages

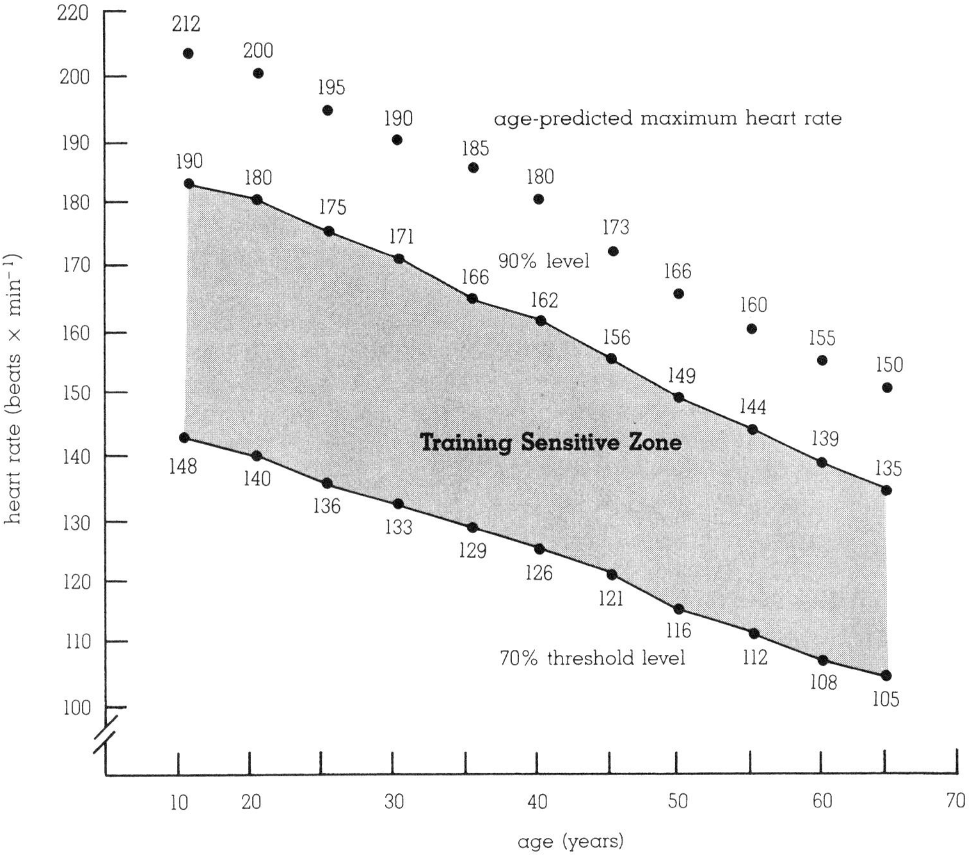

Note: From *Exercise Physiology* by W.D. McArdle, F.I. Katch, and V.L. Katch, 1986, Philadelphia: Lea & Febiger. Reprinted by permission of the publisher.

Environmental Influences

In most cases obesity relates to various environmental influences such as family eating patterns or psychological problems, including depression. Research indicates that less than 10% of children with parents who are not obese tend to be overweight; the percentage of obese children with one parent who is overweight climbs to 40%; when both parents are too fat, about 80% of their offspring are also obese. Some physicians believe that overfeeding a child, particularly a handicapped child who may not be really valued in the family, may be a subtle form of parental hostility clothed in an apparently approved form of parenting ("Please have some more cookies!").

Problems in Physical Activity

When exposed to exercises and games, overweight youngsters suffer from innumerable problems:

—lack of flexibility as folds of fat simply get in the way when children bend or engage in other actions involving the limbs and trunk.

—excess weight overloading an often weak skeletal system and resulting in knock-knees, flat feet, rounded backs, lordosis, pronation of the feet, and other divergences.

—edema in the tissues as a result of the retention of fluids around the ankles, breasts, and wrists.

—a tendency to fall and to be injured when attempting to climb, run, participate in contact sports, and so on; this kind of trauma may injure the growth centers of the long bones of obese youngsters.

—tissue damage and chafing between the legs, under the arms, or in other areas of fatty deposits that become irritated by moderate to vigorous exercise.

Interventions

Reduction of weight is not an easy undertaking and has to be supported with intelligent programming and sensitivity by a team including the physical educator, psychologist, nutritionist, physician, and parent(s).

In individual sessions the following should be pointed out to obese youngsters:

—the apparent cause of their overweight condition.

—the fact that dieting must accompany increases in exercise and work output; that one cannot simply exercise away fat. Outeating the most carefully planned exercise regime is easy to do!

—the fallacy of spot reducing; weight loss will occur over all parts of the body, and weight in a given part will be reduced to the degree that the percentage of weight in a given body part is representative of the total body weight.

—the gradual increase of exercise loads. Obese youngsters may begin, for example, with a program consisting of a half-mile or a mile walk each day.

As a weight reduction program is initiated, psychological counseling may be helpful in ascertaining what problems children have been trying to "eat their way out of," to what family pressures they may be subjected in achieving a weight loss (jealousy on the part of another obese member, a feeling of loss of control by a dominating parent, and so on), and other social, emotional, and psychological variables that may be contributing to and inhibiting efforts to reduce weight.

Exercise programs for obese youngsters should be made as pleasant as possible. In addition to detailed information concerning a reasonable diet to follow, children should not be subjected to overly strenuous or difficult initial exercise loads but should be given realistic goals for both exercise and food intake. Objective measures of weight loss, including measures of body density, skin-fold thickness, limb and trunk circumference, and total body weight loss changes, should be administered regularly. Technological advances in this area in recent years have made these measurements extremely precise and accessible. Pure recreational skills also should be encouraged to promote self-initiated activity.

One of the leading researchers in Europe who has studied body build and obesity over the past two decades has produced data indicating that weight reduction in obese children is possible through sustained, relatively intense programs lasting up to a year (Parizkova, 1977). In studying the body builds of numerous pre-school children, this same author found important relationships between parental attitudes/recreational vigor and the children's body builds, including fatty deposits. Parents who encourage activity, and who themselves are models of vigorous activity, tend to produce children who are likewise thin and fit. Sedentary parents, on the other hand, provide negative fitness models and produce children who may show obesity rather early in life (Parizkova, 1984).

Clearly, people who maintain an active life style, coupled with a reasonable diet, maintain a more desirable level of body composition than those who do not. As applied to handicapped populations, more effort may be required to achieve desirable life-style changes. As with very young normal children, many retarded and otherwise handicapped individuals simply do not perceive the long-range goals of what may be somewhat stressful and even painful exercise regimens. If their families do not support these efforts, the challenge is further magnified.

The concern of these children only with their immediate, "here and now" feelings is at odds with strenuous cardiovascular or aerobic programs. Therefore, the physical educator should introduce handicapped children to moderate overloads of pleasurable and motivating physical activities. The daily increase of caloric output when engaged in this type of activity is likely to have a long-term positive effect upon weight maintenance and even reduction. Failure of many handicapped people to engage in regular (even if moderate) physical exertion invariably will lead to gradual, stifling weight gains.

OTHER DIMENSIONS OF FITNESS

Fitness implies more than simply controlling obesity. The word denotes a positive group of qualities that permit optimum physical participation in recreational activities, competitive sports, and other aspects of life requiring movement. One may have to search diligently to find a Southern Californian who does not jog daily! The popularity of racquetball and other physically taxing sports is paralleled only by the sale of sporting goods equipment and clothing.

Concern for the fitness of handicapped children and youth has undergone a similar dramatic resurgence. Impetus for the fitness and physical education of retarded people was spurred by establishment of the Special Olympics for the Retarded in 1968. This program now includes many sports and involves hundreds of thousands of children and youth in the United States and several foreign countries. Other special programs for adults and youngsters with spinal cord injuries and other physical disabilities have flourished ever since World War II.

Unfortunately, the push for fitness of both atypical and normal persons has not been accompanied by a parallel devotion to scientifically based programs that (a) denote just what kind of fitness should be promoted, and (b) provide guidelines for improving children's capacities to move vigorously. The President's Council on Physical Fitness, however, has published numerous helpful reviews of the literature and has promoted workshops aimed at encouraging people to work toward meaningful, safe physical fitness.

Before proceeding further, *fitness* should be defined in the context of this discussion. In general, fitness is a multidimensional concept that refers to an increased capacity to move with force, to endure for sustained periods of time in an activity, to exhibit reasonable flexibility in the joints, and to perform muscular skills that permit participation in individual and group sports. For the most part, the discussion here is confined to the first three of these dimensions: improving muscular force (and speed, with equal power), endurance, and increasing range of motion at the joints.

The levels of fitness that may be exhibited and gained differ greatly according to an individual's capacities and potentials. The asthmatic person may be unable to acquire endurance without stress. This is also true of the child with a cardiac problem. On the other hand, suppressed levels of fitness (cardiovascular or muscular, or both) in retarded people and in those with sensory handicaps (the deaf and the blind) are likely a result of lack of exposure to and experience with vigorous sports rather than built-in constitutional problems. Exercise programs usually benefit these individuals. Thus, any program intending to promote various dimensions of physical fitness must be carefully crafted to meet the needs and capacities of each participant rather than being applied in a blanket manner.

Recently work physiologists have formulated four groups of tasks based upon the types of "energy pathways" (basic mechanisms) that undergird their execution. They are based upon time as well as the force/power required. This concept is elaborated upon in Figure 17.3.

When attempting to condition both normal and atypical populations, this categorical arrangement has several important implications:

1. Conditioning activities should be specific to the type of tasks they are intended to improve (endurance activities will aid endurance; power/strength actions will enhance power/strength capacities).

2. Special precautions and cautions must be taken when subjecting various atypical populations to any of the categories. For example, stressful power/strength activities should not be introduced suddenly into the physical program of a child with muscular dystrophy the subject of chapter 16), and special cautions should be adhered to when exposing diabetics to anerobic/endurance activities (see chapter 24).

3. A comprehensive conditioning program probably should include tasks from both the strength/power category and the endurance category, depending upon the individual one is dealing with.

4. Special care must be taken when introducing all youngsters to, and training them for, tasks within the power/endurance classification (e.g., middle-distance running and swimming, about 1-2 minutes in duration).

Socioemotional/Psychological Dimensions of Fitness

When discussing the concept of fitness from an academic standpoint and when operationally designing programs, various psychological, emotional, and social dimensions should be considered:

1. Very young children, those who are emotionally disturbed, and mentally retarded youth may have little or no concept of *why* they should pursue some physical activity. They do not understand long-range goals and benefits. They are affected only by the emotional

Figure 17.3 Categories of Tasks Based Upon Predominant Energy Pathways and Duration of Performance

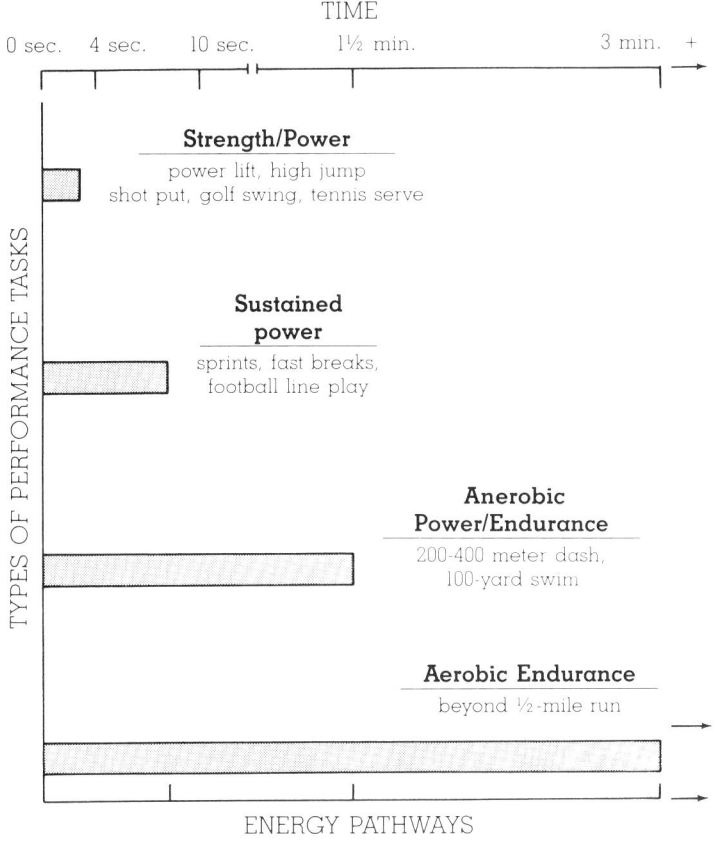

Note: Adapted from *Exercise Physiology* by W.D. McArdle, F.I. Katch, and V.L. Katch, 1986, Philadelphia: Lea & Febiger. Reprinted by permission of the publisher.

impact of the here-and-now, the concrete manner in which an activity impinges on them. Thus, exercise programs for them should incorporate immediate rewards and satisfactions.

2. To encourage the less mature or less able to participate in physical activity at all may be difficult. Overloading them with stressful, uncomfortable, and even painful experiences should be avoided to capitalize on whatever motivation they may be able to muster. Highly stimulating situations that foster self-motivated participation should be introduced. A well thought-out obstacle course, for example, can be used with success with these students, as opposed to the less interesting exercise station approach.

3. The youngster's feelings not only about the surroundings but also toward the personality of the tester or teacher may greatly influence the effort expended and the meaning attached to the entire proceedings. This factor should be taken into consideration.

4. The distractibility level, maturity, and emotional stability of the child or youth markedly influence both testability and the absolute scores of fitness measures of various atypical groups. Any record of scores should be accompanied by statements concerning the emotional tone of the testing situation.

5. An atypical child or youth may be beset with problems related to muscle tone that are not a result of a lack of exercise but, rather, subtle neurological defects that involve maintenance of muscle tone. A naive tester might interpret a fitness deficiency as stemming from laziness or lack of motivation rather than from the organic problem that is at the root of the low score. Physical educators should be knowledgeable about these neurological "soft signs."

6. Some moderately to severely emotionally disturbed children manifest an "effort syndrome"—signs of fatigue and discomfort prior to, during, and following exercise—when emotional exhaustion rather than physiological fatigue (as reflected in tissue impairment) is the true cause. Physical educators should look for signs of emotional disturbances in noting the "effort syndrome."

Thus, both the evaluation of physical fitness qualities and participation in programs intended to enhance these qualities may be markedly influenced by factors other than physiological ones. Physical educators should be aware of these mitigating factors and refer suspect students to the appropriate specialist if warranted.

Causes of Unfitness

A number of variables, acting together or alone, may influence the manner in which a child or youth performs on various tests purportedly evaluating physical fitness:

1. Lack of opportunity to play, because of an absence of available peers, rejection by neighborhood children, or lack of space (as in some apartment settings). The problem compounds itself as the child forms an extremely poor self-concept, which in turn discourages the child from participating in play situations.

2. Cardiorespiratory deficiencies that result in lowered capacities for vigorous exercise. Chronic asthma, among other conditions, falls into this category.

3. Neuromotor problems, reflected in poor coordination or awkwardness, that make these children less acceptable as play companions and discourage them from attempting new group or individual sports and recreational activities.

4. Overprotective parents who may infantilize their children, for whatever reason, by keeping them from competing with (and thus losing to) their peers. This "social-psychological contract" between parent and child may reduce the child's capacity to play, achieve, and maintain fitness. The effect has been termed *learned helplessness.*

5. Subtle parental hostility of a parent toward a child (often the case with handicapped children) to which the parent may overcompensate by overfeeding or in other ways detracting from fitness.

6. Genetic predisposition toward unfitness, with possible susceptibility to infectious disease, which limits play and exercise.

7. Poor nutrition or lack of sleep, both of which preclude vigorous physical participation. (I constantly attempt to discourage youngsters from watching TV after midnight!)

8. An aversion to perspiring, open shower arrangements, or other aspects concomitant to physical exercise that are viewed negatively.

Although locating so-called absolute scores (or minimums) purportedly denoting baseline levels of muscular strengths and endurance among various populations is not difficult, relatively few valid guidelines are available in these measures for normal children, in contrast to atypical children. Thus, I have resisted the temptation to advance these kinds of absolutes.

Rather, the pages that follow set forth *sensible principles* governing exercise, particularly for handicapped children, and suggestions for implementation programs, which also reflect general rather than specific guidelines. This possibly nebulous, eclectic approach is warranted because of (a) the lack of clear-cut criteria for the measurement and attainment of fitness in normal children, as well as sub-populations of handicapped children and youth, and (b) the incredible variations of physical capacities and personality factors within and among various populations in the amorphous territory of the handicapped.

As a note of preface, the physical education teacher should seek and follow the advice of a physician before instituting any stressful exercise program with a child who has been identified as handicapped in some way. Further, discomfort of any kind, observed by a teacher or reported by a child, should be heeded during the course of the program.

IMPROVING FITNESS: THREE GROUPS OF QUALITIES

A sensible way to measure a given kind of effort intended to improve fitness is to place it on a scale rather than to suggest that some absolute quality is being improved. This scale is represented on one end by an activity that requires total endurance or cardiovascular effort for a sustained period of time. On the other end of the scale is the effort a child or adult may manifest in a single effort—a pure-strength task (or test). Thus, the determination of how much an individual may lift (in a prescribed way) in a single effort may be placed on one end of the scale.

Most of life's activities, in contrast to these two extreme types of efforts, lie somewhere in the lower middle, middle, and sometimes the upper regions of such a scale. Accordingly, most fitness tests and the subsequent tasks prescribed to improve one's scores reflect the notion of attaining *degrees* of both strength and endurance. Exercises usually consist of tasks one is required to engage in 6, 8, or 10 times.

On the pages that follow, activities and guidelines for the evaluation, improvement, and maintenance of three interacting and related qualities are set forth: cardiovascular *endurance,* muscular *strength,* and *flexibility.* The chapter ends with activities that may improve a variety of fitness qualities.

Endurance

Endurance activities generally are those promoting the quality of the heart (cardio) and lung (respiratory) systems. The capacities of these two organs working in concert reflect marked changes in normal children aged 5 to 12 years. For example, as the child gets older and the body weight increases (approximately threefold during this period of life), a similar threefold increase occurs in (a) the volume of air the lungs process in a single breath, (b) the volume of blood the heart pumps in each cycle, and (c) the maximum amount of air the child inhales in a single breath.

Moreover, in normal children the heart not only beats faster at rest (gradually slowing as a function of age) but also reaches rates generally higher than those of adults when subjected to extreme exercise loads. In adults, the maximal heart rate tops off at about 180 beats per minute; in normal younger children heart rates under exercise stress can exceed 211 per minute. When attempting to improve cardiorespiratory function in normal children, one must both raise the heart rates slightly higher than is true among adults and encourage the children to maintain the elevated heart rate for slightly longer periods of time than for adults.

But the *ratio* of oxygen consumption at rest to consumption at work and the ratio between heart rates under the two conditions are highly similar in adults and children. Oxygen consumption of both adults and children during strenuous exercise is about 20 times over resting levels, and cardiac output (stroke volume times heart rate) may differ in both adults and children. When resting output is compared to output during strenuous exercise, the ratio is 1:7 (during exercise the heart pumps approximately 7 times more blood in both adults and children than it does during rest).

If one exposes healthy children in early and middle childhood to exercise that elevates their heart rates over 200 beats per minutes and requires them to sustain this rate for 10 to 20 minutes, this is comparable, in terms of work carried out by their smaller and less efficient (per stroke) hearts, to the effort of adults whose hearts are beating more slowly.[1]

A number of methods may be used to encourage children and youth to elevate their heart rates for sustained periods of time to promote cardiorespiratory endurance and efficiency. The key word in the last sentence is *encourage,* because selecting good motivation devices for hard work is the key to any exercise program.

1. Children may be asked to see how far they can travel (walk, run, run-walk, swim, cycle) in a given amount of time. This "how far can you get" approach, especially if arranged so the children are not in direct competition with each other, is a good beginning activity because the children usually can readily understand what they are to do and it may be used as a periodic check to determine the amount of improvement derived from another type of endurance program.

2. Children could be asked to traverse a given distance (walk, run, run-walk, swim, cycle) while the physical educator determines the time required to do this. This is the standard method used in track meets, of course. A distance of a mile and longer constitutes a training goal rather than an initial assessment. In general, the distance should not be too far when working with children 4 to 6 years (about half to three quarters of a mile).

3. Interval training, during which a series of short distances are traversed in a paced time, about one half to three fourths maximal capacity, may be conducted. For example, children may be asked to do six to ten 50-yard runs in 7 seconds each. The term *interval* means that the time between runs either is kept constant or the heart rate during the interval is monitored with an attempt to maintain a constant starting tempo for the heart prior to each exercise stint within the interval. For instance, the heart rate may be checked at about 60%-70% over resting heart rate just prior to each interval. Older and more able children and youth may be taught to monitor their own heart rates, placing the tips of the first three fingers at the carotid artery on the neck.

---

1. For further information regarding children's exercise capacities and characteristics, see chapter 12 in *Perceptual and Motor Development in Infants and Children* (3rd ed.) by B.J. Cratty, 1986, Englewood Cliffs, NJ: Prentice-Hall.

Interval training may be made increasingly stressful by:

—increasing the number of sprints (e.g., 100-yard dashes) from six to ten in number, or requiring faster times for each.
—decreasing the time between intervals.
—increasing the length of each effort (e.g., 100- to 200-yard dashes).
—some combination of the above stresses.

Generally, healthy children's heart rates may be maintained (at the termination of each interval) at 120-140 beats per minute. Research has indicated that preadolescent children who are exposed to endurance training do not suffer ill effects and may be better prepared for endurance tasks when they are adolescents or older (Chausow, Riner, & Bolidean, 1984). Following each interval, the healthy child's heart rate should climb from 180 to 200 beats per minute.

Swimming a given distance is far more taxing on the cardiorespiratory system than is running the same distance. A 100-yard swim is roughly equivalent to a quarter-mile run when comparing the duration of time required for each.

Strength

Pure strength is measured in the pounds of pressure one is able to exert in a single effort, usually in a static manner. Placing the task within an exercise program, however, may not be motivational enough for children who are handicapped, because the student is unable to perceive any results from the efforts. Seemingly no real work is accomplished as children push against or pull on immovable obstacles. Therefore, most fitness programs purporting to improve strength in children contain activities that are dynamic rather than static in nature (isotonic rather than isometric) and tap endurance as well as strength. Typically, these consist of 6, 8, 10, or more repetitions of a movement involving one or more parts of the body.

A primary emphasis in improving muscular strength should be placed on the so-called anti-gravity muscles—those that tend to support the body in an upright position against the forces of gravity. These include the musculature of the upper back and rear of the neck, the erector spinal group at the lower back, and the muscles that extend the legs and flex the ankles. Likewise, in many younger Americans the muscles of the upper limbs and shoulders are in need of strengthening, as are the abdominal muscles. Any exercise program should incorporate eight to 10 different movements performed against resistance, involving muscle groups in all parts of the body.

When working with the physically handicapped, the physical education teacher should take care not to increase strain on the joints or produce trauma to musculature that may already be deficient, or to increase any spasticity present by overexercising muscles that already are hypertonic and instead should be exposed to relaxation techniques (these may include applications of heat or cold, or both). Prior to and during administration of any program intended to promote muscular strength, the judicious physical educator should:

—obtain sound medical advice from the child's physician, as well as additional pertinent information from the physical therapist and any other medical personnel involved.
—blend and augment existing programs rather than formulating a program in isolation or remaining oblivious to what else might be going on.

—be extremely sensitive to observable signs of muscular strain or pain (particularly when working with moderately retarded children and those who lack adequate expressive language).
—heed comments from class participants about their physical condition, particularly specific complaints.

Apparatus for exercising the handicapped encompasses all the usual devices found in body-building salons (strength machines, barbells, etc.), as well as devices that have been designed exclusively for various handicapping conditions, such as the Hartwell carrier, in which nonambulatory cerebral palsied children may be suspended while learning to walk. With most younger groups, however, simple ways of adding to muscular resistance may be the most productive and safe. Loading and unloading barbells is not a very safe undertaking for students who lack the mental ability or emotional stability to perceive what is going on. Less sophisticated approaches to exercise, in which the child's own body parts, another child's pressure, or simple implements act as resistance, not only are easier to apply but also may constitute a more emotionally satisfying, "real," and concrete experience for the child.

Some simple ways to increase muscular strength are described in the next paragraphs. These are arranged in order of difficulty. If the reader wishes a detailed weight-lifting program, the publications listed in the Additional References at the end of the chapter may be helpful.

Trunk Muscles   The trunk muscles—primarily the abdominals, the transverse abdominals that flex the trunk, and the erector spinae group that extends the back—are critical muscle groups to improve. They provide a solid base from which the child is able to run, throw, and otherwise exert force with the limbs in innumerable activities including swimming and running. A weak trunk section is shown by a floppy child when running and a wobbly child in water. The hips twist and shoulders turn inefficiently when striking the water, as well as when alternately placing the feet on the ground in running.

Back extensions against resistance, including the upper body's own weight, are helpful in increasing the strength of the erector spinae group. Shifting the arms from a position along the side to an arms-out position like airplane wings (as pictured) and to an arms-in-front position increases the difficulty. If the feet are not held, it is sometimes harder. The child should be told to rise slowly from this prone position, as a back injury can occur if the head-shoulder lift is too rapid. Resistance may be increased by gently pressing downward at the upper back as the child extends and rises. (With proper instruction, another child could substitute for the teacher.)

Finally, the child may be positioned over the end of the bench for additional work. The anterior portion of the pelvis should be on the bench and the heels held or strapped down. This exercise should not be given to a weak child or to one who has a history of back problems or other muscular problems, including hernia. The position should be held for a 2- to 4-second count, and then the body should be gently lowered. Lifting upward should be done slowly.

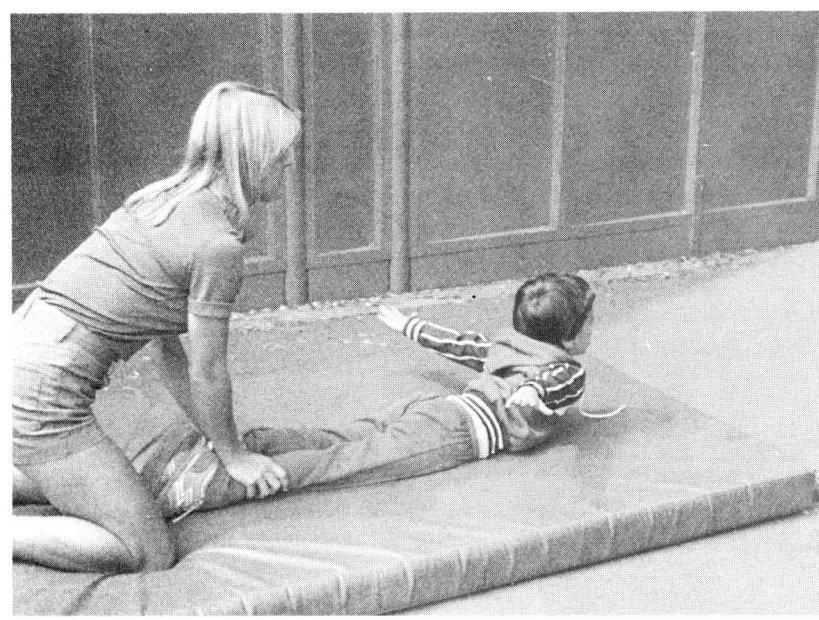

Back extensions against resistance help increase the strength of the erector muscles of the spine.

Back extension of this type should be included in all exercise programs, where permitted, for handicapped children. Six to 10 repetitions are suggested, and when these are exceeded, the next most difficult position should be attempted. Two to three sets of this exercise should be used in a 20- to 30-minute exercise program.

Abdominal Muscles   An initial abdominal tightener can consist of simply lifting the head off the mat, with the knees flexed (a 90° angle or more at the knee). This is illustrated in photo A. Then the child may be assisted in sit-ups (photo B). The teacher (or another child) should offer decreasing assistance as the participant becomes able.

If the child has more strength, the arms may be thrown rapidly from an overhead position to a forward position in attempting the sit-up (photo C). An alternative is to grip the rear of the upper leg (photo D) and pull the body upward.

Then the arms may be extended forward, without a throwing or ballistic action, in attempting the sit-up. Also, one hand, or both, may be placed behind the head (photo E), moving the center of mass toward the head and thus making the sit-up more difficult. Finally, the feet may be elevated for more resistance.

Sit-ups should be performed without a hand pushing off the mat. If the child pushes off, the next simpler sit-up should be attempted. Twisting (e.g., left elbow to right knee), while affecting the transverse abdominals, may result in muscle strain in some handicapped children. Knee-lifts are helpful if the knees bend as they are drawn toward the chest. Straight-legged leg lifts (or holds) are not recommended, as the work required is dependent on leg length and weight and could result in a hernia. Two to four sit-ups, six to 10 per set, are recommended.

A

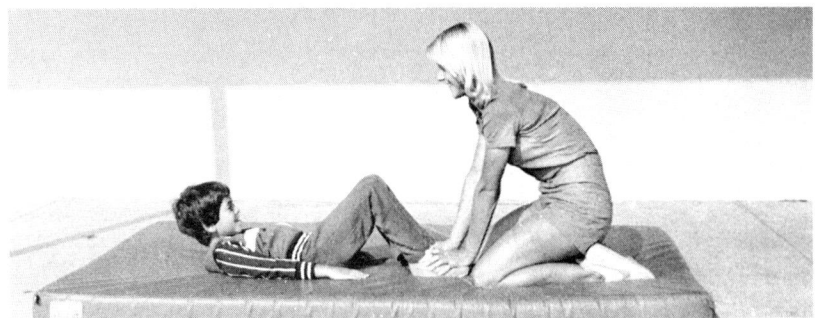

B

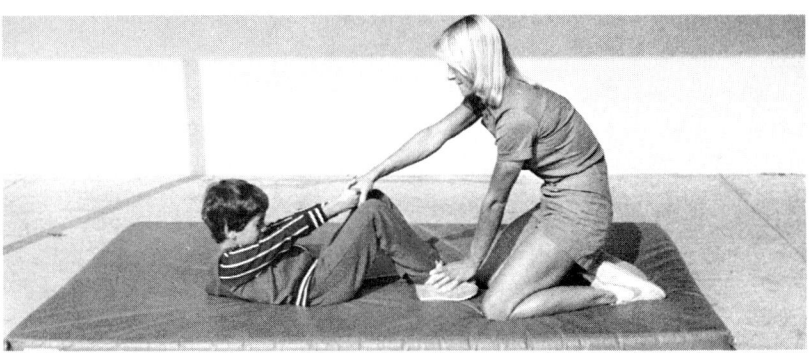

C

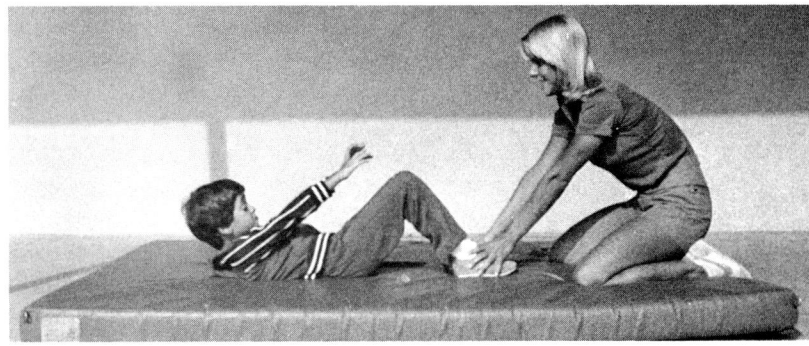

Children may begin abdominal work by lifting the head from the mat while lying with knees flexed (A). They may be assisted in sit-ups (B). Decreasing assistance should be offered as they become able to sit up by throwing the hands forward from above the head (C) or gripping the upper leg (D), . . .

D

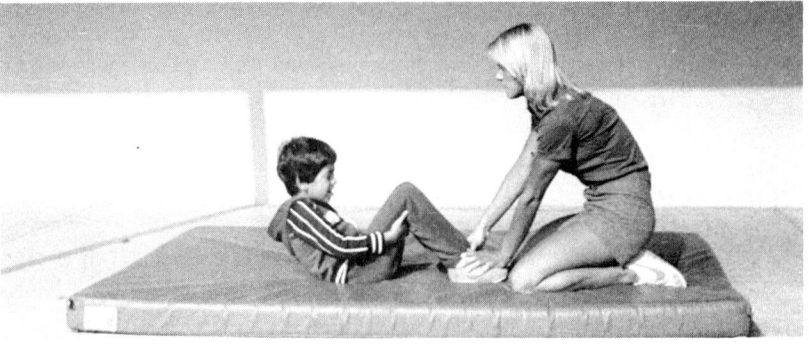

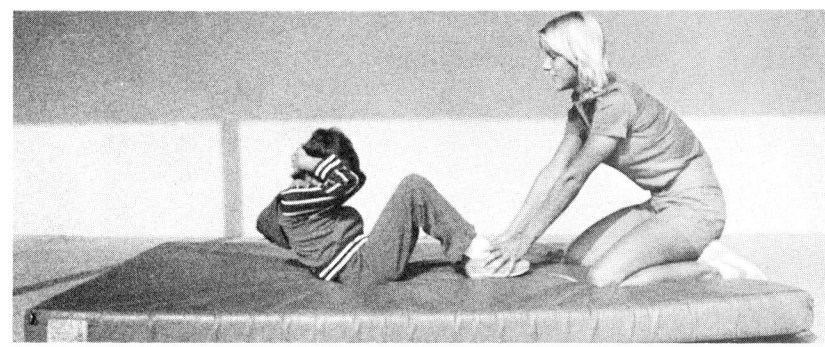

*. . . and later by
by placing a hand
behind the head (E).*

Pulling   A number of both easy and difficult pulling activities may be carried out with the help of a teacher, an aide, or another child. Again, resistance may be varied. The participant should be offered maximal resistance for six to 10 repetitions.

Pulling involves the rear deltoid (the muscles of the upper back) and the flexors (biceps, brachialis) of the elbow. Pulling is an essential exercise for children with a forward head (kyphosis). The exercises may be graded in difficulty. Simplest is pulling from a seated position, as shown in photo F, with the feet remaining on the floor or ground and assisting the arms, if needed.

F

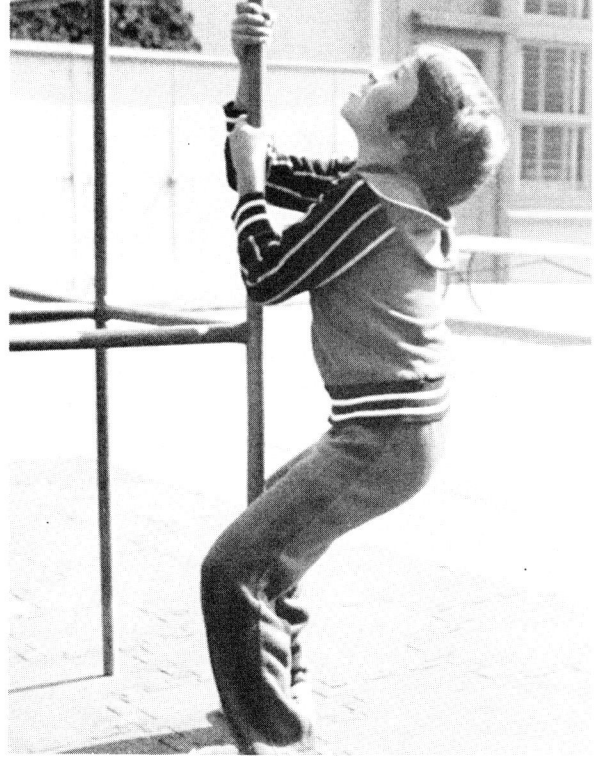

*Pulling up from a seated position is a simple
beginning exercise for children with weak
arms and shoulders.*

G

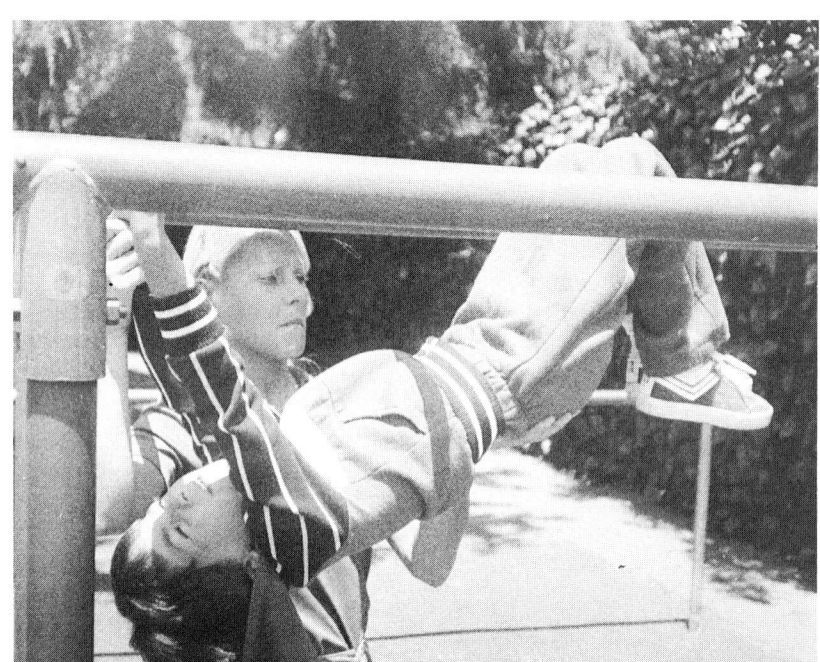

*Pull-ups may be
executed with
assistance on an
overhead bar.*

Modified pull-ups are helpful, as a complete pull-up off the ground is difficult for preadolescent boys and virtually impossible for pre- and post-adolescent girls with normal strength. With the feet remaining on the ground and the body straight, the child may pull up on a bar that is chest high.

Using an overhead bar, a pull-up may be executed as shown in photo G. The child's hands must be "jammed" against the bar by the instructor-spotter. The child's knees are hooked around the bar two or three rungs ahead.

H

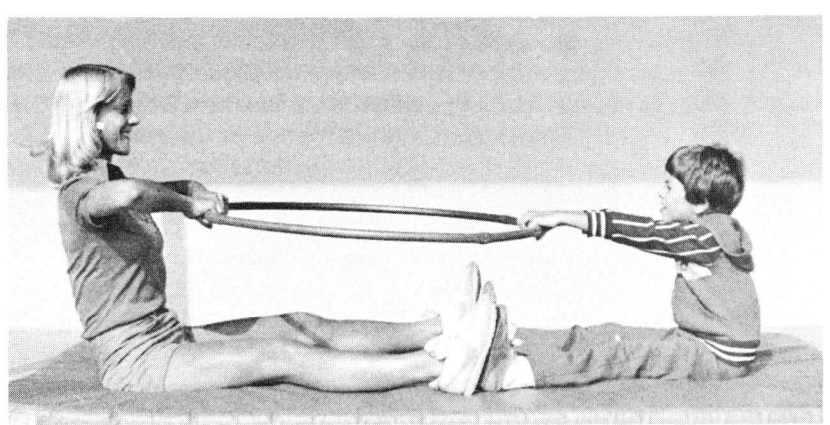

Pulling exercises . . .

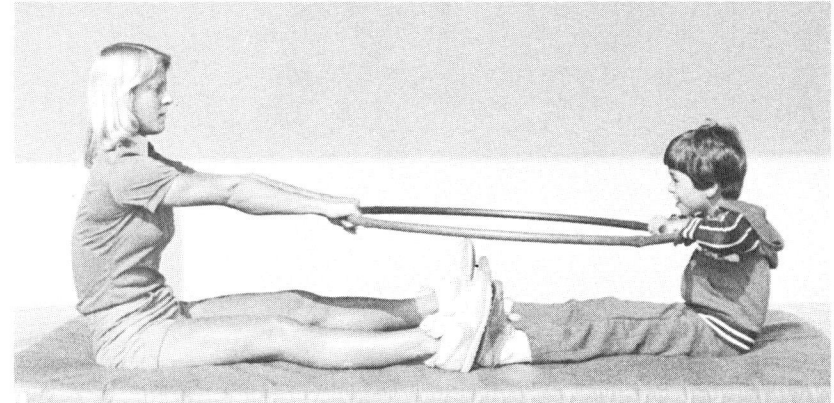

I

. . . strengthen
the arm flexors.

Many pulling exercises may be done on a mat with a partner. Two children, or a child and an instructor, as pictured in photos H and I, can face each other, bottoms of the feet touching and knees straight. Care should be taken so that the children do not lean back using the muscles of the lower back but merely alternate in pulling a rope, towel, or hoop toward each other, using the arm flexors only.

Pull-ups off the ground may be begun by having the child jump into each pull-up as the feet barely touch the ground. Also, braking strength may be gained as a half pull-up is held for increased periods of time (see photo J).

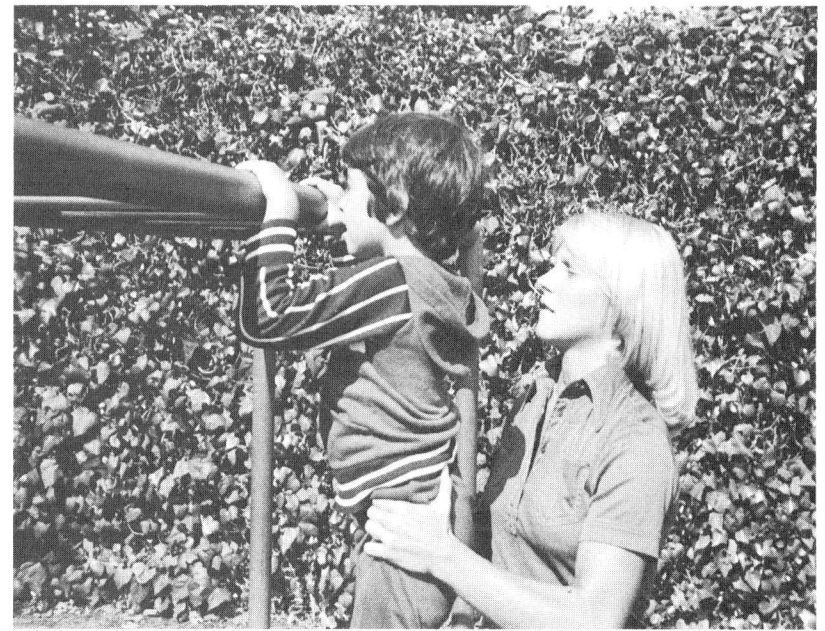

J

Half pull-ups held for
increasing periods
improve braking
strength.

K

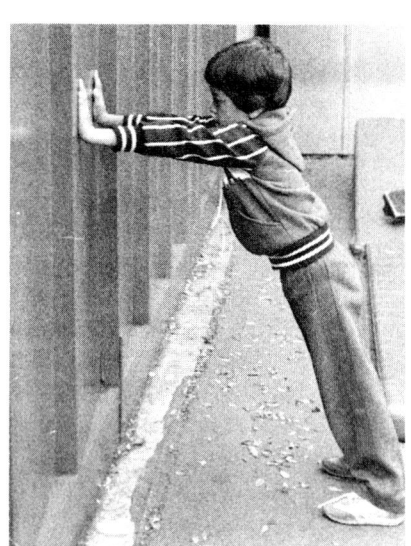

Exercises to strengthen the upper body muscles often begin with wall push-offs.

Pushing   The pushing muscles of the upper body are often tight and overdeveloped, causing round shoulders. Thus, pushing movements should be completely executed. The simplest movement, shown in photo K, is a wall push-off. The arms should be shoulder width apart so the triceps, front deltoid, and pectoralis muscles are in balance. A wider grip employs the chest (pectoral) muscles more, while a narrow grip utilizes the triceps and anterior deltoid more vigorously.

Push-ups may be graded in difficulty by gradually changing the relative height of the arms and feet if a straight-body push-up is desired. A knee push-up, often recommended, is of moderate difficulty, but its execution presents a coordination problem for many handicapped children. The tendency is to bend the body at the hips rather than to keep a straight line when executing it from the knees to the shoulders.

Leg Strength   Handicapped children often have weak leg extensors. Their knees suddenly hit the mat when they are asked to bend them slightly in preparation for a front roll, for example. A number of exercises may be employed to strengthen leg extensors.

Flat-backed squats may be executed to a seated position, as pictured in photos L and M. The final down position should be with a 90° angle at the knees. A padded landing surface should be provided. Extra strain on the extensors is obtained if the child is encouraged to keep the back in a near vertical position while arising. The ascent may be terminated by an additional movement up on the toes to influence the muscles extending the ankle at the calf.

Children may be encouraged to push against foam rubber bolsters or balls while on their backs or on their knees. The teacher should control the resistance and movement. (See photo N.)

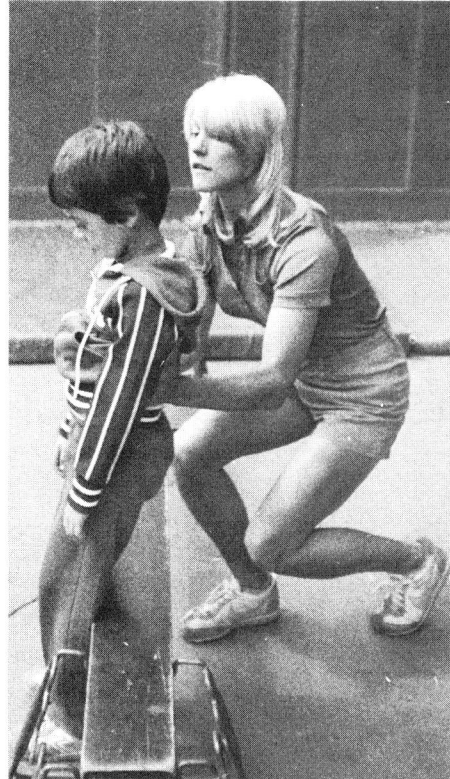

L

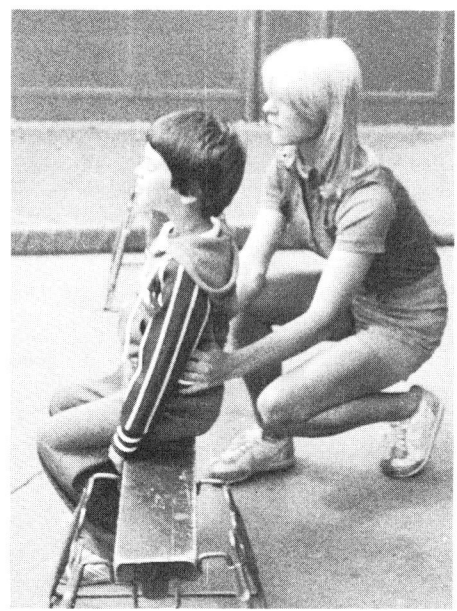

Flat-backed squats   **M**
strengthen leg extensors.

N

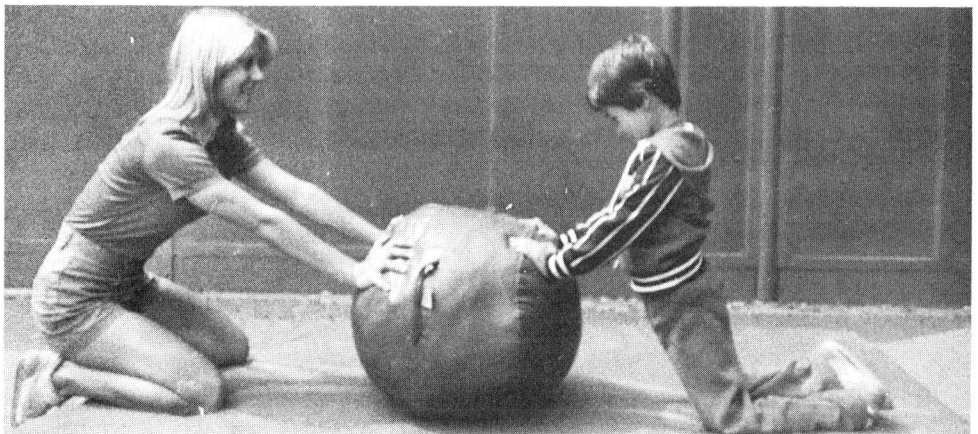

Pushing a bolster or ball against resistance can strengthen arm muscles

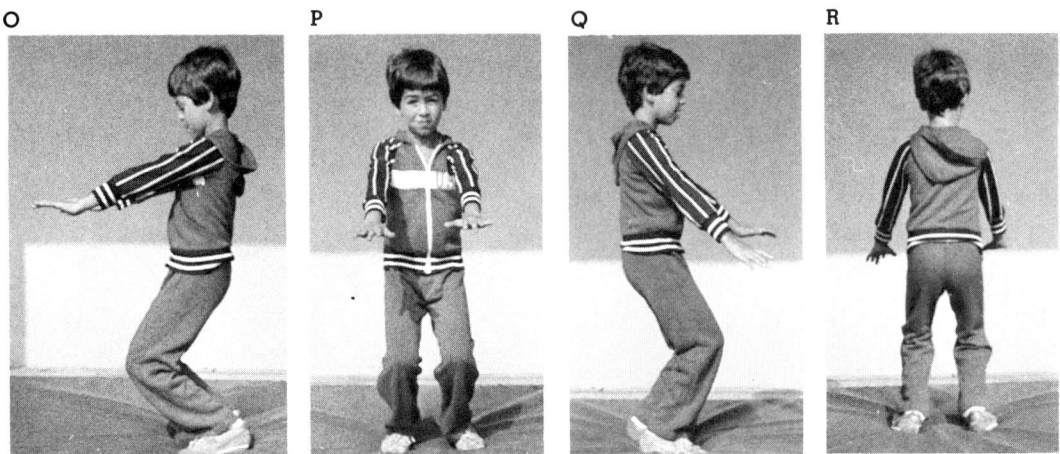

Static strength of leg extensors may be enhanced with half-turn and quarter-turn jumps in a one-quarter position.

Jumps with half-turns and quarter-turns in a one-quarter position (quarter eagles) also may aid in static strength of the leg extensors. The arms are held to the front. The commands "Left!" "Right!" may aid in establishing left-right concepts. Photos O-R illustrate some of these jumps.

Other leg extension work may be instituted on a bench with the legs over the end and resistance applied manually to leg extension. This is illustrated in photo S. Leg strength also can be increased through most games involving locomotion (see chapter 28).

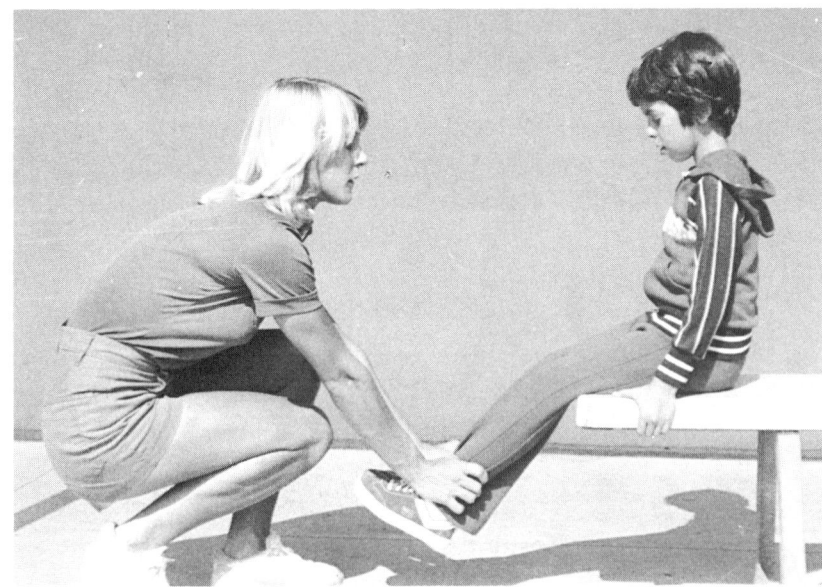

Leg extension may be carried out against resistance.

Activities with Sock Dumbbells   Socks filled with sand make reasonably good dumb-bells in adding resistance to movements when working with younger and atypical children. These are harmless (unless swung at another child!) and soft to the touch, may be graded in weight with little trouble (one simply adds or subtracts sand), and are inexpensive to produce. Various colors of socks may be used, with each child having his or her own col-or. Weights may range from 1-2 pounds through 5 and 10 pounds, depending on the children's abilities.

Using these weights, a variety of activities influencing the musculature of limb move-ment may be introduced. Resistance may be applied in the following exercises, to cite only a few:

1. Deltoid and arm extension strength may be improved by alternately raising the sock dumbbells overhead, as shown in photo T. The legs of the socks make excellent handles.

2. With the child in a bent-over position, the rear deltoid and upper back muscles are involved when the socks are raised to the sides, as shown in photo U. The back should be parallel to the floor.

3. Arm curls, alternately executed, may be carried out as shown in photo V. This exer-cise impacts the flexor muscles of the elbow.

T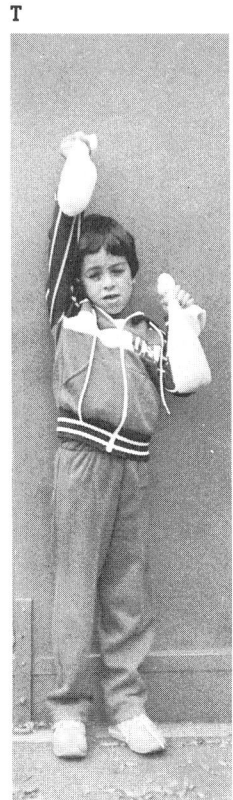

U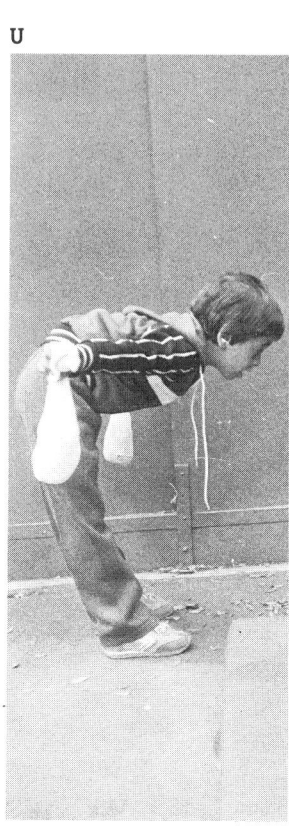

V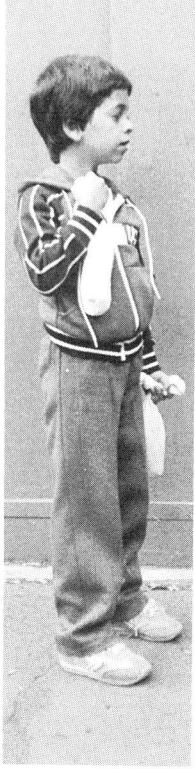

Sock dumbbells may be used to strengthen deltoid and arm extensor muscles (T), rear deltoid and upper back muscles (U), and flexor muscles of the elbow (V).

W

X

Y

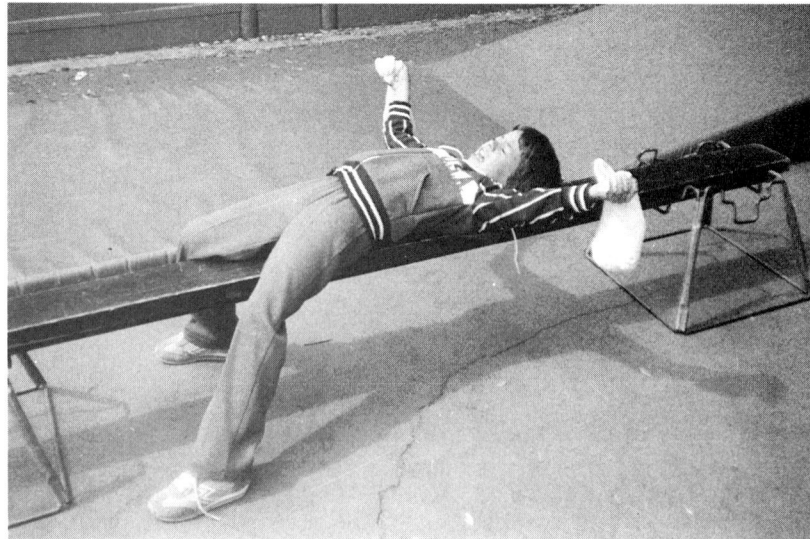

Placed behind the head, they add resistance to sit-up movements (W). Supine presses (X) and lateral raises (Y) may be executed while lying on a bench.

298

4. Alternately raising the dumbbells to the front while in a standing position aids strength in the upper back, deltoid, and arm flexors.

5. When the socks are placed behind the head, as shown in photo W, additional resistance may be applied to sit-up movements.

6. Supine presses, with effects resembling push-ups, may be done on a bench with the socks, as shown in photo X.

7. Lateral raises in the same position (photo Y) are helpful for strengthening the chest muscles. Care should be taken to bend the elbow slightly during the movements and to use light dumbbells (weighing not over a pound or two) with younger children.

Flexibility

Stretching is important, not only prior to an activity but also to elicit maximal range of motion at all joints that are vigorously called into play during running, arm/shoulder activity, and sports skills, including kicking, batting, and the like. Primary stretching exercises should be slow, and the movement should be held for a period of seconds, permitting maximum stretch to occur reflexively. A bouncing stretching movement, commonly seen, is not likely to elicit maximal ranges of motion and may actually damage tissue, impeding the development of flexibility. The problem with the held movements, however, is that they involve discomfort and stress. The benefits of these movements should be explained to students, particularly those who are very young or who are handicapped mentally.

Stretching movements should be done at the beginning of a session and interjected between strength and endurance activities in a total work-out. Some suggested stretching exercises to promote flexibility are briefly discussed in the next few paragraphs.

Hamstring and lower-back flexibility may be improved with either held seated stretches toward the feet, with the knees straight, or in a standing position with the hands extended toward the feet. Another good exercise is to squat, place the hands under the front of the feet, and slowly straighten the legs. Improvement in these and other stretching activities may be measured in units (How close to the feet can the fingertips come?), in duration of the maximal stretch held, and in the number of 5- and 8-second held stretches executed.

Hanging and stretching exercises increase the flexibility of the shoulder girdle. Initial stretching of this kind should be done with the feet on the ground as the child is squatting down and stretching away from the hands holding the bar. Later, if the child has enough strength, the feet may be raised off the ground.

In a front-leaning position, upper body parallel to the ground, shoulder (front deltoid) flexibility may be improved by placing the hands on a waist-high bar and then pressing downward with the shoulders, keeping the knees straight. Two participants, their arms interlocked as shown, also may engage in this type of stretching movement.

The lower back may be stretched in an all-fours position by arching the back like a cat, and then returning the back to a normal position. This is modeled by the boy in the accompanying photos.

If care is taken not to stress the neck unduly, the hamstring group and lower back may be stretched by bringing the feet in back of the head while in a back-lying position. Hand-held sock dumbbells weighing less than a pound may give impetus to stretching movements, with arms in rhythmic swinging positions, circling both ways.

Shoulder flexibility may be improved through mutual stretching exercises.

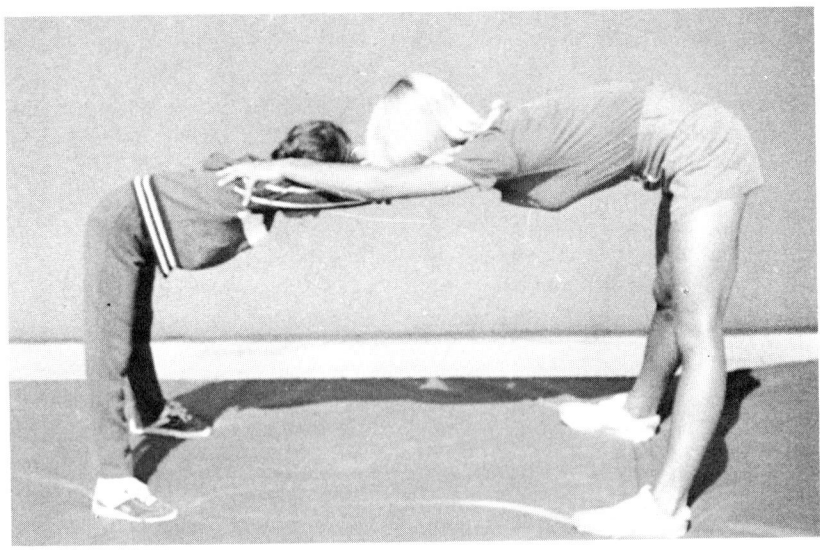

The lower back may be stretched by alternately arching the back and returning to a normal all-fours position.

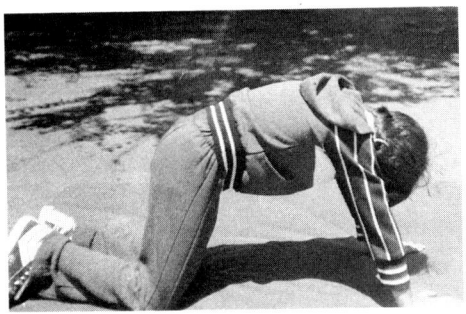
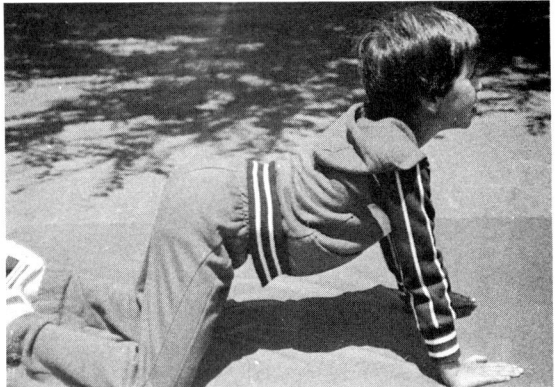

A FITNESS CIRCUIT

Various training circuits in the U.S. combine jogging for endurance with periodic stops for exercise. These circuits are useful insofar as they develop a number of abilities at the same time and, via the exercise stops, tend to maintain a level of heart rate that promotes cardiovascular endurance. Many of the circuits are badly planned, however, having, for example, a leg-tightening isometric in the middle of a course in which the intent is to keep the legs loosened up for running. Training circuits also may contain abdominal exercises that are bunched too close together and could herniate the less fit participants.

Endurance training is best accomplished without the exercise stops contained in these courses but with the interval training described previously in this chapter. At the same time, strength training may best be instituted without the great cardiovascular overloads

Figure 17.4 Sequence of 1,500-Meter Exercise and Fitness Course

START ▼ 100-meter walk (exaggerated arm swing)

Station **1** Forward stretch

▼ 100-meter walk (exaggerated knee-lift)

2 Trunk twist, stretch

▼ 125-meter normal walk

3 Shoulder stretch

▼ 100-meter jog

4 Modified or regular push-ups

▼ 200-meter jog

5 Traveling jumps

▼ 100-meter jog

6 Legs-apart stretch

▼ 200-meter jog

7 Modified or regular pull-ups

▼ 100-meter jog

8 Stretch overhead

▼ 200-meter jog

9 Sit-ups

▼ 125-meter brisk walk (warm down)

10 Bent-knee raises

▼ 100-meter walk, own pace (warm down)

11 Seated reach, stretch

▼ 100-meter walk (warm down)

12 Balance walk and step up-down

FINISH

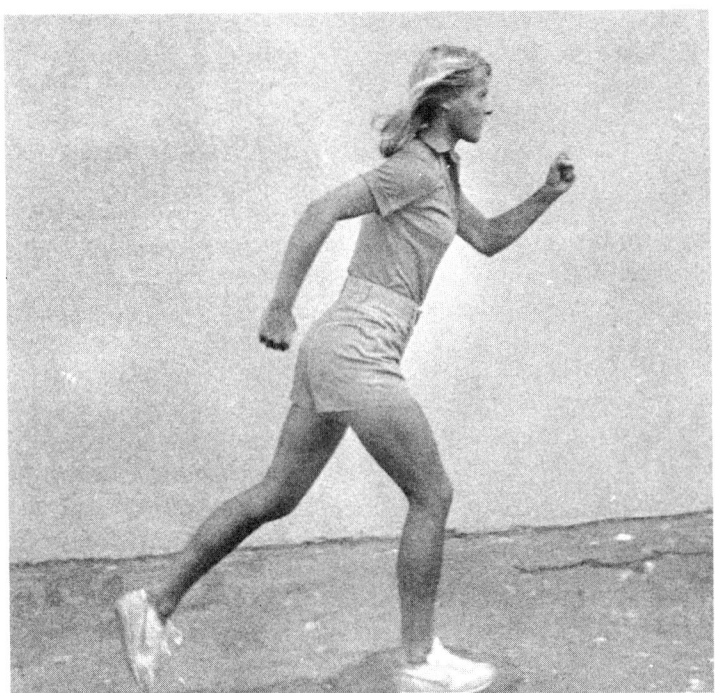

A 100-meter walk with exaggerated arm swinging precedes the exercise and fitness course.

represented by the jogging between exercise stations. To obtain the combined benefits of flexibility, arm/shoulder strength, and leg power and strength, as well as cardiovascular overloads, a course of the type sequenced in Figure 17.4 and represented photographically is useful and, if well planned and in pleasant surroundings, may be highly motivating to participants.

The 12-station course has been laid out over a 1,500-meter distance. The distance between stations may be reduced by half to make a short course, or stations may be eliminated if space, equipment, or finances do not permit construction of the entire course. Many of the exercise stops may be modified for use by wheelchair participants. Preceding Station 1 is a 100-meter walk with exaggerated arm swing.

The course has been designed to promote endurance as well as muscular strength and flexibility of the abdominal muscles, legs, and shoulder-girdle. Intervals between stations gradually warm up the participants and, toward the end, gradually warm them down.

Additional load may be obtained by attempting the course in decreased times, by attempting additional repetitions at each station, or by traversing the course more than one time. Lighter loads may be obtained by interpolating more walking between stations, by omitting stations, by shortening the course, or by reducing exercise repetitions at each station. For substitute actions that may be used with nonambulatory handicapped people, see chapter 19.

Station 1 *Forward stretch*
With knees straight in standing position, reach slowly for feet, arms extended, hold 5 seconds, stand 5 seconds, breathe, repeat six, eight, or 10 times (photo A). An exaggerated knee-lift walk (photo B) follows.

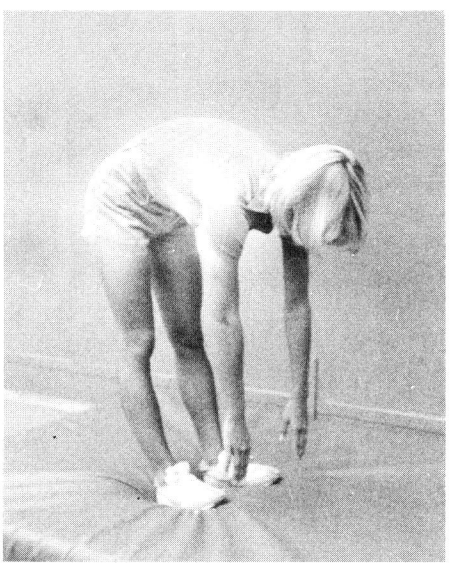

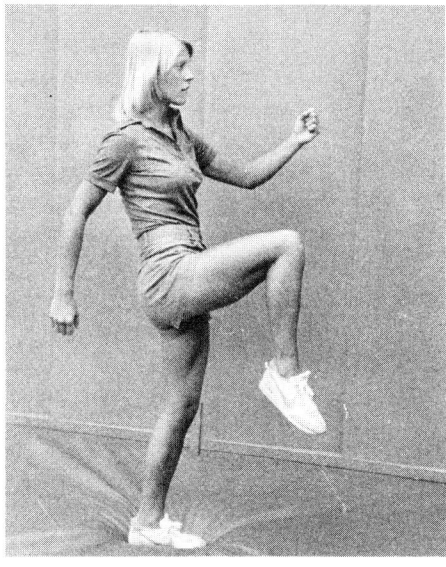

A   **B**

Station 2 *Trunk twist, stretch*
Standing, feet farther than shoulder width apart, twist slowly, touching hand to opposite foot. Hold for 2 to 3 seconds, stand, breathe, and repeat to opposite side. Repeat six, eight, or 10 times.

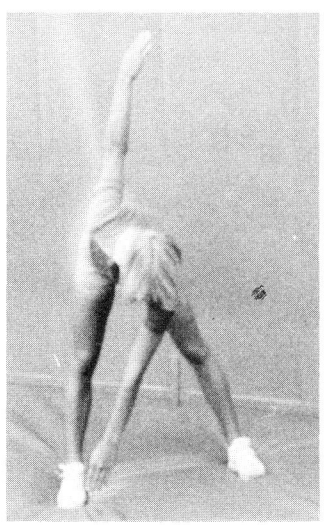

Station 3 *Shoulder stretch*
Standing, bent over at waist at 90°, hands on waist-high bar, arms straight, press downward at shoulders, stretching 2 to 3 seconds; hold, relax, and repeat six, eight, or 10 times, after a 2- to 3-second rest.

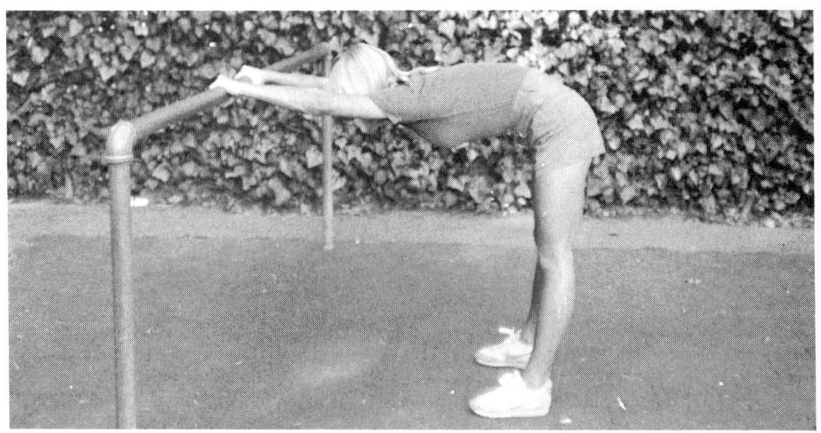

Station 4 *Modified or regular push-ups*
Perform knee push-up (photo A), push-up (photo B), or raised push-up (photo C), as able. Repeat six, eight, or 10 times, as able.

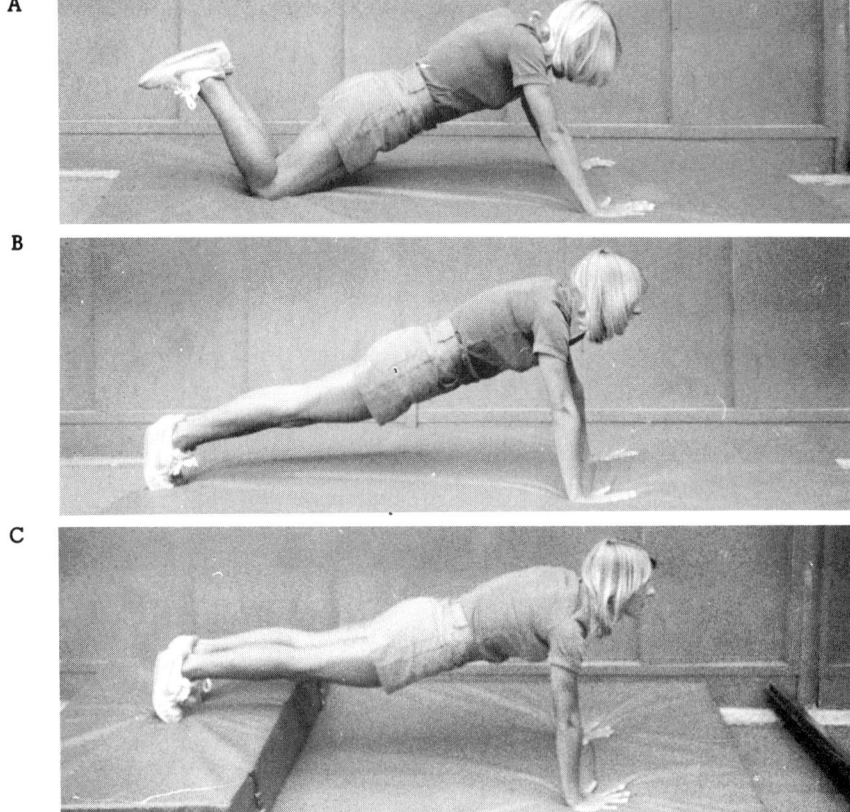

Station 5 *Traveling jumps*

Do repetition jumps, over bars or beams. Use six beams, 4'' x 4'', with 18'' between beams. Complete two, four, or six trips, with 20 seconds' rest between each trip.

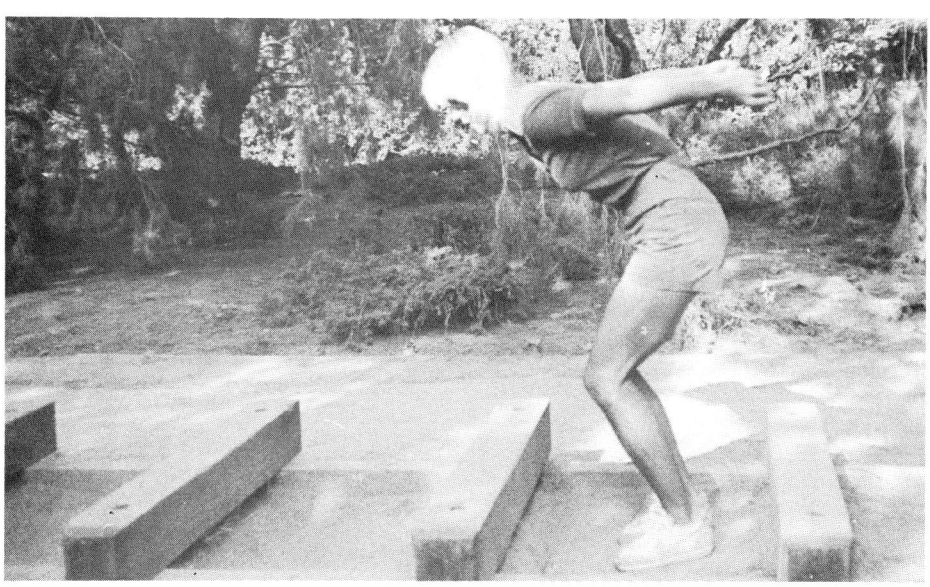

Station 6 *Legs-apart stretch*

Stand, legs apart, and stretch inward on adductor muscles on one side. Hold 2 to 3 seconds; change to the other side, body erect, hands on hips.

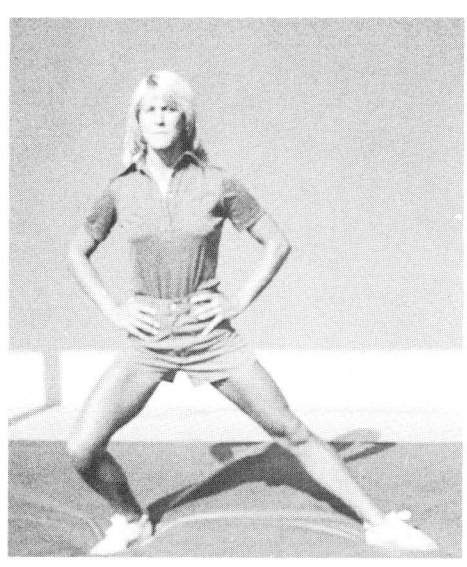 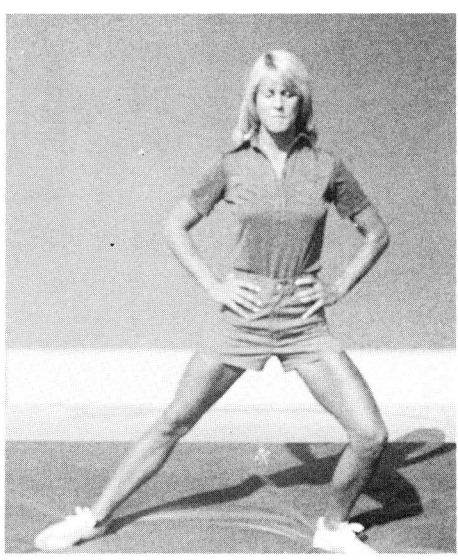

Station 7 *Modified or regular pull-ups*
With bars at chest height or overhead, perform pull-ups as able. Hold positions two, four, or six times.

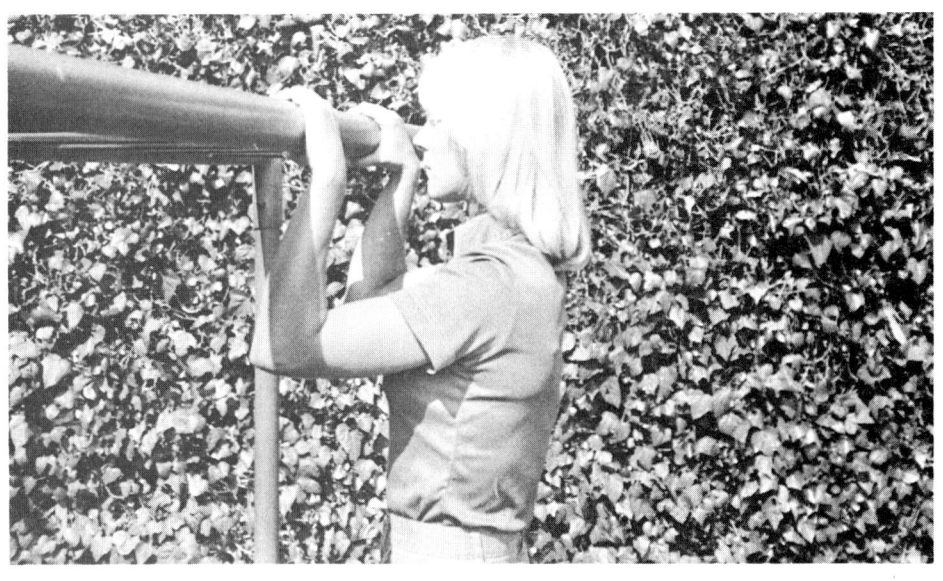

Station 8 *Overhead stretch*
Hang and stretch, as shown, on bar or ring placed so that feet just touch ground. Circle body two, four, or six times, or if on bar, stretch downward 2 or 3 seconds, hold, and repeat four, six, or eight times, after 2 to 3 seconds of rest between each.

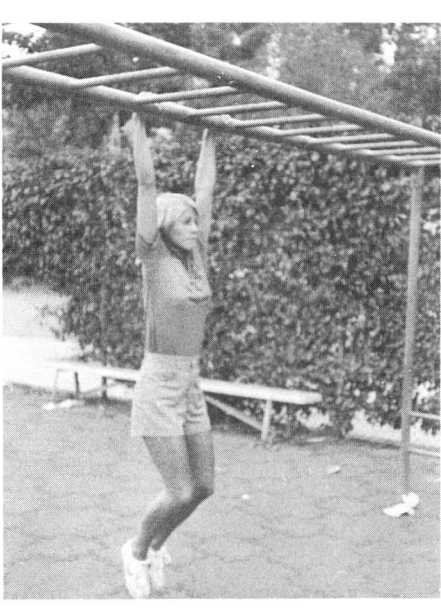
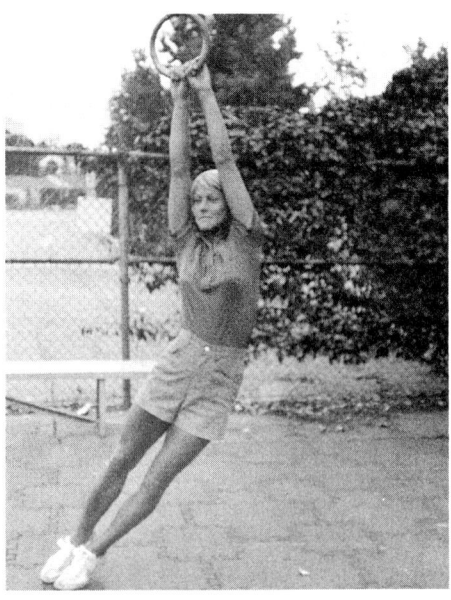

Station 9 *Sit-ups*
Using apparatus as shown, perform eight, 12, or 16 bent-knee sit-ups, hands forward or behind head, as able.

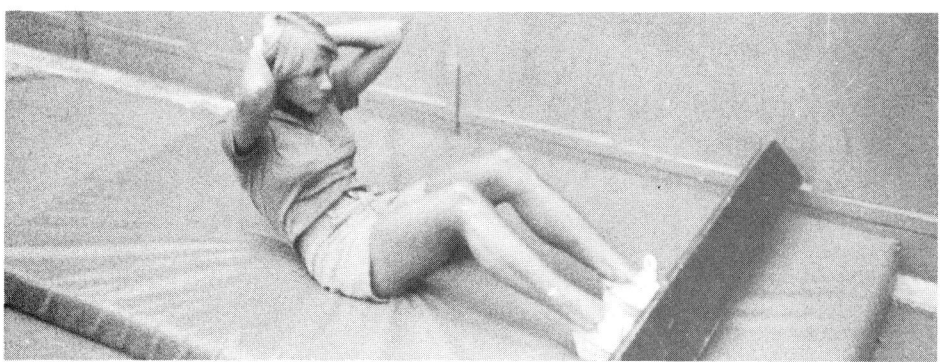

Station 10 *Bent-knee raises*
With body in supine position, slowly bend knees and raise to the chest, keeping hips on the ground; raise slowly. Hold 2 to 4 seconds, return, and rest 2 to 4 seconds between each. Repeat six, eight, or 10 times, as able.

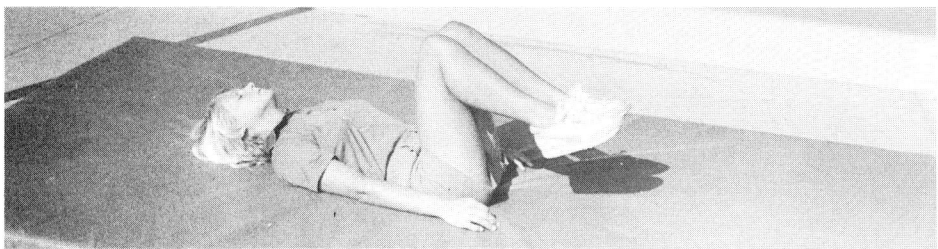

Station 11 *Seated reach, stretch*
In seated position, reach toward feet and hold for 2 to 4 seconds; sit back and relax 2 to 4 seconds between each, repeating six, eight, or 10 times, as able.

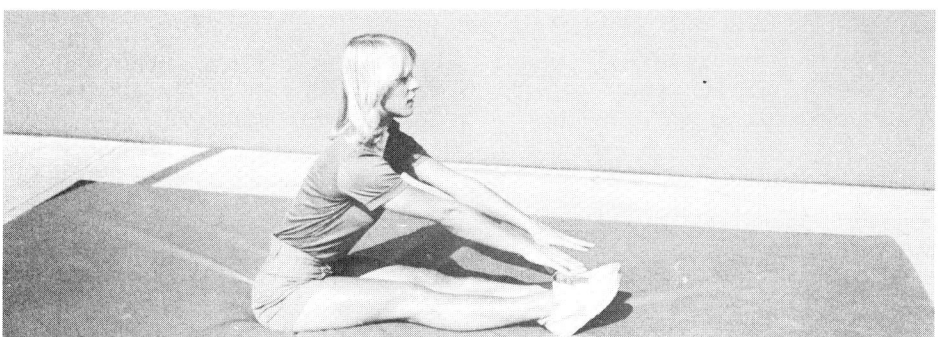

Station 12 *Balance walk, with step-ups and step-downs*
Traverse balance beam, stepping down and up, alternating sides and feet. Traverse two or four times.

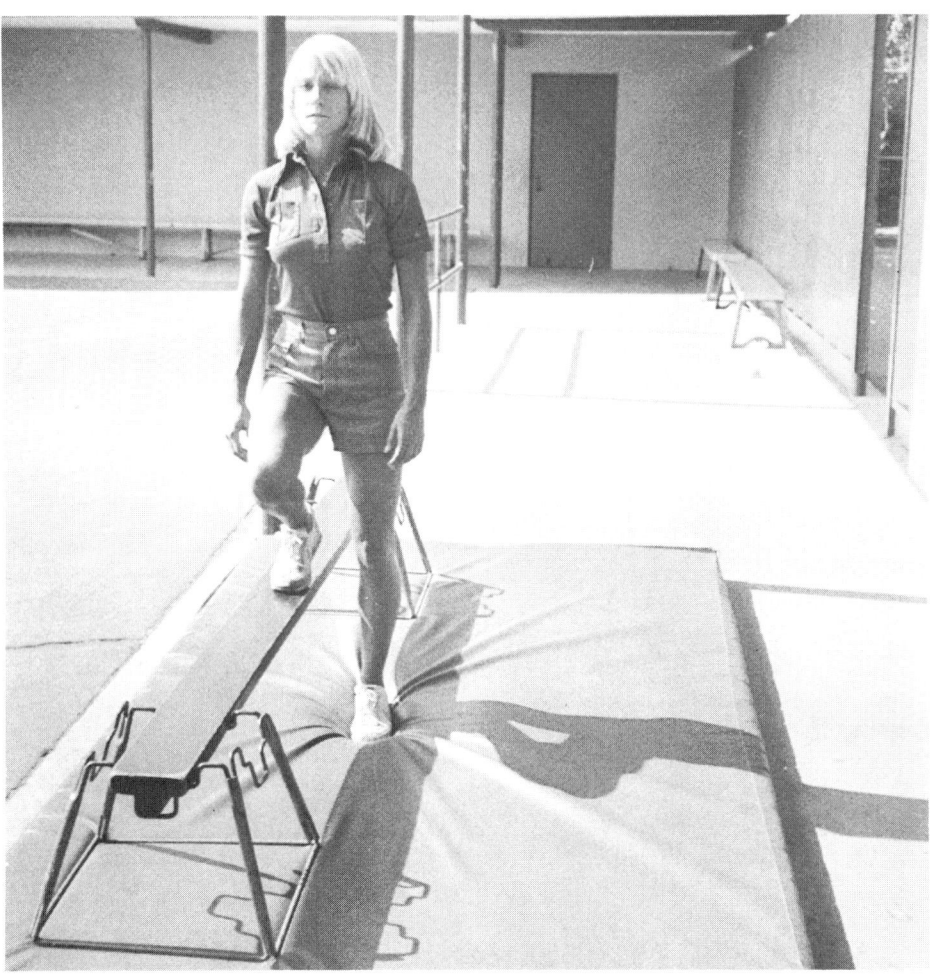

MOTIVATIONAL TECHNIQUES

The most productive way to encourage full participation in often repetitive fitness activities is to formulate individual goals via graphs and in written form and, with charts, plot the increments by which a child approaches these goals. When children and youth are intellectually capable, these goals should consist of (a) immediate goals (number of trials, sit-ups, time to traverse a given distance, etc.), to be achieved in a week or two, and (b) long-term goals, stated in the same terms but consisting of what a child is projected to reach within 3 or 6 months. These goals should place children in competition with themselves—not necessarily with other children or youth in a group. In all the previously described fitness activities, this type of goal setting is possible and desirable. As short-term goals are attained, some adjustments may have to be made in long-term goals, either raising or lowering them, as necessary.

At times a pair of children may be placed in competition if their personalities seem to be able to withstand competition and if their abilities are relatively equal. If possible, fitness testing should be carried out individually with handicapped children, or the children should participate in somewhat different tests so competition will not be excessive.

Helpful motivational devices include graphs, charts, and other presentations depicting a child's improvement. The teacher and student should agree in advance whether these are to be kept private or be available for inspection by others.

In her excellent text on adapted physical education and recreation, Claudine Sherrill (1986) recommends an extensive program of fitness counseling for children and youth who are expected to participate in a physical improvement program. She points out that a child's propensity to work on exercises for self-improvement is a function of the child's total personality and is often a reflection of the emotional strengths or weaknesses that may be present.

Teachers should listen to unfit children relative to their perceptions of the shape and condition of their bodies. Quite often, objective measures of children's physical capacities diverge markedly from their own feelings about these qualities. Psychological counseling, together with fitness counseling, is indicated when children or youth have distorted feelings and concepts about their bodies and exercise capacities, fail to perceive the need for general exercise and specific remedial activities pertinent to their personal needs, and are reluctant to participate in fitness activities intended to enhance their physical effort and overall appearance. If handled carefully, photographs taken at various angles may be used to advantage. In this way, children may obtain a more objective picture of the shape and appearance of their bodies.

Marked difficulties present themselves when younger or less intellectually able children are expected to participate fully in an exercise program. These children may be turned on by physical games and recreational skills more than by formal exercises. In any case, participation in active games is one of the best instigators of cardiovascular fitness in all children and youth.

Younger or disturbed children may be encouraged to work harder physically by (a) arranging highly stimulating conditions, such as an obstacle course or a large play area presenting colorful and motivating movement situations, and (b) instituting a reward system incorporating principles of behavior modification. The reward system should be carefully explained in advance, and rewards should be tendered when real effort and improvement occur. Judicious management of conditions and environmental stimuli, coupled with the teacher's own enthusiasm and sensitivity, will help to encourage these youngsters to exert effort in some of the activities.

SUMMARY

Obesity is a pervasive problem within "developed" countries of the world. Although a portion of this problem is attributable to glandular and other medical conditions, for the most part it stems from undesirable eating habits and environmental influences. In obese persons, both the number and size of fat cells are increased. Because the number of fat cells is influenced even before birth and continues throughout childhood, instilling proper dietary intake as early as possible in a person's life is important.

Physical activity is a vital adjunct in reducing obesity. Obese people, however, often are not highly motivated because the excess weight in itself inhibits exertion. Without question, research has supported the efficacy of exercise and movement components in a total program (including nutritional aspects) to reduce obesity.

Promotion of fitness is vital in all segments of the population, obese and slender, handicapped and nonhandicapped. Handicapped persons, however, pose special problems relative to the stresses they can tolerate when exercising, their understanding of long-term goals, and special equipment that may be needed. Handicapped youngsters in this country must have an individualized education program (IEP) suited to their unique needs. Asthmatics, children with heart disorders, and those subject to seizures, in particular, can be overstressed through exercise. Programs for students with diagnosed medical conditions should be carried out in cooperation with physicians and other medical support personnel.

Fitness has been defined as an increased capacity to move with force, to endure for sustained periods of time in an activity, to exhibit reasonable flexibility in the joints, and to perform muscular skills that permit participation in individual and group sports. The three basic groups of fitness qualities discussed here are endurance, strength, and flexibility, with specific exercises to promote these qualities. In addition, a socioemotional/psychological dimension impacts fitness. Physical educators should attempt to understand *why* a child is not fit and what environmental factors are impacting on the child's body. This awareness can contribute to an overall program that will maximize the child's physical potential while leading to increased self-esteem and the pure enjoyment of participation in a fitness program.

REFERENCES

Abraham, S., & Johnson, C.L. (1980). Prevalence of severe obesity in adults in the United States. *American Journal of Clinical Nutrition, 33,* 364-376.

Beasley, C.R. (1984). Effects of a jogging program on cardiovascular fitness and work performance of mentally retarded adults. *American Journal of Mental Deficiency, 86,* 607-613.

Brook, C.G.D., & Lloyd, J.K. (1973). Adipose cell size and glucose tolerance in obese children and effects of diet. *Archives of Disabled Children, 48,* 301-310.

Chausow, S.A., Riner, W.F., & Bolidean, R.A. (1984). Metabolic and cardiovascular responses of children during prolonged physical activity. *Research Quarterly for Exercise & Sport, 55,* 1-7.

Cratty, B.J. (1986). *Perceptual and motor development in infants and children* (3rd ed.). Englewood Cliffs, NJ: Prentice-Hall.

DeVries, H.A., Wiswell, R.A., Bulsulian, R., & Moritani, T. (1984). Tranquilizer effect of exercise. *American Journal of Physical Medicine, 60,* 186-190.

Di Natale, J., Lee, M., & Ward, G. (1985). Loss of physical condition in sightless adolescents during a summer vacation. *Adapted Physical Activity Quarterly, 2,* 144-150.

Gehlsen, G.M., Grisby, S.A., & Winant, D.W. (1984). Effects of an aquatic fitness program on the muscular endurance of patients with multiple sclerosis. *Physical Therapy, 64,* 653-657.

Glaser, R.M., & Sawka, M. (1984). Exercise program for wheelchair activity. *American Journal of Physical Medicine, 60,* 67-75.

Gortmaker, S.L., & Dietz, W.H. (In press). Childhood obesity. *American Journal of Diseases of Children.*

Jackson, H.J., & Thornbecke, P.J. (1982). Treating obesity of mentally retarded adolescents and adults. *American Journal of Mental Deficiency, 87,* 302-308.

Kelly, L.E., Rimmer, J.H., & Ness, R.A. (1985). Obesity levels in institutionalized mentally retarded adults. *Adapted Physical Activity Quarterly, 2,* 167-176.

Larsson, B., Bjorntorp, P., & Tibblin, G. (1981). The health consequences of obesity. *International Journal of Obesity, 5,* 97-116.

La Vau, J. (1977). Reliable photomicrographic method of determining fat cell size and number: Application to dietary obesity (Proceedings). *Society of Experimental Biological Medicine, 156,* 251-260.

McArdle, W.D., Katch, F.I., & Katch, V.L. (1986). Obesity and weight control. In W.D. McArdle, F.I. Katch, & V.L. Katch, *Exercise physiology* (pp. 531-660). Philadelphia: Lea and Febiger.

Mulholland, J.R., & McNeil, A.W. (1985). Cardiovascular responses of three profoundly retarded multiply-handicapped children during selected motor activities. *Adapted Physical Activity Quarterly, 2,* 151-160.

Parizkova, J. (1977). *Body-fat, and physical fitness.* The Hague, Netherlands: Martinus Nijhoff.

Parizkova, J. (1984). *Growth, fitness and nutrition in pre-school children.* Prague, Czechoslovakia: Charles University Press.

Sherrill, C. (1986). *Adapted physical education and recreation: A multidisciplinary approach* (3rd ed.). Dubuque, IA: Wm. C. Brown Co.

ADDITIONAL REFERENCES

Getchel, B., & Anderson, W. (1982). *Being fit: A personal guide.* New York: John Wiley & Sons.

Godfrey, S. (1974). *Exercise testing in children: Applications in health and disease.* Philadelphia: W.B. Saunders.

Wallis, E.L., & Logan, G.A. (1966). *Exercise for children.* Englewood Cliffs, NJ: Prentice-Hall.

QUESTIONS FOR DISCUSSION

1. What are the causes of obesity? How can it be described clinically? How might it be prevented in infancy?

2. What is the "training-sensitive zone?" What is its significance?

3. By what three qualities can fitness be defined? Give examples of exercises for each quality.

4. What kind of fitness exercises might be best for younger and mentally retarded students? Why?

5. What range of fitness activities might be contained in a program for a mainstreamed class?

6. What criteria might be used when planning endurance activities for various handicapped groups?

7. What modifications in fitness activities and motivational strategies might be incorporated when working with handicapped children and youth of varying developmental ages?

STUDENT PROJECTS

1. Design, on paper, an obstacle course of fitness activities appropriate for individuals in wheelchairs with little or no use of the lower limbs but adequate use of the upper limbs.

2. Discuss fitness activities with a physical education teacher. How often are these activities applied? What special health and motivational problems are encountered? How might a general fitness program be individualized for these children?

3. Assume that you are faced with

developing an individualized program including a goal of reducing obesity in a child? Suggest some specific short-term objectives (and exercises). What additional input (from whom) is needed? What are some ways to elicit the child's cooperation and motivation?

RESOURCES

Institute for Aerobics Research
12200 Preston Rd.
Dallas, TX 75230

President's Council on Physical Fitness
450 Fifth St., N.W.
Washington, DC 20001

18 Body Build and Posture

The overall feeling and picture youngsters have of their bodies form one of the major components of their self-concept. And, conversely, their emotional tone feeds into both dynamic and static aspects of their posture. Studies reflecting concern about posture (particularly standing or static posture) were much more prevalent 30 to 40 years ago than they are at present. Fox (1959), for example, found that 33 articles were published on this subject in the *Research Quarterly* from 1930 through 1939, while only four to six articles were published in the same journal in each of the two decades that followed.

Often both adults and children have concepts about their bodies that are markedly different from how others perceive them and from measurable components of their own body, its size and parts. Thus, youngsters should be counseled thoroughly about the more objective aspects of their body build, posture, and weight. This counseling should seek to discover individuals' perceptions of themselves and the degree to which their perceptions may differ from objective reality, and then to inform them how positive changes may be made in the body, weight distribution, and posture. Prior to counseling, however, the physical educator should establish a philosophy of what constitutes a bodily abnormality and evaluate thoroughly several aspects of youngsters' posture and body build.

Instructors' philosophies concerning postural measurements and what constitutes acceptable individual differences in body build should involve examination of personal feelings about (a) what constitutes true postural divergence,[1] (b) whether a moderate to mild postural divergence that does not interfere with functional movement should be attended to, (c) whether some kind of postural or weight correction program is likely to succeed, taking into consideration inherent and familial tendencies that may be present, (d) what constitutes measures that are reasonable and ethical for physical education teachers to employ, and (e) what information should be obtained from others (e.g., orthopedists, endocrinologists, psychiatrists) to form a comprehensive picture of youngsters' body build, weight distribution, and posture.

In this chapter we will first survey some contemporary ways in which body build is looked on and evaluated. This section is followed by a discussion of posture, postural divergence, and corrective exercises. Both *dynamic* posture, reflected in movement, and *static* (standing) posture are considered.

BODY BUILD (SOMATOTYPES)

Since the beginning of the century, scientific attention has been directed at the evaluation of physique and its possible relationship to other variables including personality traits and tendencies toward delinquent behavior. Kretschmer (1925) proposed that three types of physiques exist: *asthenic* (lean), *athletic* (muscular), and *pyknic* (fat and round).

---

1. Alderman (1966) found that high school girls displayed some divergences; most common were forward head (63%), round shoulders (36%), lateral asymmetry of the shoulders (31%), and hollow-back (29%).

Perhaps the most famous work in this field was carried out by Sheldon and his colleagues (Sheldon, Dupertuis, & McDermott, 1954; Sheldon & Stevens, 1942). Like Kretschmer, Sheldon proposed three types of physique, but unlike the German, he also suggested that within each individual, each of the three types is represented to varying degrees and that the degree to which each is represented may be rather precisely indicated by an index number. Using photographic techniques from which measurements of limb girth and the like were obtained, Sheldon and his co-workers designated three-digit index numbers reflecting the degree to which an individual evidenced muscularity (termed *mesomorphy*), thinness (*ectomorphy*), and fat-roundness (*endomorphy*). Sheldon expanded his work in later publications, attempting to prove that body build was related to personality types and also to delinquent behavior.

Physical educators should be aware of the manner in which they may informally classify the body builds of children in their classes. More recent techniques, notably a method developed by Heath and Carter (Carter, 1970, 1974, 1975), enable someone with relatively little training to engage in accurate somatotyping. The Heath-Carter method, used worldwide, is based entirely on anthropometric measures (including height, weight, four skinfold thicknesses, and the diameters of the humerus, femur, bicep, and calf). Referring to the charts from their 1975 publication, plus combinations of the above measurements, a three-part index number may be easily obtained. The techniques also utilize a photograph of the subject.

For the most part endomorphy is based on several measurements of skin folds (summed). Mesomorphy is reflected in the diameters of the humerus, femur, bicep, and calf. Ectomorphy is based on a height-weight ratio. Figure 18.1 graphically depicts the differences in these three body types. Physical educators and others working with children and youth may use these techniques to obtain rather exact somatotypes and formulate performance norms and skill expectations.

Longitudinal studies of children carried out over periods of time from 3 to 8 years have indicated that children's somatotypes do not tend to remain the same (Parizkova & Carter, 1976). With age, a larger, mesomorphic component usually emerges. If measured well, changes in physique and in degrees of fat, muscle, and linearity as they appear and disappear with increasing age and exposure to programs of exercise, physical education activities, and competitive sports may be charted. Physical educators should be particularly sensitive to (a) the limitations of predominantly endomorphic children relative to endurance activities, (b) the probable high energy levels and tendencies toward hyperactivity of predominantly mesomorphic children, and (c) the potential for endurance activities on the part of those evidencing high linearity.

Moderate to slight relationships also have been found between various body-build classifications and posture. Using 122 Springfield College men (majors in physical education), Cureton (1941) found that mesomorphs, ectomorphs, and ecto-mesomorphs evidenced the best shoulder positions. Mesomorphs and meso-endomorphs had the the least lordosis (abnormal forward curvature of the spine). Hip positioning was best for ectomorphs and endomorphs.

Surveying relationships between body alignment and somatotyping assessments based on Sheldon's techniques, Brown (1959) found only slight positive relationships between

Figure 18.1   Sheldon's Three Body Types (Somatotypes)

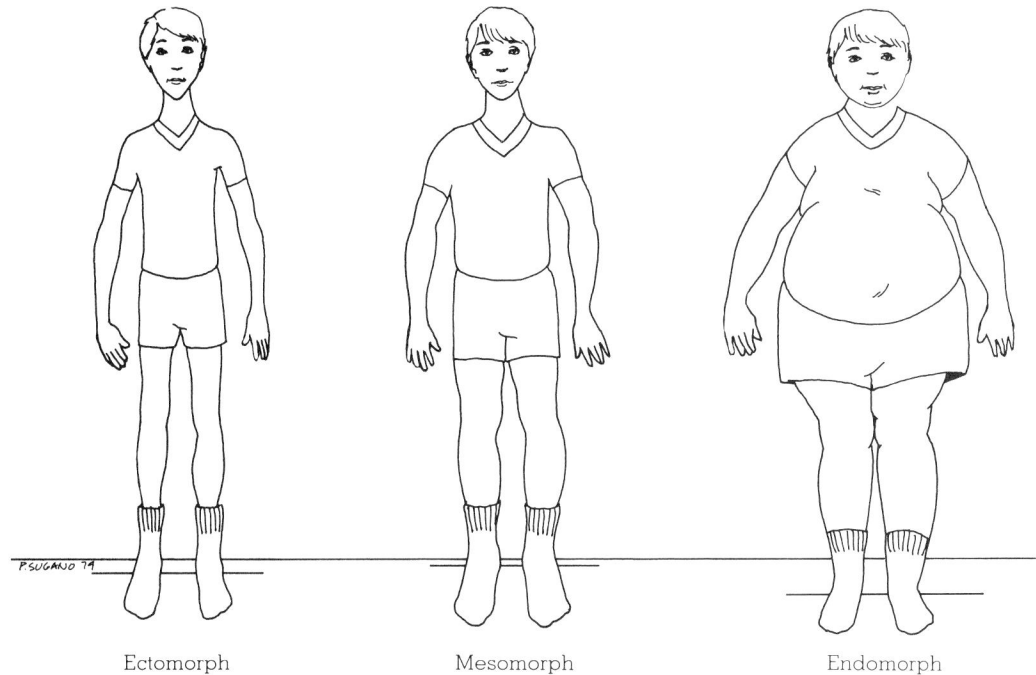

Ectomorph   Mesomorph   Endomorph

body alignment and mesomorphic tendencies. Vertical alignment, measured with a plumb bob dropped from the forehead to the pubic area, had moderate relationships to all somatotype components.

Studies of superior athletes generally indicate that a predominantly ectomorphic type is found in endurance activities. In sprints and other skills in which power must be displayed for a relatively short time, the body builds that excel are not as clearly delineated; the thick-set, as well as the linear, may be good sprinters, both in swimming and on the track.

The tools of the somatotyper include a thorough knowledge of the rationale and techniques involved plus the necessary charts from Carter's (1975) publication. Specific equipment needed includes skin-fold calipers, sliding calipers, a flexible tape, and a good height scale. The somatotyper's vocabulary includes the terms:

—*anthropometry*: the measurement of the dimensions of a person.
—*anthroposcopy*: the visual observation of physical traits that may not lend themselves to exact measurements, including form of the hair, skin color, nose, eyelids, and so forth; i.e., visual examination of the body.
—*dysplasia*: uneven distribution of tissue in the body. A gymnast with larger muscles in the upper body is said to have upward mesomorphic dysplasia, for example. Some data indicate that women may evidence more dysplasia than men. Dysplasia scores are based on individual somatotyping done on four to six body parts.

—*photoscopy*: measurements of the physical characteristics of a somatotype as obtained via a photograph.

POSTURE: EVALUATION AND REMEDIATION

Posture and postural divergences may be considered from several viewpoints:

1. Posture may be considered from an *asthetic* standpoint. Remediations may be applied to make children and youth look better!

2. Posture may be dwelt on from a *functional* standpoint, in which case efforts may be made to evaluate and correct postural problems so that (a) internal organ functioning improves and (b) permanent structural changes do not occur.

3. Posture and *biomechanics* may be dealt with almost interchangeably. Efforts may be made to analyze and improve dynamic posture (the manner in which the body moves with efficiency) and in optimum ways when moving against the pull of gravity, as well as when working and playing.

Posture may have an interrelated, but not causal, relationship to innumerable components of the children's physical and emotional make-up. For example, 31 physical and emotional variables were studied in 57 intermediate-grade girls in two groups by Moriarity and Irwin (1952). The Iowa Test of Dynamic Posture (Lee & Wagner, 1949) was employed as a criterion measure. Eleven of the variables measured indicated differences between those judged to display "good" versus "poor" posture. Those with good posture were found to be freer from disease, heart defects, hearing defects, and asthma, and less fatigued, less self-conscious, less fidgety, less restless, and less underweight than those with poor posture.

Figure 18.2 gives a typical posture chart. Criteria for the various body parts are specific, which makes scoring easy.

Goldthwaite (1952) and others have suggested that good circulation in the vital organs is hampered by a slumped chest because of resultant poor breathing and mechanical blockage. Ulcerated stomach, gastroenteroptosis, and enteroptosis in some cases may be caused by poor posture. The opposite also may be the case; generally run-down or unhealthy children may slump and have poor posture rather than their posture causing health problems and conditions.

Physical educators may take several approaches to the evaluation of posture and the remediation of deviancies. One instructor might become highly concerned with relatively minor divergences, such as a shoulder that is lower than the other shoulder by an inch or two, and institute immediate exercises to correct this abnormality. A second teacher—and this is seen more frequently in recent years—is less concerned with minor problems and concentrates instead on problems that call attention to individuals' physique and stature or reflect some potential or existing functional disturbance when children attempt to carry out movements connected with work, play, and other activities of life. I align myself with the second approach, and the material that follows reflects this philosophy. Physical education teachers should become familiar with and easily differentiate structural problems that are severe and require accommodation and modification in physical education classes from postural defects that lend themselves to possible improvement through exercises that may be applied within adapted physical classes (with the concurrence of an orthopedist or other medical specialist).

Figure 18.2 Typical Posture Chart

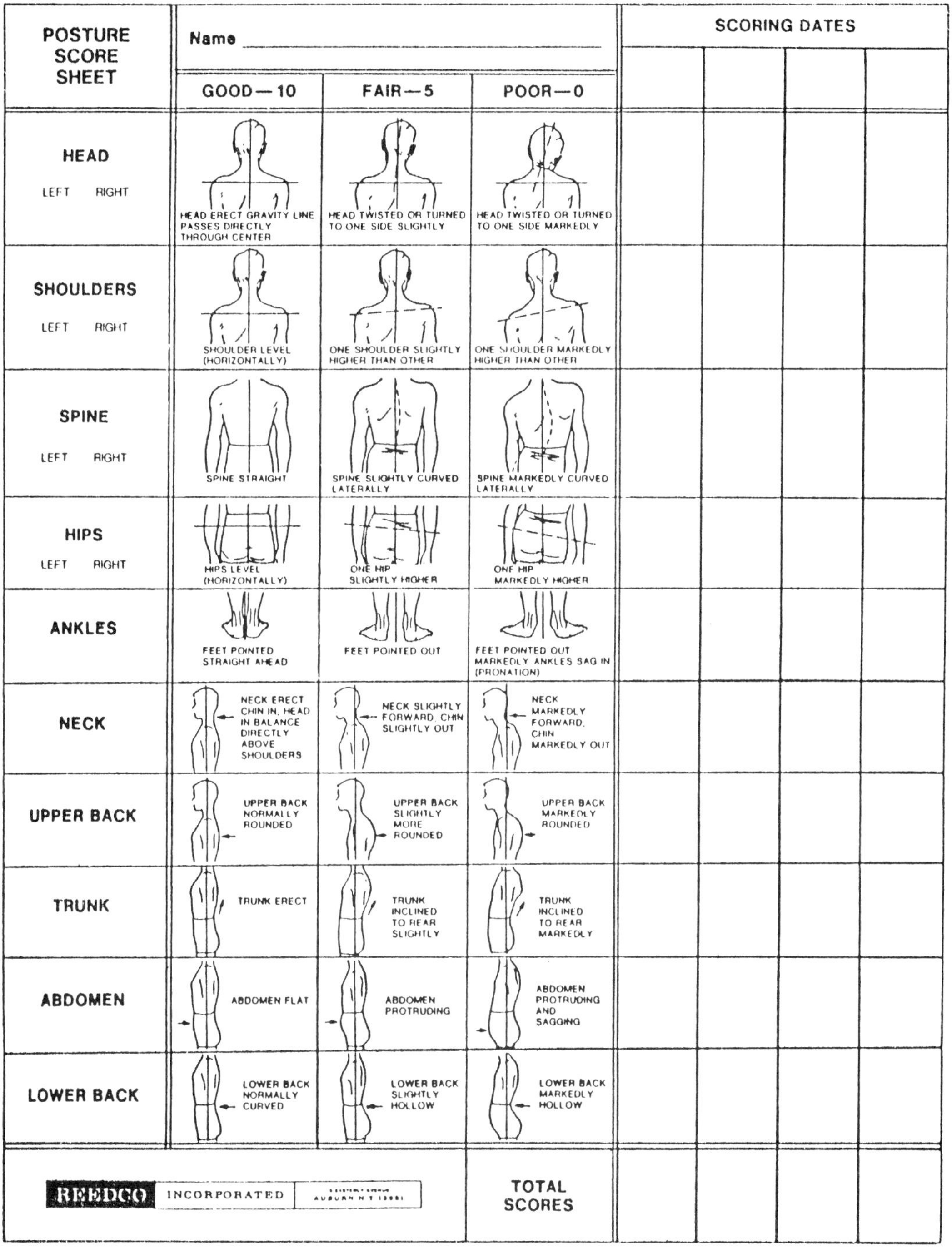

POSTURE SCORE SHEET	Name			SCORING DATES			
	GOOD — 10	FAIR — 5	POOR — 0				
HEAD LEFT RIGHT	HEAD ERECT GRAVITY LINE PASSES DIRECTLY THROUGH CENTER	HEAD TWISTED OR TURNED TO ONE SIDE SLIGHTLY	HEAD TWISTED OR TURNED TO ONE SIDE MARKEDLY				
SHOULDERS LEFT RIGHT	SHOULDER LEVEL (HORIZONTALLY)	ONE SHOULDER SLIGHTLY HIGHER THAN OTHER	ONE SHOULDER MARKEDLY HIGHER THAN OTHER				
SPINE LEFT RIGHT	SPINE STRAIGHT	SPINE SLIGHTLY CURVED LATERALLY	SPINE MARKEDLY CURVED LATERALLY				
HIPS LEFT RIGHT	HIPS LEVEL (HORIZONTALLY)	ONE HIP SLIGHTLY HIGHER	ONE HIP MARKEDLY HIGHER				
ANKLES	FEET POINTED STRAIGHT AHEAD	FEET POINTED OUT	FEET POINTED OUT MARKEDLY ANKLES SAG IN (PRONATION)				
NECK	NECK ERECT CHIN IN, HEAD IN BALANCE DIRECTLY ABOVE SHOULDERS	NECK SLIGHTLY FORWARD, CHIN SLIGHTLY OUT	NECK MARKEDLY FORWARD, CHIN MARKEDLY OUT				
UPPER BACK	UPPER BACK NORMALLY ROUNDED	UPPER BACK SLIGHTLY MORE ROUNDED	UPPER BACK MARKEDLY ROUNDED				
TRUNK	TRUNK ERECT	TRUNK INCLINED TO REAR SLIGHTLY	TRUNK INCLINED TO REAR MARKEDLY				
ABDOMEN	ABDOMEN FLAT	ABDOMEN PROTRUDING	ABDOMEN PROTRUDING AND SAGGING				
LOWER BACK	LOWER BACK NORMALLY CURVED	LOWER BACK SLIGHTLY HOLLOW	LOWER BACK MARKEDLY HOLLOW				
REEDCO INCORPORATED AUBURN N Y 13021			**TOTAL SCORES**				

Note: Used by permission of Reedco Corp., Auburn, NJ.

Historically, methods for and approaches to the evaluation of posture have been chaotic. In analyzing the literature, Fullilove (1969) cited problems in the limitations of subjective tests, the meaninglessness of composite additive scoring, and the absence of adequate norms. The most popular methods of evaluating posture are:

1. *Postural silhouette.* One of the earlier methods employed, the postural silhouette is now sometimes used in conjunction with other procedures. The individual's silhouette is compared to silhouettes arranged from poor to good in both side and front views.

2. *Gravitational line.* The subject stands sideways behind a posture frame, or screen, containing a grid or is photographed against a blank wall, and a line is dropped (or is drawn on the photograph) through five landmarks (lobe of ear, middle tip of shoulder, middle of hip, a point behind the kneecap, and a point in front of the outside ankle bone). Deviations from these landmarks purportedly indicate misalignment in the posterior/anterior plane. Although 80% agreement in the judgments of scorers has been reached using this method, analysis by Hellenbrandt, Riddle, and Fries (1952) pointed out that measurable body sway occurs from the body's gravity constantly shifting, which contributes some unreliability to such measures.

3. *Conformateur.* The conformateur apparatus consists of an upright board through which a number of dowels may be slid and which, when placed just touching the vertebral processes down the length of the spine, provides a picture of the back's conformations. Studies by Cureton (1941) and others indicate that the conformateur is among the most reliable of the instruments available and is more valid than subjective inspections of posture by trained observers.

4. *X-ray.* X-rays help trained personnel to determine whether, for example, scoliosis is structural or functional.

Types of Problems

Primarily, posture problems are reflected by exaggerated curves, convexities, and concavities in the spinal column. These abnormalities may be further divided into those that are viewed from the side (e.g., lordosis, kyphosis) and those that are viewed from the rear (scoliosis). Other postural problems involve the alignment and functioning of the legs, feet, head, and neck. Winged scapula, for instance, usually accompanies a curve in the upper spinal column.

Side-View Abnormalities   Abnormalities of the spinal column may be viewed from the side by taking photographs of youngsters or having children stand with their side to a posture screen. Side views may reveal slight to marked divergences in posture reflected in exaggerated or atypical flatness in the spinal column.

Forward Head   A forward head may be present to a mild or severe degree. If pronounced, this condition is accompanied by *dorsal kyphosis*, a compensatory adjustment of the cervical spine (hyperextension) and the thoracic spine (an increasing dorsal convexity). As is true with other conditions to be described, a forward head (a) never appears in isolation and is accompanied by compensatory adjustments in other body parts; (b) may differ from child to child in severity and some structural accommodations; and (c) may result from a combination of tight musculature (in this case, the neck flexors, or sternocleidomastoids) and flaccid musculature in the antagonistics (i.e., weak head extensors in the rear of the neck, head, and lower back). If the condition persists, the combination of muscular imbalances makes remediation difficult.

Remediation of a forward head (as of other conditions) should begin with attempts to help people gain awareness of the problem by inspecting themselves in photographs and mirrors and through a posture screening. With conscious effort expended over time, individuals sometimes can correct the problem themselves. One way is to carry a book or beanbag on the head, as pictured, preferably while observing themselves in the mirror. Exercises to stretch the head and neck flexors include slowly looking up and directly backward and holding the position, then rotating the head slowly in an attempt to touch the chin to each shoulder in turn.

Head/neck extensors may be strengthened by having someone supply resistance to the rear of the head as the person with the problem sits and attempts to push the head backward, as shown in photo A on the next page. Placing the head face down over the end of a bench and attempting to look up as high as possible strengthens and stretches head and neck muscle groups at the same time. Also effective are more vigorous bridging movements to the back of the neck, in a supine position, as shown in photo B.

Kyphosis A term applied to an unusual convexity of the upper back, kyphosis is a condition of the intervertebral disks or of the epiphyseal areas of the vertebrae. *Pott's disease* (or tuberculosis of the spine) may cause this condition, as may early disturbance in the normal growth of the vertabrae, known as juvenile kyphosis or *Scheuermann's disease*. This latter condition is similar to Perthes' disease and may undergo an active phase during which exercise is not indicated and children should be protected with a head-neck brace.

Frequently kyphosis is accompanied by weak upper back extensors, including the trapezius, and excessively tight anterior intercostals and pectorals. The sternum often is depressed, and a general slumping posture is created by malposition of the internal organs of the lower abdominal cavity. Kyphosis tends to be accompanied by a forward head and hollow chest; shoulder flexibility may become limited, and a compensatory concavity within the lumbar region may appear.

Exercises to strengthen the muscles that can correct functional kyphosis include extensions of the upper body in a prone position with the legs held, as pictured on page 321 in photo A. These reverse sit-ups should be done slowly and through a complete range of motion. This exercise may be varied in intensity and might include raising the upper body and arms only a few inches off the mat for a few seconds at a time, as well as more vigorous exercises raising the upper body up and down while in a prone position with the lower part of the body strapped to a low bench.

In efforts to stretch the antagonistic muscle groups, individuals might stretch backward slowly, with elbows up to the side, and attempt to place the scapulae together, as shown on page 321 in photo B. Various hanging and stretching activities from an overhead bar, as pictured in photo C, also may be done.

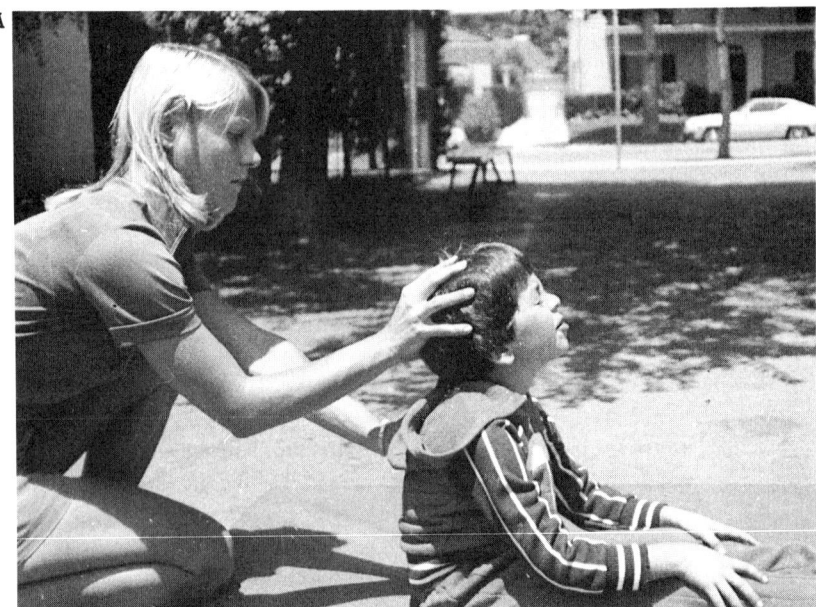

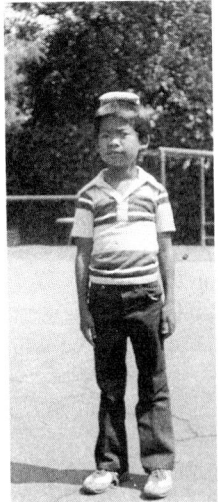

Placing a beanbag on the child's head may help improve posture.

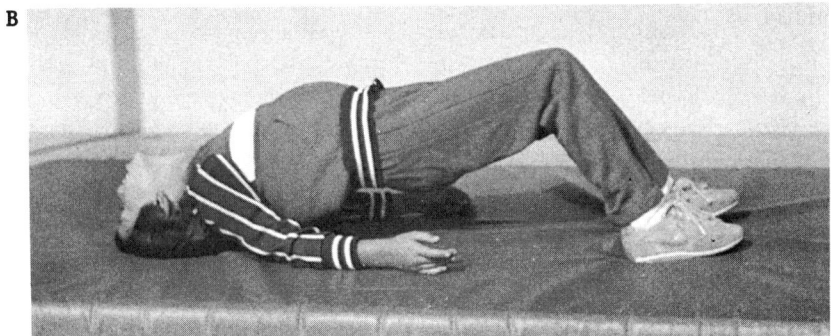

Exercises to stretch and strengthen the head and neck muscles include pushing against resistance (A) and bridging movements (B)

Round Shoulders A forward deviation of the shoulder girdle, including separation of the scapulae in back, this condition is found at times in those who bend over desks all day and in some athletes—notably those whose arms are involved in vigorous activity in front of the chest, as in baseball and basketball. Freestyle swimmers and those who swim the butterfly may evidence this condition.

Overall there is an imbalance between the muscles that rotate the shoulder forward (the pectoralis minor and serratus anterior) and the muscles that pull the shoulder back (the rhomboids and the trapezius). Pulley exercises requiring backward and upward motions are good. Any exercise or activity that stretches the upper chest group, including swimming the back crawl stroke, is helpful, as are exercises intended to strengthen the muscles that flatten the upper back.

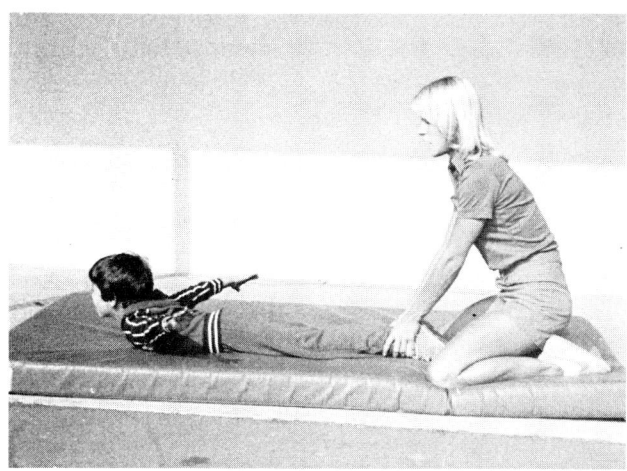

A

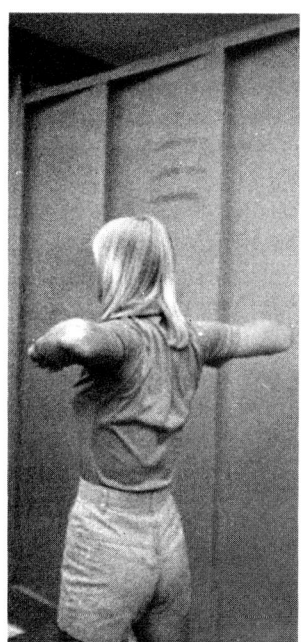

B

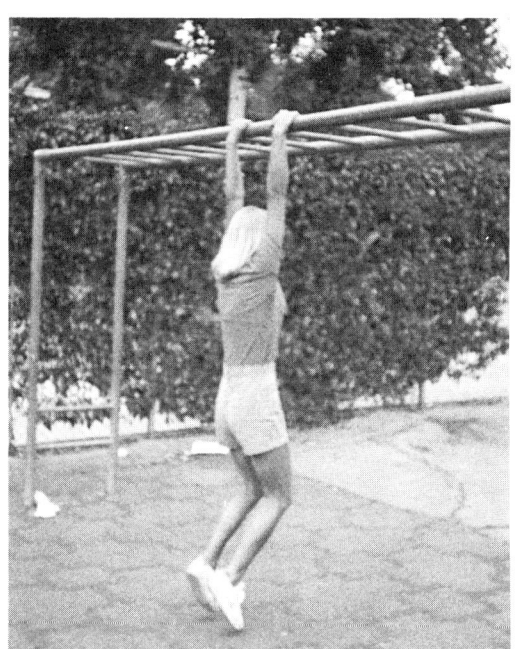

C

Exercises to help correct kyphosis include reverse sit-ups (A), stretches to move the scapulae together (B), and various hanging and stretching activities on an overhead bar (C).

Head Tilt   Often indicative of a vision or hearing impairment, a head habitually held in a tilted position requires first that the child perceive the problem through the use of mirrors and then begin slow, static stretching exercises for the muscles in the neck on the side toward which the head is tilted. These exercises may be self-applied or undertaken with the help of another person.

Torticollis   Sometimes called *wryneck*, torticollis is caused by a shortening of one of the sternocleidomastoid muscles. If the condition is not congenital, slow stretching is recommended. The condition sometimes is accompanied by compensatory changes to the spinal curvature in the cervical region or the thoracic portion of the spine.

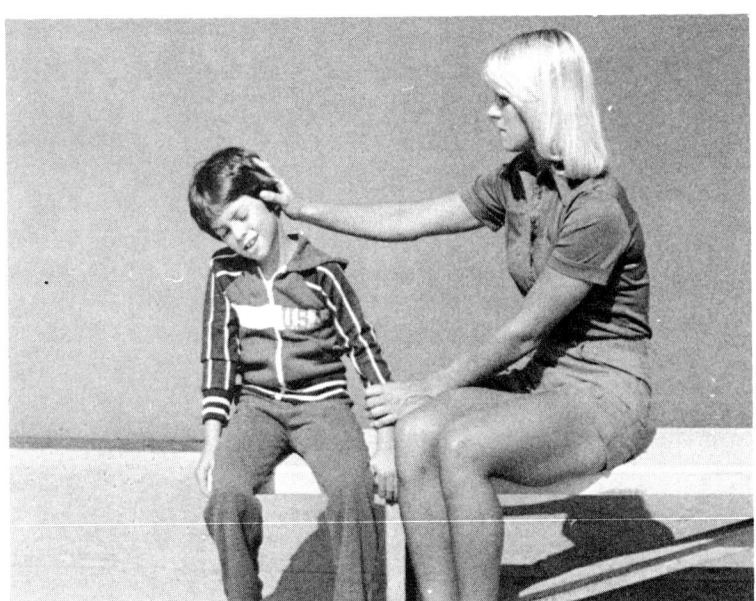

Slow, static stretching exercises to correct head tilt may be undertaken with the help of another person.

Lordosis   A swayback or hollow-back condition sometimes is seen ın relatively well functioning youth and even in superior athletes. The pelvis is tilted, with the anterior portion lower in front. The condition may be attributable to inherited traits or to muscular immaturity. Another cause may be an imbalance between the muscles that pull the pelvis up in front (the abdominals, primarily), tight hip flexors that pull the hips down in front, and tight lumbar extensions that pull the pelvis up in back. Remedial exercises should concentrate on strengthening the usually weak abdominals and muscles that stretch the lumbar extensors.

Flexibility exercises for the lower back include alternately and slowly arching and depressing the middle of the back while in a hand-knee position. Attempting to flatten the lower back against the floor while lying flat with legs bent and feet on the floor, and standing toe-touches with the knees held straight, if held, are other helpful stretches for the lower back.

The shape of the spinal column in young infants and children undergoes several changes from birth to middle childhood and adolescence. At birth the spinal column is in a flexed C-shaped curve. Prior to walking—and probably because of supine and prone kicking and stretching done naturally—rudimentary cervical and lumbar curves begin to appear by the fourth or fifth month. As children begin to walk at the beginning of the second year of life, an increased lumbar curve appears. By the time children enter pre-school, the lumbar curve may be exaggerated, but with normal maturity and the strengthening of the abdominals in play and with exercise, the curve lessens by middle and late childhood. When evaluating the severity of lordosis, these developmental guidelines should be kept in mind.

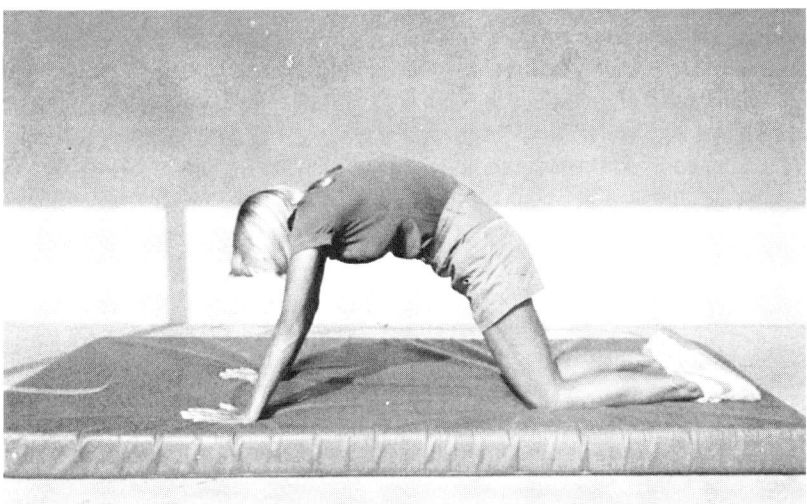

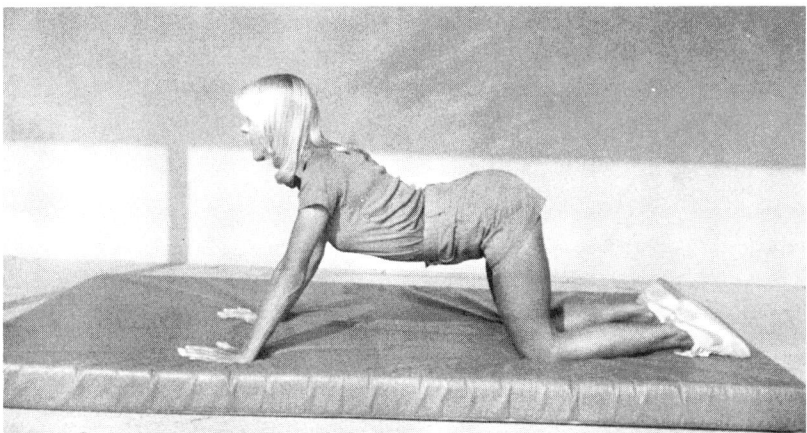

Alternately and slowly arching and depressing the middle of the back is recommended for lordosis.

Flat Back A condition that is the opposite of lordosis is flat back, a decrease or absence of the normal anteroposterior curve in the spinal column. The pelvis is inclined less than normal and is held in a continuous posterior tilt. The buttocks do not protrude as would be expected. The lower back muscles may be weak, as may be the hip flexors. After individuals are made aware of the condition through evaluation instruments, photos, and a mirror, exercises may include (a) stretching the lower back downward while in a hands-knees position and (b) hyperextension of the lower back in a front-lying position to stretch the back extensors.

Loose Abdominals (Ptosis) Much of the time a lack of tonus in the abdominal musculature accompanies lordosis. In infants and youngs children the condition is normal, but by age 5 exercise and vigorous running activity, which require that the pelvis be stabilized by tight abdominal muscles, usually result in a flattening of the abdominal wall. If the abdominal wall remains too relaxed, for a variety of reasons including lack of exercise, internal organs may be displaced. Extreme displacement of the abdominal organs resulting from an abdominal wall that is too relaxed has been termed *visceroptosis*. Researchers including Shephard (1972) contend that "surprisingly large" displacements of abdominal organs can occur without adverse effects. Many contemporary observers believe that the main justification for improving a slack stomach is aesthetic and cosmetic.

To rectify ptosis, a variety of abdominal exercises are recommended to act on the four main muscles in several layers: (a) the rectus abdominis, which flexes the lumbar vertebrae from the pubis to the bottom of the rib cage; (b) the external oblique muscles, which act most strongly when performing twisting exercises; (c) the internal oblique muscles, which also are brought into force during flexing and twisting movements of the trunk; and (d) the transverse abdominal muscles, which both flex and twist the trunk.

In general, when exercising the abdominal muscle group, care should be taken so that other hip flexors (notably the psoas major) are not brought into forceful action, causing hyperextension of the spine and possible pain. When performing most abdominal exercises, the legs should be partially flexed at the hips and knees to avoid lower back pain and to place the stress directly on the desired muscle groups.

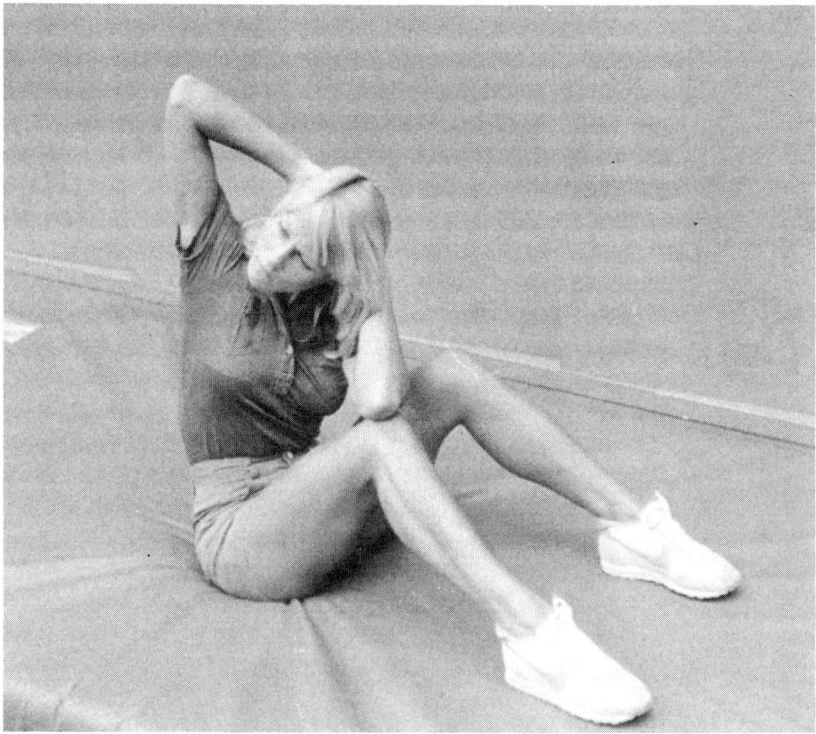

The entire abdominal muscle group, including the obliques, may be tightened by twisting sit-ups.

In addition to the variety of sit-ups described in chapter 17, other abdominal exercises, including those involving locomotion, may be used. An exaggerated knee-lift when walking, by pulling each knee in turn to the chest, will activate abdominal muscles, as will a flutter kick at the end of a swimming pool or propelling a kickboard across the pool.

Abdominal exercises should be performed with regular inhalation and exhalation of breath. Breath holding, while affording a column of air against which more resistance can be applied, is not desirable or healthy. Children and youth should be encouraged to attempt a regular breathing pattern at each repetition, or to whistle or otherwise relax the area enough to take in air regularly when exercising. This kind of regular breathing also mitigates against hernias when exercising. Twisting sit-ups are desirable to work all the abdominal muscles.

Knee raises are preferable to leg raises, particularly with the handicapped. The poor leverage applied to the lower abdominals in stiff-legged raises may pull and tear the muscle attachments or cause a hernia. Knee raises not only may improve appearance and help support important abdominal organs but also may help relieve excess stomach gas, lessen the discomfort of menstruation, and improve local circulation.

Rear-View Abnormalities: Scoliosis   Deviations that may be viewed from the rear of a child include both C- and S-shaped curves in the spinal column. These are made clear by placing a mark (using a black grease pencil) on the spinal processes of each vertebra and comparing the line they make to a plumb line dropped from the center of the back of the head.

Scoliosis, lateral curvature of the spine, may begin with a single primary curve in the upper back and a compensatory curve in the lumbar region. At times the curve begins with a C shape and progresses to an S shape. Remediation of this problem is relatively easy in early childhood but can become progressively severe and should be referred to a physician, as it can become a serious problem if it progresses from a functional condition (caused only by muscular imbalance) to a structural one (accompanied by changes in the shape of the vertebrae) (Cailliet, 1975; Keim, 1972). Surgery and bracing are done later in life in the more pronounced cases.

Differentiation between functional and structural scoliosis may be determined by having children assume an "Adam's position," bending forward as shown in the photo. If in this position the curve tends to disappear, scoliosis is still functional, but if the curve remains, the condition is assumed to be either transitional or structural.

Scoliosis is accompanied by these additional postural adjustments:

1. The spinous processes rotate toward the concavity of the curve.

2. If functional, the vertebrae assume a wedge shape, stamping in the curve, or S.

3. Maladjustment of the chest musculature occurs, including lateral displacement of the trunk toward the side of the convexity. The ribs in front may bulge out on the convex side of the curve, and the rib cage may lose its flexibility.

4. Movements or movement capacities (e.g., side bending) are freer to the concave side than to the convex. Forward flexibility of the spine may be limited as a natural protective mechanism of the body against further deformity. Muscles on the concave side become increasingly tight with maturation, while those on the convex side are stretched and become weaker.

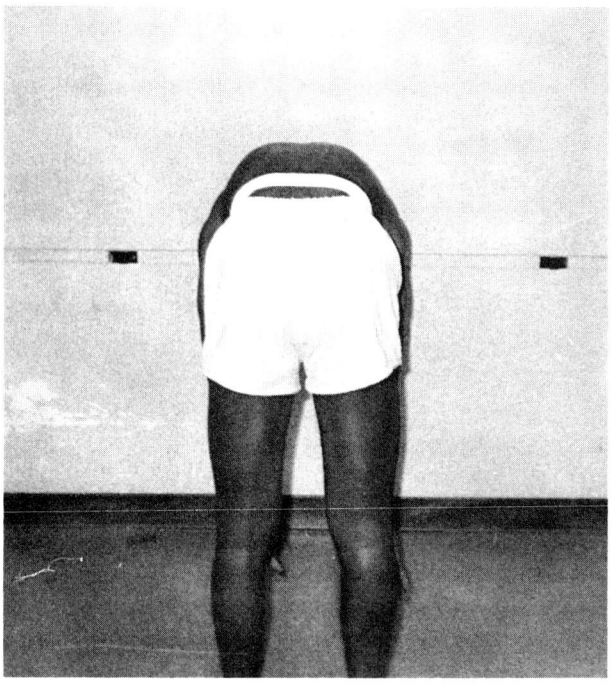

Functional and structural scoliosis may be differentiated by having the child assume an "Adam's position."

5. Other adjustments include a possible head tilt in a direction opposite from that of the shoulders, as well as differences in hip height, slanting in a direction opposite from that of a possible deviation in shoulder height.

Various forms of scoliosis, accompanied by compensatory shifts in shoulder heights and hip alignment, are shown in Figure 18.3. Slight, but observable, lateral asymmetries of posture are prevalent. In an x-ray study by Klein (1973) of 830 schoolchildren, 93% of the 8- to 12-year-old boys had some degree of scoliosis. Although the condition seemed to increase with age in boys, it appeared to decrease with age in girls.

Over a period of 3 years, Klein studied the effects of inserting heel lifts in the shoes of elementary school boys evidencing pelvic tilt. The lifts were inserted in the shoes of the experimental groups for a 6-month period. Although none of the control subjects improved, 80% of those with heel lifts did improve in the degree of pelvic tilt. Klein and others have cautioned, however, that lateral pelvic tilt may be caused by conditions, other than a short leg, including knee angulation, foot pronation, flat feet, pelvic asymmetries, and extreme rotational patterns while walking.

If the curvature does not disappear when the child lies down or assumes the Adam's position, he or she should be immediately referred to a physician, who may classify the child as having (a) mild scoliosis, marked by a deviation of 15°-30° from the major or

Figure 18.3   Various Forms of Scoliosis

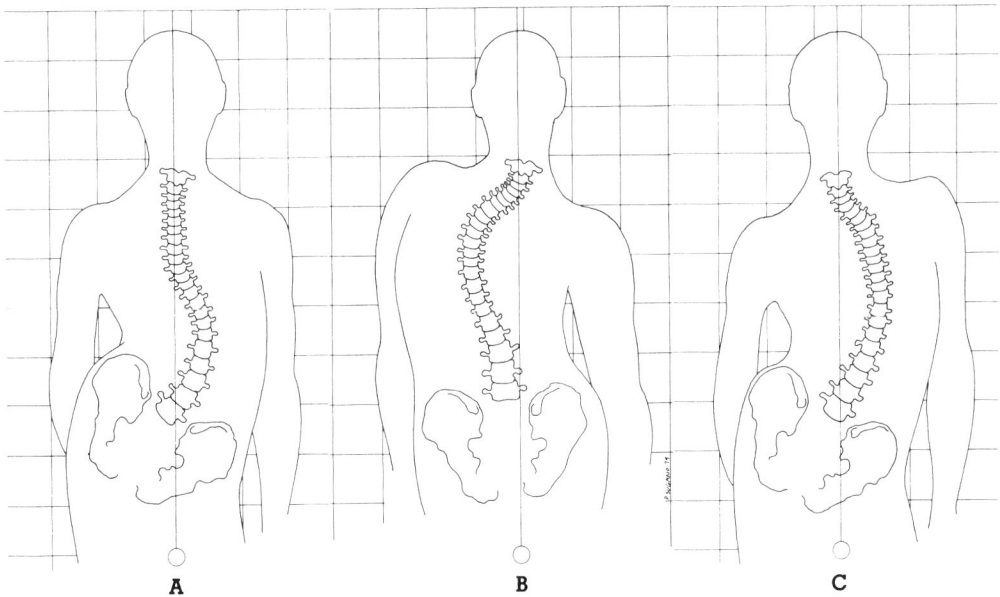

C curves in the: lumbar region (A), cervical region (B), and total spinal column (C)

ordinary curve from the normal; (b) moderate scoliosis, a deviation of 35°-75°; or (c) severe scoliosis, represented by deviations of 75°-150°. A number of medical interventions, such as a cast with a turnbuckle that can be gradually adjusted, or other bracing techniques, are used to correct the problem. Among the symmetrical exercises that may be used are stretching forward in the Adam's position and hanging and stretching from a high bar. Asymmetrical exercises are those intended to tighten the muscles along the convex side of a C-shaped curvature while loosening the muscles along the opposite side of the trunk. These should be prescribed and supervised by a physician.

Deviations of the Hips, Thighs, and Feet   Deviations of the hips, thighs, and feet are similar to and often interact with each other and with the previously discussed postural conditions. Pigeon toes, for example, may be attributable to overly tight ligaments at the hip joint. Some conditions to be discussed are structural, probably inherited, and do not readily lend themselves to correction by exercise. Other abnormalities in the hips and lower extremities are amenable to change via strength building and stretching exercises.

Like deviations of the spine, upper back, and head/neck, some of the so-called postural problems involving the hips and lower extremities are found not only in physically well functioning individuals but also in superior athletes. Some jumpers in track and field and vaulters in gymnastics, for example, are unable to touch their knees together while standing with their ankles touching. Some flat-footed individuals (in whom the longitudinal arch has fallen downward) are among the fastest runners on a track team. Therefore, prior to moving ahead with an exercise program, orthopedists who have evaluated the youngsters should be consulted.

Postural problems stemming from functional or structural abnormalities of the hips and thighs are closely associated and are classified according to three types:

1. Deviations reflecting excess inward or outward rotation of the femur as it articulates with the hip socket.

2. Unusual angulations of the neck of the femur, causing either a knock-kneed or a bow-legged effect.

3. Femoral shaft descending from the hip at angles that prevent good mechanical efficiency (e.g., a too wide-hipped effect for good forward thrust, particularly in running; this explains the loss of running efficiency in some girls as they mature in adolescence).

Femoral Torsion   Lack of flexibility in the hip rotators may indicate femoral torsion, also called *anteversion*. This twisting or bending forward of the femur is seen most often in infancy, and it often corrects itself with maturation. Individuals who are restricted in rotation are capable of much more inward rotation (from 60° to 80°) than outward rotation (about 20°). Those who are restricted in the ability to rotate outward at the hips have great difficulty in assuming the five positions in ballet without an extended program of slow stretching exercises.

Toeing Inward/Outward   The tendency to toe inward or outward may stem from imbalances in the strength of muscles that rotate the hips. Toeing inward usually is caused by the inward rotators', including the gluteus minimum and gluteus medius, being stronger than the outward rotators. These inward rotators may be stretched by attempts to assume the basic ballet positions and other foot positions that rotate the thigh outward.

Toeing outward is caused by greater strength in the six muscles to the rear of the hips (sacrum) than in the inward rotators. To correct the tendency to toe outward, exercises include walking and standing with inward rotating movements instigated by placing one's feet into paper footprints pasted on the floor, and resisting manual inward rotation of the feet while lying on one's back.

Hyperextended Knees   A "shock-kneed" stance may appear infrequently in children or youth, particularly those who are thin and, therefore, whose knee-joint musculature permits hyperextension. The condition may be accompanied by lordosis. If habitual, the chances for knee injury are increased. Forward stretching exercises should be avoided because they tend to exaggerate the condition. Exercises to strengthen the hamstring group, the hip extensors, and the knee flexors are helpful.

Bow-Legs   Bow-legs usually are structural and congenital in nature. Many times they do not impede function. The weight is placed on the outward part of the foot. Exercise may be useful in rectifying the condition only if it is functional. Before instituting a program, however, a diagnosis should be obtained from an orthopedist.

Knock-Knees   Knock-knees, usually congenital, is a condition often accompanied by obesity and by increased stress on the collateral ligament of the inner (medial) aspect of the knee. This condition makes youth susceptible to knee injury, particularly if they participate in football, in which blows to the outside of the knee are frequent. Pronation of the feet and weakness in the longitudinal arch often accompany this condition. Among the muscle groups that may need strengthening are the sartorius and medial hamstrings passing over the knee joint to insert on the tibials and the outward rotators of the hip joint. Thus, muscles on the lateral part of the leg (peroneal group) should be stretched, if possible.

Tibial Torsion   A chronic inward rotation of the tibia or of the entire leg, tibial torsion often is more marked in one leg than in the other. If the child has had a condition that has not permitted normal weight bearing in childhood, tibial torsion can develop. A short leg on which weight has not been borne also tends to rotate inward by middle or late childhood. Various compensations by ligaments in the joints of the feet and knees may require surgery to correct. With the help of an orthopedist, exercises should help children or youth strengthen and stretch muscles that permit normal weight bearing by the leg(s) rotated inward. Exercises for pronated feet and flat feet also may be helpful.

The important foundations on which movement takes place—the feet—can severely impede efficiency of the entire body if they are misaligned, deformed, or malfunctioning. Deviations of the feet may even produce chronic pain, which prevents comfortable locomotion. Many conditions of the feet are not easily remediable through exercise. Others are closely related to overall postural divergences and alignments.

The foot contains two arches—the *longitudinal arch* and the *transverse arch*. The longitudinal arch extends along the foot from the calcaneus to the far end of the first metatarsal. It is held in place primarily by three bowstring ligaments. Normally the arch is flexible and absorbs shock during running and walking. The height of the arch seems independent of its strength. An abnormally high and inflexible longitudinal arch is termed *hollow foot* (pes cavus) and constitutes an abnormality. It is usually congenital and not amenable to corrective exercise but may be aided with gentle stretching.

The transverse (metatarsal) arch is a concavity on the underside of the front portion of the foot formed by the five metatarsals. The cupping and releasing action of this arch gives the foot its main springing motion. Foot pain often accompanies a drop in this arch, as nerves are pinched between the metatarsals.

Fallen Arches   Fallen arches may be acute or chronic. These two conditions—termed *traumatic sprains*—are caused by some trauma to the foot. Acute sprains are accompanied by pain, swelling, and discoloration. Like any sprain, these are treated with cold, followed by local heat, strapping, and total rest of the foot for a period of time. A medial or lateral heel lift may be used to relieve tension. The foot usually is wrapped or taped prior to physical activity for several months following a drop or sprain. Chronic arch sprain, depending on how often it has occurred, is difficult to treat satisfactorily.

Arches that are permanently low because of elongated ligaments are termed *static sprains*. An overweight condition can cause the ligaments to fail to support the metatarsals in their proper positions. A job that requires long hours on the feet or vigorous exercises without proper conditioning also can permanently strain the foot's arches. Most of the time arch supports and strapping are more helpful than exercises in remediating static sprain.

Flat Feet   Some infants are born with a flattened longitudinal arch. Members of the black race seem particularly susceptible to this condition. If the arch falls straight downward without any foot misalignment, functioning may not be impaired and the condition may not be considered abnormal. In infants the longitudinal arch develops as the result of walking and other exercise. When tibial torsion, knock-knees, toeing outward, or pronation of the foot accompanies flat feet, functional stresses and problems occur.

Exercises for flat feet involve strengthening the muscles, ligaments, and tendons on the medial portion of the foot by inversion exercises and stretching the tight muscles, ligaments, and tendons on the lateral side of the foot.

Pronated Feet   Commonly found in children and youth, this condition is likely to produce malfunctions in walking, jumping, and running. The foot is habitually turned upward and outward, with the weight borne on the inner edge of the foot. Subsequent stretching of the bowstring ligaments that support the longitudinal arch results in pain to the arch and calf muscles.

Lifts in the medial border of the shoe can be used to force the weight to the outer border of the foot. Children wearing these lifts should not change to tennis shoes or go barefooted without consulting their orthopedist.

Corrective exercises include flexing the foot inward, using the arch, by sitting and pulling a towel, as pictured, toward oneself. Also helpful are various toe-curling movements (e.g., picking up small objects with the toes). Children or youth with pronated feet should avoid activities that forceably exert the feet.

Club Foot   Accounting for about 75% of all congenital foot defects, *talipes equinus* often is totally correctable in infancy through surgery and proper bracing. Later, however, these children may be considered lagging in physical development because of the months during which bracing has been imposed.

Morton's Toe   A painful tumor within the area between the third and fourth metatarsophalangeal joints, *plantar neuroma* is sometimes experienced by athletes. Surgery corrects the condition, and physical activity must be terminated for a period of time following surgery.

Metatarsalgia   Caused by prolonged physical activities that place stress on the ball of the foot (e.g., jogging incorrectly on hard surfaces and not heeling enough when running), metatarsalgia is accompanied by severe pain. Massage and exercises to increase the flexibility of the front of the foot and cessation of jumping and springing may be required for several months. Supports under the metatarsal arch may be helpful in relieving the pain.

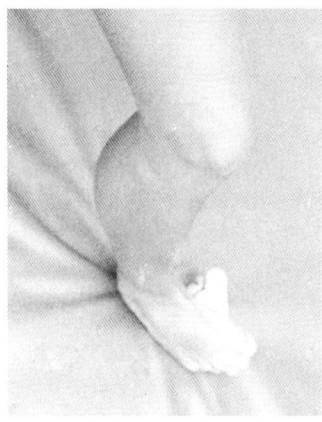

Flexing the foot inward can help to correct pronation of the foot.

Calluses Usually caused by improperly fitting shoes, the pain of calluses may be reduced by changing shoes, inserting pads to shift weight-bearing surfaces, buffing down the calluses, and applying lotions. Properly fitting shoes that are well broken in help to avoid the problem altogether.

Papillomas Known as plantar warts, papillomas are a form of benign skin tumor growing inward. They are treated by x-ray, surgery, or chemicals. Weight-bearing activities may be painful for some time after treatment.

Syndactylism Extra, webbed, or absent toes are part of the inherited condition called syndactylism. Webbing of the toes can be corrected surgically, and extra toes may be removed. A missing big toe creates a severe mechanical disadvantage in running and jumping, in which the foot acts as a lever.

Hallus Valgus In hallus valgus the big toe is deviated inward over the first metatarsal. If the bursa enlarges, it is called a *bunion*. When it is inflamed, it is termed bursitis. Bursitis in the foot is caused by improperly fitting shoes for the most part. It is treatable medically and with proper footwear. Ill-fitting shoes also can cause an associated condition in which the toes overlap; the fourth toe most often overlaps the fifth.

SUMMARY

Modern methods of categorizing body build permit the classification of children into body types in ways that may be helpful in ascertaining how much and what kind of physical activity should be undertaken. Feelings about bodily conformation and deviations should be given special consideration and attention when dealing with youngsters who deviate from the norm.

Interest in the measurement and correction of postural deviations and problems has tended to wane over the past several decades. Physical educators, however, may be called upon to conduct posture screenings and to prescribe strategies and exercises that will help to correct problems of body alignment, as well as of deviations of the hips, legs, and feet. These problems generally may be classified as structural (involving changes in bony structures) or functional (modification in the balance, tension, and construction of the muscles). The correction of postural problems may have both physically and psychologically positive effects. Standing straight and tall helps elevate one's mood, and proper body alignment also facilitates biomechanically correct ways of moving.

REFERENCES

Alderman, M.K. (1966). *An investigation of the need for posture education among high school girls, and a suggested plan of instruction to meet these needs.* Master's thesis, University of Texas, Austin.

Brown, G.M. (1959). *The relationship between body types and static posture of young adult women.* Master's thesis, State College of Washington, Pullman.

Cailliet, R. (1975). *Scoliosis: Diagnosis and management.* Philadelphia: F.A. Davis.

Carter, J.E.L. (1970, December). The somatotype of athletes: A review. *Human biology, 42,* 527-569.

Carter, J.E.L. (1974). Somatotype, growth and physical performance. In J. Vague & J. Boyer (Eds.), *Regulation of the adipose tissue mass* (Proceedings of the International Meeting of Endocrinology, Marseilles). Amsterdam: Excerpta Medica.

Carter, J.E.L. (1975). *The Heath-Carter somatotype method* (Monograph). San Diego: San Diego State University.

Cureton, T.K. (1941, May). Bodily posture as an indicator of fitness. *Research Quarterly, 12*(2) (Supplement), 348.

Fox, M. (1959). Body mechanics. In American Alliance for Health, *Research methods in health, physical education and recreation* (2nd ed.). Washington, DC: Author.

Fullilove, M.A. (1969). *A critical analysis of the problems encountered in posture research.* Master's thesis, University of North Carolina, Greensboro.

Goldthwaite, J.E. (1952). *Body mechanics* (5th ed.). Philadelphia: Lippincott.

Hellenbrandt, F.A., Riddle, K.S., & Fries, E.C.R. (1952, March-April). The influence of posture sway on stance photography. *Physiotherapy Review, 22*(2), 143.

Keim, H. (1972). *Scoliosis.* Summit, NJ: Ciba Pharmaceutical Co.

Klein, K.K. (1973, February). Progression of pelvic tilt in adolescent boys from elementary through high school. *Archives of Physical Medicine & Rehabilitation, 54*(2), 57.

Lee, M., & Wagner, M.M. (1949). *Fundamentals of body mechanics* (p. 156). Philadelphia: W.B. Saunders.

Kretschmer, E. (1925). *Physique and character* (W.J.H. Sprott, Trans.). New York: Harcourt, Brace.

Moriarity, M.J., & Irwin, L. (1952). Study of the relationship of certain physical and emotional factors to habitual poor posture among school children. *Research Quarterly, 23*(2), 221.

Parizkova, J., & Carter, J.E.L. (1976, March). Influences of physical exercise on stability of somatotypes in boys. *American Journal of Physical Anthropology, 44*(2), 327-339.

Sheldon, W.H., Dupertuis, C.W., & McDermott, E. (1954). *Atlas of men, a guide for somatotyping the adult male at all ages.* New York: Harper & Bros.

Sheldon, W.H., & Stevens, S.S. (1942). *The varieties of temperament.* New York: Harper & Bros.

Shephard, R.J. (1972). *Alive man: The physiology of physical activity.* Springfield, IL: Charles C Thomas.

ADDITIONAL REFERENCES

Basmajian, J. (Ed.). (1978). *Therapeutic exercise.* Baltimore: Williams & Wilkins.

Lindsey, R., Jones, B.J., & Van Whitley, A. (1974). *Body mechanics—Posture, figure, fitness.* Dubuque, IA: Wm. C. Brown Co.

MacEwen, G.D. (1974). *Spinal deformity in neurology and muscular disorders.* St. Louis: C.V. Mosby.

QUESTIONS FOR DISCUSSION

1. What influences might body build have on the emotional/social make-up of youngsters?

2. What signs might indicate that children's perceptions of their bodies differ from objective measurements of their bodies? What influences might such distortions produce in children as they participate in a physical activity program?

3. What postural divergences seem most amenable to change via exercise? Which types seem most resistant to modification through exercises? Why?

4. Are children's body builds relatively fixed throughout their life, or do they seem to change with time?

5. What is the difference between dynamic and static posture? What assessment tools might be used to evaluate various aspects of static posture? What tasks might be observed to evaluate dynamic posture?

STUDENT PROJECTS

1. Inspect a physical education class. Through observation, classify the children into three groups: mesomorph, ectomorph, and endomorph. What differences do you see in the physical ability of children in the three groups? In their attitudes during vigorous activity in the class? What program modifications, if any, has the teacher provided to accommodate different body builds?

2. Visit a physical education program and interview the teacher about static posture. If the teacher thinks it is important, why? What methods, if any, does the teacher use to evaluate both static and dynamic posture?

3. Obtain some height/weight tables. What limitations, if any, might such tables have? What advantages might a formal somatotype have over the application of a height/weight table in assessing a child's body build relative to optimum development?

4. Using the Heath-Carter method, formulate a somatotype for a youngster. What difficulties, if any, did you have obtaining the index number? Can another observer, using the same methods on the same child, obtain the same results?

19 *Orthopedic Impairments*

Orthopedically impaired individuals have handicaps or deformities that interfere with the normal use of muscles, bones, or joints. The picture most often conjured up in the minds of the lay public in reference to the handicapped are orthopedically handicapped people in wheelchairs or those who move only with the aid of supporting canes or crutches. Actually, the broad heading of orthopedic impairments encompasses, in addition to the more obvious structural impediments such as clubfoot and spina bifida, conditions including poliomyelitis, osteomyelitis, arthrogryposis, tuberculosis of the bones or joints, and other diseases that may not have immediately noticeable orthopedic symptoms. Although cerebral palsy presents some orthopedic characteristics, it is classified as a disorder of the central nervous system (see chapter 13).

Orthopedic handicaps may be differentiated by conditions that are relatively permanent and those that are transitory. Among the latter are scoliosis, Legg-Perthes disease, slipped capital femoral epiphysis, Osgood-Schlatter disease, and numerous rare problems. A text of this type cannot cover the myriad conditions that might be classified as causing some bone, joint, or muscular malfunction. This chapter (a) describes characteristics of some of the most prevalent conditions; (b) discusses common emotional and social problems of the orthopedically handicapped; (c) presents some ways in which physical programs can be optimized for these children; (d) gives cautions that should be observed in physical activity; and (e) includes strategies and ideas for mainstreamed classes.

PHYSICAL CHARACTERISTICS

Permanent Orthopedic Conditions

Perhaps the term *relatively fixed* is a better word than *permanent* to describe the various conditions that seem somewhat static, having arisen from congenital defects or from trauma later in life. They often are aided with carefully planned programs of physical activity and recreation. Moreover, the mental and emotional outlook of individuals with the conditions described here can be improved through success in physical skills, which in turn encourages them to strive harder in other endeavors.

Persons with apparently irrevocable conditions differ not only in the emotional strengths and weaknesses they bring to the play arena arranged by physical education teachers but also in the amount of courage and fortitude with which they attack new sports and developmental activities and pursue more familiar ones. Children and youth with medically the same apparent orthopedic problem react in markedly different ways when confronted with challenging and difficult tasks.

The problems described do not represent the totality of conditions that might be called relatively fixed orthopedic problems.[1] Rather, they are conditions that educators tend to encounter most frequently.

Myelomeningocele, Meningocele, and Spina Bifida   One of the more serious handicaps in children is caused by open defects in the spinal column resulting from abnormal fetal development. This type of deformity occurs in from .1 to 4.13 of 1,000 births and may appear as any one of three related conditions. *Myelomeningocele* is a protrusion of the spinal cord through the back of the vertebral column when the bones have failed to form correctly. This disorder is five times more common than *meningocele,* which is a similar protrusion, but only of the *coverings* of the spinal cord, and not the cord itself. *Spina bifida occulta* occurs when the back arches of the vertebra fail to form and the bony defect is covered by skin. Figure 19.1 illustrates this. These three spinal conditions are caused by failure of the neural tube to develop completely and to close during the first 20 days of pregnancy.

Figure 19.1   Spina Bifida

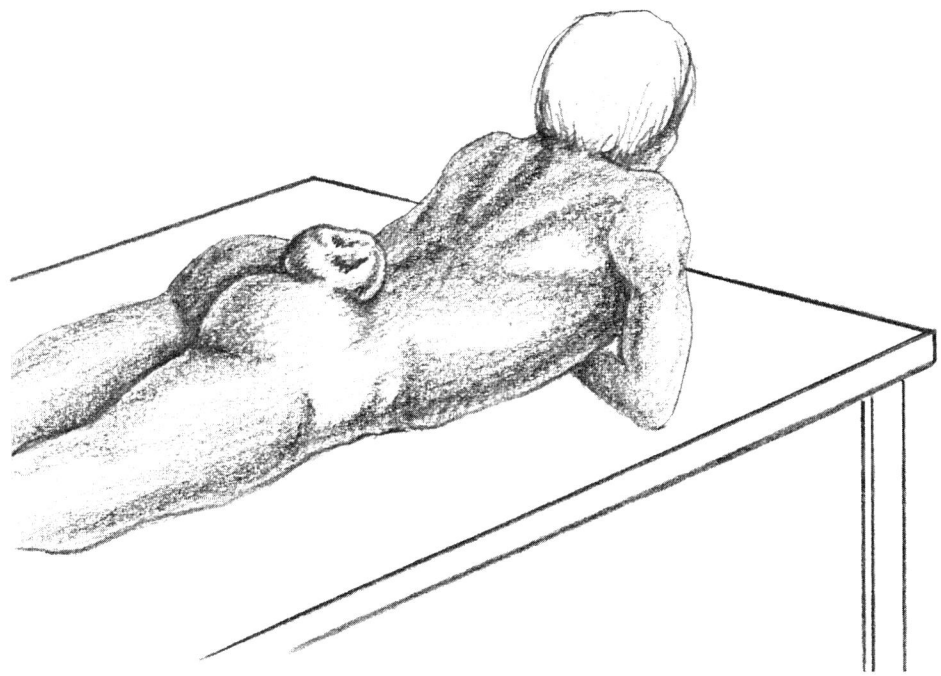

1. A multitude of rare and exotic conditions may cause various types of impairments to the skeletal-muscular system. Teachers of orthopedically handicapped youngsters should be aware of these rare syndromes and seek medical intervention for the children when appropriate.

Figure 19.2   Hydrocephalus Condition with Shunt

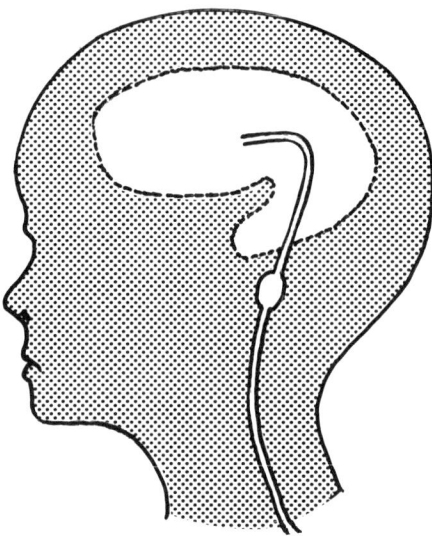

Hydrocephalus is an associated condition in over 90% of children with myelomeningocele. Excess fluid collects in the brain's ventricles because of blocked spinal fluid circulation to the brain. This enlargement of the ventricles results in compression of brain cells and nerve fibers, which ultimately may lead to intellectual retardation, spastic paralysis of the lower limbs, or seizures. Hydrocephalus is controlled by placing tubes (shunts) consisting of plastic tubing between the brain's ventricles and the neck artery, as shown in Figure 19.2, or the abdomen, which acts as a drain, relieving pressure on the brain. This surgery has to be repeated at intervals as the child grows.

Children with spinal defects may be afflicted with associated conditions. They may experience partial to complete loss of skin sensation to pain, temperature, or touch in the lower part of the body, in which case they may have to be taught to inspect their skin and shift their sitting positions frequently to avoid tissue damage from pressure. Bladder and bowel paralysis can cause problems in urination and at times a backing up of urine, which enlarges the renal pelvis. As a result, bladder and kidney infections are frequent. Bowel paralysis also is common, resulting from partial paralysis of the rectum and anal muscle (sphincter). Sometimes behavioral strategies can be introduced to help empty the bladder (e.g., crying, turning, laughing, sneezing, or manually pressing the lower abdominal wall have all worked in specific individuals). Mechanical draining devices (a condom-like collection system) may be used with boys. Girls usually use diapers. Although individuals with spinal defects of this type are treated early with closure surgery to avoid life-threatening infections such as meningitis, the surgery does not reduce paralysis.

Problems in motor planning have been assumed to be associated with these spinal defects, but the data do not always confirm this (Brunt, 1984). Neverethless, care should be taken to present motor information to these children at a rate at which they can assimilate a skill without undue effort.

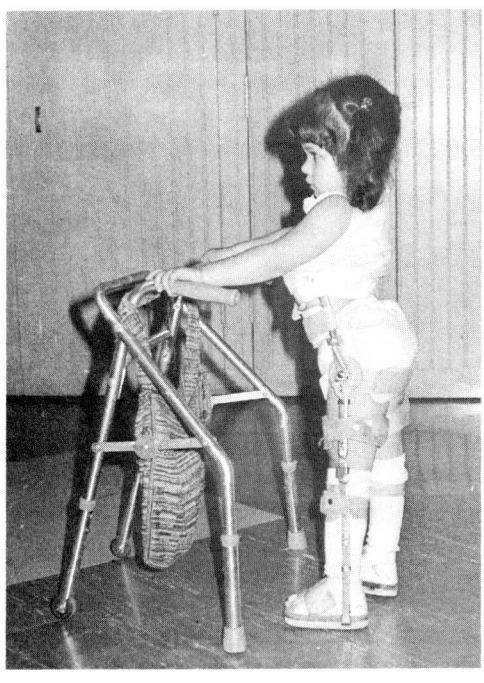

Young girl with spina bifida has a carryall bag
on her walker.

Courtesy, Special Education Branch, Los Angeles City Schools

Early use of self-standing braces may help the child walk. If the trunk muscles are weak or paralyzed, both a trunk support and long leg braces with locked hip joints are used. If the trunk musculature is not paralyzed, only leg braces may be employed. Many children use crutches for support. Those who have both trunk and hip paralysis use wheelchairs for most activities. In general, the acquisition of useful walking depends on the level of paralysis. With involvement above the 12th thoracic level, no practical walking can be accomplished. Involvement from the 12th thoracic to the fourth lumbar level means that partial household walking with crutches and braces is possible. When involvement is confined to the fourth lumbar to the second sacral levels, walking is possible.

In an unpublished 1972 survey referred to by Bleck (1975), 80% of the 100 patients surveyed over the age of 12 could walk successfully; 28% used crutches or braces; 20% were in wheelchairs. Bowel control was established in 65%, but only 35% had good urinary control. Hydrocephalus was arrested in 38% and about half had ventriculoatrial shunts. An IQ of 80 or higher was found in 89% of those tested; 75% had graduated from high school; and 27% had a college degree or were in their fourth year of college.

One promising contemporary device has been employed successfully to help in the ambulation of those with spina bifida. This device, called the *reciprocal gait orthosis,* allows some who would otherwise be wheelchair-bound to become ambulatory (McCall & Schmidt, 1986). The device is a cable assembly that regulates and controls hip joint motion. Tension is adjusted to prevent bilateral hip joint flexion while the person is standing. As the individual advances one lower extremity by flexing the hip, the cable provides stability to the other hip. Alternate hip stability and advances then are possible, producing a hesitating gait pattern. The person may control a cable release device that permits bilateral hip flexion necessary for sitting.

As might be expected, children and youth with this condition may suffer from emotional "overlays" of various kinds. Of course, they vary greatly in their emotional make-up because of many factors including environmental and family surroundings. Some patterns, however, have appeared with some consistency, particularly in children who have hydrocephalus. These children have been described as even-tempered early in life, although sometimes irritable in strange environments and overly sensitive to noise. Some researchers have observed the spina bifida infants tend to be passive and do not always display the intellectual curiousity usually seen at this age in normal children (Anderson & Spain, 1977).

If spina bifida children are pressured during exposure to academic work, thay may become more apathetic, cautious, and moody. One reason for this may be that they no longer can depend on their social and verbal skills previously learned but must begin to rely more heavily on motor and perceptual skills. Surveys of spina bifida children in the first grades of school indicated that they tended to resent correction and were unresponsive. Data collected in middle childhood indicated that a number of them had poor concentration and were fearful of new things. Few, however, were viewed by their teachers as anti-social or overly aggressive.

Adolescents with spina bifida were found to be more socially isolated, had lower self-esteem, and evidenced some depression, as contrasted with their normal peers (Blum, 1983). Moreover, the concerns of adolescents in this study involved feelings of sexual inadequacy and, for that matter, of mastery and adequacy in social situations in general. A further finding was that the adolescents' parents were largely unaware of their teenagers' negative feelings.

Spinal Cord Injuries   Spinal cord injuries have been increasing in a society that encourages off-road vehicles and has condoned the combination of alcohol and driving. In general, the higher in the spinal cord the trauma or severance is, the more severe is the limitation of movement. Lesions are classified according to the region of the spine affected—*cervical, thoracic, lumbar,* and *sacral*—and the specific vertebra affected.

C-4 refers to the fourth cervical vertebra and is the highest lesion that can be sustained after which life can be maintained. A C-4 injury implies use only of the neck, diaphragm, and shoulder-girdle muscles. An injury from T-2 to S-5 influences only the use of leg muscles, and individuals who have been affected in that way often participate in wheelchair athletics. Persons with L-5 injuries, and below, may be able to walk reasonably well. Figure 19.3 presents the classification system graphically.

Each spinal cord injury is manifested individually, and the extent of physical participation is impacted also by level of motivation, age at which the injury occurred, and previous exposure to vigorous physical activity. When working with spinal cord cases, the following possible problems should be considered:

1. Youngsters with spinal cord lesions tend to get infections involving the kidneys and urinary system. Signs of infection (a flushed face, for example) should be a signal to cease exercise until the child is evaluated further.

Figure 19.3   Classification System for Spinal Lesions

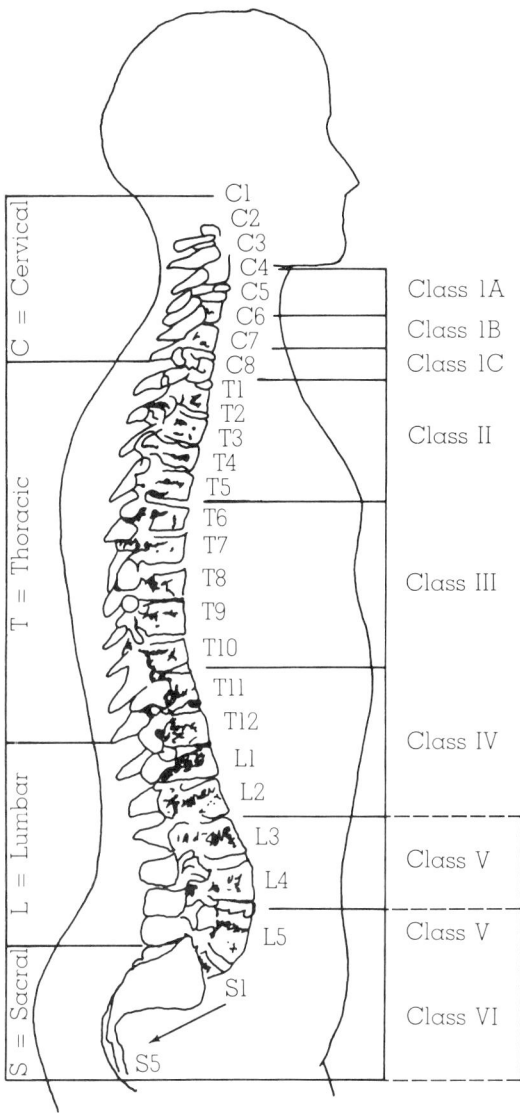

    2. Special problems are encountered with a lesion at the sacral level, which interferes with bowel and bladder control. The affected individuals must wear bags or use catheters even when swimming. If an ileostomy or colostomy has been performed, the bag is removed and the opening covered with a water-repellent bandage while swimming.

Paraplegics can and do participate in a number of vigorous activities—many involving the upper body (weight lifting and the like). These individuals should be exposed to comprehensive conditioning programs to build muscular strength and improve upper and lower limb flexibility, as well as activities that promote cardiovascular endurance. These qualities are needed from the standpoint of improving and maintaining a strong, positive self-concept and also because these strengths are needed daily in the management of crutches and wheelchairs.

Table 19.1 gives the classification system used to determine groupings for participation in the various wheelchair sports (National Association of Sports for Cerebral Palsy, 1979). This system is useful for the classification of those with spinal cord injuries in addition to individuals with cerebral palsy.

Arthrogryposis   About 500 children in the United States are born each year with a condition that involves one or several fixed, rigid joints. The condition is not accompanied

Table 19.1   Classification System for Wheelchair Sports

Class I
Individuals who:
- are quadriplegic
- are wheelchair-bound—cannot ambulate a long distance without assistance
- have poor functional strength and severe control problems in the upper extremities and torso
- move wheelchair with their arms during track events

Class II
Individuals who:
- are quadriplegic
- are wheelchair-bound, cannot ambulate without assistance
- have poor functional strength and severe control problems in the upper extremities and torso
- propel wheelchair using feet during track events

Class III
Individuals who:
- are quadriplegic or triplegic
- ambulate with assistive devices without personal assistance and/or need to use a wheelchair at all times or for regular daily activities
- have fair functional strength and moderate control problems in the upper extremities and torso
- propel wheelchair with arms during track events

Class IV
Individuals who:
- are paraplegic or triplegic (two legs and one arm or possible quadriplegic)
- ambulate with assistive devices without assistance and/or need to use a wheelchair for convenience in daily activities
- have good functional strength and minimal control problems in the upper extremities and torso (upper extremities may have exaggerated reflexes)
- move wheelchair with arms during track events

Note: Adapted from National Association of Sports for Cerebal Palsy, 1979, *Constitution, Rules Classification, and National Records Sports Manual,* New Haven, CT: National Association of Sports for Cerebral Palsy.

by pain and involves the lower limbs more often than the upper ones. When several limbs are involved, the condition is called *multiple congenital contracture*. The cause is unknown, but the contractures may be observed relatively early in fetal life because of a primary muscle disease or a spinal cord disease with muscle contraction.

Although the limbs may be fixed in any position, in the usual form the shoulders are turned in, elbows are straight and extended, forearms are turned with the palms outward (pronated), wrists are flexed and deviated upward with the fingers curled into the palms. The hips are bent and turned outward (externally rotated), the feet usually are turned in and down, the limbs are small in circumference, and the joints appear large and do not allow the full range of motion. Scoliosis of the spine (see chapter 18) often is evident. Figure 19.4 depicts how a child with arthrogryposis might appear.

Children with arthrogryposis usually have normal intelligence, but associated physical conditions can include congenital heart disease, urinary tract abnormalities, respiratory problems, abdominal hernias, and facial abnormalities. These children may walk indepen-

Table 19.1   Continued

Class VA
Individuals who:
- are quadriplegic athetoid (or similar involvement)
- ambulate without assistive devices during regular daily activities
- will compete in track events on their feet without assistive devices
- have moderate to severe control problems in all extremities and torso
- may use a chair for stabilization in non-track events

Class VB
Individuals who:
- are spastic paraplegic (or similar involvement)
- utilize cane or crutches in regular daily ambulation
- will compete in all events on their feet utilizing assistive devices (canes/crutches)
- have good functional strength and minimal control problems in the upper extremities and torso (upper extremities may have exaggerated reflexes)
- may use a chair for stabilization in non-track events

Class VI
Individuals who:
- are quadriparetic athetoid with moderate to minimal control problems
- ambulate without assistive devices during daily activities
- will compete in track events on their feet without the use of assistive devices
- have moderate to minimal control problems in three or all extremities and torso
- may not use a chair for stabilization in non-track events

Class VII
Individuals who:
- are hemi- or monoplegic (one arm, possible very minimal quadriplegic)
- ambulate without assistive devices during daily activities and are capable of running and jumping freely
- will compete in all events on their feet without assistive devices
- may not use a chair for stabilization in non-track events

Figure 19.4 Manifestations of Arthrogryposis

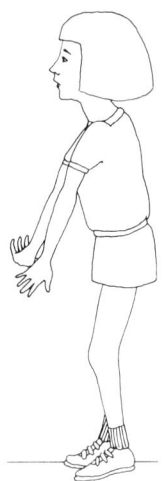

dently, but at times stiffly, or they may depend on wheelchairs. Surgery often can correct hip conditions and knee and foot deformities and sometimes can increase elbow and wrist flexibility.

Despite this overwhelming number of possible problems, these children have a great deal of potential for participation in adapted sports and associated skills. Their condition does not deteriorate, and their intelligence, sense of humor, and motivation may remain intact. As willing participants to the limits of their ability, these children may be seen to throw a small ball well and accurately in a back-handed manner, arm pronated with the palm turned outward from the body.

Congenital and Acquired Amputations   Congenital amputation means being born without a limb or with only part of a limb. Acquired amputation refers to the removal of a limb, in part or in total, by accident or by surgery, in a child who was normal in that respect at birth. Amputations of both kinds are classified by site and level of absence. Figure 19.5 gives some of the terminology used to describe types, levels, and sites of amputation.

Not only may these children engage in physical activities according to their level of functioning, but their potentials also can be increased through the use of *prostheses* (artificial devices). Early attachment of a false limb encourages infants and young children to incorporate the appendage into the body schema more readily than later introduction of prostheses.

For the most part, the intellectual ability of children who have congenital or acquired amputations is unrelated to the disability. Some have above-average academic achievement, possibly as a compensation for their physical limitations in certain cases. Using projective tests and other means, Centers and Centers (1968) and others have attempted to obtain clues to amputees' feelings about their disabilities. Generally the drawings of amputee children

Figure 19.5   Terms to Describe Amputation of Limbs

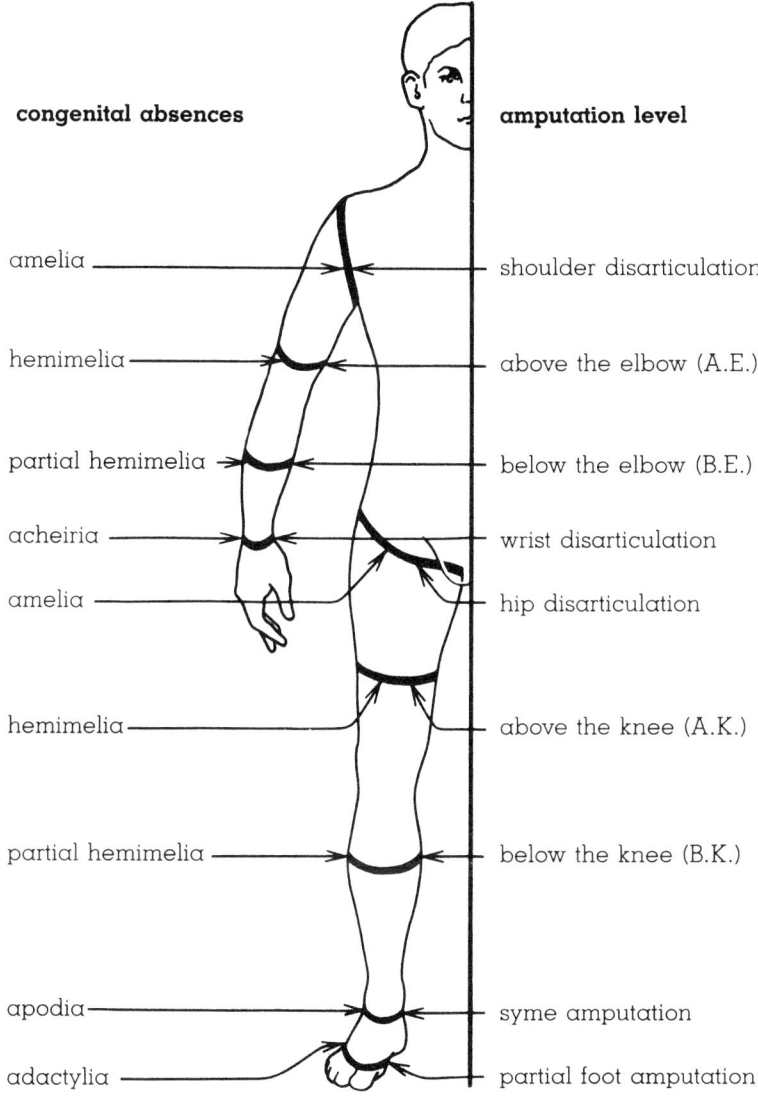

congenital absences   **amputation level**

amelia ——————————————→←—————— shoulder disarticulation

hemimelia ——————————→←—————— above the elbow (A.E.)

partial hemimelia —→←————— below the elbow (B.E.)

acheiria ——————————→←——— wrist disarticulation

amelia —————————————— hip disarticulation

hemimelia ——————————→←—— above the knee (A.K.)

partial hemimelia ——————————→←— below the knee (B.K.)

apodia —————————————→←— syme amputation

adactylia ———————————— partial foot amputation

Note: From *Physically Handicapped Children* by E. Bleck and D. Nagel, 1975, New York: Grune & Stratton, p. 17. Used by permission of the publisher.

have been found to accurately reflect differences between themselves and normal individuals, without undue anxiety or apprehension. Analysis of these drawings has not revealed any marked differences in emotional health between amputeed and normal children and adolescents.

   Above-the-knee and elbow amputations are more difficult to compensate for than are those below the joints. Children usually discover what works best for them. With the proper aids, above-the-knee amputees can walk, run, swim, ski, and participate in many other physical activities. Because some have a tendency to become sedentary, amputees might be exposed to one or two activities in which a reasonable level of proficiency can be achieved rather than to a wide range of physical activities, some of which may be too difficult and reduce their motivation.

Osteogenesis Imperfecta (Brittle Bone Disease) Osteogenesis imperfecta is a condition marked by weak bones and elasticity of the joints, ligaments, and skin. It most often is inherited, although at times it seems to be caused by *mutation* (spontaneous changes in the genes). The defect is in the collagen fibers of the bone, which arrange themselves in a net-like mesh rather than the normal linear pattern.

The bone formations of children with this defect are illustrated in Figure 19.6. In many ways they are like those in the developing fetus. The immaturity is caused by a deficiency

Figure 19.6   Bone Formations of Osteogenesis Imperfecta

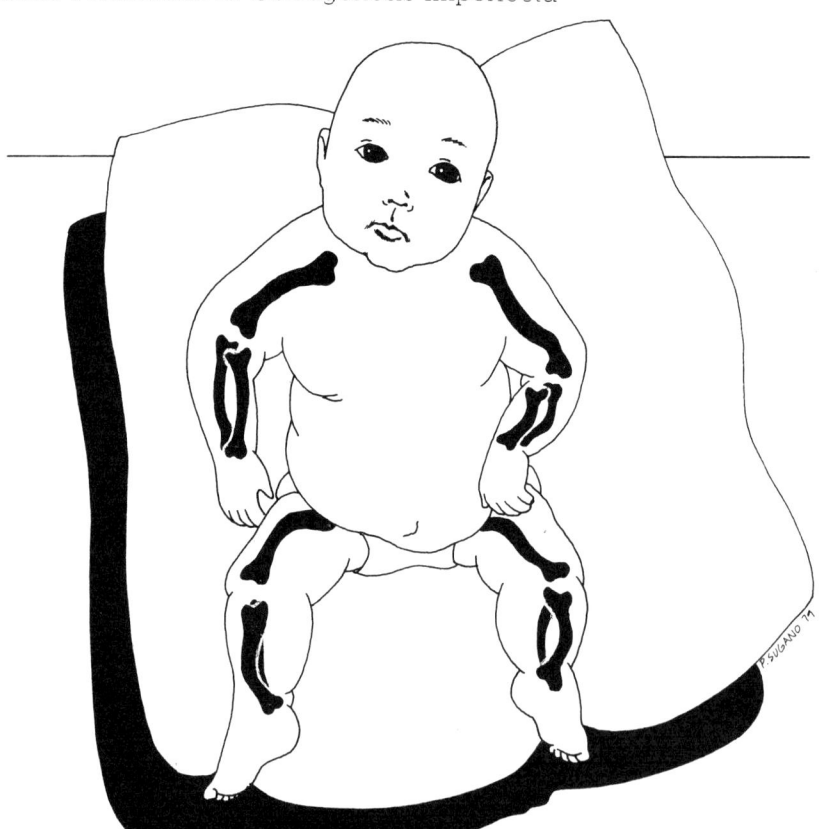

in bone salts (calcium and phosphorus) rather than a defect in the calcification mechanism. The underlying layer of the eyeball (choroid) shows through as a blue discoloration.

The two main types of osteogenesis imperfecta are *congenital* (at birth) and *tarda* (late onset). At birth children with this condition have short, deformed limbs, many broken bones, and a soft skull, which tends to grow into a triangular shape, broad at the forehead and narrow at the chin. Many babies with this condition die at birth.

Brittle bone disease occurring later in life usually produces mild symptoms but may be recognized by the blue "whites" of the eyes. As growth continues in individuals with both forms of the disease, the limbs tend to become bowed from numerous fractures. The spine is rounded backward as in kyphosis (see chapter 18). The teeth are in poor condition, easily broken, discolored, and prone to cavities. The joints are excessively flexible, so that children easily give the impression of being double-jointed (e.g., able to bend the thumb back to touch the hand).

No known chemical substance or nutrient has been shown to correct the condition. The most satisfactory treatment is the surgical insertion of a steel rod between the ends of the long bones, as shown in Figure 19.7. This treatment, plus bracing, permits some individuals to walk some of the time. Many need a wheelchair at least part of the time, and the most severely involved persons require a wheelchair exclusively.

Figure 19.7   Surgical Treatment for Brittle Bone Disease

(1) sectioned

(2) rodded

(3) healed

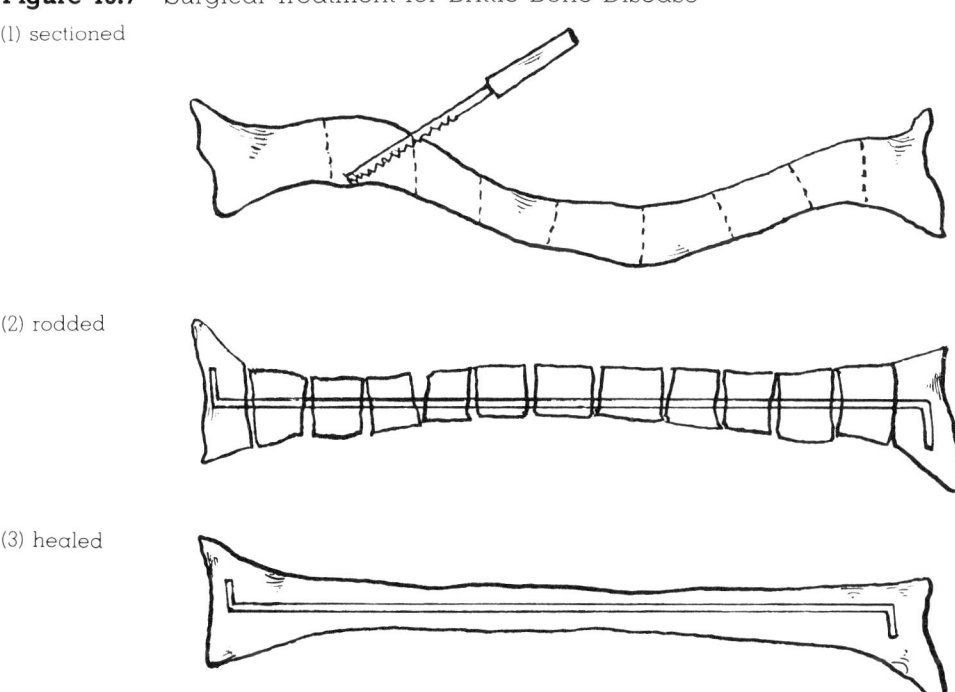

Children with this disease are of normal intelligence. They are very verbal and learn easily. Deafness may develop as they age—a problem to which teachers should be sensitive. Visual disorders also can occur later in life.

Although some authorities have ruled out physical activities for this population, others suggest that those who have been "rodded" (surgery of the type described) may participate in specialized programs in aquatics and activities taking place in specially padded gymnasium settings. As they grow older, the condition of those who have had surgery tends to stabilize; they incur fewer fractures and can attend a regular school.

Miscellaneous Conditions   Other relatively fixed orthopedic conditions include the rare *osteodystrophy* (Morquio's disease, a progressive spinal deformity resulting in skeletal malformations usually not seen until several months after birth), dwarfism, and rickets, among others.

Dwarfism   A congenital condition, dwarfism is reflected in immature physical growth and manifested in over 100 syndromes characterized by abnormally short stature. The type of dwarf usually seen in physical education classes is afflicted with achondroplasia, has normal intelligence, and does well academically. Dwarfs are restricted only by their size, so they can participate in most physical activities.

Rickets   Rickets is characterized by an abnormal bowing of the longer bones of the body. It is caused by nutritional problems, inborn metabolic anomalies, or congenital kidney impairment. The latter two causes are by far the most prevalent in the United States at this time. Children with bowed limbs are aided by passive exercises in which strenuous weight bearing is not required. Exercising outdoors to obtain vitamin D from sunlight is often helpful.

Post-Burn Victims   In recent years post-burn victims are seen more often in physical education classes. Thick hypertropic scar tissue causes contractures and limits the range of motion across joints. As these children age, the scar tissue thickens and becomes more dense, often requiring additional surgery to enhance joint motion. Jobsts (rigid plastic braces) and elastic supports, often worn under clothing, tend to reduce thickening of scar tissue. Splints are worn at times to apply additional pressure to scar tissue and reduce its size.

Burn cases are rehabilitated with extensive physical therapy to prevent contractions and the resulting limitation of movements. Therapists use gentle stretching and assistive activities. Tasks involved in daily living, together with ambulatory activities, also are included in post-burn rehabilitation (Helm, Lushbaugh, Pullium, Head, & Croones, 1982).

Working in swimming pools and in warm environments is helpful. Attempts to increase the range of motion via exercise should be accompanied by frequent consultations with the children's physician. Work in direct sunlight tends to dry, and at times, crack, scar tissue that is forming. Therefore, indoor activities are preferable, according to most authorities.

Transitory Orthopedic Conditions

A number of conditions that physical educators may encounter involve relatively transitory but disabling orthopedic problems. Some of these are caused by trauma to the bony structure or the joints, even as a result of the continued strain of competitive sports. Others are caused by various viral infections, ill health, malnutrition, hormonal problems, or heredity. At times the causes are unknown.

For the most part, these problems affect the maturation of bones in the "growth plate" at their ends. By age 25 (earlier in girls), the end plate and the bone fuse unless some disorder causes delayed closure, premature closure, or other interruption in the growth process. Collectively, disorders of the growth plate are termed *osteochondrosis.*

Under a physician's direction, these conditions have been helped by having children or youth rest in bed with the legs in braces that hold them wide apart so that the hip (a joint often affected) fuses and becomes weight-bearing. Alternatively, to avoid removing children from the mainstream for 2 to 3 years, physicians prescribe immobilization of the leg with a special brace or sling or cast that permits the child to walk with crutches—albeit with an unusually wide gait. Surgical treatment is advised in some cases, involving bone grafting in the growth center to speed up the repair processes or change the shape of the hip joint, permitting a more stable union with the head of the femur.

Generally, children with these conditions should be kept in relatively passive sports, often suited for those in wheelchairs. Undue speed or weight bearing, even if the child is ambulatory, is not recommended. Swimming is sometimes a helpful component of the physical education program.

Through improved nutrition, rest, and other treatments, transitory orthopedic conditions often are corrected within 2 to 3 years. During that time physical educators should (a) provide motivating maintenance activities, with the physician's concurrence; (b) avoid subjecting the youth to excessive stress and trauma to a weakened bony system; and (c) when they are able, help children back to normal participation in careful sequences of activities involving gradually increased stress.

Some specific transitory conditions are described briefly in the following paragraphs. They include Legg-Perthes disease, Osgood-Schlatter disease, slipped capital femoral epiphysis, and congenital scoliosis.

Legg-Perthes Disease   Between the ages 4 and 8 a destruction of the growth center (epiphysis) at the hip end of the thigh bone (femur) sometimes occurs in children. It is diagnosed by x-ray. This condition can be caused by rare metabolic diseases, by blood diseases (including sickle cell anemia), by low-grade infections (sometimes associated with tuberculosis), and from complications stemming from from various medications such as cortisone. If the cause of this hip condition is not apparent and not attributable to any of these factors, it is called Legg-Perthes disease. Accompanying symptoms include diminished blood supply to the hip joint.

The condition is reversible and usually repairs itself by laying down new bone. If only a portion of the growth center is involved, the repair takes place more quickly. Figure 19.8 illustrates Legg-Perthes. Protection of the growth center while repair is taking place is advocated, together with bracing and, at times, bone grafting. Boys are more frequently affected than are girls.

Osgood-Schlatter Disease   Another type of growth plate disorder is caused by trauma and first manifests itself in swelling and tenderness just below the knee joint. Upon ruling

Figure 19.8   Legg-Perthes Disease

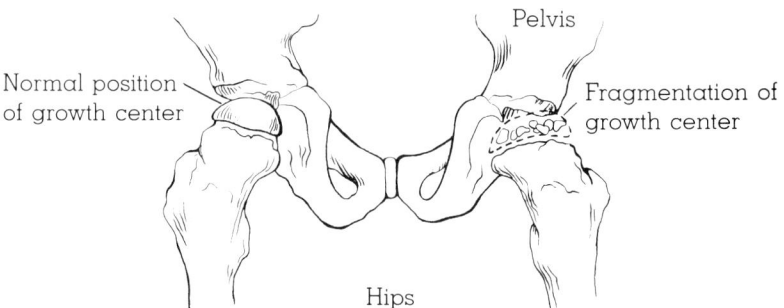

Pelvis

Normal position
of growth center

Fragmentation of
growth center

Hips

Note: From *Physically Handicapped Children* by E. Bleck and D. Nagel, 1975, New York: Grune & Stratton, p. 196. Used
by permission of the authors and the publisher.

out other causes, such as a tumor, the condition usually is diagnosed as Osgood-Schlatter
disease. Sometimes x-rays show an irregularity of the bone at the insertion of the tendon
of the knee. The cause of the condition, however, is a tearing away of the bone at the point
where the tendon from the kneecap (patella) attaches to the front (anterior-forward) part
of the leg bone (tibia).

Depending on the diagnosis, treatment of the condition may take several forms. Restriction in activities—particularly those involving forceful extension of the knee joint by the
large thigh muscle—is advocated. Running, jumping, bicycle riding, long-distance walking, and other active sports sometimes are suspended for as long as needed.

If the condition is severe and the bone is lifting up a great deal at the attachment of
the tendon, children and youth may be immobilized in a cast that limits knee motion for
a period of weeks. This condition is seen primarily in youth ages 14-19. It tends to subside
in adults. Adults engaging in vigorous sports occasionally complain of symptoms, however,
and would do well to rest.

Slipped Capital Femoral Epiphysis   Slippage of the growth center at the upper end
of the thigh bone where it joins the pelvis sometimes is seen in adolescents during the
time of rapid growth between ages 11 and 16. Normal and slipped growth centers are illustrated in Figure 19.9. This condition usually occurs later in boys than in girls because
girls' skeletons mature earlier. Additionally, boys may engage in more vigorous sports more
often and stress this joint area further, increasing the incidence among males.

Sometimes during rapid growth the angle at which the femur joins the hip changes
from a horizontal position to a more vertical plane. This is thought to be a major cause
of slipped capital femoral epiphysis. Hormonal problems also are believed to be a major
cause.

Although the problem is in the hip, children may complain of pain in other areas,
including the thigh and knee, and may begin to limp as a result. If not diagnosed correctly
and soon, the condition may become aggravated and develop into a major slip, particularly

Figure 19.9   Slipped Epiphysis Compared to Normal Growth Center

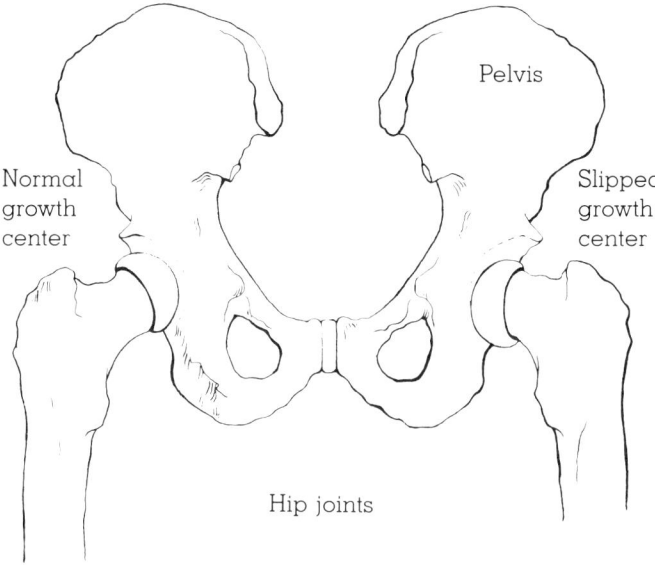

Note: From *Physically Handicapped Children* by E. Bleck and D. Nagel, 1975, New York: Grune & Stratton, p. 198. Used by permission of the authors and the publisher.

after a fall. The problem may require a bone graft or pins to keep the hip in proper position. Other times major surgery is required.

After recovery, children or youth with this condition should be gradually introduced to active sports. More than a year should be taken to assume a full level of activity. Swimming is often helpful because of the freedom from physical stress that accompanies this water sport. Both physicians and physical education teachers should be sensitive to possible slippage of the other hip and also to possible postural problems (e.g., scoliosis) that may accompany this asymmetrical hip condition.

Congenital Scoliosis   Scoliosis is dealt with in chapter 18. It also belongs in this discussion because it is a major nonpermanent orthopedic condition. Its common cause is improper formation or segmentation of the bones of the spine, resulting in a curve that does not necessarily progress to a serious structural deformity. Congenital scoliosis also occurs in association with other conditions, including asymmetrical fusion of two or more bones making up the spine, as well as abnormal spinal cord development (meningomyelocele). Idiopathic (meaning cause unknown) scoliosis is most common, however, and is seen more often in girls than in boys. It is often exaggerated when children reach adolescence and undergo a growth spurt.

The type of treatment is based on the severity of the condition and its potential for becoming exaggerated. Although the condition formerly was believed to become stabilized following the growth of adolescence, more recent long-term studies now indicate that increases of 20° to 30° in curvature may occur after skeletal maturity has been reached.

Treatment includes the use of bracing and exercises. X-rays are taken frequently to determine the effects of treatment. The braces commonly are used from 2 to 4 years, and sometimes exercises are prescribed while the person is in braces. If bracing and exercise do not improve the condition, surgery involving internal fixation of metal devices sometimes is done to achieve greater correction. While encouraging moderately active recreational sports for children while they are in a brace, most physicians do suggest that, for the rest of their lives, these individuals completely avoid activities that may jar the spinal cord.

Other Temporary Conditions   Other conditions that temporarily affect the body structure and functioning include broken bones and trauma from sports, affecting the bones (e.g., shear fractures), tendons (torn or traumatized), and cartilage. Sometimes children complain of pain and discomfort in the knee. This may be diagnosed as *chondromalacia*, a softening of the cartilage. It may be caused by a blow to the knee or by an inflammatory disease. Chondromalacia may be corrected by increasing nourishment to the cartilage, through movement of the knee joint without undue pressure, so that the cartilage will heal itself. Initial treatment sometimes consists of leg raises and isometric tightening of the muscles attached to the kneecap. Later, more vigorous activities such as bicycling are encouraged.

Inflammatory conditions are treated in a variety of ways including anti-inflammatory drugs (aspirin is one), other medicines, a cast to immobilize the region, exercises, and surgery. When working with these children, physical educators should (a) initially consult with the physician concerning the degree of stress, if any, that might be applied via physical activities and recreational sports; (b) talk with the child continually to ascertain if any exercise causes pain; and (c) further consult with the physician to determine when the condition seems to be terminating and what increase, if any, in the vigor of exercise is allowable.

SOCIAL/EMOTIONAL CHARACTERISTICS

One advantage that orthopedically handicapped persons have when encountering others in society is that the nature of their condition is usually obvious. If reared in warm, accepting families, most orthopedically handicapped youngsters have come to grips with their disabilities to a large extent by mid-childhood. They often have devised ways to circumvent problems and strategies to optimize social, recreational, and academic functions. In contrast, children or young adults with more subtle problems, including emotional disturbance, minimal neurological defects, and the like, are not as obviously impaired. Their peers and others are not likely to be as tolerant of these subtle incapacities as they are of overt orthopedic handicaps.

Despite surveys of the literature indicating that orthopedically handicapped people often are reasonably well adjusted, they may be reluctant to enter and compete in new social situations. Also, some may have secondary handicaps including speech and language difficulties, perceptual and conceptual problems, as well as behavior disorders and overcompensations stemming from the primary disability.

Individuals react in various ways to handcapped persons. When confronted with orthopedically impaired individuals, the primary social/psychological error is to take an overly solicitous attitude—to exude pity rather than to offer truly constructive help and support. In contrast to some other handicaps, such as mental retardation, however, the orthopedically handicapped are more frequently accepted socially by normally functioning individuals.

More and more, mainstreamed orthopedically handicapped children are being accepted by their normal peers in physical education classes. The duration of time handicapped and nonhandicapped children are exposed to each other in a class may make a difference. Likewise, the type of aid (e.g., crutch or wheelchair) may make a difference relative to acceptance (Eason & Schuler, 1979). Normal children as young as 6 years of age have been taught to be assistants for physically handicapped children mainstreamed in physical education classes (Cecconi & Rothenberg, 1980).

A most striking individual variation within populations of the orthopedically handicapped is the difference in determination and courage with which they attack physical activities and sports skills. I will never forget the day I saw a slender boy, his leg amputated at the hip, playing tackle football with boys twice his size. His stump was jammed into a single wooden crutch, and he attempted a tackle on each play. On bouncing off ineffectually, he would crawl slowly to the crutch, with which he usually had parted company, jam the stump into the crutch again, and line up for the next play!

Educators should consider whether the best interests and needs of the orthopedically handicapped are being served. Does the school day present them with opportunities to interact and compete with normal children and youth in using social and academic abilities that permit them to succeed? Physical education classes should be specially designed so that their abilities are nurtured and not crushed. In addition to the mainstreamed class, two alternative settings for moderately to severely impaired students are (a) a special class of similarly involved youngsters taken from the total school or from several neighboring schools, and (b) a special class in which student volunteers from the nonhandicapped population act as aides and recreational helpers to encourage the youngsters to participate as vigorously as possible and with as much enjoyment as in activities modified and adapted for their special needs and capacities.

The self-concepts of many physically handicapped individuals are quite intact. One recent study found that individuals with spinal cord injuries posted reasonably high scores reflecting their moral, social, and personal self-concepts. Only in responses reflecting their *physical* self-concept were the scores lower (Green, Pratt, & Griggsby, 1984).

The problems—physical, social, and emotional—of orthopedically handicapped youth are highly individualistic. Before teachers of these children interact with a youngster having an orthopedic disability, they should thoroughly understand both the obvious and the subtle manifestations of the condition and the unique social and emotional problems that may be associated with it. As with the blind and others, the orthopedically handicapped should have the opportunity to earn the respect of their nonhandicapped classmates, particularly for their efforts and striving to improve themselves physically and for whatever successes they demonstrate as a result of their attempts in self-improvement.

PHYSICAL EDUCATION PROGRAMMING

As is apparent on surveying the types and conditions represented among the population of orthopedically handicapped, their problems are highly diverse and differ from individual to individual. Therefore, programs of physical activity must be carefully planned and also must be flexible enough to accommodate individual differences. Not only must a variety of activities be available, but the equipment and settings in which these activities take place may also differ from school to school. With implementation of the laws described in chapter 2, orthopedically handicapped youngsters may be placed in situations that require them to interact with normal students, or they may be placed in relatively homogeneous groupings with their handicapped peers. Placement of orthopedically handicapped children in a regular physical education class requires adjustment by instructors as well as peers.

Trends in Physical Activity

Emphasis is being placed increasingly upon the inclusion of physical activity—even strenuous exercise and competitive sports—in programs for the physically handicapped. Experts are recommending more intense physical training for physically handicapped children (Dresden, deGroot, Mesa-Mead, & Bauman, 1985). One reason is that persons with spinal cord injuries tend to become obese with inactivity (Winnick & Short, 1984). Also, cardiovascular efficiency can be improved through interval training with wheelchair-bound children (Glaser & Sawka, 1981). This type of activity can include races in wheelchairs—an activity that improves both emotional and physical attributes in the physically handicapped (Madorsky & Madorsky, 1984).

This kind of training is reflected in the enlargement of competitive sports programs for the physically handicapped, which in turn has engendered positive attitudes toward sport on the part of the disabled (Cooper, Sherrill, & Marshall, 1986). Facilitating this rush toward competitive sports is the production and invention of a broad range of devices enabling the disabled to perform a variety of sports including swimming, shooting, cycling, and running (Rubin & Fleiss, 1984). Using modern aids, a majority of those with below-knee amputations can now attain a true running pattern (Enoka, Miller, & Burgess, 1982).

With each passing day, more and more activities formerly thought to be within the sole purview of the physically able are being taken up by the physically handicapped, with accommodations in rules or equipment. Modifications of tennis, skiing, and all events in the Wheelchair Olympics are open to orthopedically handicapped children and adults. Wheelchair basketball long has been a staple in the exercise diet of those with spinal cord injuries that prevent full use of the lower limbs. Horseback riding has evolved from a recreational activity into a serious therapeutic intervention (Fox, Lawlor, & Luttges, 1984). Horses are being trained as "moving therapy tables," with the child placed in various positions on the horses' backs in ways that stimulate vestibular and motor activity and improvement.

Moreover, participation in vigorous competitive sports tends to broaden the psychological vistas of participants. The anger they may direct at their condition can be transferred into positive physical performance (Henschen, Horvat, & French, 1984). Care is being taken to instill confidence rather than to reinforce feelings of helplessness in these children (Wool & Siegel, 1980). Specific programs of confidence training used with the handicapped have significantly improved self-confidence and reduced helpless behaviors (Gouvier & Richards, 1985).

In the 1980s careful attention is being paid to the ways physical skills are taught to the handicapped. Systematic reinforcement schedules used by therapists to aid motor activities are being taught to parents so that continued teaching and progress can take place in the home (Manella & Varni, 1984). In this day and age physical education teachers are well advised to pay attention to the devices and locomotor "tools" needed and used by physically handicapped students in their charge. For example, Butler, Okamoto, and McKay (1984) have found that children as young as 2 can be taught the skills needed to use a motorized wheelchair. These skills may be incorporated into a lesson in physical education and transformed into game forms. Instructors should become familiar with the nature of devices available, how to use them, activities that can be carried out while using these devices, and the types of assistance and adjustments needed for a specific child (Frederick & Fletcher, 1985).

Activities for the Orthopedically Handicapped

On the pages that follow are examples of activities in three categories:[1]

1. Developmental activities suitable primarily for more physically handicapped youngsters.

2. Games and activities suitable for mixed groups of normally functioning children and those with orthopedic problems.

3. Versions of traditional games and sports, modified so that they can be played by those with various physical handicaps involving the skeletal-muscular system.

Participation in various games for the exclusive development of orthopedically handicapped youngsters is predicated on answers to the following questions:

- Are the children ambulatory, or are they in wheelchairs?
- If they are ambulatory, what use do they have of the upper limbs, and how fast and safely can they move with crutches, walkers, or other aids?
- If they are in wheelchairs, what are their capacities?
  —severe impairment with difficulty in head control?
  —fair head control but no use of the arms?
  —good head control with fair use of one arm?
  —head control with good use of one arm?
  —head control with the use of both arms in a minimal way?
  —head and trunk control with the good use of both arms?
- What energy and emotional limitations do the children have?
- What limits and capacities might they have in understanding the game rules and their complexities?

Upon gaining the answers to these questions, instructors should attempt to (a) survey what games or activities the children may have participated in previously; (b) determine what new activities might aid in their development; and (c) determine how the students may be introduced to new activities in positive ways. Initially, it is most important that

---

1. Illustrations are from *Educational Games for Physically Handicapped Children* by B.J. Cratty and J.E. Breen, 1972, Denver: Love Publishing.

the students achieve success, even if this means an activity that requires very little effort or movement.

Developmental Activities   Individuals who have marked problems could participate in activities that simply require them to hold a ball in their laps while being wheeled through a game, as illustrated.

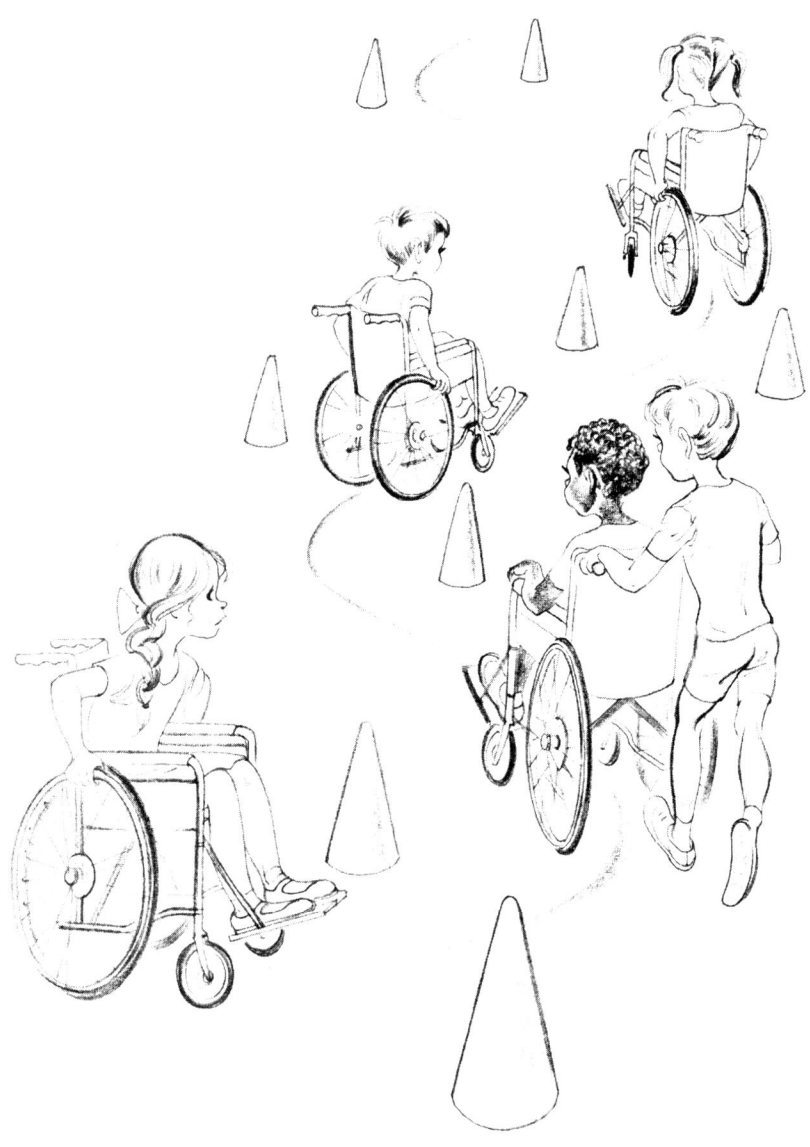

Further interest may be added to a relay game by having teammates pass the ball to one another. Children may move themselves or be moved.

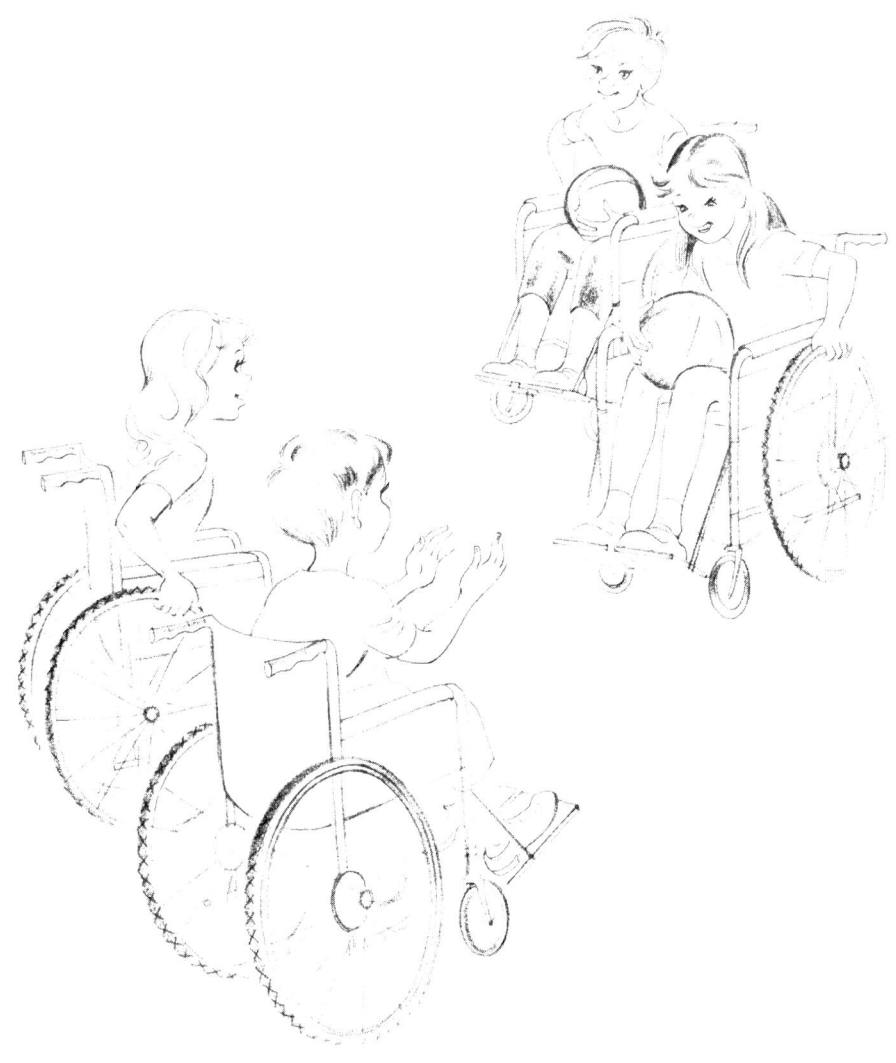

With chairs in a tight-knit circle, children may pass a ball among themselves. For variety, different types of balls may be used, or the direction in which the ball is passed might be changed.

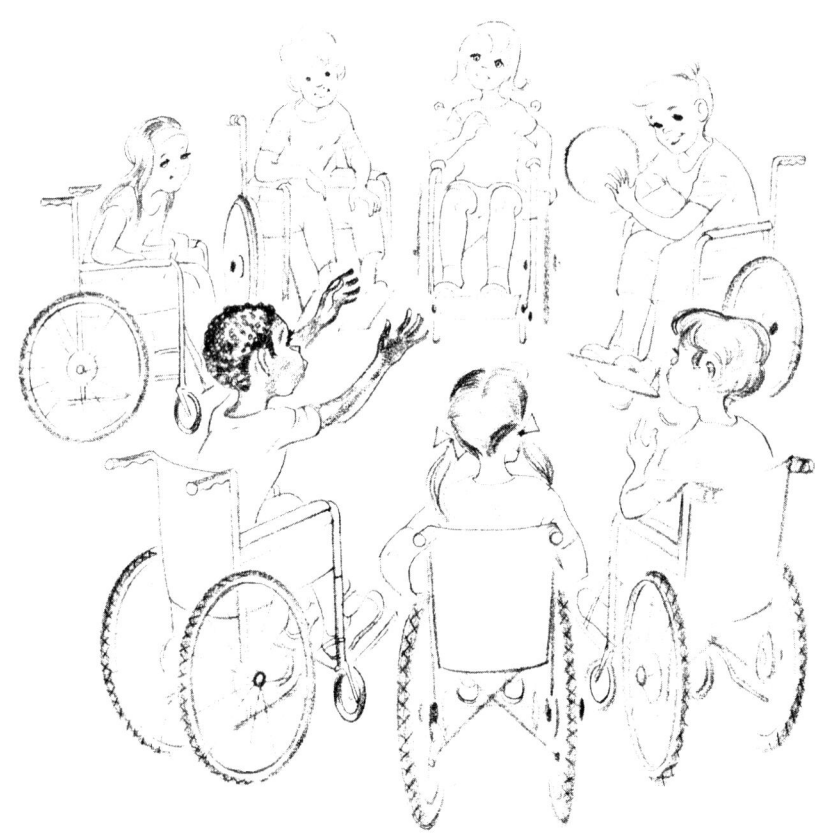

Later, simple exercises involving picking up balls while in a wheelchair, bouncing or throwing them to each other, or projecting a beanbag connected by a string to their chairs may be introduced. Initially, retrieval of the beanbag may be as developmentally helpful as throwing it. Picking up a ball while seated in a wheelchair is difficult. Children may practice "walking" the ball to and up onto the footrest or lap (A). Or two children—one with a beanbag and one with a suspended ball—may play together (B). A suspended ball also may be passed from child to child (C).

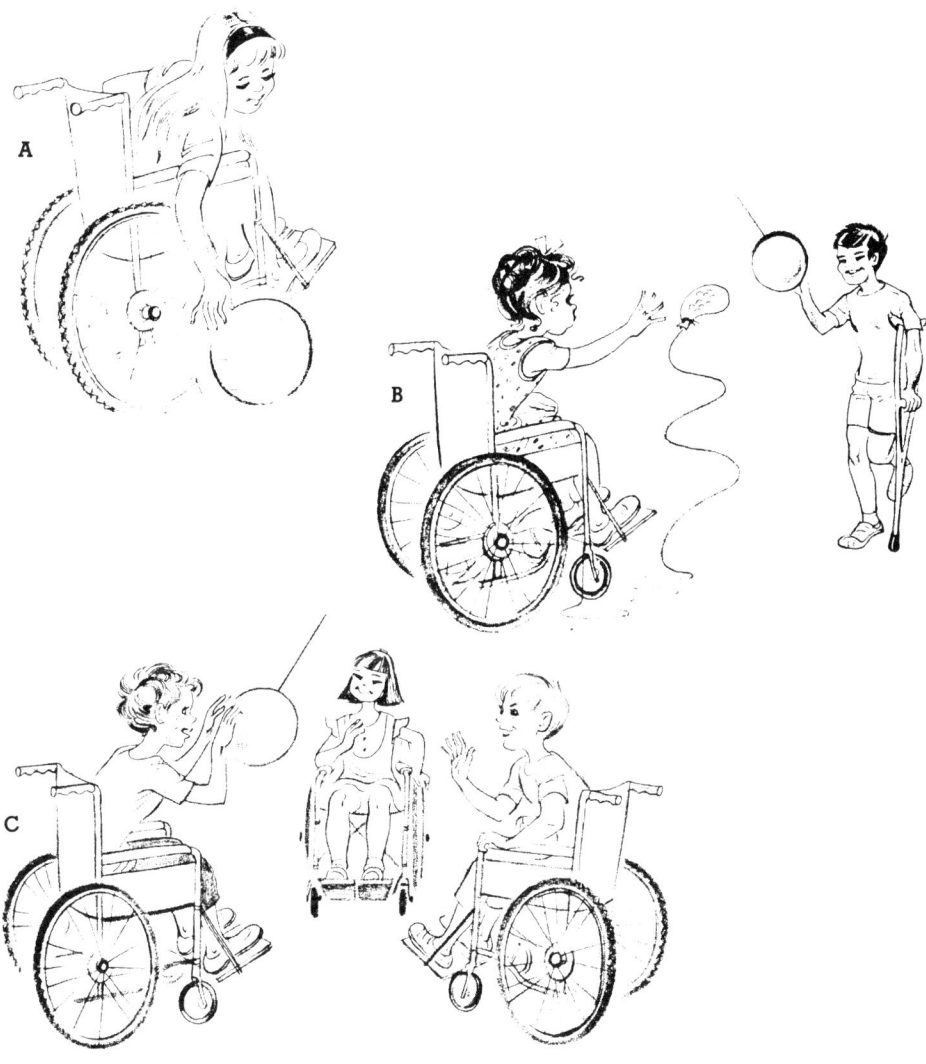

If participants' movements are extremely limited, simple adjustments of their weight in the wheelchair may prove developmentally useful and aid their seated balance. For example, to move balls or other round objects through the mazes, as illustrated, children have to shift their knees and their upper bodies. Maze box games also challenge children intellectually. Players can work alone (A) or in groups, cooperating or competing (B and C).

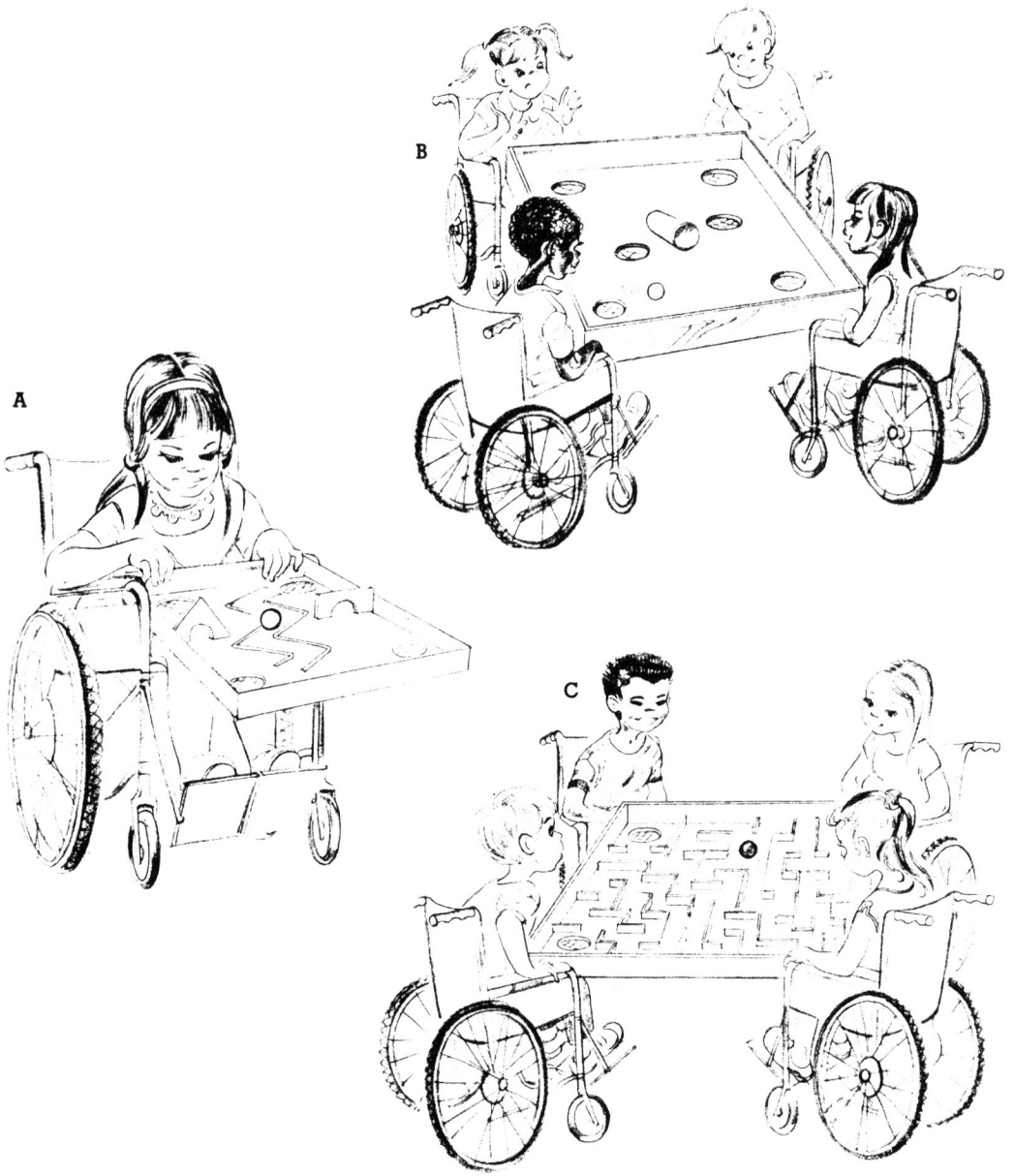

Various gymnasium activities, modified as shown in the photos, challenge the abilities of the orthopedically handicapped. The instructor should first determine whether the brace or assistive device may be removed or must be worn during activities, how much muscular exertion the child is allowed, and whether the muscular actions are contraindicated by therapeutic programs prescribed by medical personnel. In one possible activity (A), a rope tied securely 6″-8″ above the floor challenges the child to pull himself along by his arms. In another activity (B), a smooth beam is used to help this physically handicapped girl exercise the shoulder girdle.

A

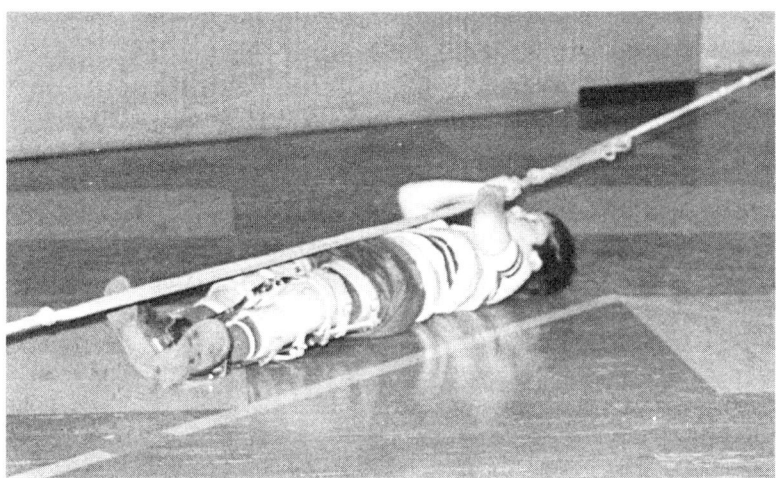

B

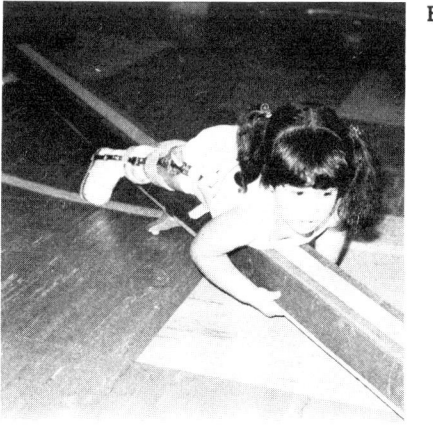

Gymnasium activities may be combined in interesting obstacle courses that appeal to the handicapped as progressively faster scores (time reduction) are recorded from day to day. Moreover, normal youngsters may compete with the handicapped when the latter have practiced the course extensively. At times the handicapped youngsters come out ahead!

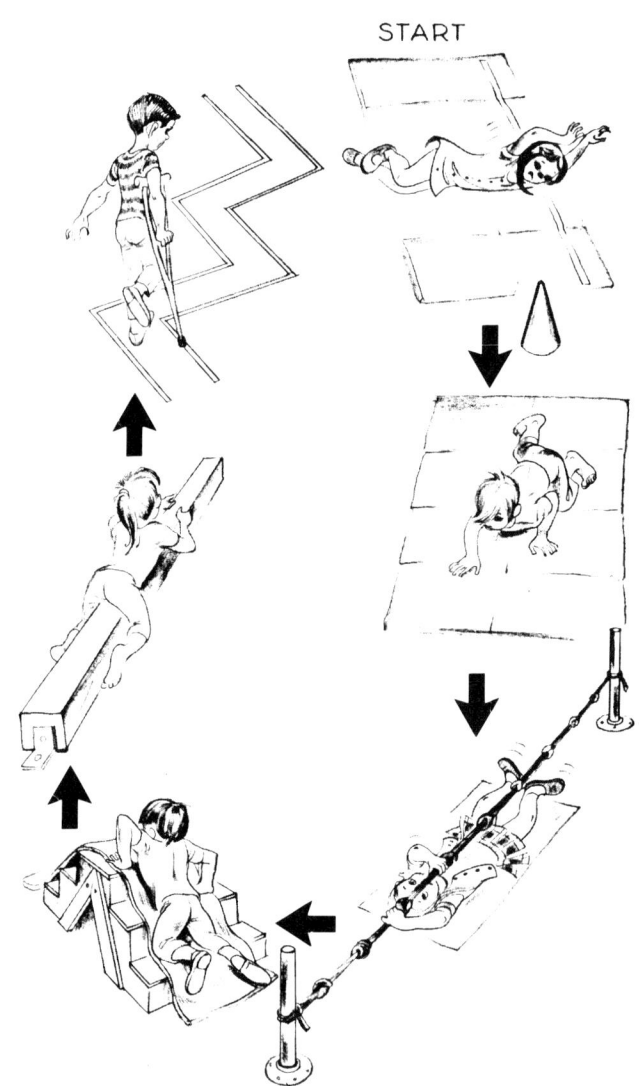

START

Outdoor obstacle courses can be marked off with paint or colored string. The course could be used for weekly progress evaluation.

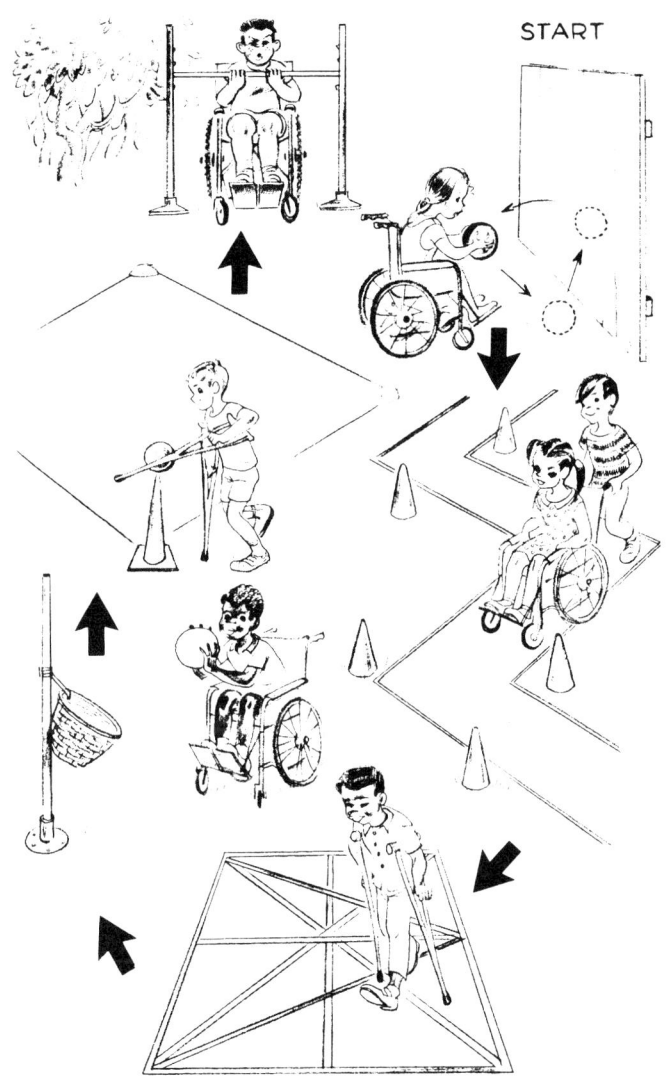

The orthopedically handicapped can play many table games. These are made possible with slight modifications to tennis tables or other tables similar in size. One game is a simple one- and two- bounce catch (A). With more complex modifications, surfaces can be tilted, and balls made to follow different courses (B). Again, normal youngsters can compete with handicapped children who have become somewhat proficient with practice.

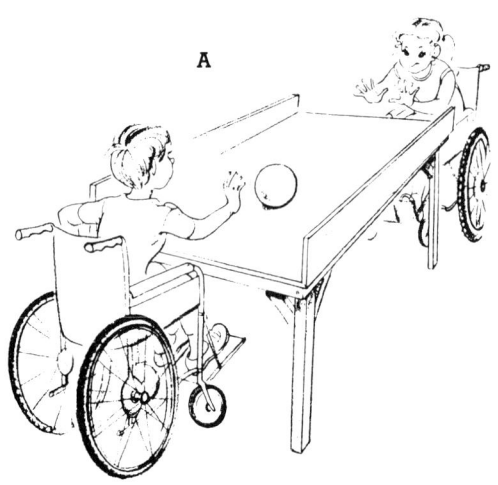

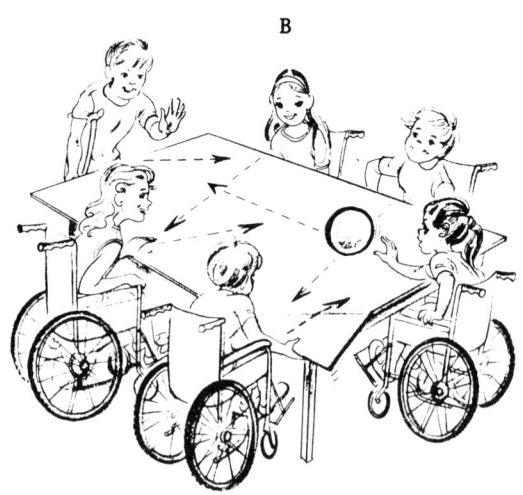

Activities for Mixed Groups   Handicapped and normal youngsters may participate at the same time in many activities. In these activities able youngsters substitute their skills for those of the handicapped, and both work together to achieve some aim in the game. An example of this is having a normal child and a child in a wheelchair play ball in the outfield together. When the ball is hit in their direction, it is first retrieved by the normal youngster, who places it in the lap of the handicapped youngster and then pushes the handicapped child to a position that permits the child to throw the ball in the direction of the base runner.

Base games can be modified so that the able and the handicapped may participate together. Movement from base to base may be assisted by the able. The total number of bases reached, rather than the number of complete runs, could be the criterion for success. Or the game may have a base path that is marked shorter than that for nonhandicapped players. Additional modifications in base games could involve various ways of a batter's projecting a missile. Normal youngsters may be required to kick the ball as it is rolled to them; children with minimal handicaps might be required to kick the ball from a spot in front of them; and more handicapped children may be required to use a crutch to hit a softball from a one-bounce pitch, as illustrated.

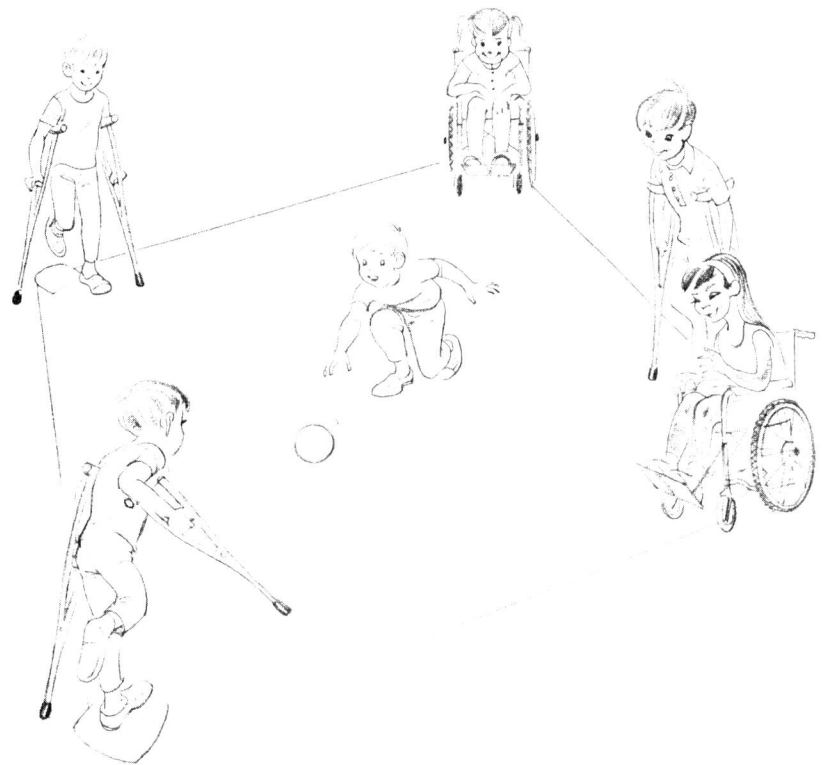

Modified Traditional Sports and Games   Observers of adult wheelchair basketball usually are amazed at the extremely high skill level achieved by participants, many of whom are spinal cord victims of armed conflicts. Younger handicapped children in wheelchairs usually enjoy participating in "lead-up" activities with the goal of taking part in this type of sport as they get older.

An initial game might involve bouncing a ball against a wall and attempting to catch it, and upon gaining more proficiency, playing a form of handball with an individual of similar ability (A). With appropriate apparatus, children in wheelchairs can propel themselves or be wheeled toward a basket and shoot the ball (B). A centrally located target permits children to take various positions around it and shoot baskets (C). In zone basketball, children are assigned to zones, passing and shooting over the outstretched arms of their opponents (D).

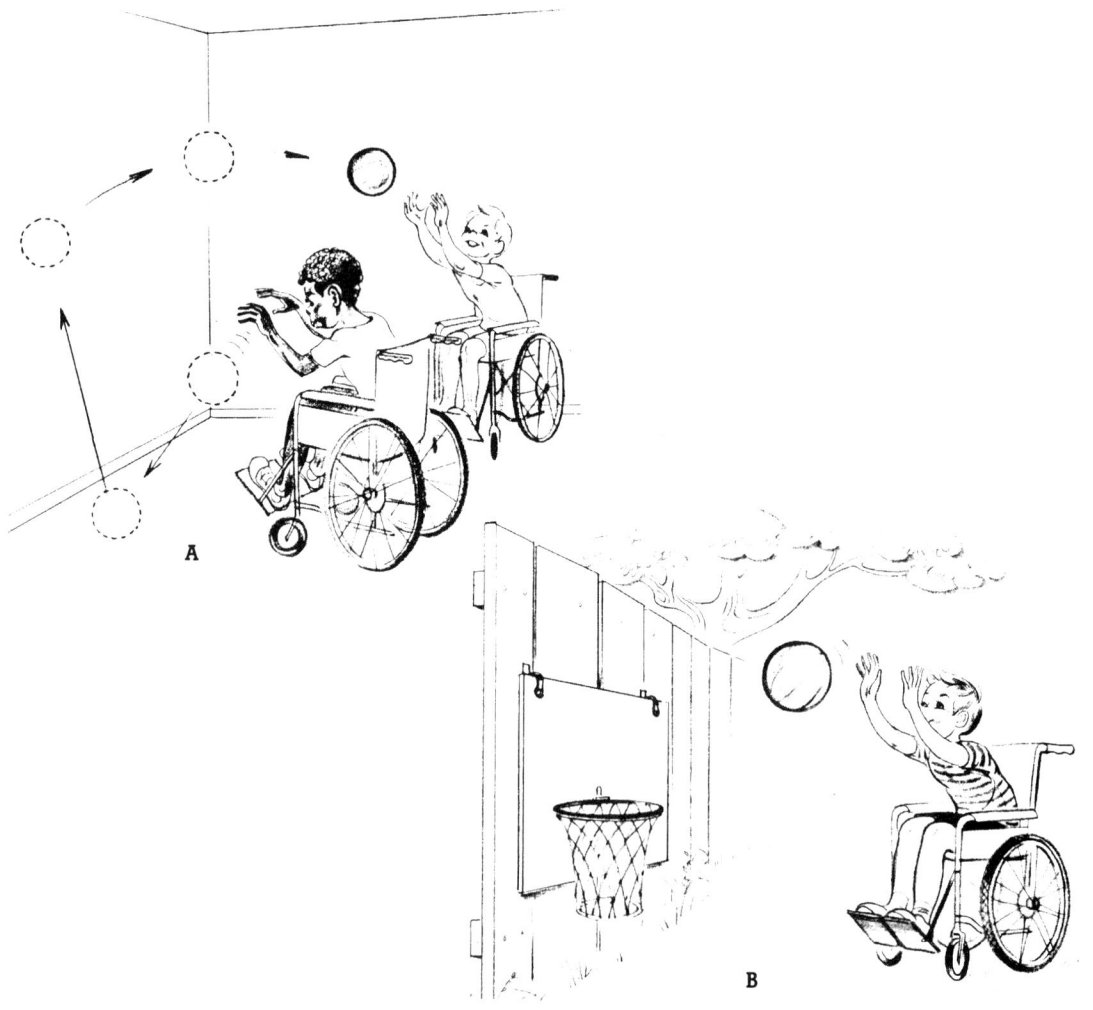

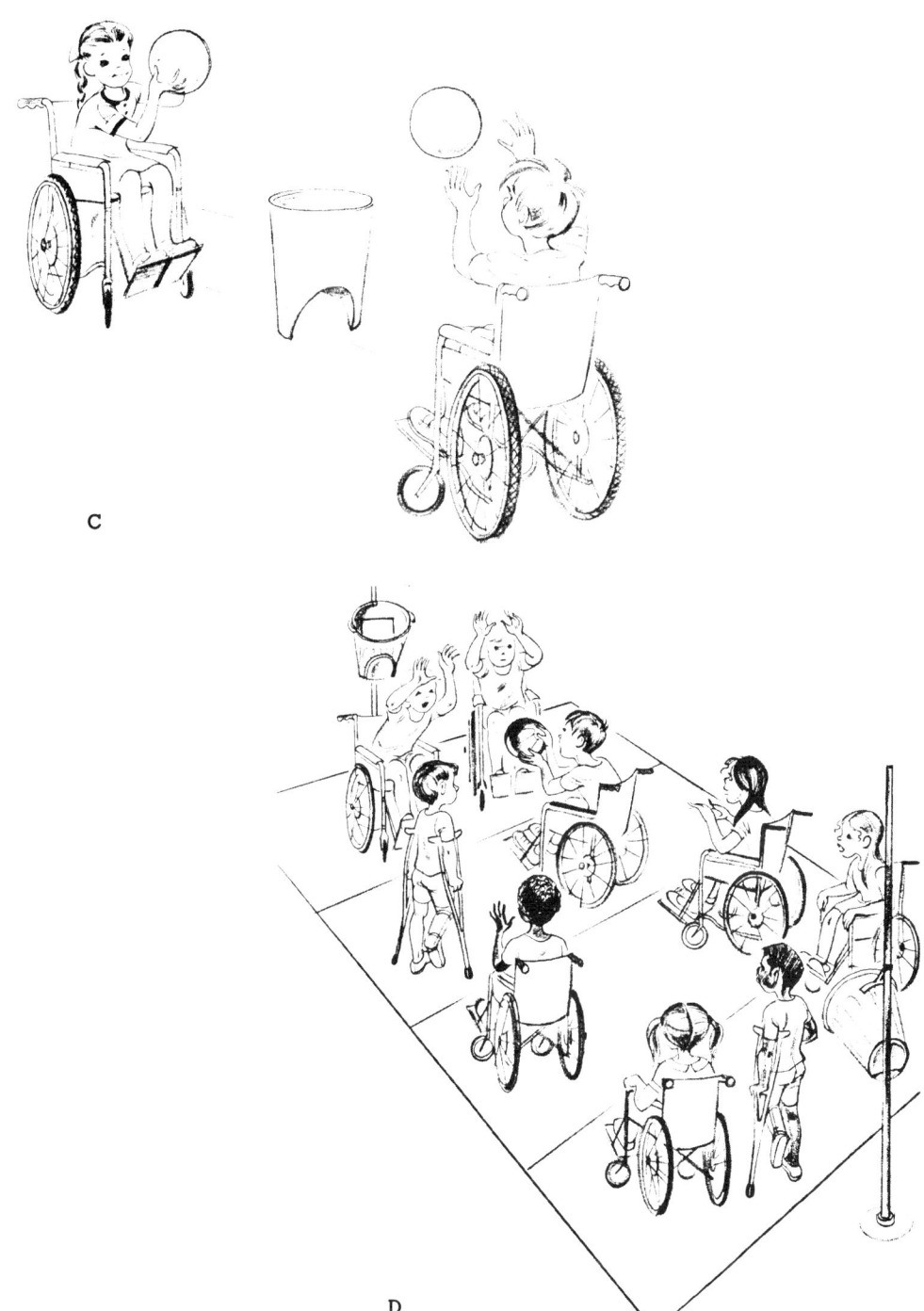

C

D

Volleyball also may be practiced in modified forms, as illustrated. One or more children positioned at either end of an overhead cable can propel a ball tied to the cable over the line (A). Or a tetherball attached to a horizontal cable can be used to play a modified form of volleyball (B).

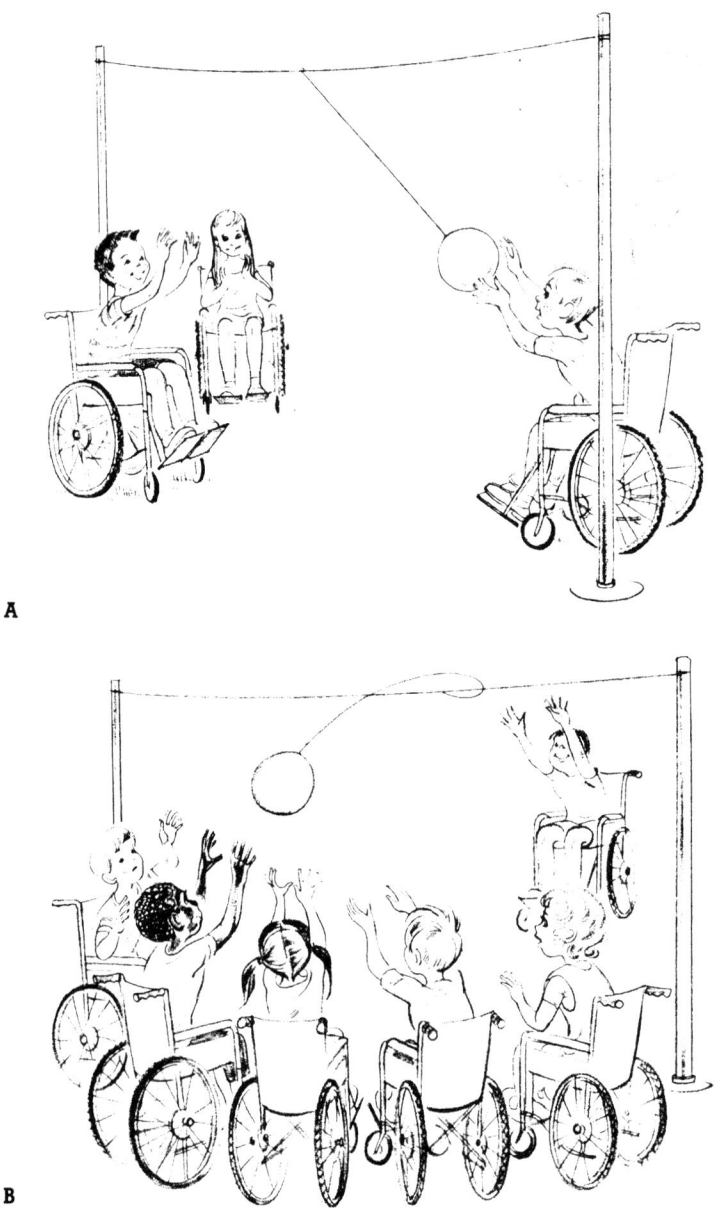

A

B

Field soccer and similar activities may be modified for handicapped children. Children may play a simple form of soccer by bumping a ball with their footrests to push the ball through an opponent's goal (A). After children have mastered two-player soccer, more players and goals may be added to the game (B).

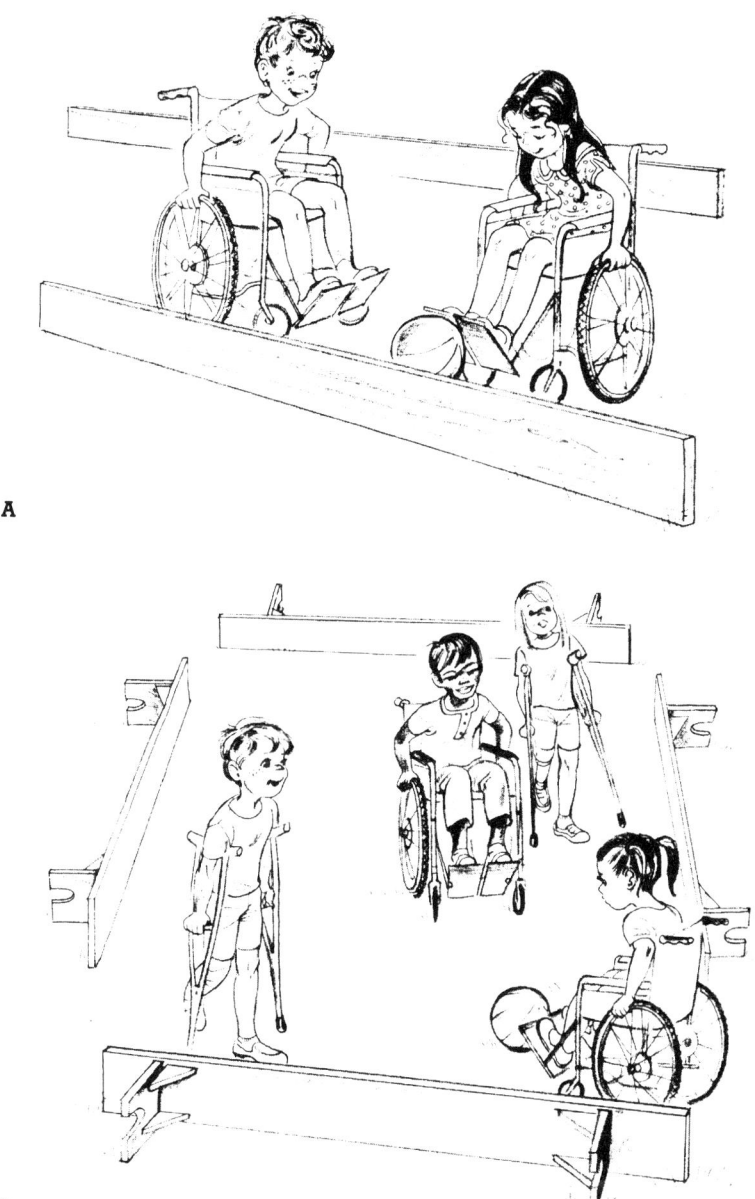

A

B

Following World War II various kinds of wheelchair athletics have been initiated in the United States. Well over 10,000 individuals participate in these sports in this country. In conjunction with the Special Olympics, the ParOlympics is held annually for paraplegics. The events in this competition are numerous and include archery, darts, modified track and field events, precision javelin throwing, fencing, and a variety of swimming and weight lifting events.

SUMMARY

Children and youth with orthopedic impairments have disabilities ranging from slight and possibly transitory to severe and relatively fixed, or permanent. Because of the wide variety of conditions and their innumerable manifestations, physical educators have a large task in devising, modifying, and implementing appropriate activities for these students, many of whom are in mainstreamed physical education classes.

Physical educators must work closely with consulting physicians and paramedical personnel, including occupational and physical therapists, in the rehabilitation and physical development of these youngsters. All efforts should be complementary in the child's total program.

Programming and instructional principles that should be helpful in working with the orthopedically handicapped include the following:

1. Special means might be required to encourage children to participate in activities that are new to them. Taking their picture next to a piece of apparatus, for example, may be helpful initially.

2. Activities should not be too difficult or contraindicatory to prescribed programs, while still offering some challenge and potential for improvement.

3. Activities should be self-sustaining and should not require constant monitoring or assistance by the physical education teacher.

4. Physically handicapped children mainstreamed into a normal class should receive modifications that will allow them to participate with their peers rather than being relegated to a different role, such as score keeping.

5. Orthopedically handicapped children and youth should be introduced to individual as well as team sports. Of particular worth are activities in which they may participate after their school years are over.

6. Equipment may have to be modified, and new equipment and apparatus introduced to optimize the participation of physically handicapped students. This chapter illustrates several ideas.

REFERENCES

Anderson, E.M., & Spain, B. (1977). *The child with spina bifida.* London: Methuen.

Bleck, E.E. (1975). Myelomeningocele, meningocele, spina bifida. In E.E. Bleck & D.A. Nagel, *Physically handicapped children: A medical atlas for teachers* (ch. 17). New York: Grune & Stratton.

Blum, R.W. (1983). The adolescent with spina bifida. *Clinical Pediatrics, 22,* 331-335.

Brunt, D. (1984). Apraxic tendencies in children with meningomyelocele. *Adapted Physical Activity Quarterly, 1*, 61-67.

Butler, C., Okamoto, G.A., & McCay, T.M. (1984). Motorized wheelchair driving by disabled children. *Archives of Physical Medicine & Rehabilitation, 65*, 95-96.

Cecconi, C.M., & Rothenberg, S.P. (1980). Model instructional program for mainstreaming handicapped children. *Physical Therapy, 60*, 1022-1025.

Centers, L., & Centers, R.A. (1968). A comparison of the body images of amputee and non-amputee children as revealed in figure drawings. *Journal of Projective Personality Assessment, 27*, 158-165.

Cooper, M.A., Sherrill, C., & Marshall, D. (1986). Attitudes toward physical activity of elite cerebral palsied athletes. *Adapted Physical Activity Quarterly, 3*, 14-21.

Dresden, M.A.W., de Groot, G., Mesa-Mead, J.R., & Bauman, L.N. (1985). Increased training intensity recommended for handicapped children. *Archives of Physical Medicine & Rehabilitation, 66*, 302-306.

Eason, J., & Schuler, J. (1979). *Changes in social attitudes toward disability following integration of handicapped children* (Monograph). Minneapolis: University of Minnesota, Dept. of Physical Medicine.

Enoka, R.M., Miller, D.I., & Burgess, E.M. (1982). Below knee amputee's running gait. *American Journal of Physical Medicine, 61*, 66-74.

Fox, V.M., Lawlor, V.A., & Luttges, M.W. (1984). Pilot study of novel test instrumentation to evaluate therapeutic horseback riding. *Adapted Physical Activity Quarterly, 1*, 30-36.

Frederick, J., & Fletcher, D. (1985). Facilitating children's adjustment to orthotic and prosthetic appliances. *Teaching Exceptional Children, 17*, 228-230.

Glaser, R.M., & Sawka, M. (1981). Exercise program for wheelchair activity. *American Journal of Physical Medicine, 60*, 67-75.

Gouvier, W.D., & Richards, J.S. (1985). Behavioral modification in physical therapy. *Archives of Physical & Medical Rehabilitation, 66*, 113-115.

Green, B.C., Pratt, C.C., & Griggsby, T.E. (1984). Self-concept among persons with long-term spinal cord injury. *Archives of Physical Medicine & Rehabilitation, 65*, 751-754.

Helm, P.A., Lushbaugh, M., Pullium, G., Head, M.I., & Croones, G.F. (1982). Burn injury: Rehabilitation and management. *Archives of Physical Medicine & Rehabilitation, 63*, 6-16.

Henschen, K., Horvat, M., & French, R. (1984). Visual comparison of psychological profiles between able-bodied and wheelchair athletes. *Adapted Physical Activity Quarterly, 1*, 118-124.

Madorsky, J.G., & Madorsky, A. (1984). Wheelchair racing: An important modality in acute rehabilitation after paraplegia. *Archives of Physical & Medical Rehabilitation, 64*, 186-187.

Manella, K.J., & Varni, J.W. (1981). Behavior therapy in a gait training program for a child with myelomeningocele. *Physical Therapy, 61*, 1284-1287.

McCall, R.E., & Schmidt, T.W. (1986). Clinical experience with the reciprocal gait orthosis in myelodysplasia. *Journal of Pediatric Orthopedics, 6*, 157-161.

National Association of Sports for Cerebral Palsy. (1979). *Constitution, rules classification, and National Records Sports Manual*. New Haven, CT: Author.

Rubin, G., & Fleiss, D. (1984). Devices to enable persons with amputations to participate in sports. *Archives of Physical Medicine & Rehabilitation, 64*, 37-40.

Winnick, J.P., & Short, F.X. (1984). Physical fitness of youngsters with spinal neuromuscular conditions. *Adapted Physical Activity Quarterly, 1*, 37-51.

Wool, R.N., & Siegel, D. (1980). Task performance in spinal cord injury: Effect of helplessness training. *Archives of Physical Medicine & Rehabilitation, 61,* 321-325.

ADDITIONAL REFERENCES

Altman, K., Haavik, S., & Higgins, S.T. (1983). Modifying the self-injurious behavior of an infant with spina bifida and diminished pain sensitivity. *Journal of Behavior Therapy & Experimental Psychiatry, 11,* 165-168.

American Academy of Orthopaedic Surgeons. (1972). *Symposium on myelomeningocele.* St. Louis: C.V. Mosby.

Brasile, F.M. (1986). Wheelchair basketball skills proficiencies versus disability classification. *Adapted Physical Activity Quarterly, 3,* 6-13.

Cull, C., & Wyke, M.A. (1984). Memory function of children with spina bifida and shunted hydrocephalus. *Developmental Medicine & Child Neurology, 26,* 177-183.

Gonnella, C., Hale, G., Ionta, M., & Perry, J.C. (1981). Self-instruction in a perceptual-motor skill. *Physical Therapy, 61,* 177-184.

Kegel, B., Jeffrey, J.C., & Burgess, E.M. (1980). Recreational activities of lower extremity amputees. *Archives of Physical Medicine & Rehabilitation, 61,* 258-264.

McCarthy, G.T. (1984). *The physically handicapped child.* London: Faber & Faber.

QUESTIONS FOR DISCUSSION

1. What conditions are not permanent? How might physical educators deal with these children physically so that their conditions become better sooner?

2. What special bracing is seen on various handicapped children? What precautions should be taken in the physical education of these children?

3. What special problems do youngsters with spina bifida bring to the physical education class? How might these problems best be dealt with in programming for these youngsters?

4. What traditional team games may be adapted for the handicapped? What special playground markings might be useful for the orthopedically handicapped? What individual sports may be modified, and in what ways?

5. What kinds of equipment might be made in shop programs that will facilitate the physical development of orthopedically handicapped youngsters?

6. How might one formulate a useful situation-specific instrument with which to assess the physical competencies and recreational skills of the orthopedically handicapped? What items might appear on such a device?

STUDENT PROJECTS

1. Interview a parent of an orthopedically handicapped child. Discuss the child's social and emotional adjustment in the classroom and in the physical education program. Does the child seem to differ in the two environments?

2. Observe a class in which children with orthopedic handicaps have been mainstreamed. Describe the programming, teaching methods, and general social-emotional tone.

3. Interview a physical therapist active in

working with the orthopedically handicapped. What special problems does the therapist encounter in working with the children, their parents, and the school administration? How has the therapist provided input for the child's individualized education program?

4. Attempt to interview an orthopedic surgeon. Discuss recent operations, the prognosis for improved function arising from such operations, and the manner in which various kinds of physical exercise can either impede or aid progress.

RESOURCES

American Wheelchair Bowling
  Association
2424 North Federal Hwy., Suite 109
Boynton Beach, FL 33435

American Wheelchair Pilots
  Association
3953 West Evans Dr.
Phoenix, AZ 85023

Canadian Amputee Sports Association
18 Hale Dr.
Georgetown, Ontario
Canada L7G 4C2

Canadian Wheelchair Sports
  Association
333 River Rd.
Ottawa, Ontario
Canada K1L 8B9

International Medical Society of
  Paraplegia
E & S Livingstone
43-45 Annandale St.
Edinburgh, EH7 4AT
Scotland

International Sports Organization for
  the Disabled
Stoke Mandeville Sports Stadium
Harvey Rd.
Aylesbury, Bucks
England

National Easter Seal Society for
  Crippled Children and Adults
2023 West Ogden Ave.
Chicago, IL 60612

National Spinal Cord Injury
  Foundation
369 Elliot St.
Newton Upper Falls, MA 02164

National Wheelchair Basketball
  Association
110 Seaton Bldg.
University of Kentucky
Lexington, KY 40506

National Wheelchair Marathon
369 Elliot St.
Newton Upper Falls, MA 02164

National Wheelchair Softball
  Association
P.O. Box 737
Sioux Falls, SD 57101

Ontario Wheelchair Sport
  Association
585 Tretheway Dr.
Toronto, Ontario
Canada M6M 4B8

Paralyzed Veterans of America
4330 East-West Hwy., Suite 300
Washington, DC 20014

Wheelchair Motorcycle Association
101 Torrey St.
Brockton, MA 02401

Wheelchair Sports Foundation
c/o Benjamin H. Lipton
40-24 62nd St.
Woodside, NY 11377

20 *Arthritis*

Millions of people in the United States suffer from one of several forms of arthritis. This inflammation of the joints may appear in many forms. The most common symptoms are swelling, tenderness, and limitations of motion at the joints, together with some atrophy.

Although arthritis usually is thought of as a condition of the middle-aged or aged, juvenile rheumatoid arthritis may afflict children as young as 6 weeks. Estimates of the number of children in the United States afflicted with this condition vary from 100,000 to 300,000. Most important, however, is that 60%-70% of the children will be free of the active disease after about 10 years. With good care and therapy only about 10% of all children afflicted with arthritis will retain any functional problems or disorders in later life. The length of time a child will remain arthritic is not predictable and varies from a few months to years. Therapy extended to youngsters should be predicated on the assumption that permanent remission will occur.

Arthritis is not considered to be an inherited disease, although its exact causes are unknown. The inflammation is believed to be a result of an immunologic attack on normal body materials. Abnormal antibodies—proteins that may destroy various materials needed for protection against joint inflammation—strangely appear in the blood. The appearance of these abnormal substances does not seem to be related to diet, climate, or pattern of living.

In this inflammation the synovial cells of a joint become infected. The joint then swells and may become granulomatous, resulting in scarring. In juvenile arthritis the swelling may affect the bone growth plate and cause a growth disturbance. It may result either in an increase in the rate of bone growth, causing longer bones, or premature closure of the bone growth plate, causing bones to be shorter. The arthritic process also can lead to destruction of joint surfaces (articular cartilage), which eventually may undergo bony bridging.

TYPES OF ARTHRITIS

Although over 100 causes of joint inflammation have been identified, three major categories account for two thirds of all arthritis: *rheumatoid arthritis, osteoarthritis* (degenerative joint disease), and *nonarticular rheumatism,* including arthritis of psychogenic origin. Because the primary type found in school-age children is juvenile rheumatoid arthritis,[1] the following discussion concentrates on this variation. This juvenile affliction is illustrated in Figure 20.1. It takes one of three forms:

1. *Polyarticular rheumatoid arthritis.* From 50% to 60% of all children with arthritis contract this form, which involves inflamed joints, most often of the knees, ankles, and wrists. Initially the pain in the knee joint is minimal, but after onset other joints may become involved and the pain sometimes becomes acute. Among the symptoms of this form of arthritis are painful joints, flexion contractures, and muscle atrophy resulting in muscular

---

1. Other common types of juvenile arthritis include those caused by known infectious agents, abnormal joint stresses including fractures, torn ligaments, and the like, rheumatic fever, and gout.

Figure 20.1   Juvenile Manifestations of Rheumatoid Arthritis

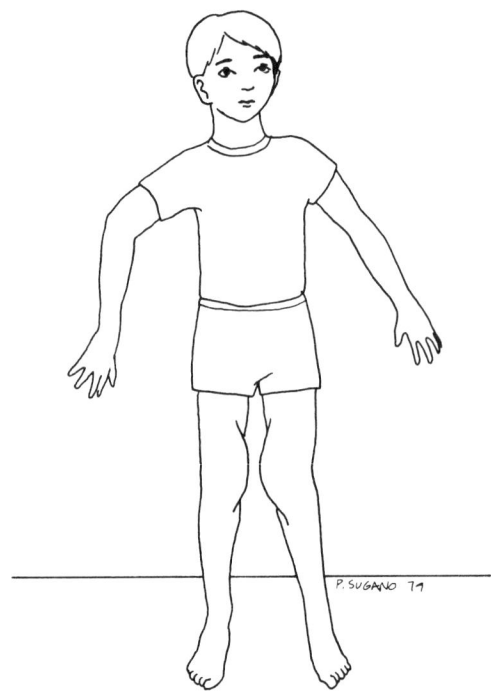

weaknesses. A decreased range of motion results in stiffness. If the disease occurs early in life, it interferes with both growth and sexual maturation. The afflicted youngsters may be compelled to sit in a flexed position for comfort.

2. *Systemic rheumatoid arthritis.* This is the least frequent form of arthritis, affecting about 20% of children diagnosed as arthritic. It is characterized by high, spiking fevers once or twice a day during onset of the disease. The child usually shows fatigue, anemia, a high white blood cell count, and other nonspecific signs of general inflammation. The arthritis itself may appear several months after these symptoms, and extensive tests should be carried out during the interim to rule out the possibility of other serious infections. At first the diagnosis may be difficult, unless the triad of symptoms—a rash, a fever curve, and eventual appearance of joint soreness—is recognized. These attacks may last for months, disappear, and then recur months or even years later. Children with this systemic type of arthritis may go on to evidence polyarticular symptoms.

3. *Pauciarticular rheumatoid arthritis.* Children with four or fewer painful or swollen joints are assumed to have contracted pauciarticular rheumatoid arthritis. They do not have systemic signs, nor do they look or feel ill, except for soreness in the joints involved. They may have only one swollen joint, but after some months more and more joints may be affected, resulting in a diagnosis of polyarticular arthritis. These children may suffer in-flammation of the iris and muscles controlling the lens of the eye, which may lead to blind-ness. Thus, they should be seen immediately by an ophthalmologist.

Children with arthritis may have various emotional problems including loss of self-esteem (Brewer, Giannini, & Person, 1983). They also may experience anger, denial, social withdrawal, self-imposed starvation (anorexia) or uncontrollable eating and obesity. They often are insecure and at times uncooperative, showing passive forms of aggression (Geist, 1966; Rothermich & Whisler, 1985). Children with less severe symptoms, and thus less obvious forms of the condition, might be subjected to more social criticism from others, as it seems that they are simply lazy rather than suffering from a debilitating joint prob-lem. Difficulties in the classroom may be diminished if the child is permitted to move around frequently and is given the time to take medication when prescribed.

SPECIFIC AND GENERAL COMPLICATIONS

The degree to which cartilage and other joint structures go untreated will determine the amount of permanent damage. Most children respond to good therapy. Because some damage to the cartilage is inevitable, the presence of juvenile forms of the disease may be seen later in arthritic conditions reflecting the wear and tear of old age.

Some complications arise from medicants. Cortisone and related drugs should be ad-ministered only when a child's life or eyesight is threatened. Unfortunately, medicants sometimes are given too frequently, producing side effects such as a blunting of long-bone growth, a puffing up or "moon face," brittle bones, and a decrease in resistance to severe infection.

Atypical functioning of the total body may result from pain and decreasing mobility in various joints. For example:

1. Pain in the knee joint encourages the child to walk with a knock-kneed gait and with a slight limp. This mode of walking may in time result in some atrophy of the muscles extending the knee.

2. Pain in the feet may make wearing shoes uncomfortable and lead to various minor to moderate foot deformities including pronation, flat feet, and general muscular rigidity.

3. In the wrist and hand, pain and swelling may lead to an abnormal union of bones whose interjacent cartilages have been destroyed, to muscular atrophy, and to reduction of normal grip strength and limitations of range of motion of the fingers when opening and closing.

4. The deltoid muscles sometimes atrophy, at times causing a shoulder drop and sometimes deformities in the head and neck of the humerus.

5. Arthritis in the hip and spinal column usually affects one joint more than the other and limits the range of movement in the hip. The rearward swing of the thigh becomes limited during walking, and unequal leg length and lordosis may occur. Stiffness and loss of mobility in the spinal column are experienced. Sometimes trunk flexion resembles kyphosis (see chapter 18). If the condition is prolonged, vertebral bodies atrophy, longitudinal ligaments become calcified, pectoral muscles shorten, and the rib cage becomes rigid, mak-ing deep breathing difficult. Hyperextension braces sometimes are prescribed for the spine.

IMPLICATIONS FOR PHYSICAL EDUCATION

Physical educators encounter arthritic children and youth only when they are in remission. By that time, however, the children's immobility and their lack of movement experiences may have exerted a profound effect on their capacities. They are likely to suffer recurring joint tenderness along with a variety of residual symptoms. Physical educators should incorporate the following information and suggestions when planning programs for these children:

1. With the aid of the attending physician and therapist, an extensive program of passive stretching exercises should be implemented daily. These exercises should be carried into the home, if possible.

2. Strength should be maintained, and any atrophy of various muscle groups should be counteracted with daily exercises.

3. Further flexion contractures might be prevented by emphasizing exercises that strengthen the extensors while stretching the flexors. Also, exercises should be devised to strengthen the pronators and stretch the supinators, to exercise the abductors while stretching the adductors, and to promote a range of motion and strength in the internal rotators.

4. During early stages of remission, children may need help in planning motor activities needed to arise from a chair, to dress, to be seated without trauma, and to otherwise carry out daily life activities.

5. Often, gait reeducation is needed. Bars with arm support and a movable walker can be used, with the advice and aid of a physical therapist. Gait training on level surfaces may be progressively advanced to ascending and descending stairs with low risers.

6. Moist heat may be prescribed to accompany exercise. Hydrotherapy often is useful in such cases, when prescribed by a physician.

7. Frequent use of aspirin can have short-term effects on hearing in arthritics. This loss of hearing disappears when aspirin treatment is stopped.

8. Physical educators should expect periodic mood fluctuations in children after a good or bad night relative to the joint pain experienced.

9. A phenomenon known as "jelling" may occur after children arise in the morning and have difficulty initiating movements in stiff joints, and at various times during the day. Physical educators should encourage frequent changes of position by arthritic children and permit them sufficient time to move around during a class period, particularly if the child has had a period of immobility between movement activities.

10. Physical education teachers (as other teachers) may be in a position to detect vision problems in children who have an insidious onset of iridocyclitis. This should be cause for immediate referral to an ophthalmologist.

11. The physical education program offered to arthritics, even when the condition is in apparent remission, should omit activities that tend to jar the bony frame and joints. Hopping, leaping, and tasks that involve contact with others and objects (e.g., football, soccer, gymnastics, roller skating) should be avoided.

12. Rhythmic stretching activities such as modern dance, relaxation exercises, and modified forms of water ballet and swimming are suitable and are not likely to cause further joint trauma. Quiet recreational games also are helpful and socially satisfying.

SUMMARY

Juvenile rheumatoid arthritis affects from 100,000 to 300,000 youngsters in the United States. Approximately 60%-70% will be free from the symptoms after 10 years or so. The amount of time children will evidence the condition is difficult to predict, and the exact causes of arthritis are unknown, although it is thought not to be inherited. It is marked by the appearance of abnormal antibodies in the blood, which destroy materials needed by the body for protection against joint inflammation.

Of children with juvenile arthritis, most have *polyarticular arthritis*, which most often affects the knees, ankles, and wrists. Contractures develop, and the joints lose flexibility. Other types are *systemic arthritis*, which is manifested in joint soreness accompanied initially by a high, spiking fever, and *pauciarticular arthritis*, which affects relatively few joints.

Conditions accompanying arthritis include atrophy of various muscle groups, postural and gait abnormalities, and possible effects from prescribed medication. A physical education program for these youngsters should consist of gentle stretching exercises, attempts to maintain strength, and heat and hydrotherapy applications for pain relief.

REFERENCES

Brewer, E.J., Giannini, E.H., & Person, D.A. (1982). *Juvenile rheumatoid arthritis*. New York: W.B. Saunders.

Geist, H. (1966). *The psychological aspects of rheumatoid arthritis*. Springfield, IL: Charles C Thomas.

Rothermich, N.O., & Whisler, R.L. (1985). *Rheumatoid arthritis*. Orlando, FL: Grune & Stratton.

ADDITIONAL REFERENCES

Calabro, J.J., & Wykert, J. (1971). *The truth about arthritis care*. New York: David McKay.

Jeremy, R., Schaller, J., Arkless, R., Wedgwood, R.H., & Healey, L.A. (1968). Juvenile rheumatoid arthritis persisting into adulthood. *American Journal of Medicine, 45,* 419-434.

National Foundation, March of Dimes. (1972). *When your child has rheumatoid arthritis*. Washington, DC: Author.

Schaller, J., & Wedgwood, R.J. (1972). Juvenile rheumatoid arthritis: A review. *Pediatrics, 50,* 940-953.

QUESTIONS FOR DISCUSSION

1. What types of juvenile arthritis are likely to be encountered? How do their symptoms vary? What are common symptoms?

2. What special precautions should be taken with arthritic children in a physical education class?

3. What might a special program of phys-

ical activity consist of for a child with arthritis? What specific exercises might be useful? What exercises or activities are harmful?

4. What are some side effects of medication taken to reduce arthritic symptoms?

STUDENT PROJECTS

1. Review applicable literature and describe how juvenile rheumatoid arthritis differs from various arthritic conditions in the aged.

2. Design an ideal program of physical exercise for a specific child with juvenile arthritis. Ask a physician to inspect and evaluate the program.

3. Observe an arthritic child, recording his or her daily movements, including those at play and in physical education class. Note the incidence of apparent pain, constriction of joints, and possible occurrences of jelling. After making these observations, plan an ideal day for the child, attempting to maximize physical comfort and enable him or her to function most effectively in all phases of life.

RESOURCES

Annals of the Rheumatic Diseases
Arthritis and Rheumatism Council
   for Research in Great Britain
   and Commonwealth
B.M.A. House
Tavistock Square
London WC1H 9JR

Arthritis and Rheumatism
   Bulletin on the Rheumatic Diseases
American Rheumatism Association
1212 Avenue of the Americas
New York, NY 10036

Arthritis Foundation
3400 Peachtree Rd., N.W.
Atlanta, GA 30026

21 *Heart Disease*

Heart malfunctions in childhood are classified into two main types: congenital and acquired. Congenital heart disease is 20 times more prevalent than acquired types in childhood, while acquired heart conditions occur far more frequently in adults. Approximately 6 of every 1,000 live births are accompanied by some heart abnormality. The largest proportion of these infants die within the first month of life, and many within the first year. The prevalence of children with these conditions by age 10 is 1 or 2 per 1,000.

CONGENITAL HEART CONDITIONS

The causes of congenital heart conditions are largely unknown. Only a relatively small percentage (estimated at about 5%) can be traced to an identifiable chromosomal abnormality. Down syndrome is the best known of these. Although most causes of congenital heart conditions are difficult to determine, mothers who contract German measles (rubella) during early pregnancy are more likely than others to give birth to infants with problems of the heart or its associated vessels.

Figure 21.1 Normal Blood Flow Patterns of the Heart

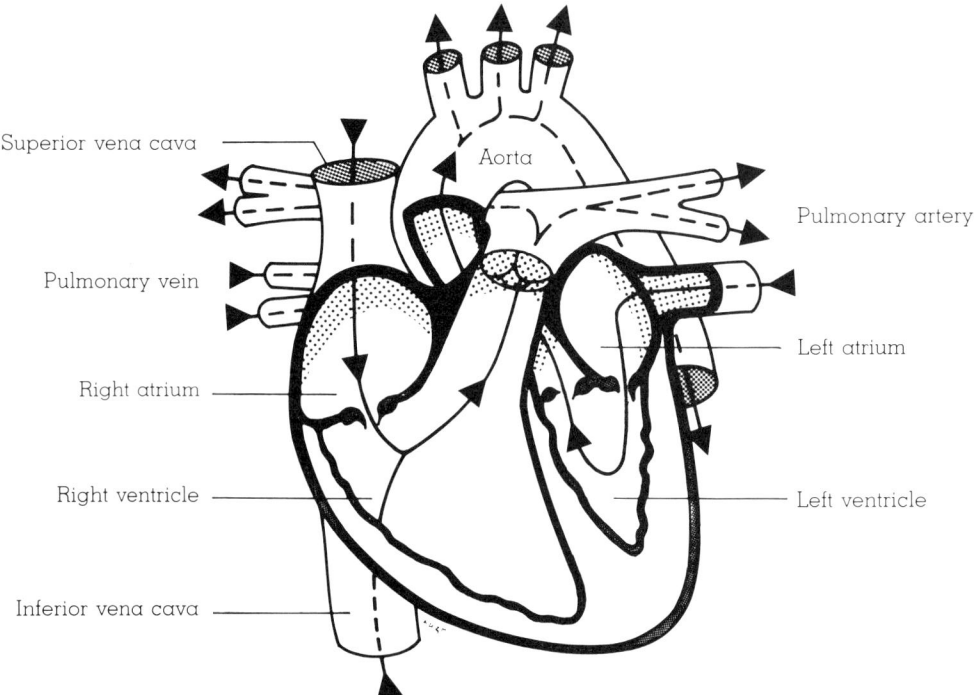

Superior vena cava

Aorta

Pulmonary artery

Pulmonary vein

Left atrium

Right atrium

Right ventricle

Left ventricle

Inferior vena cava

The child's heart condition may be diagnosed at birth from obvious signs (e.g., a "blue baby") or signs encountered during a physical examination given early in life (e.g., a heart murmur). Modern surgical techniques often can correct the condition in infancy, so that little or no residual malfunction remains by the time the child enters school. Problems that remain sometimes can be reduced by medication. Certain children with early malformations of the heart and associated structures, however, need continual monitoring throughout their early lives, including careful control of the type and intensity of physical activity in which they engage (Rudolph, 1974). Figure 21.1 shows the major parts of the heart and the path of normal blood flow through it.

Patent Ductus Arteriosis

Prior to birth a duct exists between the two large arteries arising from the heart—the pulmonary artery and the aorta. Normally, with inflation of the lungs after birth, this duct closes after a few weeks. When it remains open, however, an extra load is placed on the heart as some of the blood from the aorta is shunted back to the lungs through this passage. The heart must pump harder to supply the body, as well as providing the extra blood needed to pass through this open duct. This condition, patent ductus arteriosis, is illustrated in Figure 21.2.

The operation to correct this condition is performed early in life. It is a simple one, in which the duct is tied off. The result is normal circulation. At times this defect can lead to an infection called *bacterial endocarditis*. Thus, prior to surgery, the child receives antibiotics.

Ventricular Septal Defect

Sometimes a baby is born with an opening through the tissue (septum) separating the two ventricles of the heart, as shown in Figure 21.3. If the opening is small, little malfunction will occur, and only a murmur will be heard. If the opening is large, the same problem occurs as with children who have patent ductus arteriosis. Both ventricles must pump large

Figure 21.2 Patent Ductus Arteriosis   **Figure 21.3** Ventricular Septal Defect

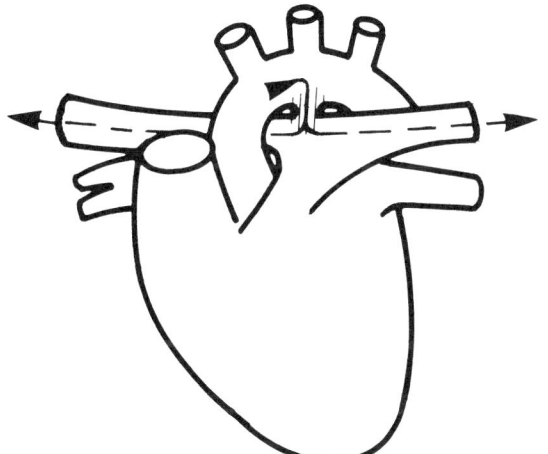
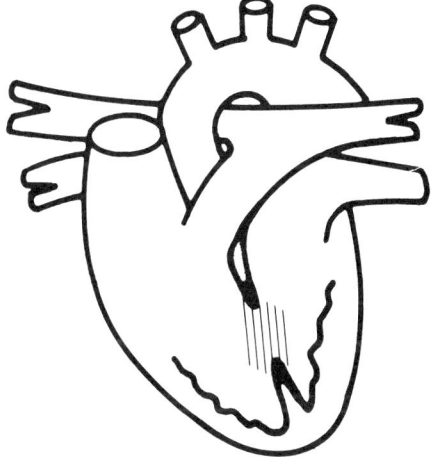

amounts of blood through the system, supplying a sufficient amount to the total body and additional blood through the opening in the septum.

If the condition persists over time, the heart will enlarge. The child can do reasonably well in spite of this abnormality if compensatory mechanisms are adequate, but growth will be slower and the body will be malnourished. Youngsters with large defects of this type are more likely to have infections of the lungs, as well as pneumonia. If a younger infant with a large defect contracts pneumonia, heart failure can result. Surgery can correct the condition when the symptoms, including repeated infections, become a persistent problem. Children who grow up with uncorrected ventricular septal defects are prone to bacterial endocarditis, so antibiotics may be prescribed during childhood.

Atrial Septal Defect

Holes also occur in the atria, or the septum separating the receiving chambers of the heart. This is depicted in Figure 21.4. In contrast to an opening in the septum between the ventricles, the only symptom of atrial septal defect is a slight heart murmur, which may not be detected until middle childhood. If the problem is acute, it usually is diagnosed between ages 4 and 10.

Abnormal heart rhythm and heart failure are more prevalent later in the lives of these individuals, during their 20s and 30s, if the condition is not corrected. Inflammations and infections (bacterial endocarditis) usually are not a problem later in life.

Tetralogy of Fallot

Infants born with this condition are often referred to as "blue babies" because four associated heart malfunctions result in the mixing of a portion of poorly oxygenated blood returning from the body (systemic venous return) through the ventricular septal defect in the left ventricle with oxygenated blood returning to the lungs. This causes *cyanosis*, a bluish discoloration. Figure 21.5 illustrates tetralogy of Fallot. Other structural conditions that

Figure 21.4   Atrial Septal Defect   **Figure 21.5**   Tetralogy of Fallot

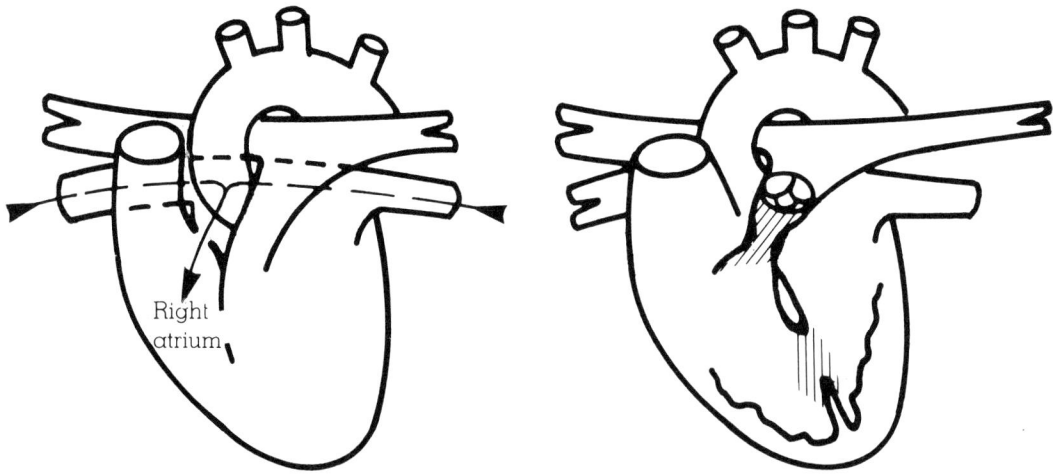

Right
atrium

evolve include hypertrophy of the right ventricle, because of overwork, and an overriding or straddling of the ventricular septal defects by the aorta. This child usually develops cyanosis of the lips, mucous membranes, and nail beds. When the condition is present in extreme form, the infant may hyperventilate and faint.

Total correction of this condition is not frequent. When it is not feasible, temporizing operations can be carried out to increase blood flow to the lungs, thus improving the child's overall condition and decreasing the possibility of further hypoxic spells. Early correction of the condition often results in great improvement in growth and development. Because the possibility of bacterial endocarditis remains, antibiotics should be used to prevent recurring infections.

Transposition of the Great Vessels

This condition, one of the more dramatic and fatal malformations of the heart, is shown in Figure 21.6. Locations of the aorta and pulmonary artery are reversed or transposed. Without surgery 90% of affected infants succumb within the first year of life because of reduced oxygen and heart failure.

Surgical procedures include enlarging interatrial communication by passing a catheter with a small deflated balloon from left to right through the atria. If this fails, the atrial septal opening is enlarged surgically. This strategy permits general improvement and growth. For further correction, a baffle is inserted in both atria. This diverts the systemic venous blood to the left ventricle and pulmonary artery for oxygenation while directing the oxygenated blood returning from the lungs to the right ventricle and aorta for distribution to the body. Although not totally satisfactory, these procedures do result in some improvement, but the children always may have to restrict their activity level.

Aortic Stenosis

In aortic stenosis a congenital obstruction of the aortic valve, caused by a deformity of the valve itself, forces the left ventricle to pump at higher pressures to force blood through

Figure 21.6 Transposition of the Great Vessels   **Figure 21.7** Aortic Stenosis

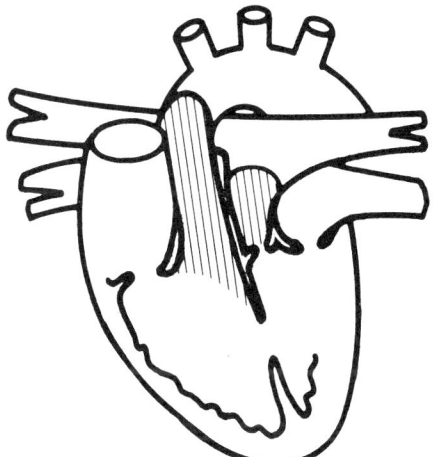
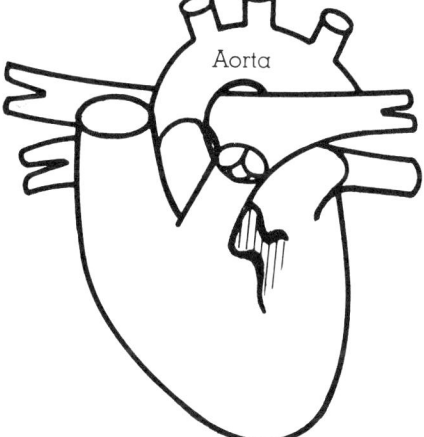

the narrowed aorta. Figure 21.7 illustrates this abnormality. If the condition is severe, the wall of the left ventricle hypertrophies. If demands on the ventricle are too great, heart failure may occur.

This condition sometimes is found in active children who outwardly seem normal. Unless they report chest pain, no symptoms may be apparent. After diagnosis, parents often have difficulty accepting the reality of this condition and its concomitant risks. When working with these children, physical educators, under the advice of a physician, should restrict the children from competitive athletics and permit them to rest when they have chest discomfort, shortness of breath, or unusual fatigue.

Enlargement of the obstruction may be accomplished surgically, but the child often is left with residual deformity of the valve, resulting in some leakage back into the left ventricle. Because correction via surgery is not considered ideal, it is advised only when the obstruction is reasonably severe. Children with this condition are susceptible to bacterial endocarditis and require the usual precautions, including administration of antibiotics.

Coarctation of the Aorta

At times the aorta is constricted at the point where the large arterial branch to the left arm arises. If severe, this narrowing (or coarctation) interferes with delivery of the blood to branches beyond. Coarctation of the aorta is illustrated in Figure 21.8. Although collateral vessels are present, an extra load is placed on the left ventricle. High blood pressure may develop in the arms and legs, but unless the condition is considered severe, corrective surgery is postponed until after the child is 4 or 5 years old.

Valvular Pulmonic Stenosis

Narrowing of the pulmonary valve imposes an extra work load on the right ventricle to generate increased pressure, as illustrated in Figure 21.9. The walls of the ventricle thicken (hypertrophy). If the obstruction is severe enough to produce high pressure, the valve may

Figure 21.8 Coarctation of the Aorta

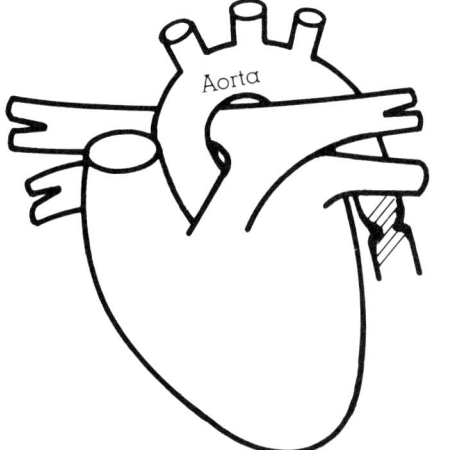

Figure 21.9 Pulmonary Stenosis

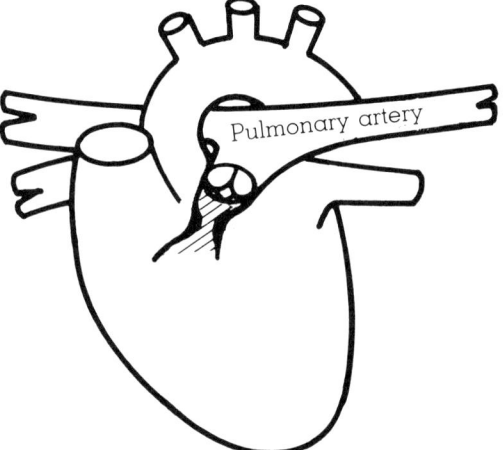

be opened surgically. The results of this procedure usually normalize the child's heart function. As in similar conditions, the danger of later infection suggests the administration of antibiotics following the operation.

One half of all congenital heart problems are classified under three of the conditions described: ventricular septal defect, patent ductus arteriosis, and tetralogy of Fallot. The other conditions discussed account for about 30% of the remaining heart conditions present at birth.

ACQUIRED HEART CONDITIONS

Rheumatic Fever

An estimated 500,000 children and youth between the ages 5 and 19 have contracted rheumatic fever. Associated heart disease constitutes one of the primary causes of death for individuals in this age group, occurring in about half of all youngsters who have had rheumatic fever.

The disease is caused by a *streptococcus* infection. The characteristic inflammation is caused by an allergic reaction to the antibodies that develop to fight the streptococcus bacteria. This overall reaction results in the formation of what are termed *Aschoff bodies* in the joints, lungs, tissue under the skin, and in the brain and the heart. These microscopic bodies form and disappear quickly, but scar tissue remains. If an excess of scar tissue is built up in the heart, heart disease occurs. At times the condition is temporary and disappears in a year or so. In other patients it is recurring, in which case the individual must receive continuous antibiotic prophylaxis.

The valves of the heart most frequently involved are the mitral (between the left atrium and the left ventricle) and the aortic (between the left ventricle and the aorta). Damage to the heart and valves makes the individual susceptible to bacterial endocarditis, and surgical correction sometimes is needed. This is seldom necessary before adulthood. In addition to inflammation of the valves, the wall of the heart may become enlarged and inflamed (myocarditis), as may the outer lining (pericarditis).

A heart murmur may accompany the condition, as may tenderness in one or more of the joints. Motor awkwardness and tics, when seen in children with rheumatic fever, indicate inflammation in part of the brain. In more severe cases, small subcutaneous nodules develop over the elbows, knees, shins, and backs of the forearms or wrists.

At one time children with this condition were subjected to prolonged bed rest, but more recently they may be ambulatory in a few weeks and able to participate in moderate exercise to overcome the effects of physical restriction. Because the disease may recur, continual monitoring of symptoms is necessary, together with regular ingestion of penicillin to prevent further inflammation. Even in adulthood individuals who have had rheumatic fever as children may be susceptible to pericarditis, myocarditis, and endocarditis.

Hypertension

Infrequently, signs of elevated blood pressure are seen in children, usually as the result of kidney or endocrine disease. The severity, as well as medication needed to control the symptoms, must be considered when prescribing exercise for children with hypertension.

Innocent Murmurs

Innocent or insignificant murmurs sometimes are heard during a medical examination. These are not necessarily associated with a heart condition. Follow-up diagnosis, taking into consideration the child's history and evidence from a chest x-ray and electrocardiogram, may preclude the presence of any serious condition. Innocent murmurs are relatively common in childhood, and when they occur, the family should not be unduly concerned without reason.

IMPLICATIONS FOR PHYSICAL EDUCATION

Recent case studies have revealed that, on an individual basis, carefully planned programs of physical activity may have a positive effect upon children who have heart conditions. The program should be uniquely suited to the youngster and approved by the physician (Frazee, Brunt, & Castle, 1984). Some parameters for the physical educator are as follows:

1. Many post-cardiac patients, particularly those with corrected congenital difficulties, need no restriction in physical activity later in childhood or young adulthood.

2. Each case must be considered individually. No overall guidelines for all children are useful.

3. A child with severe involvement, whose heart is pumping hard against a restricted aortic valve or because of leakage in the mitral valve, should be carefully monitored. Exercise will not correct conditions of this type. A program of passive exercise, lying down, or leisure sports such as archery or shooting, should be substituted for more vigorous activities.

4. Aquatic activities may be useful if not engaged in too vigorously. Water can be supportive and relaxing, but attempting to swim rapidly may be much too taxing for a child with a heart problem or recovering from one.

5. Exercise loads that prevent the heart from returning to its normal rate in 2 to 3 minutes should be reconsidered and reduced, with a physician's concurrence.

6. Physical educators should pay attention to any child who reports chest pain or shows any signs of overexertion, and refer the child to proper experts.

7. Activities in which the child has a choice of the intensity, duration, or number of sub-tasks involved allow flexibility.

8. Competition in sports, even passive recreational ones, should encourage children to exceed their own norms rather than those of others.

9. Obviously, children with diagnosed heart conditions should participate in any physical education program only with the input and continued awareness of a physician.

SUMMARY

Two types of heart condition influence cardiovascular functions in children—those that are acquired and those that are present at birth (congenital). The latter is 20 times more prevalent. Although many types of of congenital conditions are correctable through surgery during the early weeks of life, some persist. Their presence suggests various precautions in intensity of physical exercise to which these children are exposed. Medications to reduce symptoms may also cause restrictions in the amount and type of physical exercise desirable for children with heart conditions.

Acquired types of heart conditions include rheumatic fever, hypertension, and innocent murmur. The latter is not considered serious if tests do not reveal a true condition. About half of all children who contract rheumatic fever eventually acquire a heart condition, because of scar tissue remaining after the disease has abated. Children who have rheumatic fever and other acquired conditions may be susceptible to inflammatory diseases of various parts of the heart, including the pericardium and valves, for the rest of their lives.

Moderate exercise is recommended for many youngsters with heart conditions (Fletcher & Cantwell, 1974). A post-cardiac child whose congenital difficulties have been corrected in early childhood may need no special restriction in physical activity. Children with persistent conditions should receive individualized programs, under the advice and supervision of medical personnel. Aquatic activities may be helpful. Unduly strenuous exercise loads are not recommended. Children should be encouraged to explore their own limits without undue stress to push themselves.

REFERENCES

Fletcher, G.F., & Cantwell, J.D. (1974). *Exercise and coronary heart disease.* Springfield, IL: Charles C Thomas.

Frazee, R., Brunt, D., & Castle, R.F. (1984). Exercise tolerance of a young child with congenital heart disease associated with asplenia syndrome. *Adapted Physical Activity Quarterly, 1,* 332-336.

Rudolph, A.M. (1974). *Congenital diseases of the heart.* Chicago: Year Book Medical Publishers.

ADDITIONAL REFERENCES

American Heart Association. (1970). *If your child has a congenital heart defect.* New York: Author.

American Heart Association. (1970). *An introduction to your child who has congenital heart disease.* Loma Linda, CA: Loma Linda University, School of Medicine.

Ross, J., & O'Rourke, R. (1976). *Understanding the heart and its diseases.* New York: McGraw-Hill.

Zohman, L.R., & Tobias, J.S. (1970). *Cardiac rehabilitation.* New York: Grune & Stratton.

QUESTIONS FOR DISCUSSION

1. What kinds of congenital heart conditions seem most amenable to early corrective surgery? Which conditions seem most likely to persist into middle childhood?

2. What are the symptoms of heart disease arising from rheumatic fever? How might children who have had rheumatic fever be dealt with through physical activity in later years?

3. When formulating a program of physical exercise, what kinds of special precautions must be taken with a child diagnosed as having a heart condition?

4. What social problems might children with chronic heart conditions have when interacting with normal peers at play and in other situations?

STUDENT PROJECTS

1. Interview a physical educator who has planned and executed a program for a child with a heart anomaly. What important information was needed prior to formulating and implementing the program? Who provided input?

2. Review the literature on heart conditions (see Additional References) and compare approaches in programming physical activity for children with a congenital heart condition and cardiac rehabilitation for older individuals who have suffered a heart attack.

RESOURCES

Aeorobics Center
12100 Preston Rd.
Dallas, TX 75230

American Heart Association
7320 Greenville Ave.
Dallas, TX 75231

National Foundation, March of Dimes
1275 Mamaroneck Ave.
White Plains, NY 10605

22 *Hemophilia and Sickle Cell Anemia*

The two conditions discussed here are unrelated, but they both reflect abnormalities in the composition of the blood. Hemophilia and sickle cell anemia are the subject of this chapter, together with their implications for physical education.

HEMOPHILIA

Characteristics and Prevalence

A hereditary condition, hemophilia is a disease in which the blood clots very slowly or not at all. When the skin is broken, excessive blood is lost. Even more of a problem is internal bleeding, occurring within organs and joints, which is difficult to bring under control.

Hemophilia is an inherited condition, transmitted by the female, who has about a 50% chance of passing the disorder to male offspring. The mother also may pass the gene to a female child, but that child, like her mother, will become a *carrier* and not be afflicted with the disease herself. The National Heart and Lung Institute (1972) reported that the prevalence of hemophilia was 20,000 in the United States. According to later statistics from the National Hemophilia Foundation, the incidence is 1 in 4,000 live births.

Although many different bleeding disorders are associated with anomalies in the blood's *platelets* (small bodies that float in the blood), the most common forms are *classic hemophilia* and *parahemophilia*. Normal clotting of the blood occurs when (a) vascular contraction provides a slowing of the flow, which in turn allows time for a firm fibrin clot to be generated, and (b) platelets adhere to tissue surrounding the break, plugging the opening and preventing blood loss (the term *platelet plug* is used to denote this process).

Normal platelets function in two other important ways: (a) to release chemical mediators, which cause smooth muscles around the blood vessel to attract more platelets to the area, and (b) to release enzymes, which aid in the formation of a firm fibrin clot. In hemophilia a poor quality clot forms—one that is easily dislodged. As a result, a small cut will bleed for days unless the bleeding is arrested.

One of the major problems in children with hemophilia is continual bleeding into the joints (hemarthrosis), which results in a thickening of the joint lining (synovium). Recurrent bleeding in the joint causes extensive destruction of the smooth cartilage of the lining of the joint, and degenerative arthritis may result. As a result, hemophiliacs may develop crippling joint diseases in early adulthood.

Joint function in the child and young adult is more likely to deteriorate within various weight-bearing joints, including the knees and hip. Joint bleeding is relatively easy to recognize and is signaled by pain after some kinds of physical exertion. Bleeding within internal organs is more difficult to ascertain and presents serious problems to the child afflicted with hemophilia. Internal bleeding can cause especially serious complications in the head and neck region. Trauma that causes bleeding in these two areas may be fatal.

It produces signs including headache, sleepiness, nausea, and vomiting and requires immediate medical attention.

Organs contained in the thorax are relatively well protected and are not likely to incur bleeding from some blow or trauma. Abdominal organs are more likely to be susceptible to injury and subsequent internal bleeding. If a kidney is injured, the urine may be dark brown or red—a sign that a physician should be consulted immediately.

Implications for Physical Education

Although this disease necessarily limits physical activity, hemophiliacs should be encouraged to participate in sports that maintain their strength and endurance. Swimming (but not diving) usually is recommended, as is modern dance, if no leaps are involved. Passive recreational sports, stretching exercises on soft mats, and hiking may be good physical activities. Sports to be avoided include all that have the potential to cause joint trauma or a blow to any part of the body. Contact sports and those in which hard balls are thrown should be totally eliminated.

Studies have produced data showing that exercise for children with hemophilia improves muscular development and decreases the frequency of bleeding. One of these investigations demonstrated that lack of exercise in hemophiliac children resulted in poorer fitness levels when contrasted with the fitness levels expected in normal children (Koch, Galioto, Kelleher, & Goldstein, 1984). The hemophiliacs were poorer in measures of endurance, including pulse rates at peak exercise loads. The authors of this investigation recommend individually applied "exercise prescriptions" for these youngsters. They further suggest that exercise and fitness are important to the emotional development of younger hemophiliacs.

Physical educators should be sensitive to subtle signs—a small bruise that does not heal, changes in color of the urine, and the like—when working with hemophiliac children. Youngsters with this condition should be exposed to sports that permit them to engage in normal social interaction, as sensitivity about their own condition may have adverse effects on their self-concept.

If a child does receive a blow to the body, limbs, or abdomen, immediate treatment should be sought. Medical advances have greatly aided hemophiliacs. For instance, medications now facilitate blood clotting after trauma has produced internal or external bleeding.

SICKLE CELL ANEMIA

Characteristics and Prevalence

Sickle cell anemia first was identified by James Herrick in 1910. While evaluating a black boy, he noted that the child's red blood cells had an unusual cylindrical shape. After this initial report, many physicians noted the same condition among black patients suffering from anemia (Kempe, Silver, & O'Brien, 1970; Wintrobe, 1967).

According to the latest figures from Howard University, in which this condition has been studied carefully, about 1 in 500 newborn black children have this condition. Its prevalence within the overall black population ranges from 1 in 400 to 1 in 600. It is rarely found in racial/ethnic groups other than blacks, and when it is, it usually is found in those whose backgrounds stem from people living around the Mediterranean Sea.

The condition has been postulated to reflect a reaction tending to ward off malaria and is found in many peoples from areas of the world in which malaria is found, including West Africa. Malaria is not found in the United States at this time, and sickle cell anemia is seemingly becoming less prevalent, as the sickle cell adaptation no longer is useful.

Normal blood cells are round and very flexible. Chemically, the hemoglobin they contain binds and carries oxygen to all areas of the body. Iron contained in the hemoglobin is related to the properties of a normal red blood cell to hold, and thus transport, oxygen. If sickle hemoglobin is present in large amounts, the amount of oxygen in the iron diminishes, and the abnormal molecules become less flexible and change from the normal round disk shape to a long, rigid shape.

A normal red cell lives about 120 days and, when removed, is quickly replenished by new red blood cells constantly being formed in the bone marrow. The process of producing new red cells may become inadequate in the presence of sickle-shaped cells, whose lifespan is only 15 to 25 days. The body tends to destroy these unusual cells rapidly, causing a reduction in hemoglobin and *jaundice*, seen as a yellow cast to the "whites" of the eyes—a sign that the anemia is present.

Because sickled red cells are inflexible, they often are unable to pass through small blood vessels easily and tend to jam, depriving some tissues of proper blood flow. This kind of vasoocclusive action may deprive organs and tissues of normal blood supply, causing pain and, in some cases, cellular death. These phenomena result in the following clinical signs in youngsters with sickle cell anemia:

1. Children under age 3 may have swelling and pain in the hands and feet as a result of vasoocclusion of the bones. The bones may become fragile because of poor blood flow. The symptoms may last for days or weeks. Treatment includes analgesics, bed rest and, at times, intravenous fluids.

2. This same vasoocclusion occurring in the intestines may result in severe abdominal pain, producing symptoms similar to those of appendicitis. The same problem can occur in the spleen and over time may worsen, making breathing difficult and preventing the spleen from performing its filtering function. Incidents of pain may increase. Similar vasoocclusion in the liver, manifested by a distended abdomen, loss of appetite, and lethargy, may produce nausea and jaundice in the child.

3. Vasoocclusion in the brain may result in sudden loss of function in an arm or leg (hemiplegia), or even coma in extreme cases.

4. Vasoocclusion of the lung (pulmonary thrombosis) can cause chest pain, fever, coughing, and rapid respiration.

5. Some patients with sickle cell disease have an *aplastic crisis*: The manufacture of red blood cells suddenly stops. As the life span of sickle cells is from 15 to 25 days, a crisis situation such as this is serious and requires immediate medical attention. The onset of this crisis is marked by weakness, lethargy, and a sudden rise in the heart rate, with possible fainting spells.

Implications for Physical Education

Children and youth with sickle cell anemia should be exposed to moderate exercise with caution. Increased utilization of oxygen from the blood may bring on a sickling episode. Marked overheating of the skin during vigorous exercise may precipitate an attack in the sickle cell child. This may involve severe and sudden pain in certain joints and bones, particularly the rib cage and abdomen. Vasoocclusion stresses weight-bearing joints. All exercises thus require a physician's approval and direction.

Individuals with sickle cell *trait*—who may never experience symptoms of the condition—are less prone to various sickling phenomena because their red cells contain normal hemoglobin, which does not interact with sickle hemoglobin. In these persons severe oxygen depletion or severe *acidosis* must occur before any significant sickling will occur. They may participate fully in most vigorous activities and games but should avoid mountain climbing at extreme altitudes (over 6,500 feet), flying in planes without pressurized cabins, and underwater swimming and other breath-holding activities of this type.

SUMMARY

The two unrelated blood conditions discussed in this chapter are hemophilia and sickle cell anemia. The former is an inherited condition characterized by an abnormal amount of internal bleeding, or external bleeding when the skin is pierced. It is a disorder involving abnormalities in the blood's platelets and may result in bleeding within the joints, which in turn causes chronic joint impairment. Internal bleeding in the head and neck may prove fatal unless given immediate medical attention.

Those afflicted with hemophilia should be encouraged to participate in physical activities to maintain strength and vigor, but these should consist of swimming, passive recreational sports, and slow rhythmic and stretching activities such as those found in modern dance. Activities that involve possible joint trauma, falling, or sudden stresses should be avoided.

Sickle cell anemia is characterized by unusual crescent-shaped red blood cells whose proliferation results in swelling and pain in the joints, fragile bones, and at times severe abdominal pain and loss of function of an arm or leg, at the extreme. Sickle cell crises should be referred for immediate medical attention.

Physical educators should expose children and youth diagnosed with sickle cell anemia to moderate, not vigorous, exercise. Exercises should be carried out only under the direction of a physician, because of the possibility of overheating and trauma to the joints.

REFERENCES

Kempe, C., Silver, H.K., & O'Brien, D. (1970). *Sickle cell anemia.* Los Altos: Lange Medical Publications.

Koch, B., Galioto, F.M., Jr., Kelleher, J., & Goldstein, D. (1984). Physical fitness in children with hemophilia. *Archives of Physical Medicine & Rehabilitation, 65,* 324-326.

National Heart and Lung Institute. (1972). *Blood resources studies: Pilot study of hemophilia treatment in the United States* (Vol. 3). New York: Author.

Wintrobe, M.M. (1967). *Sickle cell disease, thalassemia and the abnormal hemoglobin syndromes.* Philadelphia: Lea & Febiger.

ADDITIONAL REFERENCES

Mengel, C.E., Frei, E., III, & Nachman, R. (1971). *Hematology principles and practices.* Chicago: Year Book Medical Publishers.

Owen, C.A., Jr., & Walter, E.J., et al. (1969). *The diagnosis of bleeding disorders.* Boston: Little, Brown.

QUESTIONS FOR DISCUSSION

1. How is hemophilia transmitted?

2. What are the signs that a child with hemophilia may be bleeding internally?

3. What are the characteristics of sickle cell anemia?

4. What physical activities should youngsters with sickle cell trait avoid?

5. Discuss exercise intensity and stress in sports in relation to the two conditions described in this chapter.

6. What psychological and emotional overtones might be seen in youngsters with either of the two conditions described?

STUDENT PROJECTS

1. Formulate an ideal week-long program of physical activity for a child with sickle cell anemia.

2. Discuss with a parent of a hemophiliac child the kinds of problems the youngster has in daily living. What kinds of constraints does the disease impose on the child's play in the neighborhood?

RESOURCES

Center for Sickle Cell Disease
College of Medicine
Howard University
2121 Georgia Ave., N.W.
Washington, DC 20001

National Hemophilia Foundation
110 Green St.
New York, NY 10018

23 Asthma and Other Respiratory Conditions

Respiratory disorders are among the more prevalent handicaps found in children and youth in the United States. Asthma, hay fever, and allergies account for almost one third of all chronic diseases in children under 17 years of age. Bronchitis, sinusitis, and similar conditions account for another 15% of chronic diseases within this same age group.

ASTHMA

As compared to other debilitating conditions, asthma has been judged to cause the largest number of days absent from school. Over a million and a half children and youth suffer from the disease in the United States. The condition formerly was considered only debilitating, but as many as 7,000 deaths may be attributable to asthma in the United States annually. Whether this figure is tied to increased air pollution or other factors is difficult to determine. In areas where high pollution is likely to occur, however, physicians have advised that people with severe asthma not engage in heavy exercise. Fortunately, many individuals tend to outgrow asthma following their teens.

Asthmatic children and youth in physical education classes pose a challenge to their teachers. Physical educators should be thoroughly aware of the causes, degree of severity, and symptoms of asthmatic attacks before prescribing exercise loads that are appropriate to asthmatic students and allow them to exercise to their optimal level with a minimum of discomfort.

Causes and Symptoms

In essence, asthma is caused by biochemical imbalances, particularly in the control of adrenalin and nerve fibers that liberate acetylcholine, which in turn causes changes in the flexibility of the lining of the bronchial tubes. These deficits result in hyperirritability of the bronchi to various stimuli including smoke, changes in body temperature, air pollutants, animal fur, dust, and numerous others. Various infections can affect the delicate homeostasis needed to prevent constriction of the bronchial tubes. Spasms of the bronchial tubes, swelling of the linings, and excessive secretions of mucus cause coughing. An asthma attack may last a few minutes or several days.

Excitement, fear, and other emotional states that influence adrenalin production can cause an imbalance in the delicate mechanisms needed to maintain open and clear air passages in the lungs. Asthma is a product of mind-body relationships, of emotions and accompanying biochemical changes rather than a simple lack of regulation of the emotions or the physiological biochemical processes.

During an attack asthmatics have difficulty exhaling after a breath because of constriction of the bronchioles. As the next breath is attempted, more muscular effort is needed to force the air through the constricted passages into an already inflated lung. Figure 23.1 illustrates the difference between the asthmatic bronchus and the normal bronchus. As ox-

Figure 23.1 The Asthmatic Bronchus and the Normal Bronchus

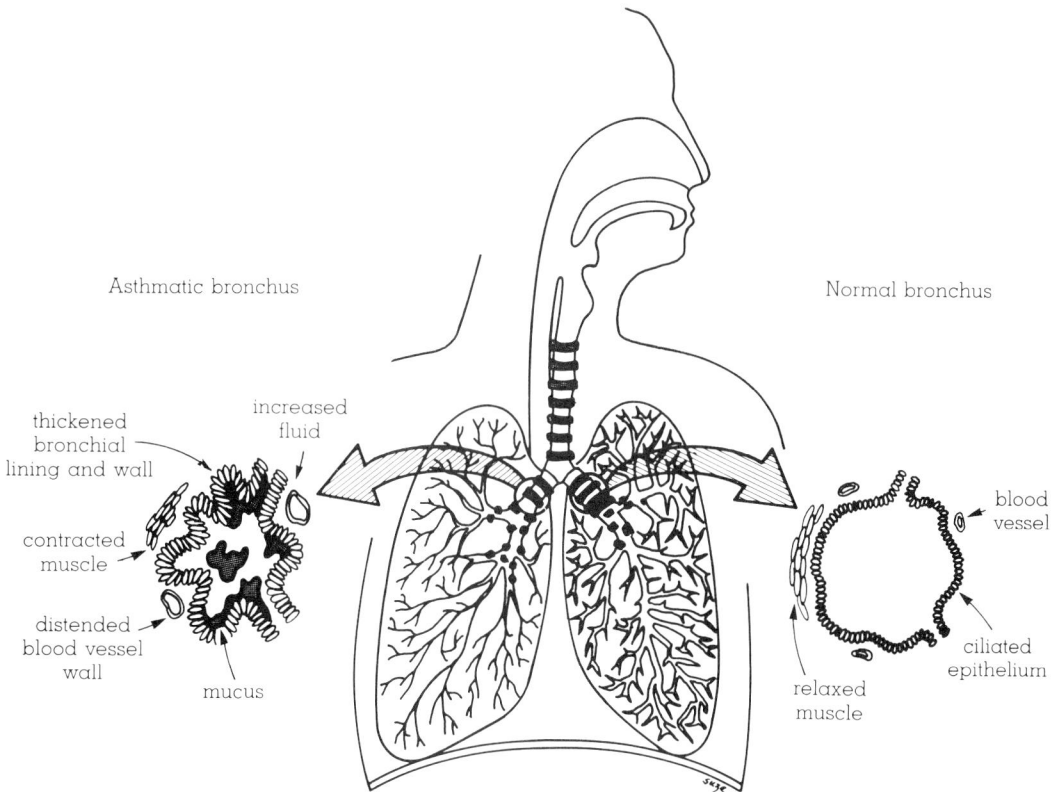

Asthmatic bronchus

Normal bronchus

thickened
bronchial
lining and wall

increased
fluid

blood
vessel

contracted
muscle

distended
blood vessel
wall

ciliated
epithelium

mucus

relaxed
muscle

ygen becomes scarce, the child tries, through increased muscular exertions of the breathing apparatus (including muscles of the upper chest and intercostals), to take in more air and thus compounds the problem. As the tension grows, so does the problem. The extreme discomfort may be relieved only through the use of various inhalants intended to dilate the bronchioles or medicines taken orally. In severe attacks, without proper steps taken for relief, the child may require immediate hospitalization, as the resulting cyanotic condition can lead to death.

Asthmatic children and youth are beset with a number of problems that tend to feed on themselves, producing a chain of events. These self-perpetuating circumstances consist of the following:

1. The child compounds the problem during an attack by attempting take in more and more air through the restricted passages.

2. Various bronchodilator drugs, although giving immediate and needed relief, if overused can cause abnormalities in blood gases, including hypoxemia, or insufficient oxygenation in the blood. This in turn makes the asthmatic susceptible to slight changes in the diameters of the bronchial passages, which increases the incidence of attacks.

3. Exercise, though it is needed and was recommended for asthmatics by the Committee on Children with Handicaps (1970) of the American Academy of Pediatrics, may trigger an asthma attack if engaged in excessively.

4. A psychological defense termed *reaction formation* has been associated with the behavior of asthmatics. This cycle of events consists of the child or youth first establishing unrealistically high goals in school or in other aspects of life and making exhaustive efforts to meet these goals. Upon failing in this, because of an asthmatic attack, he or she has a built-in excuse for failure. Thus, a cycle of aspiration, extreme effort, failure, frustration, emotional upset triggering an attack, and excuses related to the asthmatic condition is set in motion.

Types of Asthma

Asthmatic conditions may be divided into two types: dermal respiratory syndrome and allergic rhinitis asthma. Individuals with *dermal respiratory syndrome* typically have eczema in infancy, and wheezing begins within 5 years in half of the cases. Asthmatic episodes are preceded by symptoms varying from child to child. Nonspecific irritational factors such as infection, air pollutants, emotional trauma, fatigue, chilling, and medicines may trigger attacks of this type of asthma. Symptoms may include changes in appetite, abdominal pain, bed wetting, irritability, hyperactivity, or listlessness. This form of asthma is the most difficult to treat. If not dealt with effectively, the child may become a pulmonary cripple in adolescence or later.[1]

Allergic rhinitis asthma is a form of asthma contracted later in life. The inhalant allergents are relatively easy to identify and usually are airborne. Control of symptoms is simpler than with the dermal respiratory syndrome.

Asthma is termed (a) *spasmodic* if the symptoms are interrupted by long periods during which no attacks occur; (b) *continuous* if the person wheezes constantly although actual attacks are infrequent; (c) *intractable* when all symptoms (coughing, mucous formation, and wheezing) are continous; and (d) *status asthmaticus* when treatment brings little relief. An attack usually passes through several stages, beginning with coughing and progressing to moderate and then severe bronchial obstruction. If exercise has caused the attack, its discontinuance tends to allay other symptoms. If a dusty gymnasium or chalkboard seems to be the culprit, the child should be removed from these stimuli immediately.

Implications for Physical Education

Exercise programs should be carefully introduced and adjusted to levels that help asthmatic children gain and maintain cardiorespiratory fitness without triggering an attack. For example, running is more likely to precipitate an attack than is cycling, which in turn is more likely to trigger an attack than is walking (Anderson, Connolly, & Godfrey, 1971). The onset of asthma attacks as related to exercise has come to be studied heavily in the last decade. These studies have found that a number of variables bring about "exercise-induced asthma" (EIA), including vigorous exercise prolonged over 4-5 minutes, running, and hard exercise with over 75% or more of maximum oxygen uptake involved.

---

1. The main facility for the study and treatment of asthmatic children in the U.S. is the Children's Asthma Research Center, Denver, Colorado. Treatment includes breathing techniques and postural draining, among other methods, conducted by a respiratory therapist.

Recommendations concerning the asthmatic child include directing the child into games that require short running or movement distances such as those demanded by volleyball and baseball, versus soccer. Intermittent exercise periods of not more than 5 minutes also are recommended. Swimming is the preferred activity for a child who is likely to have an exercise-induced attack.

Before dealing with asthmatic children, physical educators should gain some information concerning the nature of asthma in general, as well as more specific information about the symptoms and propensities for attacks in the specific children they are to serve. Some of the passive exercises and asthma-specific exercises that are most beneficial are unlike those engaged in many normal or other handicapped populations. Information needed for an asthmatic child includes (a) the child's age and type of asthma; (b) conditions that trigger attacks in this particular child; (c) frequency of attacks, particularly during the past several months; (d) the seasonal nature of the attacks (if a seasonal pattern is present); and (e) a measure of the child's pulmonary efficiency. Three tests are most often employed to evaluate pulmonary efficiency.

1. Force expiratory volume (FEV) may be determined in 1 second through the use of a spirometer (as illustrated). This test evaluates the number of cubic centimeters (cc) of air forcefully exhaled during the first second after a deep inhalation. Normal FEV values are from 500 to 4,500 cc for boys and 350 to 3,400 cc for girls. Consultation with a physician should enable the physical educator to determine if the FEV for a particular child of a given age and size is less than appropriate. Children who are capable may be encouraged to attempt (via exercises, both passive and active) to increase their scores on subsequent FEV tests.

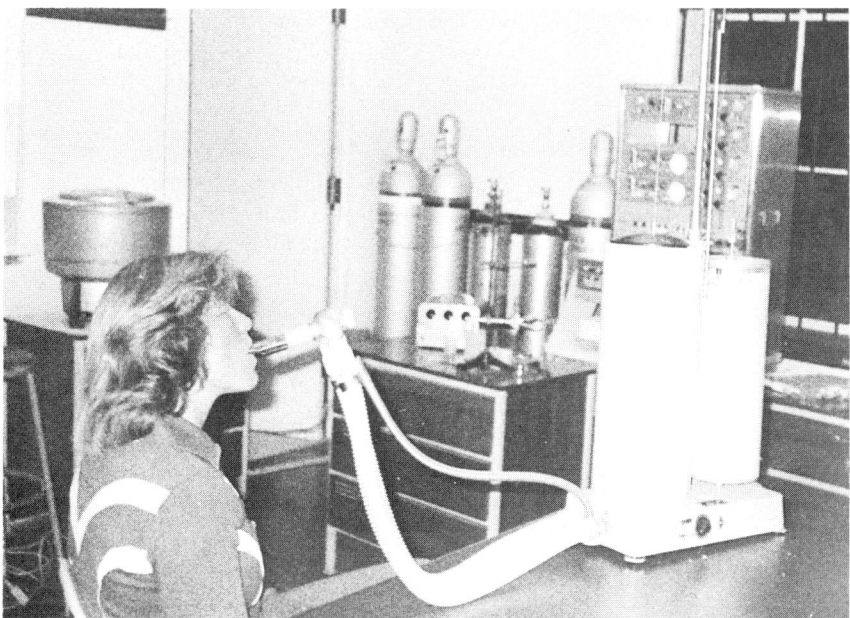

Spirometers are used to evaluate respiratory efficiency.

2. Maximal breathing capacity (MBC) also is ascertained via laboratory testing. The measure obtained is the number of liters of air per minute a child can move when asked to breathe as deeply as possible. Normal range in boys is from 43 to 155 liters and for girls is slightly below that. This test is used both to diagnose the severity of the asthmatic condition and to predict the frequency of occurrences of severe bronchial restriction (dyspnea). Again, when periodic administrations of this test are possible, improvement in values obtained (measured in liters of air) may motivate asthmatic children to work harder in special breathing exercises and adapted physical education.

3. Wright's peak flow meter is a relatively inexpensive piece of equipment that affords easily understood and measurable indices of expiration force. Improvement, measured by this helpful device, helps asthmatic children see the benefits of regular exercise.

Special Adjustments in the Environment and Facilities

To reduce the incidence and severity of attacks in asthmatic children in physical education, the physical educator should:

1. Provide game situations that are not likely to raise emotional levels to highs that might cause excessive excitement, frustration, elation, or aggression.

2. Provide the children with ample opportunities to obtain fluids during their exercise period. Lack of fluids, or fluids that are too cold, are likely to thicken mucus secretion and make its elimination more difficult. Frequent fluid intake is likely to aid the child in breathing freely during moderate exercise.

3. Provide places in which an overly tense or anxious asthmatic child may relax. The intake of many bronchiodilating drugs tends to cause hypoxemia, which in turn alters moods. Some asthmatic children taking these medications act restless, agitated, or depressed, as well as evidencing highs similar to those seen in people taking diet pills. Severe depression may accompany withdrawal from these drugs. The physical educator should anticipate and be prepared to deal with any of these conditions and should not assume the child is "bad" or emotionally disturbed.

4. Supply the child with sufficient tissue and a box for used tissue, to reduce the social stigma attached to frequent nose blowing and expectorating of mucus. The alternative is coughing, congestion, and wheezing, with possible instigation of an attack.

5. Provide a dust-free environment, particularly during high pollen count season. A clean, air-conditioned gymnasium is the best environment for an asthmatic, particularly during the hot summer months. Chalkboards, dusty mats, and dusty storage places should be avoided.

6. Establish specific goals related to the previously mentioned measures of FEV, MBC, and measures of improved diaphragmatic efficiency in breathing.

7. Introduce relaxation exercises at any point in the day when the child seems agitated or otherwise overstressed—conditions that are likely to bring about an attack.

8. Prevent, if possible, sudden alterations in body temperature (either cooler or warmer). Either sudden cold or overheated conditions can bring about attacks. If overheated, cold towels applied to the forehead or back of the neck may help.

9. Encourage children with asthma to listen to body signs, to be alert to subtle changes in breathing and note when wheezing begins to take place. When children are closely attuned to the sounds of an impending attack, various steps (stopping activity, using breathing exercises, and the like) may be undertaken.

10. Provide specific instruction on the anatomy and physiology of the breathing apparatus. Place particular emphasis on the important role of the diaphragm (the dome-shaped muscle at the floor of the chest cavity), its changing size, and its role in changing the pressure within the cavity. Most asthmatics' breathing is too shallow and involves the upper chest muscles, those attached to the neck and chest, and the intercostals.

11. Augment an academic approach to the importance of deep diaphragmatic breathing with instruction in specific exercises to promote deeper and more efficient inhalation and exhalation. Some suggested exercises are pictured and described in the following pages.

Lying back abdominal exercise. In a lying-back position, the child, with hands placed on either side of the rib cage, first breathes out slowly, while tightening the abdominal muscles. Next the child relaxes the abdominal muscles and breathes in quickly through the nose. Finally, the child breathes out quickly through the nose and mouth, again tightening the abdominal muscles. This exercise can be repeated as often as desired, keeping the hand on the lower ribs, as pictured.

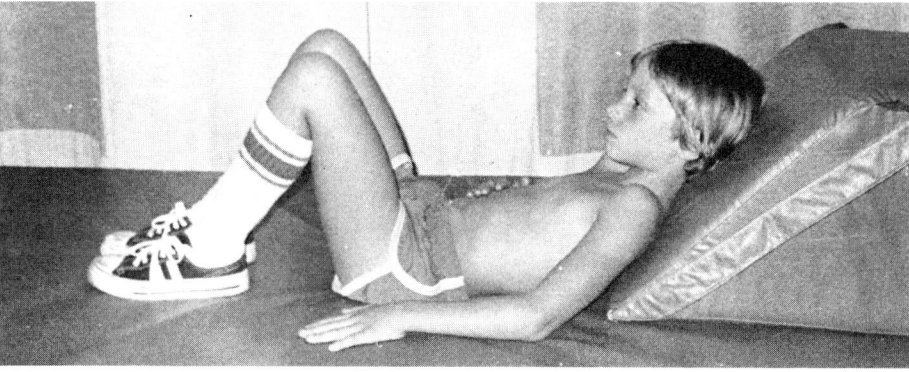

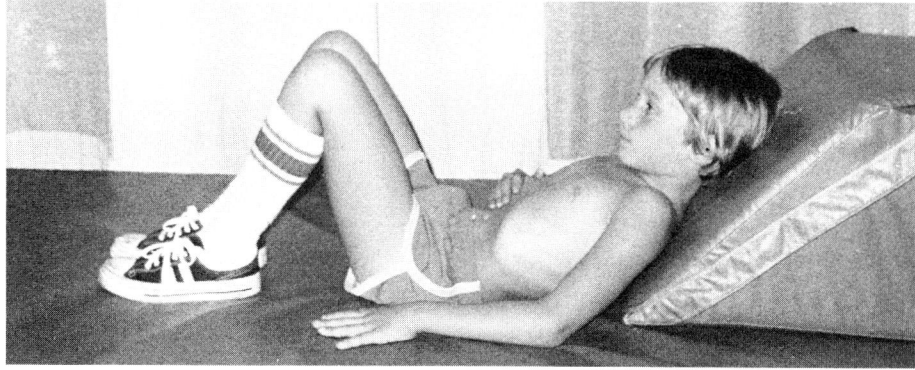

Lying-back abdominal exercise

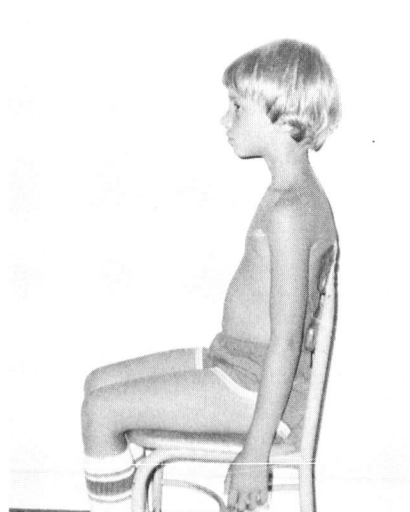
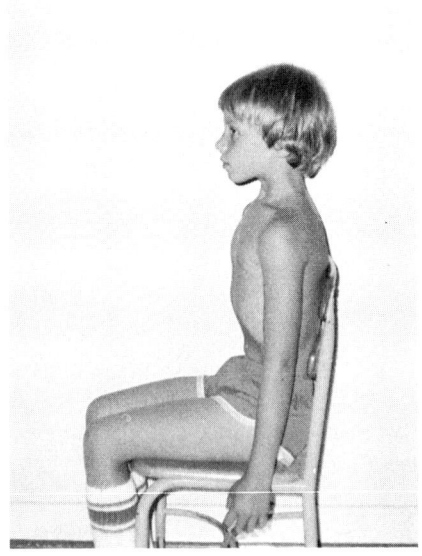

*Seated
diaphragmatic
exercise*

Seated diaphragmatic exercise. In the diaphragmatic breathing exercise, the child sits with the back resting against the back of a chair in a relaxed position and then breathes out slowly, lowering the chest and tightening the abdominal muscles. The child then relaxes the abdominal muscle while breathing in through the nose.

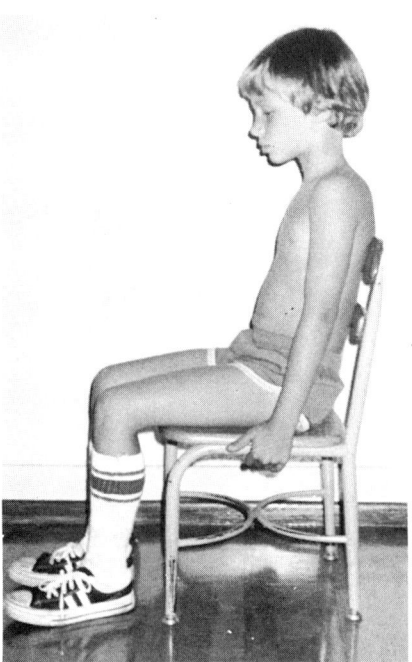
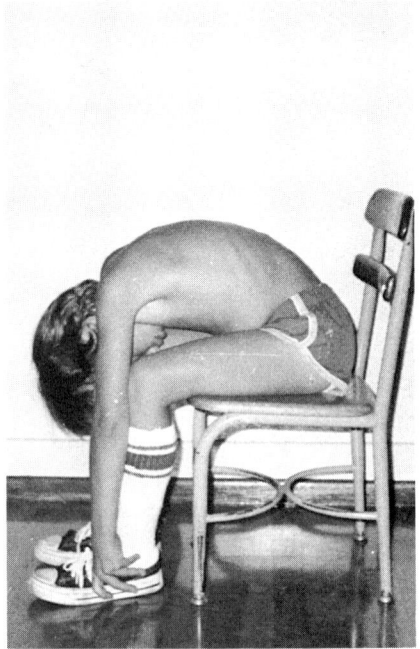

*Seated
forward
bending
exercise*

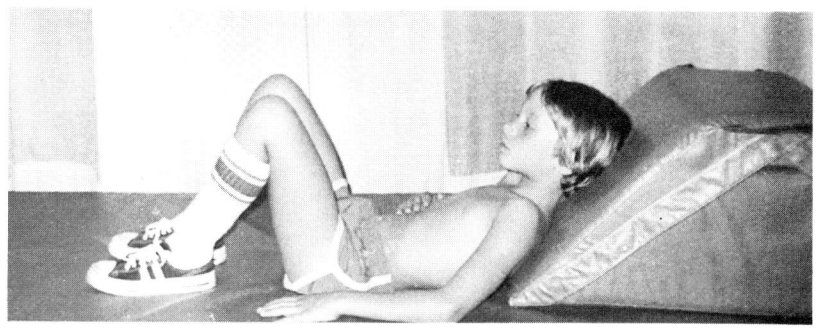

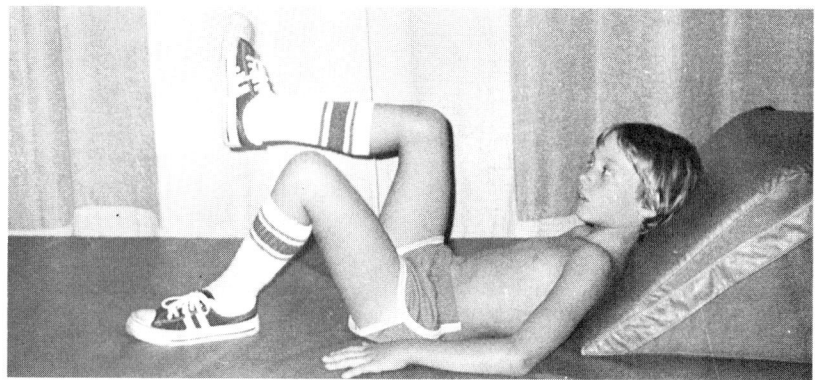

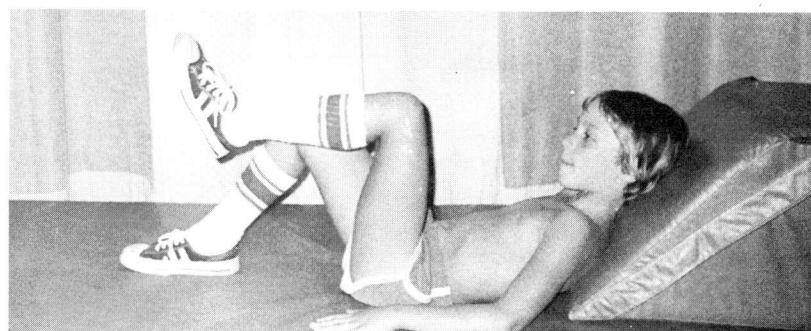

Lying-back
knee-lift
exercise

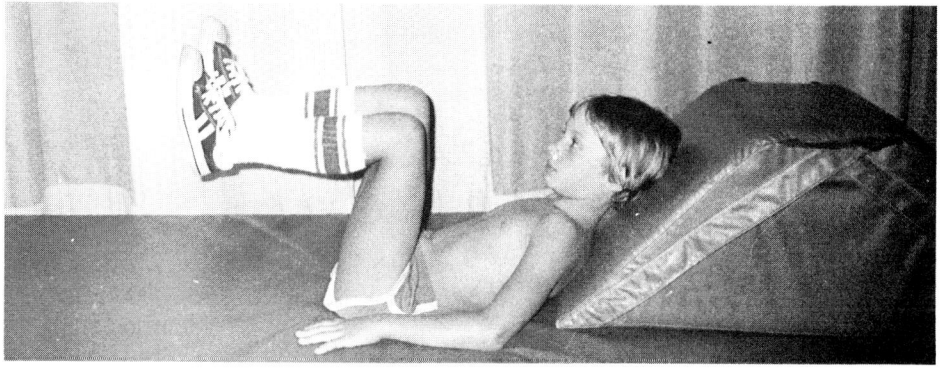

Seated forward bending exercise. In the seated forward bending exercise, the child sits with feet apart and arms relaxed at the sides. The child breathes out slowly while bending forward. First the head goes forward, then the shoulders, until the head almost touches the knees. All the while the abdominal muscles are tightening. The child straightens up while breathing in, first pushing the lower back against the chair, then the middle back, the upper back, shoulders, and finally the head. At the upright position the abdominal muscles should be relaxed and the child should take small breaths to expand the lower ribs and to relax the abdominal muscles further.

Lying-back knee-lift exercise. For this abdominal exercise the starting position is with the knees bent, feet on the floor. Keeping the arms and shoulders relaxed, the child first lifts the right knee slowly to the chest, breathing out and tightening the abdominal muscles. The child then pauses in breathing, lowers the right knee, breathes in, relaxes the abdominal muscles, and gently expands the lower ribs only. This same cycle should be repeated for the other leg, and again by bringing both knees to the chest simultaneously and lowering them from the chest, as pictured.

Standing forward bending exercise. In a standing forward bending exercise such as the one pictured, the child is positioned with the back against the wall, feet about 6″ from the wall. The child breathes out while slowly bending forward, first dropping the head, then the shoulders, and last the lower back. The arms should hang limply, and the abdominal muscles should be kept tight. The child straightens up, keeping the abdominal muscles tight and flattening the lower back against the wall. The abdominals should be relaxed, with a breath taken inward as the back is gradually straightened. The upper back

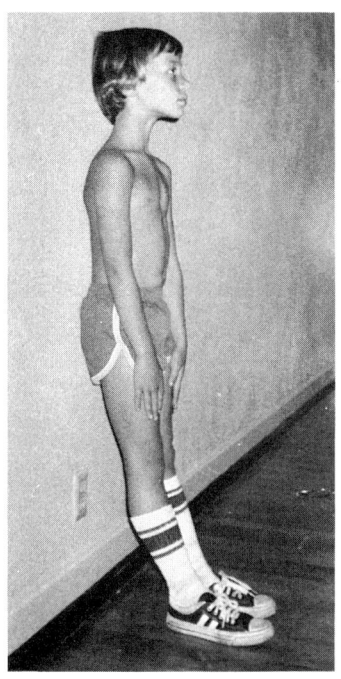 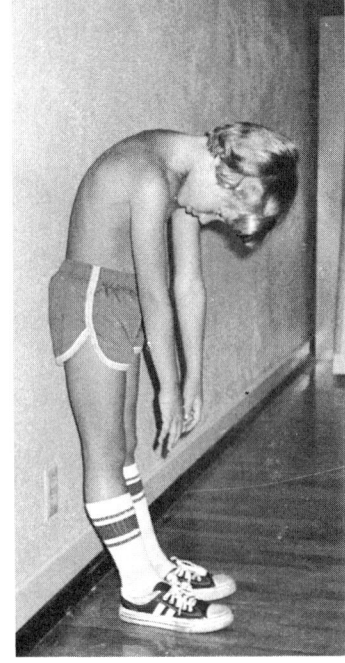 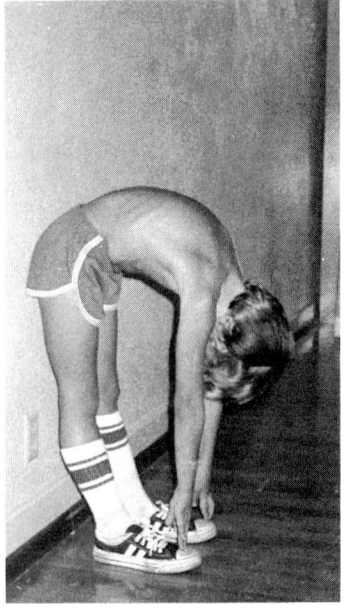

Standing forward bending exercise

and head are held against the wall. The child takes a quick breath out, tightening the abdominal muscles. This cycle is repeated after the child takes a short breath in the upright position.

Side bending rotation exercise. The side bending rotation exercise pictured begins with the child standing feet apart and breathing in while bringing the arms above the head. Then the child bends slowly to the left, letting the arms hang loosely. While bending forward, the arms and hands hang outside the left foot. As the body is rotated, the child continues to breathe out. The child then resumes the upright position, arms over head, breathing in. The exercise is repeated, but to the right side.

Other exercises, both in a seated position and a lying-back position, may be instituted on the recommendation of a physician before the child engages in physical activity. The reader is referred to Fein and Cox (1955) for more good exercises for asthmatic persons.

Additional games employing the abdominal muscles as the child breathes include those in which children are encouraged to laugh, either silently or out loud. For example:

- Children may have a laughing contest in which the object is to laugh as long as possible, either while making a laughing noise or while laughing without sound.

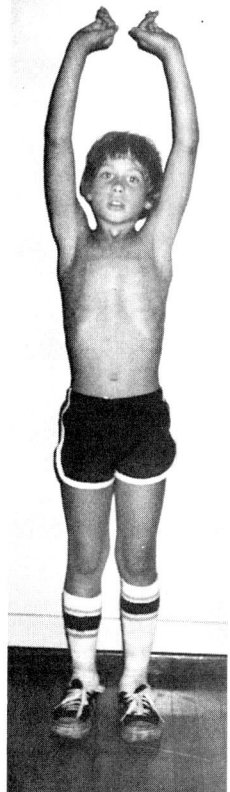

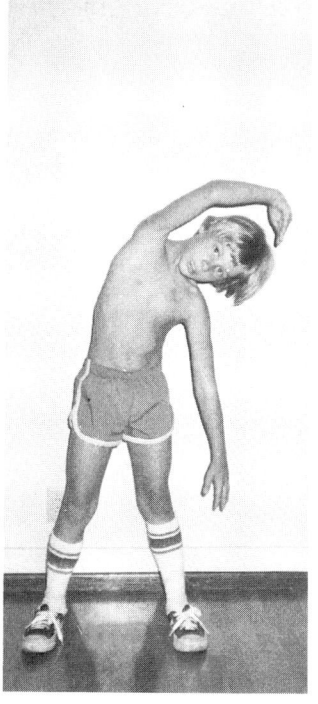

Side bending rotation exercise

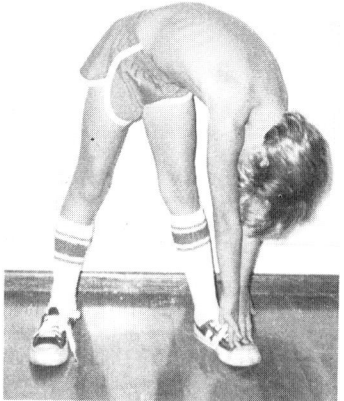

- Children might try to make other children laugh via grimaces, jokes, and so forth.
- Stop-and-go games such as "Red Light–Green Light" may be used, with laughing accompanying or being substituted for running.

Blowing games are also helpful. These might include:

- Contests to see who can blow out a candle first or from a greater distance.
- Blowing ping-pong balls along a trough or on a table.
- Keeping a balloon in the air for increased periods of time by blowing under it.

Through the use of progressively more vigorous activities of this type, Franklin (1971) found that significant changes were achieved in selected fitness measures of asthmatic children. These include tests of jumping jacks, push-ups, pull-ups, rope jumping, wind sprints, and jogging.

With proper supervision the asthmatic child can be placed in various positions in efforts to drain mucus from the bronchial tubes. The area to be drained is vigorously clapped with cupped hands to promote drainage. Figure 23.2 illustrates this.

CHRONIC BRONCHITIS AND EMPHYSEMA

Other obstructive diseases include chronic bronchitis and pulmonary emphysema. Pulmonary emphysema involves a destruction of the walls of the alveoli of the lungs, leading to overdistention of the sacs and a loss of lung elasticity. The afflicted individual must breathe about twice as rapidly as a normal person to effect the air exchange necessary, with a concomitant increase in heart rate. Smoking and other forms of pollution are suspected causes. The condition is not usually found in children.

A restriction of activity because of the fear of wheezing and coughing frequently is found in individuals with chronic obstructive pulmonary disease. This voluntary restriction results in pronounced lack of fitness. Some of the activities to promote diaphragmatic breathing, drainage, and greater volumes of exchanged air during expirations and inspirations may be helpful for these individuals, under the direction of their physicians.

Figure 23.2 A Position to Promote Mucous Drainage

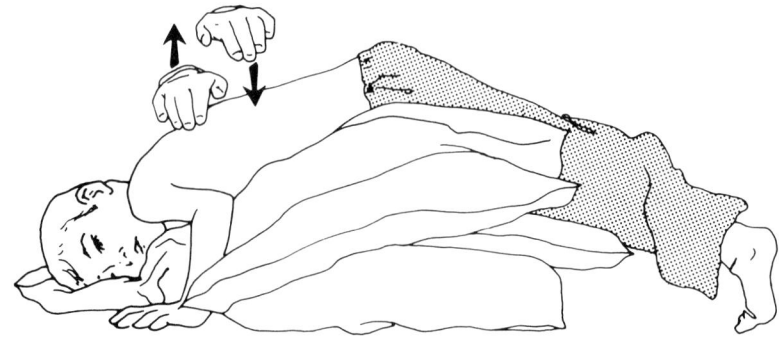

Note: From *Physically Handicapped Children* by E. Bleck and D. Nagel, 1975, New York: Grune & Stratton, p. 34. Used by permission of the author and the publisher.

CYSTIC FIBROSIS

Cystic fibrosis in childhood was not recognized as a separate disease until the late 1930s. Dorothy Anderson, a pathologist, reported on a series of infants who died within the first year of life from a lung disease accompanied by involvement of the pancreas. She further observed that the diseased pancreas contained many cysts and a great deal of fibrous scarring. She hypothesized that some disorder of the pancreas preventing the absorption of vitamin A seemed to trigger pathological changes in the lungs. Although the precise causes of the disease are not known, a combination of problems involving mucous-secreting glands of the liver, intestine, stomach, and salivary glands, as well as abnormal secretions of the sweat glands, are believed to be involved.

Cystic fibrosis is the most common cause of death from a genetic disorder in the United States. About 1 in 25 caucasians carries the gene. It occurs much less frequently in the black race and is infrequent in oriental people. A method for identifying those carrying the gene may soon be developed, using an abnormal protein isolated from the blood of children with cystic fibrosis.

In children with cystic fibrosis, the mucus secreted by the bronchial tubes is not easily expelled as is true in normal children. With the lungs poorly cleared, the mucus remains, and areas of the lungs become blocked. Like the asthmatic, the child with cystic fibrosis finds inhaling easier than exhaling—an action that makes the clogged bronchial tubes even smaller and more restricted. When enough constriction occurs, the area of the lung impacted may collapse. In addition, infection in the small bronchial tubes may occur because of poor clearance of inhaled material plus damage to areas of lung tissue.

The physical appearance of children with this condition varies depending on its severity, but, because of hyperinflated lungs, the chest usually has a large, rounded appearance. Also, because the abdomen has more gas than normal, it may be distended, and the child may need to pass a greater quantity of stools more often. The limbs may be thin, with a bulb-like, rounded look to the ends of the toes.

Because those with cystic fibrosis have trouble absorbing fat-soluble vitamins (A, D, E, K) from food, vitamin supplements are suggested. In warm weather, salt intake is increased, particularly when individuals are active and perspiring freely. Salt tablets usually are recommended following, and at times during, vigorous exercise.

As in asthma, the lungs should be kept as clear of mucus as possible. Postural drainage techniques similar to those employed with asthmatics are used. The child's upper body is lowered, and the chest is tapped and vibrated in efforts to dislodge mucus. Some physicians precede percussive and vibrative activities of this type with aerosol treatments.

At times the physician requires that a child afflicted with this condition sleep in a plastic tent filled with a fine mist, to aid breathing by thinning the mucus secretion. The most helpful method of treating this condition, however, has been through antibiotics.

With the advent of antibiotics in the 1940s and 1950s, and as more effective methods of clearing the lungs were developed in the late 1960s, longevity for individuals with cystic fibrosis has been increasing. The average age of death is in the middle teens, but some of the deaths that previously were caused by lung congestion are precipitated by secondary factors such as heart failure, liver involvement, or shock resulting from rapid loss of salt during excessive physical activity in hot weather. The upward trend in longevity continues, and now a large percentage of persons with cystic fibrosis reach adulthood and function well.

Some of the activities suggested for asthmatics may be applicable to youngsters with cystic fibrosis as well. A physician's advice, however, should be sought before initiating any physical exercise program for students who have this condition. The more general and obvious recommendations are (Scarnati, 1969):

1. Children should be encouraged to cough freely. Coughing clears the lungs and does not expel infectious materials.

2. Children may have to go to the bathroom more often than their peers, and this should be encouraged, as should increased food intake, which is characteristic of many with cystic fibrosis.

3. Children may have to be encouraged and reminded to take multiple medications during the school day, as prescribed.

4. Although children's physical stamina may be impaired, they should be encouraged not to hide the condition during play. On hot days children should be encouraged not to play as vigorously as usual and to supplement normal body salts with salt tablets because of potentially heavy perspiration.

SUMMARY

Asthma and similar conditions reflected in respiratory ailments are among the most prevalent debilitating conditions found in children and youth, affecting over 1.5 million youngsters. At times triggered by undue amounts and intensity of physical exercise, respiratory conditions also can be aided through exercise that is administered judiciously.

Asthma attacks can be brought on by infections, air pollutants, emotional trauma, fatigue, and chilling, as well as certain medications. The condition is caused by a biochemical imbalance that precipitates changes in the flexibility of the lining of the bronchial tubes. This lining becomes hyperirritable and results in constriction of the bronchioles as breath is exhaled.

The role of the physical educator is to instigate optimal amounts of exercise that does not increase emotional stress or strain physical capacities. The physical education teacher also should be alert to the signs of an impending attack and be knowledgeable of means to interrupt the chain of events and prevent a full-scale attack. Easily accessible laboratory equipment can be used to assess children's lung capacity and give some indication of the amount of exercise a child is able to handle.

In addition to providing a stress-free environment, the physical educator also should permit children with respiratory diseases, including cystic fibrosis, to evacuate mucus secretions from the throat, provide places to relax, and enlist their peers' support in exercises that can aid their respiratory function. Specific techniques and exercises, of course, should be introduced only with the advice and supervision of a physician.

REFERENCES

Anderson, S.D., Connolly, N., & Godfrey, S. (1971). Comparison of broncho-constriction induced by cycling and running. *Thorax, 26,* 396-401.

Bleck, E.E., & Nagel, D.A. (1975). *Physically handicapped children: A medical atlas for teachers.* New York: Grune & Stratton.

Committee on Children with Handicaps. (1970). The asthmatic child and his participation in sports and physical education. *Pediatrics, 45*(1), 150.

Fein, B.T., & Cox, E.P. (1955). The technique of respiratory and physical exercise in the treatment of bronchial asthma. *Annals of Allergy, 13*, 378-383.

Franklin, J. (1971). *An experimental study of physical conditioning for asthmatic children.* Unpublished master's thesis, Texas Woman's University.

Scarnati, R.S. (1969, January/February). Recreation therapy for persons with cystic fibrosis: A review. *American Corrective Therapy Journal, 23*, 7-13.

ADDITIONAL REFERENCES

Evans, H. (1979). *Lung diseases of children.* New York: American Lung Association.

Evans, H. (1979, March). What happens when a child has asthma? *American Lung Association Bulletin, 65*, 7-13.

Fisher, L. (1976, June). New frontiers in the treatment of asthma in children. *American Lung Association Bulletin, 62*, 2-5.

Fitch, K. (1975). Exercise-induced asthma and competitive athletics. *Pediatrics, 56* (Supplement), 847-850.

Ghory, J. (1975). Exercise and asthma overview and clinical impact. *Pediatrics, 56* (Supplement), 844-846.

Godfrey, S. (1972). *Handbook for the asthmatic.* New York: Allergy Foundation of America.

Godfrey, S. (1974). *Exercise testing in children: Applications in health and disease.* Philadelphia: W.B. Saunders.

Marley, W.P. (1977, July/August). Asthma and exercise: A review. *American Corrective Therapy Journal, 31*, 95-102.

Puthoff, M. (1972, September). New dimensions in physical activity for children with asthma and other respiratory conditions. *Journal of Health, Physical Education, & Recreation, 43*, 75.

Routon, J.R. (1977). *Self-concepts and attitudes toward physical education of asthmatic and non-asthmatic children.* Unpublished master's thesis, Texas Woman's University, Denton.

Schneider, M. (1977). *Intensive physical conditioning for asthmatic children and changes in selected pulmonary measures.* Unpublished master's thesis, Texas Woman's University, Denton.

Sirota, A.D., & Mahoney, M.J. (1974, July). Relaxing on cue: The self-regulation of asthma. *Journal of Behavioral Therapy & Experimental Psychiatry, 5*, 65-66.

Tuft, L., & Mueller, H. (1970). *Allergy in children.* Philadelphia: W.B. Saunders.

Verma, S., & Hyde, J. (1976, August). Physical education programs and exercise-induced asthma. *Clinical Pediatrics,* 697-705.

Williams, H.E., & Phelan, P.D. (1975). *Respiratory illness in children.* Oxford: Blackwell Scientific Publications.

QUESTIONS FOR DISCUSSION

1. What is the chain of events that seems to create a vicious circle and contribute to the distress of asthmatic children and youngsters?

2. What special measurement techniques may be applied to children with respiratory conditions to assess lung efficiency? **3.** What special precautions should be applied when working with an asthmatic child through physical activity? In what

ways might an activity contribute to, or detract from, the child's physical well-being?

STUDENT PROJECTS

1. Discuss with an asthmatic adolescent the nature of the condition, whether symptoms have abated or worsened with age, and what special stresses seem to trigger an attack.

2. Formulate the outline of a speech or pamphlet that might help explain symptoms and physiology of asthma. What might be the content of a talk to be given

to normal children in whose class an asthmatic child is about to be placed?

3. Using a fireplace bellows, explain diaphragmatic breathing.

4. Interview the parents of a child with cystic fibrosis or other respiratory condition. Attempt to ascertain what special problems they have had when working with their youngster.

RESOURCES

Allergy Foundation of America
801 Second Ave.
New York, NY 10017

American College of Allergists
2117 West River Rd. North
Minneapolis, MN 55411

American Lung Association
1740 Broadway
New York, NY 10019

Cystic Fibrosis Foundation
6000 Executive Blvd., Suite 309
Rockville, MD 20852

24 *Juvenile Diabetes*

$\mathbf{T}$he American Diabetes Association has estimated that for every 10,000 people in the United States, one person under the age of 20 has diabetes. In the older age ranges the numbers are greater. Approximately 10% of people over age 60 have some form of diabetes. This disease involves abnormalities of carbohydrates, protein, and fat and is marked by an inability of the pancreas to make insulin, which is needed for glucose to be used as an energy source to the muscles. The discovery of insulin treatment in the early 1920s has made diabetes largely controllable.

Most diabetes in children is of the type called *insulin-dependent mellitus*. A non-insulin-dependent form is referred to as Type II. This form can be treated by oral hypoglycemic agents to control the elevated blood sugar and does not require insulin injections. In another type, adult-onset diabetes, the pancreas is able to make some insulin, but the amount is insufficient for normal glucose utilization. The discussion in this chapter concentrates on juvenile diabetes mellitus, the form most commonly seen by physical educators in a school setting.

SIGNS AND SYMPTOMS

Diabetes arises in children rather quickly and does not seem to be related to anything they do or eat. When the pancreas does not manufacture insulin, the glucose level in the blood rises and the amount of glucose passing through the kidneys increases until glucose appears in the urine. This is one of the first signs of onset of the disease. Water is lost along with the glucose in the urine, and blood sugar does not reach the muscles. As a result, the individual begins to experience weakness and weight loss. This leads to a diabetic coma (ketoacidosis) and, without proper intervention, death. When diabetes first appears, this chain of events may take several weeks, but subsequently a diabetic coma may be triggered within a day or two without proper treatment and care. Figure 24.1 shows normal glucose metabolism, and Figure 24.2 depicts abnormal glucose metabolism.

Diabetes is one of the few diseases in which patients are taught to act as their own physicians. Because insulin is a protein hormone, administration by mouth would result in its being digested by the intestine and, therefore, it would be useless to the diabetic. To be effective, particularly in juvenile diabetes, it must be injected. Some of the more recent derivatives of insulin (NPH insulin or Lente insulin) act for 8 to 16 hours after their injection, so injections are needed less frequently than in past years.

If an excessive amount of insulin is injected, the amount of sugar in the blood decreases, and some organs (such as the brain) that have absolute requirements for glucose as an energy source begin to malfunction. Headaches, dizziness, irritability, blurred vision, nausea, vomiting, profuse perspiring, a fast heartbeat, and cold hands are among the possible symptoms of an *insulin reaction* (hypoglycemic episode), reflecting too low a blood sugar level.

Figure 24.1   Normal Glucose Metabolism

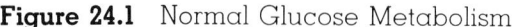

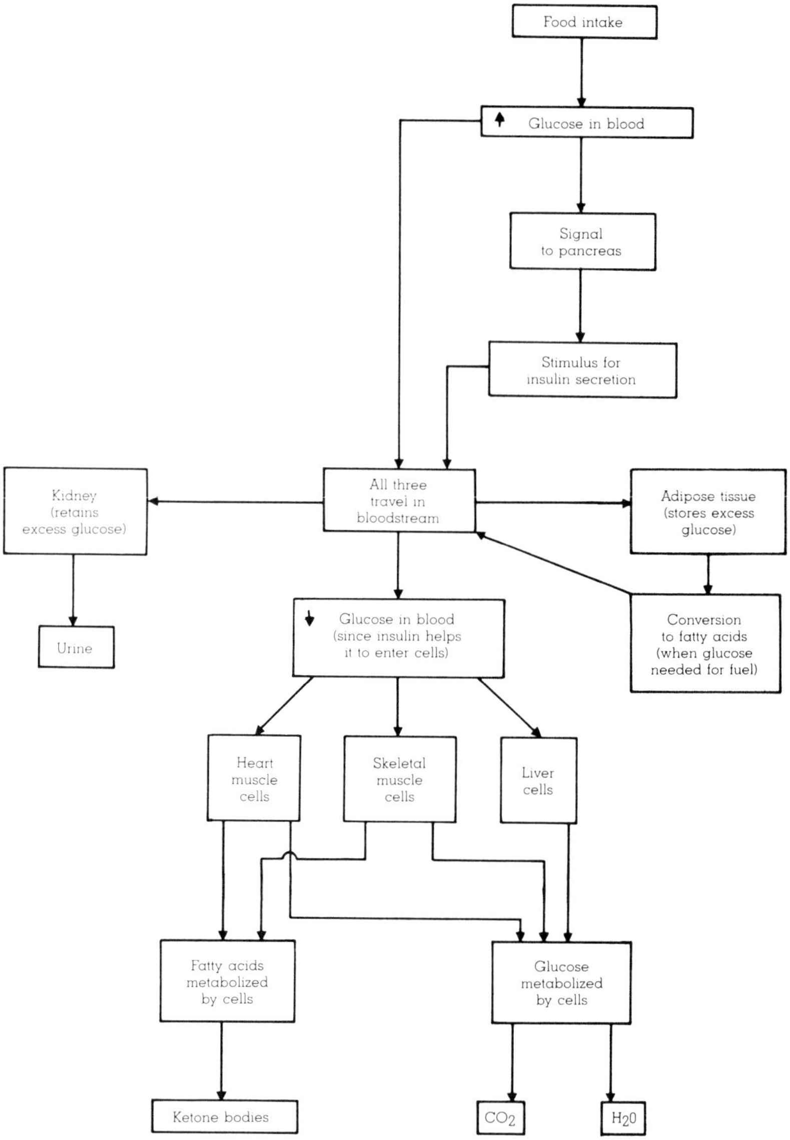

If the reaction is prolonged, convulsions, coma, and even death may result. Normally, taking concentrated sugar in some form, such as sweetened fruit juices or fruit-flavored hard candies, will terminate the insulin reaction in 2–3 minutes. If the diabetic with an insulin reaction does not ingest the sugar or vomits what is given, immediate medical attention is imperative.

Figure 24.2   Metabolism in Diabetes Mellitus

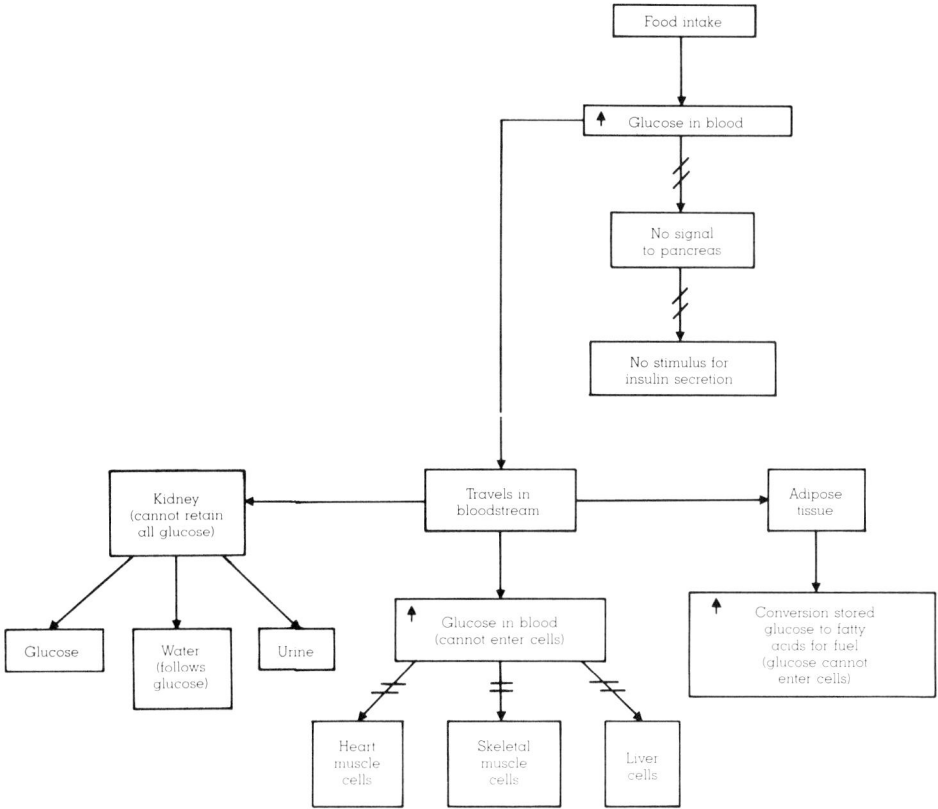

A number of conditions may accompany diabetes:

- *Macrovascular diseases*, usually involving heart conditions, turn out to be the cause of death for about three fourths of older diabetics in the United States (Steiner, 1981). This is manifested in cardiovascular disease, cerebrovascular disease, and renal disease.
- *Microangiopathy* also can occur, reflected in structural and functional problems with smaller arterioles, the venules, and capillaries (McMillan, Utterback, & LaPuma, 1978). These problems can result in renal failure, sensory deficits, partial paralysis, and blindness.
- *Hypertension* occurs to a greater degree in the diabetic population, particularly juvenile diabetics (Christlieb et al., 1981). Juveniles possibly can lower hypertensive characteristics through exercise, but this has not been proven.
- Diabetics may have higher levels of *fatty deposits* in the blood and on the walls of the blood vessels. This has not been conclusively demonstrated, although Lewis (1981) reported that cholesterol levels tend to be high in many diabetics.

• *Obesity* accompanies atherosclerosis as it is related to insulin resistance (Steiner, 1981).

CONTROL OF DIABETES

Controlling diabetes in most children who acquire the condition is relatively easy. Many, if not most, lead relatively normal lives and may participate vigorously in sports. Some have reached international levels of competition. The physical educator, as an administrator of a crucial variable, exercise, can play a critical role.

Children whose diabetes has just been diagnosed are usually hospitalized for about a week to learn procedures and facts vital to their well-being, including (a) testing of their urine, (b) the physiology and biochemistry of the disease, (c) how to administer insulin, and (d) how to adjust the dosage so that the amount taken is correct. Over 50 summer camps for diabetic chidren are offered in the United States and Canada to aid children in adjusting to and understanding the disease.

Four criteria of good diabetes control are commonly cited:

1. Children's growth, both height and weight, should be normal and comparable to that of normal peers of the same age and size.

2. The urine must contain no acetone. Ketones in the urine mean that the diabetes is out of control and fat breakdown is necessary for energy. When diabetes is in proper control, no fat breakdown should be occurring.

3. Insulin reactions should be absent.

4. The urine should not contain an excess of sugar (causing the volume to increase). Children should not have to get up at night to pass urine.

The effects of too much insulin (insulin reaction) and too little insulin (ketoacidosis) are summarized in Table 24.1.

IMPLICATIONS FOR PHYSICAL EDUCATION

In addition to careful attention to proper dosages of insulin, the diabetic person must regulate both diet and exercise. Diet should be constant from day to day. This does not mean that diabetics must have a special diet composed of the same foods but, rather, that they should be consistent in the amount and content of daily intake. The concept of exchange is employed when educating diabetics in proper eating habits. They may eat different things each day but must select foods that roughly approximate each other in quantity and content during the same meal. Additionally, diabetics usually do better if they eat more and smaller portions daily. Many diabetics eat five meals a day.

The other major factor, exercise, works like insulin. When exercising, a diabetic burns glucose but conserves insulin. The diabetic should stop exercising after each half hour to hour of play or exercise and eat a snack to cover the energy that has been expended. Usually this simple precaution is enough to prevent insulin reactions.

Moreover, the intensity of exercise should be relatively consistent from day to day so that it corresponds to the amount of insulin taken. If exercise is suddenly changed in inten-

Table 24.1 Effects of Too Much and Too Little Insulin

	Insulin Reaction	**Ketoacidosis**
Onset	Rapid (matter of minutes)	Gradual (matter of hours)
Symptoms	Headache	Tiredness
	Nausea	Fatigue
	Vomiting	Polydipsia
	Palpitations	Polyphagia
	Tremulousness	Polyuria
	Irritability	
Skin	Cold and moist	Warm and dry
Breathing	Normal or shallow	Deep (air hunger)
Urine tests	Negative glucose	4 + glucose
	Negative acetone	Positive acetone
Treatment	Sugar	Insulin

Note: From "Juvenile Diabetes Mellitus" (ch. 10) by R.O. Christiansen in *Physically Handicapped Children* by E. Bleck and D. Nagel, 1975, New York: Grune & Stratton, p. 128. Used by permission.

sity, an accurate judgment must be made in advance of the amount of insulin that will be needed. The challenge is to match exercise intensity with insulin intake.

When exposed to well designed exercise programs, diabetic children benefit in the same ways as other youngsters do. More important, exercise helps to reduce blood glucose in diabetics and helps maintain this lowered level. Muscle glycogen depletion during physical work results in prolonged stimulation of peripheral glucose utilization in diabetics (Maehlum, Felig, & Wahren, 1978). The glycogen replenishment effects of exercise on glucose metabolism may persist up to 2 days after exercise is terminated (Wahren, 1979). Inactivity lessens glucose tolerance and the diabetic state even though physical work capacities may not be lowered significantly (Coram & Mangum, 1986).

Although research has indicated that exercise therapy is an important part of diabetes control, most diabetics have reduced abilities to exercise vigorously. A number of factors can lower tolerance to exercise and efficiency in diabetics (Rubler & Arvan, 1976):

1. Lactic acid and other products of muscular fatigue rise sharply when diabetics exercise. Although the reasons for this are not clear, the assumption is that, because of the viscosity of diabetic blood, oxygen delivery to muscle tissues is impaired (McMillan et al., 1978).

2. Stiffened arteries, together with increased blood viscosity, tend to make the heart work harder during exercise (Pillsbury, Hung, Kyle, & Fries, 1974).

3. Plasma volume in exercising diabetics drops markedly during increased work loads.

4. *Microangiopathy* accompanies reduced exercise abilities in diabetics whose condition has persisted. Microvascular changes remove both protein and water from the plasma and reduce cardiac output. Diabetic blood pressure changes that are greater than in normal persons during exercise probably are a result of the presence of these changes in the smaller blood vessels (McMillan et al., 1979).

5. Diabetic neuropathy may cause paresis or paralysis and thus alter the individual's ability to exercise in biomechanically efficient ways.

Another caution of which diabetics and their teachers should be aware concerns the consequences of infection. Usually infections tend to make diabetes worse. When an infection occurs, a diabetic who has been in good control begins to excrete acetone in the urine. Extra insulin may be needed at these times. Once the infection has been eliminated, the insulin dosage must be cut back.

PRINCIPLES AND GUIDELINES

General guidelines for the physical education instructor in dealing with diabetic students include the following:

1. Monitor the program closely. Adjust the medication and caloric intake as frequently as necessary.

2. Carefully ascertain work capacities and tolerances in advance through a thorough and graded exercise testing program.

3. Keep individual goals within limits consistent with the child's psychological and physiological limits.

4. Encourage nutritional soundness and adherence to medically supervised dietary programs.

5. Avoid sports and physical programs that would encourage weight changes (e.g., wrestling, football), as sudden weight shifts may be extremely hazardous to diabetics.

6. Pay particular attention to circulation and skin care, as these are closely associated with microvascular abnormalities. Clothes should fit loosely. Tight shoes, belts, and wraps should be avoided as they may restrict the blood flow.

7. Treat all cuts, scrapes, and the like at once to avoid infection.

8. Make periodic checks for injuries, as microcirculation problems can reduce the child's pain perception.

9. Support frequent evaluations by a physician.

10. Give the feet special attention. Footwear should be well fit, and a complete foot/ankle evaluation should be conducted by a podiatrist, orthopedist, or physical therapist yearly.

11. In water sports have the child wear earplugs, and be alert to any signs of infection.

12. Refer the child for medical attention if resting blood pressure is excessive (SBP 140 mm Hg), if blood glucose changes (300 mg/100 ml), an infection is suspected, or any other unusual problem arises.

13. Keep up-to-date medical information on diabetes available for reference, both in general and specifically concerning the diabetic youngster.

14. Test urine or blood before strenuous exercise, and monitor resting blood pressure during and after exercise sessions.

15. Schedule exercise periods at about the same time each day, and keep the relationship between medicine, food, and exercise constant. Keep fast-acting sugar sources on hand.

Negative mood changes sometimes are encountered in diabetic children. These fluctuations may stem from an occasional glucose-positive urine test. Perhaps the best way to counteract any adverse reactions of classmates toward the diabetic's emotional variance is to give the class (or have the diabetic student do this) a "lesson" in the physiology of the disease, its metabolism, chemical reactions, and manifestations. An understanding of the condition may be all that is needed to engender acceptance of the diabetic.

The physical education teacher may be the one teacher at school who is in a position to observe a child administering insulin in the locker room. The educator who observes an increase of scar tissue at the site frequently used for injections may recommend that the child ask the physician to suggest other portions of the body into which the insulin may be injected.

In working with diabetic students in a physical education class,, the single most important function is to be acutely sensitive to reactions indicating that a child is receiving too much or too little insulin and, therefore, is at risk for a serious reaction. If this seems to be the case, the teacher should be prepared to take the proper steps immediately to rectify the problem.

SUMMARY

Juvenile diabetes mellitus usually becomes apparent during the first decade of life. The condition is caused by an inability of the pancreas to make insulin, which causes blood glucose levels to rise. When excessive glucose is secreted in the urine, blood sugar is prevented from reaching the muscles. If the disease is not immediately diagnosed and treated, the child begins to experience weakness and weight loss, which will lead to a diabetic coma.

Diabetes is controllable through insulin injections, but the dosage needed, exercise limitations, and dietary considerations are sensitive factors that must be closely monitored. The child should have (a) knowledge about the biochemical nature of the condition, (b) ways to self-medicate, and (c) an understanding of the signs indicating changes in insulin dosages or additional sugar needed. To prevent ketoacidosis or an insulin reaction, the diabetic child has an added responsibility of acting as his or her own physician. The four criteria of good diabetes control generally accepted are (a) normality of growth and body size, (b) lack of acetone in the blood, (c) absence of insulin reactions, and (d) lack of excess sugar in the urine.

The physical educator should be aware of the ways in which diet and exercise interact to influence the diabetic's functioning. Exercise works like insulin insofar as it burns glucose but spares insulin. The diabetic should snack every half hour or so during exercise sessions to compensate for the energy expended. Further, the amount of exercise should stay constant from day to day. If the intensity of exercise is changed, the amount of insulin taken should be adjusted accordingly.

When it is under control, diabetes may not interfere with even the most vigorous exercise. Many superior athletes have diabetes. The physical educator, however, should be continually alert to signs of an imbalance of insulin in the diabetic's body and take immediate steps to regulate the biochemical mechanisms involved when an emergency situation occurs.

REFERENCES

Bleck, E., & Nagel, D. (1975). *Physically handicapped children.* New York: Grune & Stratton.

Christiansen, R.O. (1975). Juvenile diabetes mellitus. In E.E. Bleck & D.A. Nagel (Eds.), *Physically handicapped children: A medical atlas for teachers* (ch. 10). New York: Grune & Stratton.

Christlieb, A.R., Warram, J.H., Krowlesky, A.S., Busick, E.J., Ganda, O.P., Asmal, A.C., Soeldmer, J.S., & Bradley, R.F. (1981). Hypertension: The major risk factors in juvenile-onset insulin-dependent diabetes. *Diabetes, 30*(2), 90-96.

Coram, S.J., & Mangum, M. (1986). Exercise risks and benefits for diabetic individuals: A review. *Adapted Physical Activity Quarterly, 3,* 35-57.

Lewis, B. (1981). Summary of section. *Diabetes, 30*(2), 88-89.

Maehlum, S., Felig, P., & Wahren, J. (1978). Splanchic glucose and muscle glycogen metabolism after glucose feeding during post exercise recovery. *American Journal of Physiology, 235,* E255-E260.

McMillan, D.E., Utterback, N., & LaPuma, J. (1978). Reduced erythrocyte deformation in diabetes. *Diabetes, 27,* 895-901.

Pillsbury, H.C., Hung, W., Kyle, M.C., & Fries, E.D. (1974). Arterial pulse waves and velocity and systolic time intervals in diabetic children. *American Heart Journal, 87,* 783-790.

Rubler, S., & Arvan, S. (1976). Exercise testing in young asymptomatic diabetic patients. *Angiology, 27,* 539-548.

Steiner, G. (1981). Diabetes and atherosclerosis: An overview. *Diabetes, 30*(2), 1-7.

Wahren, J. (1979). Glucose turnover during exercise in healthy man and diabetes mellitus. *Diabetes, 28*(1), 82-88.

ADDITIONAL REFERENCES

British Diabetic Association. (1969). *The effects of exercise on the young diabetic.* London: Author.

British Diabetic Association. (1970). *Social problems and the diabetic.* London: Author.

British Diabetic Association. (1972). *Introducing diabetes.* London: Author.

Sussman, D.E. (Ed.). (1971). *Juvenile-type diabetes and its complications.* Springfield, IL: Charles C Thomas.

Traisman, H.S. (1971). *Management of juvenile diabetes* (2nd ed.). St. Louis: C.V. Mosby.

QUESTIONS FOR DISCUSSION

1. Under what conditions is the diabetic likely to have an adverse reaction?

2. What special precautions should be taken when working with diabetics in a physical education program?

3. What are the four generally accepted criteria of good diabetes control?

4. In what ways does the diabetic child have to act as his or her own physician?

STUDENT PROJECTS

1. Discuss and diagram the biochemical cycles and reactions important to main-

tenance of a steady state by the diabetic.

2. Interview someone with diabetes to

learn about special control problems, how he or she learned of having the condition, and under what kinds of circumstances adverse symptoms are likely to occur.

3. From a review of the literature, what can you ascertain about the long-term effects of diabetes in the fourth, fifth, and sixth decades of life?

4. Formulate an ideal month-long program for a diabetic 17-year-old, during which you attempt to train this pupil for competitive swimming. What special precautions should you take? What kinds of consultation should you have with the youth's parents and with the family physician?

RESOURCES

American Diabetes Association
600 Fifth Ave.
New York, NY 10020

British Diabetic Association
152 Harley St.
London W1, England

Diabetes
18 E. 48th St.
New York, NY 10017

Diabetes in the News
Ames Co.
3553 W. Peterson Ave.
Chicago, IL 60659

Section VII

Interventions

25 *Infant Stimulation*

During the 1980s the moral and legal climate in the United States has increasingly promoted interest in and programs for "suspect" infants and children of pre-school age. These programs have been inspired by findings of Head Start programs from the 1960s and 1970s and by widespread acceptance of the principle that the earlier a developmental problem is detected and corrected, the better are the chances for children to maximize their potential.

Early intervention encompasses the concept of applying stimulation from birth, particularly with infants who show signs of muscular problems. Some babies are born with cerebral palsy—spasticity that may become more marked or may lessen in the months ahead. Others may show athetoid tendencies, which could change into irregular, relatively uncontrolled movement patterns without intervention. They may be in the initial stages of some kind of degenerative neuromuscular condition. Infants with neuromuscular symptoms must be thoroughly diagnosed—at times by more than one pediatric expert.

Finally there is a group of "floppy" infants who are difficult to diagnose. They are free from disease but may have muscular developmental delays from 6 months to over a year. Their condition may be labeled infantile hypotonia or other term, but the mechanisms causing the problem remain a mystery. I have developed home programs for several of these infants recently, and this chapter is directed toward this general condition, described by Eng, Koch, and Binder (1979).

High-risk infants are usually found in populations that are extremely small at birth, primarily because of prematurity. As more sophisticated efforts are being made to stimulate these high-risk infants, their later problems seem to be diminishing. For example, Astbury, Orgill, Bajuk, and Yul (1983), who for 2 years followed over 100 infants with very low birth weights, found that by the end of that time, about 85% were free of serious handicaps, but by the second year about 40% were judged hyperactive. Moreover, the development of various types of abilities may not be even. Astbury and her colleagues found, for example, that the psychomotor abilities of the infants she and her colleagues studied trailed their mental development.

Many school districts that previously had been reluctant to institute programs for children younger than the traditional school-entry age of 5 or 6 have begun to realize that enrolling "problem children" into their schools without prior attention by professionals can cause more difficulties educationally than would be the case if they were to have received sound intervention earlier. Moreover, federal legislation (PL 94-142 and PL 99-457) addresses educational services from age 3, and preferably, from birth.

Research evaluating effects of infant stimulation overwhelmingly supports the beneficial effects of early intervention, according to one recent reviewer (Ulrich, 1984). But sorting out just what effect movement/kinesthetic stimulation may have is difficult. Infants have individual differences in their needs and toleration for stimulation (Bromwich, 1977). Among the favorite movement techniques employed are: (a) manual handling by mothers and caregivers, and (b) rocking infants in special platforms, sometimes within incubators (Freedman, Boverman, & Freedman, 1966). Motorized hammocks also have been used (Rice, 1977). Waterbeds are another popular "platform" with which to stimulate infants kinesthetically (Korner, Ruppel, & Rho, 1982). Waterbeds have been used not only to stimulate infants' kinesthetic and vestibular receptors but also to preserve fragile skin, offer soft head support, and help the infant deal with gravity. Although stimulation programs focus primarily on high-risk infants and those who have obvious handicapping conditions at birth (Bricker, 1982), those who study the effects of infant stimulation are struck with the notion that normal infants may well benefit from the ideas and operations contained in them.

Although the current research provides promising beginnings, it has shortcomings. The samples used are highly diverse and at times not adequately described. The techniques and programs applied often are of a short-term nature, while the possible long-term effects of programs are not evaluated carefully. The best hope is to tailor programs to individual infants, based on proper medical evaluation, together with intelligent and perceptive therapy.

To an increasing extent adapted physical educators, acting alone or within a therapy team, have been responsible for (a) planning and carrying out program content for these young clients, (b) instituting components of parent education programs directed toward younger charges, and (c) formulating evaluation strategies directed at the movement qualities of young children.[1]

This chapter presents general principles and examples of what kinds of movement-associated problems may be detected in infants and what kinds of therapeutic strategies may be applied. The industrious physical educator should attempt to gain as wide a background as possible through close association with occupational and physical therapists and by a thorough perusal of literature focused on the stages of normal development during the early months and years of life, as well as monographs and books with practical suggestions for developmentally sound intervention programs for younger children and infants.

TYPES OF "SPECIAL INFANTS"

Infants with movement problems may be classified into two basic categories from the physical educator's perspective: those who are hypotonic and those who are hypertonic.

Hypotonic

Hypotonic infants have insufficient muscle tension. They are floppy and weak. Within this category are Down syndrome babies, along with others lacking muscle tone. Their motor development is delayed because they lack the strength to assume various positions, control the head, and move out from a crawling position. Their inability to sit without support at an appropriate age prevents them from developing the use of their hands and mastering hand-object tasks. Some hypotonic youngsters later (at about the third or fourth year) are diagnosed as having athetoid cerebral palsy. Many, however, simply lack strength and adequate tonus in their muscles. Their lack of muscle tone also may be reflected in flaccid facial muscles or half-closed, "droopy" eyelids.

---

1. The principles and techniques explained in this chapter also are appropriate when working with severely and profoundly developmentally delayed individuals of all ages.

Hypertonic

A second general grouping is characterized by an excess of muscular tension and tone. Infants' movements seem restricted as they reach and try to extend an arm, for example; they seem to be controlled by a force that refuses to let the arm extend. Often these infants and young children are diagnosed as having various forms of cerebral palsy (see chapter 13).

In some ways the remediation of hypertonicity may be more difficult than working with the hypotonic youngster. At times the hypertonic infant displays restrictive, even annoying, reflexes that usually are not seen in maturing children. For the most part, however, the overly tense baby retains "normal" reflexes too long, delaying attainment of the voluntary movements that usually emerge during the first and second years of life. These unusual and unwanted flexions and tensions must be reduced before useful, healthy movements can be encouraged. Straddling activities sometimes can accomplish this, as shown in Figure 25.1. Hypertonic infants require careful diagnosis by pediatric experts to discover what unique reflexes, flexions, and tensions are present.

Other Movement Patterns

There are other types of suspect movement patterns in infants. Some are born without limbs (congenital amputees). Others have movement abnormalities in a portion of their bodies

Figure 25.1   A Straddling Activity to Reduce Flexion and Scissoring

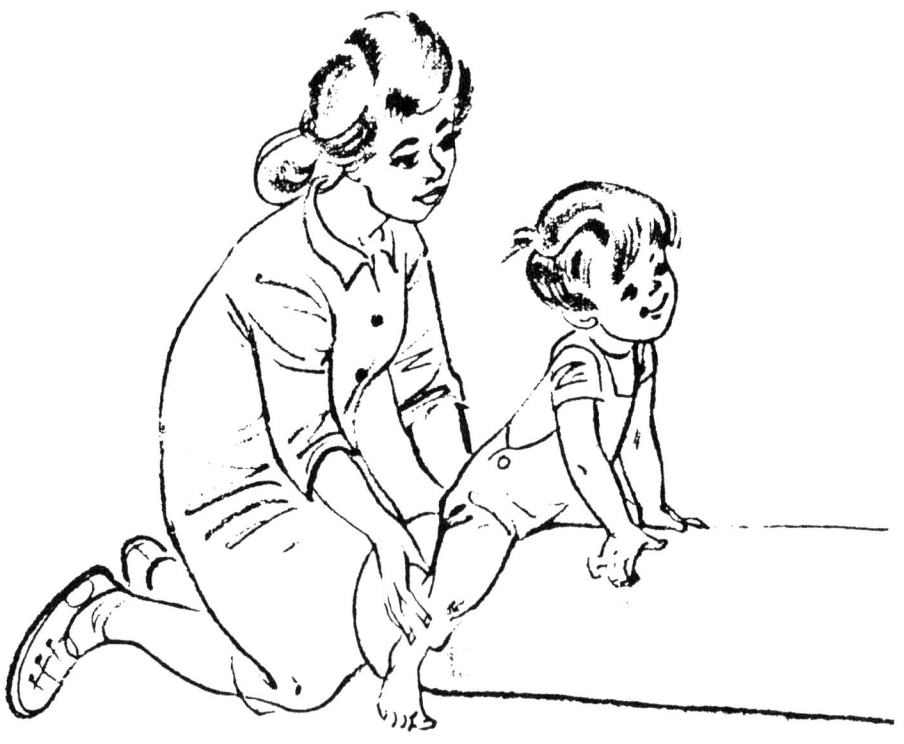

(one limb, for example) rather than displaying total patterns of hypertonicity or hypotonicity. Still others may exhibit early signs of degenerative neuromotor disorders, presenting formidable challenges for endocrinologists, pediatric neurologists, and other diagnosticians.

Several new types of stressed infants have come to the attention of medical and paramedical professionals. These infants share developmental anomalies and lags but are, in both obvious and subtle ways, different from each other. The thorough identification of developmental accompaniments to these conditions is ongoing. Organized efforts at remediation, accompanied by scientifically useful data and studies, are also in the first stages.

Leukemia in Remission   More and more infants and young children diagnosed with leukemia are being medically managed so that the remission rates are reaching over 75% (based on a 5-year period of recovery). At the same time, the chemicals (alkaloids), together with radiation that is necessary to ensure their survival, seem to be causing neuropathies that are reflected a year or two later in motor problems including mild ataxic tendencies and graphomotor disturbances (difficulty with printing and writing).

At this point in my own clinical practice, I am assessing, enriching, and following the progress of several of these children. Future efforts by oncologists to save the lives of these infants and children will surely be accompanied by equally intensive efforts to assess and stimulate motor-developmental processes that may be influenced negatively.

Drug-Using Mothers   Before the turn of the century, it was noted that maternal alcohol use negatively influenced neonatal health and capacities (Rossett & Sander, 1979). Further insults to the fetus have been documented as the result of the mother's use of tobacco and other commonly used substances (Pasamanick & Knobloch, 1966). And in the 1980s the widespread use of exotic drugs is spawning rather unique and shocking developmental signs at birth—signs that are beginning to attract the attention of researchers (Chasnoff, 1983; Golden, 1982), as well as clinicians interested in infant stimulation and developmental progress. Because the mothers of such infants often use a combination of drugs, the relationship between the effects of specific drugs and identifiable developmental syndromes is confounded. Often these mothers do not legally retain custody of their infants, so locating the children, and evaluating and stimulating them in useful ways, becomes a difficult practical/legal matter.

Generally the symptoms of each category of drug-stressed infant differ. The infant stressed with *heroin* displays vibrating, rapid, twitching movements at birth, accompanied by hypertonicity. These problems may persist through the first year; they are reflected in tense, awkward grasping movements by 9-10 months, along with hyperactivity and the inability to make useful and frequent social contact with caregivers. Although the drugs are often shown to disappear from the infants' systems by about 3 days, the symptoms that persist indicate lasting damage to the central nervous system. These pathologies are not well understood today.

In addition to the hypertonicity displayed by the "heroin baby," the infant with *PCP* often displays meaningless and slow tracking movements of the eyes. These "ramps" probably interfere with their gaining information, and they present unique problems in stimulation (Balster, 1980).

In contrast, the baby stressed with maternal *cocaine* use is floppy (hypotonic) and displays an out-of-contact visual expression, which also may prevent useful input from positively influencing development. These infants fail to display the normal and potentially useful stereotypies discussed later in this chapter. It has been hypothesized that cocaine influencing the neurotransmitters of the adult user may result in a similar interference with neurotransmission over synapses of the developing infants.

All these infants present new challenges to society in general and to those who may become responsible for their enrichment and development. Currently various researchers around the country are beginning to study these infants and to plan for their enrichment. The patterns and syndromes are still unfolding. As they are studied and tested by developmental specialists, experimentally oriented pediatricians, biomechanists, speech pathologists, and others, it will become more apparent just what one might expect from efforts at stimulation.

INTERVENTION PRINCIPLES AND STRATEGIES

One must remember that if an infant displays abnormal movement characteristics, he or she does not necessarily have intellectual deficits. When working with these youngsters, an important task is to provide appropriate stimulation so that their inabilities to deal physically with their world will not interfere with their perceptual and intellectual growth and, if possible, should promote these potentials. Interventionists must talk to them, give them things to look at and manipulate, and encourage them to use language skills in ways that often require more inventiveness than strategies applied with normally developing infants and pre-schoolers.

The strategies set forth in this chapter work with the majority of infants with movement problems. Also, specific strategies are presented for use with hypertonic and hypotonic children. These strategies must be applied individually, as the child's symptoms and needs dictate.

Good "Therapy Hands"

Good therapy hands can guide a child with movement problems through normal developmental phases. Hypotonic infants in particular must be gently guided through positions and

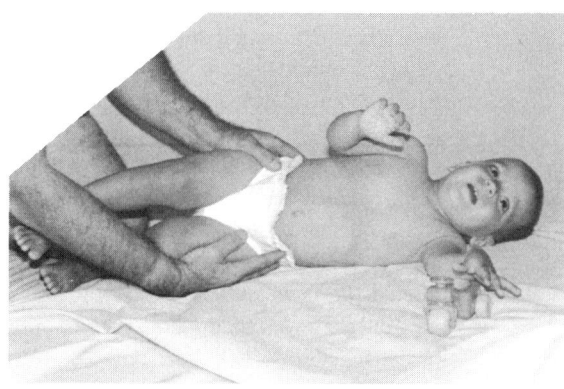

Good therapy hands guide a body derotative movement.

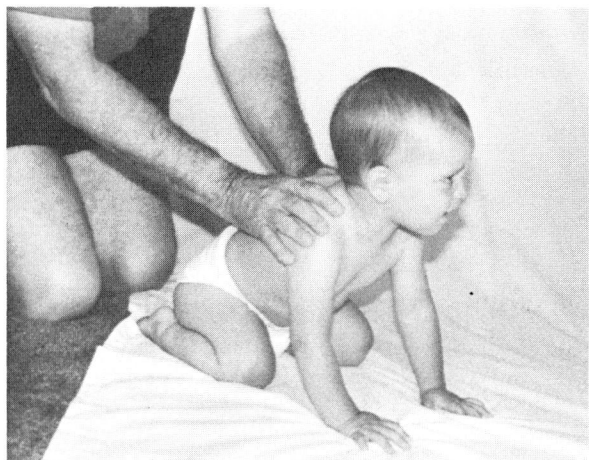

The therapist partially supports the infant in a creeping position.

movements like those seen in typical children. The infant should be moved with minimum effort on the part of the therapist and maximum involvement on the part of the infant. The therapist does not need those particular exercises—the infant does!

For example, the infant may be guided in turning from front to back by placing the hands gently at the hips as shown. When turning the infant, the therapist should hold back somewhat, allowing the infant to participate, if possible. In this example, turning the hips can elicit a body-derotative response that stimulates turning of the body and head.

Another example is to position the infant, as pictured, in a low preparatory position for creeping. The infant should be held gently by the shoulders and hips, and some of the therapist's grip pressure should be released, permitting the infant to maintain the position briefly, if possible, through his or her own efforts.

Actions of the limbs may be similarly guided, as in a reaching response. Then, later in the developmental sequence, brief efforts to stand should be permitted if the infant's strength contributes 60%-80% of the total effort (with the therapist's contribution being the remaining percent). Pulling, tugging, and placing the infant in desired movements and through various actions by an energetic therapist is likely to change little except the muscular strength of the therapist!

Objects to Motivate Actions

Infants, like all of us, need reasons to do things. Simply getting a suspect child to posture in a creeping or a standing position will not likely elicit the actions that normally stem from these positions—creeping and walking. Infants are unlikely to pull themselves from a sitting to a standing position unless some desired object is overhead to be reached for and acquired.

Blind infants often gain the same static, unmoving postures (sitting, kneeling, standing) at the same ages as the sighted do, but they lack the actions that come out of these positions. The blind child simply does not have any reason to creep and reach for something,

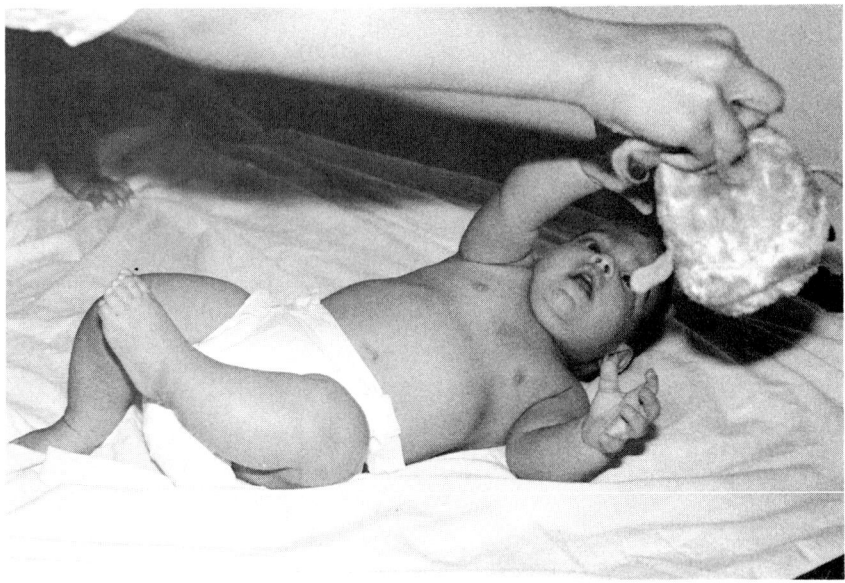

The turning response may be stimulated through the use of an object.

Reprinted from *Perceptual and Motor Development in Infants and Children* (3rd ed.) by B.J. Cratty, 1986, with permission of the publisher, Prentice-Hall.

to stand to get a better look, or to walk to some desired goal, because the child does not see those things.

Virtually all actions early in a child's development may be stimulated through desired objects. Early turning responses may be triggered by the assistance discussed, together with an object placed to one side or the other. Turning may be stimulated by moving the object across the infant's visual field, as pictured, eliciting head-turning—an action that then may promote other turning responses.

Early attempts at creeping will be enhanced by placing an object just out of reach as the infant postures in a hand-knee position, as pictured. The first reaching effort may cause the infant to collapse, but subsequent efforts may result in primitive creeping in which the arms and legs advance one at a time with little timing or patterning. Later creeping will be more rapid and with a normal cross-extension pattern (left hand advancing with the advance of the right knee).

If the child has reasons and goals, he or she will be more likely to stand, and later walk. As pictured, the child is encouraged to stand, not only because of the object but also by the rungs on the vertical surface, permitting easy hand-holds.

Walking also will be enhanced if desirable things are placed in the way of the tottering infant. The child will be more likely to persist in both standing and walking if the therapist helps the infant descend in a proper "parachute response," by bending the knees and reaching out with the hands; at the same time the head moves forward to counterbalance the downward

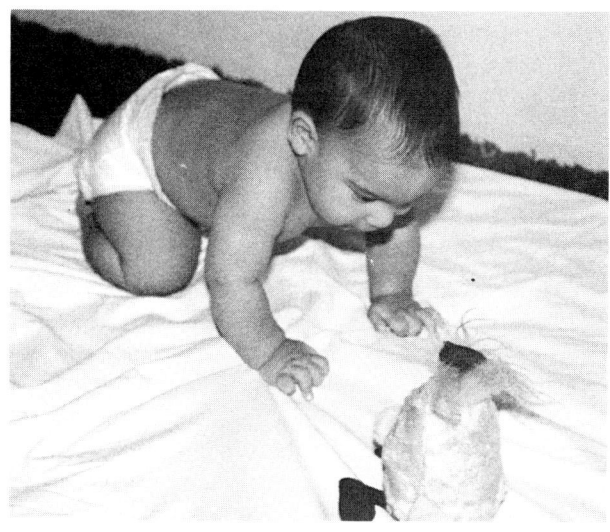

The child considers creeping to acquire an object.

Reprinted from *Perceptual and Motor Development in Infants and Children* (3rd ed.) by B.J. Cratty, 1986, with permission of the publisher, Prentice-Hall.

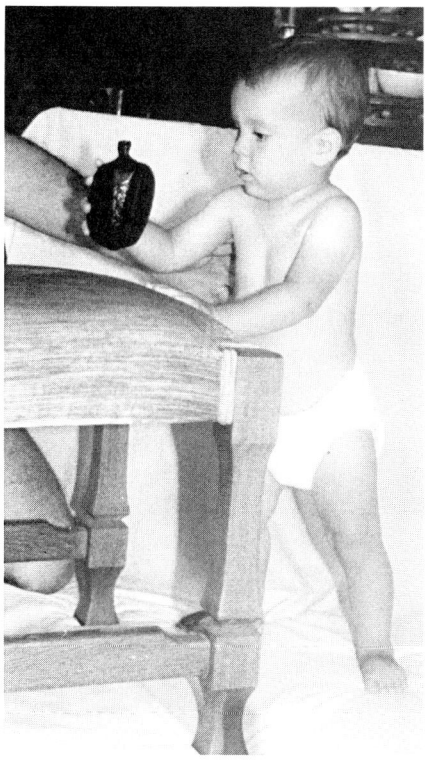

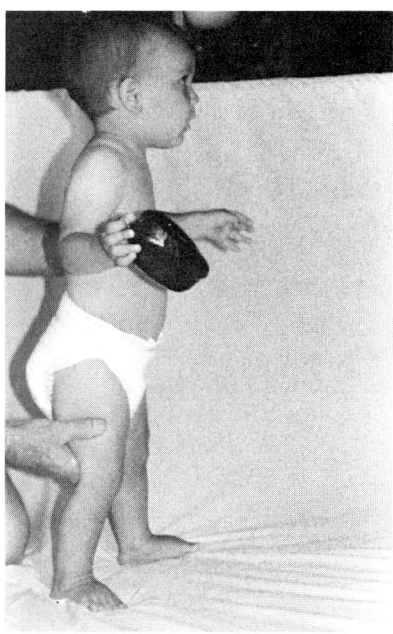

The infant is helped to descend by bending the knees and reaching out—the parachute response.

The infant stands to gain object placed on chair.

and backward movement of the hips. Training for the parachute response is pictured. If standing or walking is terminated by an unpleasant or hurtful descent to the floor, the infant will be less likely to try the maneuver again in the near future.

Rhythmic Stereotypies

Late in the 1970s a researcher in infant development at the University of Missouri, Esther Thelen, began to record and study the rhythmic actions of normal infants. These actions, which she named "stereotypies," consume about 40% of the waking hours of normal infants. They occur in various parts of the body—the face, hands, arms, and legs. These rhythmic actions also are seen in movements of the trunk while the infant is sitting, kneeling, and standing. Figure 25.2 depicts some of these stereotypies, and one of them is pictured.

Thelen and others who have researched these stereotypies postulate that they form important training tasks, facilitating establishment of neuromotor pathways imperative to the acquisition of voluntary movements used in sitting, creeping, and the like (Thelen, 1981). Recent work has further found that the timing and rhythm of these actions are not random but instead coincide with the locations and patterns of the later voluntary movements (Thelen & Fisher, 1983). Leg-kicking stereotypies, for example, are similar to the same responses seen in the same infant when he or she attempts to gain some advantage by extending the leg. Figure 25.3 compares rhythmic stereotypies seen in the arms and legs during the first year of life. Figure 25.4 depicts three types of rhythmic stereotypies seen in torso movements. The encouragement of leg stereotypies is pictured.

Figure 25.2   Rhythmic Stereotypies in Infants

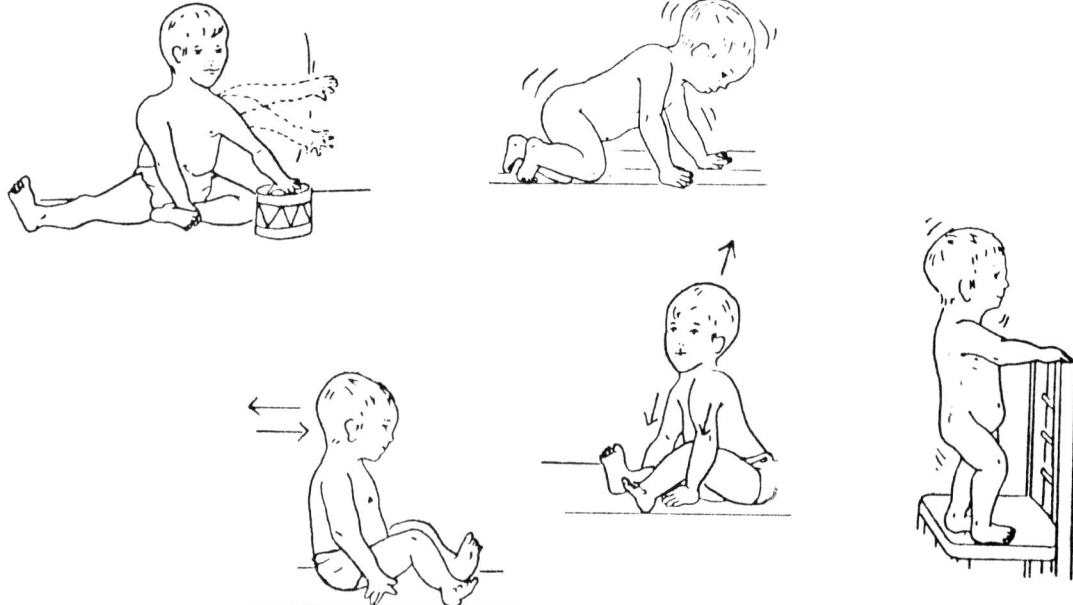

Note: From *Perceptual and Motor Development in Infants and Children* (3rd ed.) by B.J. Cratty, 1986, Englewood Cliffs, NJ: Prentice-Hall. Used by permission.

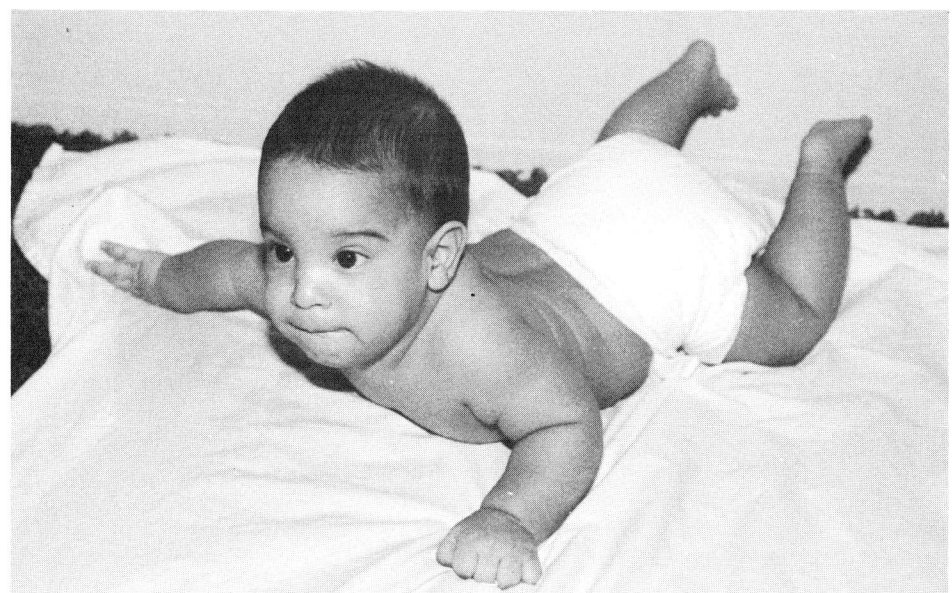

The infant engages in kicking and rocking stereotypies.

Reprinted from *Perceptual and Motor Development in Infants and Children* (3rd ed.) by B.J. Cratty, 1986, with permission of the publisher, Prentice-Hall.

Figure 25.3   Rhythmic Stereotypies of Arms and Legs During First Year

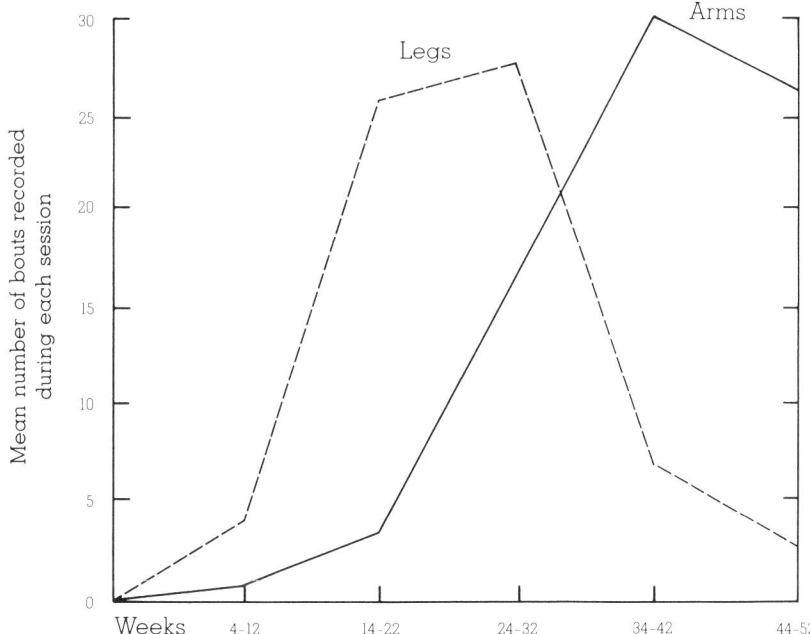

Note: Drawn from data in "Rhythmical Stereotypies in Infants" by E. Thelen, 1979, *Animal Behaviour, 27,* pp. 699-715. Used by permission of the author and the publisher, Baillière Tindall, London.

Figure 25.4   Rhythmic Stereotypies in Torso Movements During First Year

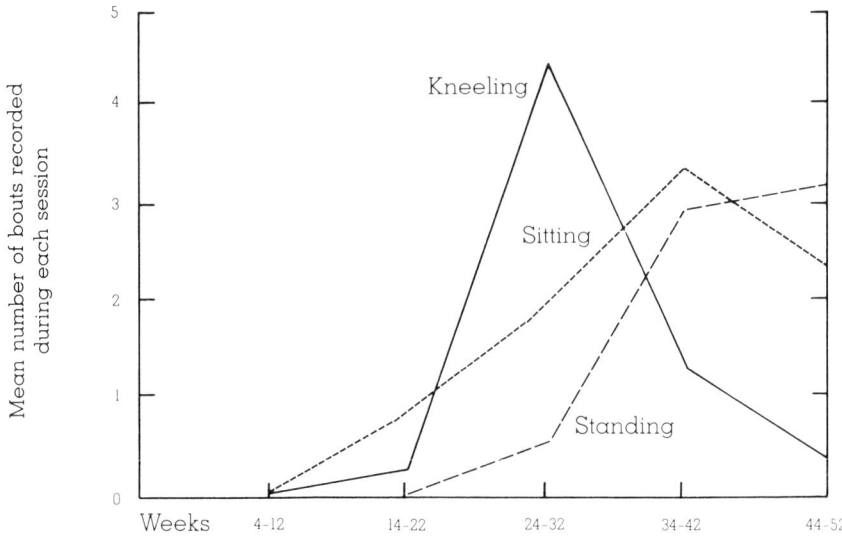

Note: Drawn from data in ''Rhythmical Stereotypies in Infants'' by E. Thelen, 1979, *Animal Behaviour, 27*, pp. 699-715. Used by permission of the author and the publisher, Ballière Tindall, London.

The following strategies are based on traditional knowledge about how infant reflexes work and the nature of stages leading toward upright locomotion, as well as relatively recent information about the role of rhythmic stereotypies in the make-up of infants. These findings and conclusions strongly suggest that specific movements should be encouraged in infants who are hypotonic, as well as some who are hypertonic.

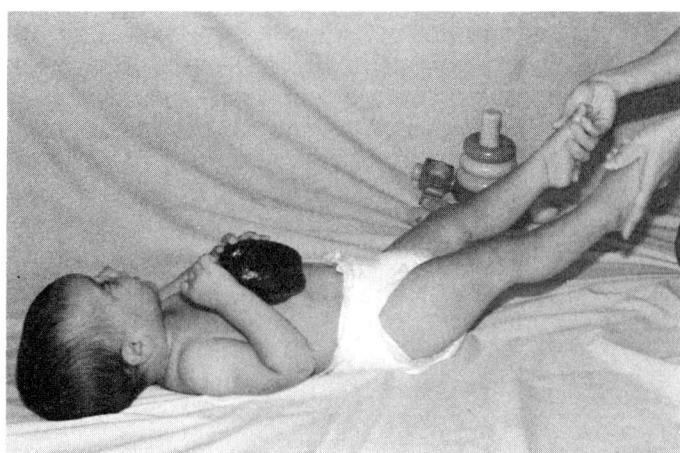

The therapist encourages leg stereotypies (alternate kicking) in an infant.

When an infant is able to support himself or herself in sitting, the therapist (or parent) might gently rock the infant back and forth and from side to side to stimulate the balance and muscular patterns needed to maintain a stable seated position. The same strategy might be employed when the infant begins to posture in a creeping position (hand-knee), and to stand. Rocking of the trunk and actions of the arms and legs might be guided during even earlier stages of development.

Care might have to be taken if a pre-schooler is suspected of being autistic, as the stereotypies seen in autistic children may be pathologically delayed manifestations of the rhythmics seen in normal children during their first year to 16 months. Autistic stereotypies, therefore, should not be encouraged by using the strategies and methods discussed and illustrated.

Positioning and Placement Strategies

Developmentally delayed infants may be positioned and placed in many ways to facilitate motor development. For example, an infant whose trunkle muscles and strength do not permit unaided sitting should be placed in positions that permit the hands to grasp and manipulate objects. A hypertonic youngster could be propped up on bolsters, as illustrated in Figure 25.5, to permit active manipulation.

The platitude often expressed that a child's gross-motor development must precede, and transfers to, fine-motor development is simply not defensible in the case of late-developing infants. Many infants whose trunkle strengths do not permit sitting and similar gross-motor skills are able to advance quite well in manipulative fine-motor tasks involving the hands.

Figure 25.5   Positioning to Allow for Exploration and Manipulation

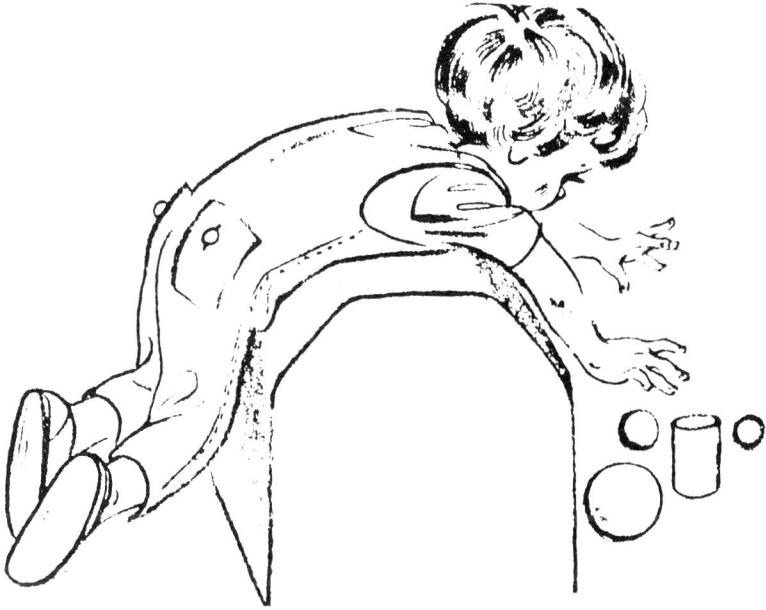

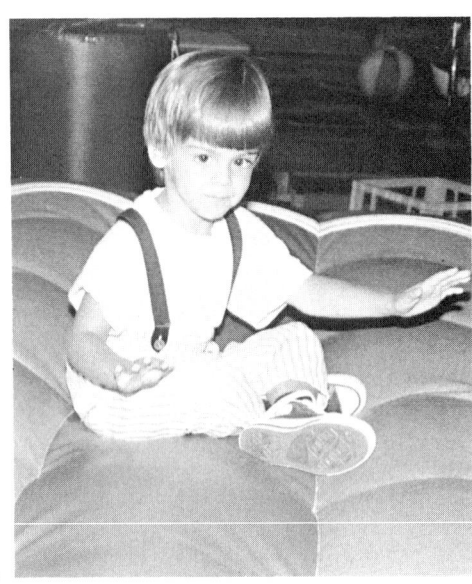

Soft surfaces help children relax.

Placement in upright positions permits the delayed infant to acquire a normal three-dimensional perspective of the visual world. This type of upright position may be accomplished at a table to help the young child feel equal to his or her normally developing peers.

The too-tense child may be aided by positionings of various kinds. A soft, giving surface helps youngsters to relax and extend their limbs before active manipulation and therapy take place, as pictured.

At times the therapist may relax excess tensions by promoting helpful reflexes. For example, an infant or child who exhibits severe flexion on one side of the body (e.g., an arm is flexed against the side with undue tension) may be helped to extend that arm by first turning the head away from the flexed side, and then trying to gently straighten out the hypertonic arm. This triggers the asymmetrical tonic neck reflex—a response that results in heightened arm-leg tension on the side toward which the head is turned and conversely results in a lessening of tension on the side away from the turned head.

This same asymmetrical reflex may prevent a hypertonic infant from turning over from front to back. As shown in Figure 25.6, turning over (a) may be facilitated by stimulating a body-derotative response (b) if the infant has a good support response (c). If the asymmetrical tonic neck reflex is too strong, however, it will detract from turning over, as the arm will act as a brake when the head turns (d). This arm's tension may be reduced by gently tapping the back of the upper arm and applying pressure to the biceps of the arm acting as a brake.

Experienced therapists have in their repertoire a large number of these strategies. They should be consulted and observed by others who are helping infants gain essential actions. The enterprising person also might consult recent writings with complete discussions of infant reflexes and stereotypies, including one of mine.[2]

2. *Perceptual and Motor Development in Infants and Children* (3rd ed.) by B.J. Cratty, 1986, Englewood Cliffs, NJ: Prentice-Hall.

Figure 25.6   Contributors and Detractors to Rolling Over

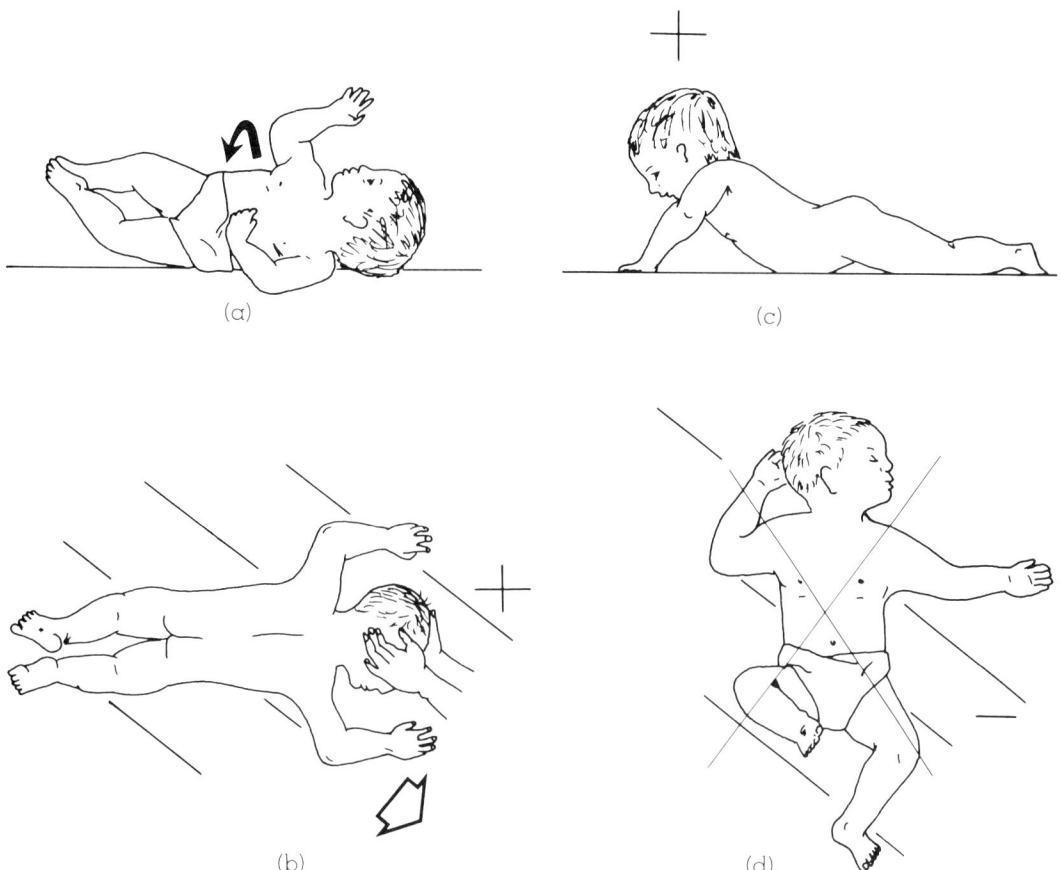

(a)

(c)

(b)

(d)

Note: From *Perceptual and Motor Development in Infants and Children* by B.J. Cratty, 1979, Englewood Cliffs, NJ: Prentice-Hall. Used by permission.

Sensory Stimulation

Movement itself involves sensations. In execution of a movement, kinesthetic receptors provide important information to the central nervous system—information that is used (if the action is slow enough) to program and then execute the next action or part of an action. As infants' actions and positions are molded, encouraged, and assisted by a therapist, important sensory information also is produced.

Formulators of content for infant intervention programs must be sure to insert special ways in which the infants may receive a variety of sensory stimulations. At the same time they must not be over-stimulated. For example, visual displays that are too complex may overwhelm or overexcite an infant looking up at them from the crib.

Developmentally, the parts of the nervous system that monitor tactile information are relatively mature near birth, and the centers of the brain that receive and organize visual and auditory information mature shortly afterward, during the first year or two.

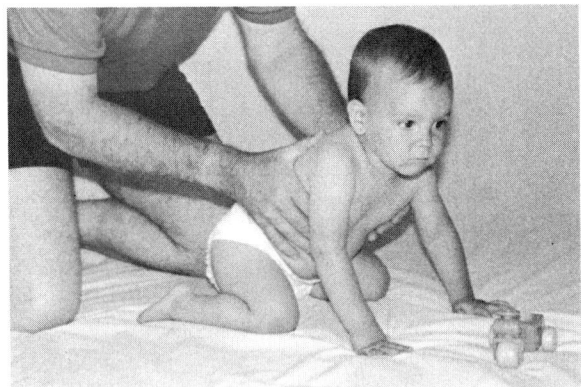

Gentle massage is often used in programs of infant stimulation.

Tactile Stimulation   Tactile stimulation often is employed in conjunction with kinesthe-tic/vestibular stimulation. Massage may be combined with rocking and work on water beds, accompanied by vocalizations (Rose & Bridger, 1979). Programs of infant stimulation abroad have emphasized the importance of gentle massage, as pictured. It is advocated that the limbs be stroked and massaged, to enhance movement capacities.

Auditory Stimulation   The most important kind of sound information emanates from the mouth of the caregiver or therapist in the speech and language of the child's culture. During the first six months of life, children babble, emitting a wide variety of sounds that are found in all language families.[3] If their hearing is normal, by about the sixth month the infant begins to echo back only those sounds heard from others—sounds important in the language of that culture.

Thus, infants, especially those with potential problems, must be talked to frequently and when appropriate caregiving tasks (feeding, diapering, dressing) are being carried out. A lack of response from "suspect" infants makes caregivers' jobs harder, as they are not being reinforced by infant responses for their communicative efforts.

Visual Stimulation   Visual stimulation is derived from stables hung over cribs, mirrors, and movements of the caregiver's face. Normal infants give close attention to facial expressions as well as to movements of the mouth of those nearby. Smiling is one of these reciprocal expressions, as pictured.

Vestibular Stimulation   Vestibular stimulation is necessary in the development of normal motor capacities. Typically, therapists spend a great deal of time providing experiences that will encourage the child's balance mechanisms to function better. The structures of the inner ear provide information about the child's relation to gravity as head control is gained, and then sitting, kneeling, and standing postures are attempted.

---

3. This apparently innate babbling is heard even in deaf infants during the same early months.

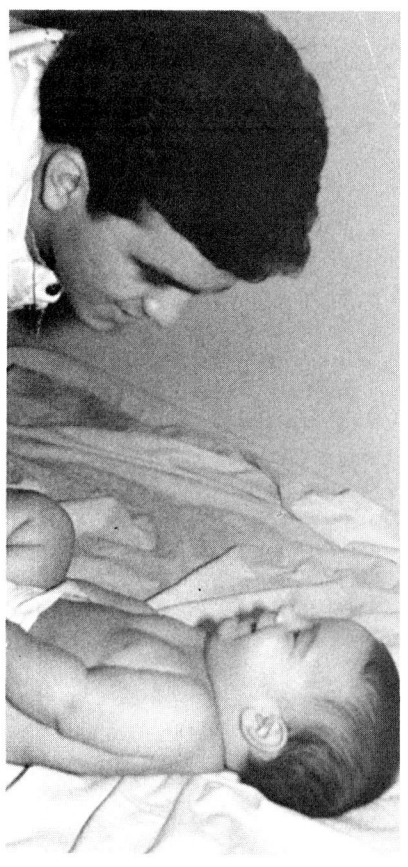

Smiling often is elicited in the presence of a smiling face hovering over the crib.

The therapist tries to trigger "tilt," or support, responses. This may be done, as pictured, by making the child unstable on a stable base. The child is gently moved from side to side in a sitting position while being helped to compensate for the movement to the left by a head shift to the right and to support the imbalance by reaching out with the hand on the side of the imbalance.

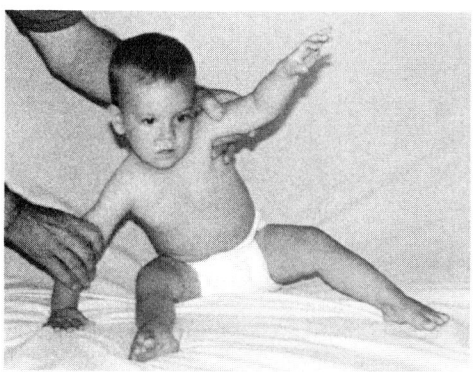

The child is being aided in the tilt response.

Figure 25.7   Unstable Surface to Stimulate Tilt Reactions

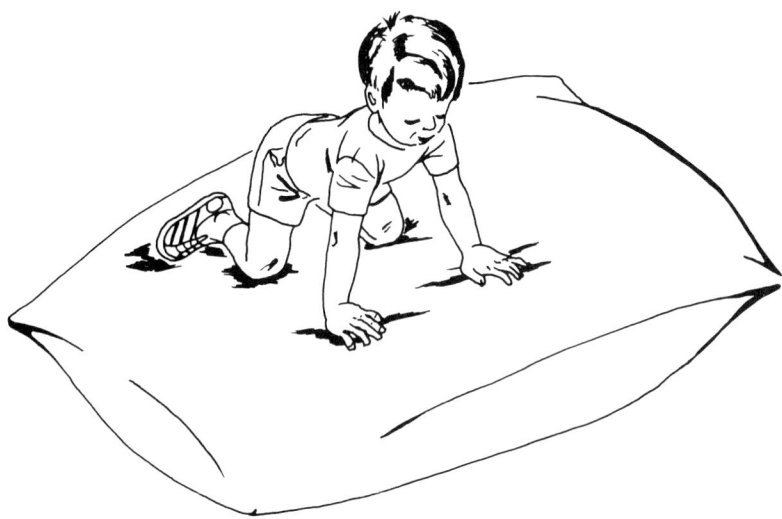

Or the base on which the infant is postured (seated, lying) may be unstable, as shown in Figure 25.7. Again, the infant is encouraged to regain balance with proper head-body alignments and limb compensation.

Third, the infant may be placed in a continuously moving platform to train vestibular functioning. The Ayres method of sensory integration (see chapter 5) emphasizes this type of experience. Care must be taken, however, so that the experience does not unsettle the youngster, causing stomach upset or even triggering seizures.

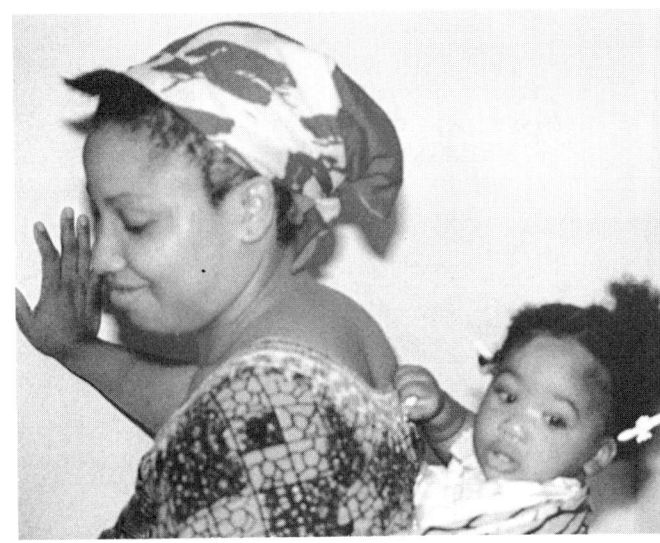

Carrying an infant provides physical contact, gives the infant an upright view of the world, and promotes good head control.

One of the more important sensory stimulation experiences is offered by carrying infants around as pictured. This provides vestibular information in an upright position; it provides touch information as contact is maintained between the carrier and the infant; it provides the infant with visual information of both a static and a moving nature; and it motivates the infant to better control the head.

The few examples given here are far from exhaustive. Special efforts to provide sensory stimulation should not be made capriciously. Mere sensory input without careful thought and planning may produce as many adverse as positive effects. Appropriate sensory input at appropriate intensity levels is advocated.

Thought and Language

When possible, movement interventions should be planned so that the child has concomitant opportunities for thought and language experiences. A program providing only for pure movement experiences is superficial and short-sighted.

The movements discussed previously should be accompanied by words, as the therapist describes for the child what is happening. In this way infants' receptive language capacities may be stimulated. For example, as the infant is assisted to assume a seated position, the therapist might say, "Now we are sitting up tall and can reach for that block there in front of you," while handing the block to the child. This provides a link between the object and the word "block."

Object manipulation provides many opportunities to pair social, intellectual, and language behaviors with actions. For example, a child who is led through various stages in the concept of object permanence may be helped to understand that objects can have an existence even when out of view. First a desired object may be partly hidden, with the child given the opportunity to recover it. Next the object may be completely hidden, as pictured. Further stages can include giving the object impetus (rolling it) behind an opaque screen, with an effort to help the infant predict the position in which it is likely to emerge from the other side of the barrier.

Many pairings of thought, speech/language, and action may be devised and incorporated into infant intervention programs in which movement may be a primary focus. For exam-

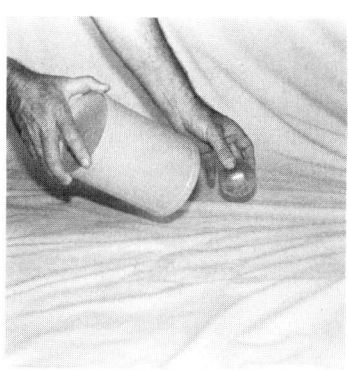

Desired object is hidden, with child observing.

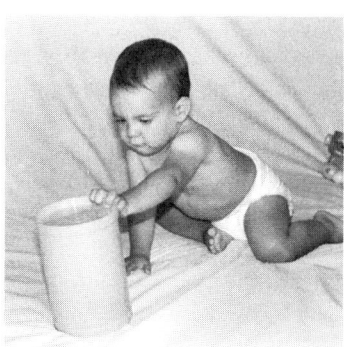

Child removes cover and obtains object.

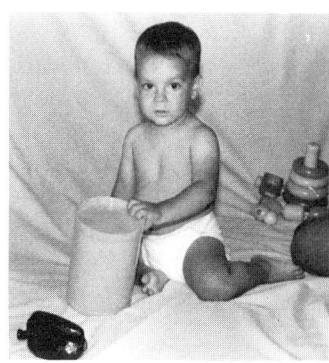

"There—I did it!"

ple, as the child gains expressive language, the therapist should name the action, and the child should be asked to repeat it before, during, and after it takes place. In the evolution of motor-speech relationships, this kind of pairing usually occurs naturally. For example, a 3-year-old may be heard to say on the playground: "Johnny (I) is going to bounce the ball." . . . "Now (as the ball is bounced) Johnny is bouncing the ball." . . . "There (after the action is completed) the ball bounced!"

Speech and expressive language should not be forced into developmental programs, however. Consultation and teamwork with a speech pathologist are essential. Overloading the child with too many language skill requirements while engaged in movement therapy of various kinds may interfere with the development of both speech and actions.

Developmental psychologists such as Bower (1974) have sought to discover important precursors to intellectual development in children. One study monitored infant-parent pairs through recording devices. It was found that later intellectual adequacy was preceded by parent-child interactions that encouraged children to try out hypotheses. As two pots are banged together, youngsters discover what makes noise. Throwing objects in a pail of water produces information about what objects are denser than others. Most hypothesis testing of this kind requires movement skills. Thus, therapists who acquire the knowledge and skills to provide intellectual and language content along with movement opportunities in programs of infant intervention are in a position to expand and promote the child's total development.

EVALUATION TOOLS AND STRATEGIES

Evaluation is a critical part of educational programs, and the infant intervention program is no exception. The instruments and measures used vary in complexity and sophistication, as well as the data upon which they are based. Two excellent instruments evaluate the complex interweaving between voluntary movements and reflexes during the first year of life. The first was developed by pediatric neurologists in Italy, Drs. Milani-Comparetti and Gidoni (1965). It is used to assess possible motor development lags and requires some background in infant reflexes and early responses. A second, more recent and slightly more complex, instrument of this same type was developed by two American physical therapists, Hoskins and Squires (1973).

Innumerable scales extending back over 50 years list developmental stages through which infants and children pass. These include the well known instruments by Arnold Gesell (Gesell & Amatruda, 1947) and Nancy Bayley (1984). The Denver Developmental Screening Test (Frankenburg, Dodds, & Fandal, 1975) is particularly useful because of its flexibility in indicating the *range* of months through which a behavior is likely to appear rather than assigning rigid, specific times (see Figure 3.3 in chapter 3). Another helpful tool was designed by Koontz (1974). Obtained from a survey of norms, it is accompanied by strategies that may be used to stimulate each of the behaviors listed. Other tools include the Inventory of Early Development by Brigance (1977) and the sophisticated rating tool by Brazelton (1973), which, in the hands of a well trained specialist, can reveal important information about the social/emotional and psychological make-up of infants.

In the 1980s two trends have become apparent relative to the early motor evaluation of both normal and at-risk infants' motor abilities. An increasing number of assessment instruments are directed specifically toward evaluating motor competencies. In contrast to earlier instruments such as the Gessell and the Bayley scales, these recently developed tools focus only on motor development and provide good guidelines for both assessment and program planning. Some of these are directed toward evaluation of suspect infants and pre-schoolers (Campbell & Wilhelm, 1985).

Observational assessments of infant motor development are becoming more objective and reliable (Harris, Halty, Tada, & Swanson, 1984), and tasks are being scored both qualitatively and quantitatively (Noller & Ingrisano, 1984). Traditional scales developed earlier to assess the interaction of infant reflexes and early voluntary responses, such as the Milani-Comparetti (Milani-Comparetti & Gidoni, 1965), now can be scored in more objective-numerical ways than in the past (Ellison, Browning, Larson, & Denny, 1983). Armed with these new assessment instruments, those who formulate programs will become better able to assess progress, develop valid programmatic objectives and components, and provide more concrete guidelines for the assisting behaviors of staff members.

GENERAL GUIDELINES

When approaching the area of infant stimulation, physical educators should be aware of the following basic issues:

- The need for proper training, together with adequate consultation and teamwork.
- Knowledge of the wide variety and differentiation of techniques and strategies to accommodate the vast individual differences within developmentally delayed populations.
- The need to optimize the amount and type of sensory stimulation in conjunction with motor stimulation.
- The necessity of communicating to parents, volunteer aides, as well as others involved with the child, the essential one-to-one manipulations involved.
- The importance of a sound, proven evaluation program to pinpoint the youngster's problem areas, which can serve as a navigation aid to formulating appropriate programs.

SUMMARY

For the most part, the methods for early stimulation described in this chapter apply to ages ranging from early infancy to about 18-20 months developmentally. The "suspect" population can be divided largely into two major groups—those who have excess muscle tension (hypertonic) and those who lack adequate muscular tone and control (hypotonic). In addition are emerging classifications of children who are being treated for early leukemia and infants of drug-abusing mothers. Intervention strategies stem from knowledge of reflex functions of the normal child and rhythmic stereotypies seen in infants during their first 18 months of life.

Among the strategies and principles covered are (a) good therapy hands, which means using the appropriate amount of assistance physically to enable the youngster to proceed through the sequential stages of turning, sitting, kneeling, creeping, standing, and walking; (b) using objects and tasks to increase the probability that infants will advance from static postures; (c) encouraging the rhythmic stereotypies that are found naturally in infants; (d) various placement strategies to free the hands and arms for manipulative activity; (e) sensory stimulation (visual, auditory, tactile, and vestibular); and (f) exploring ways in which movement tasks may be combined with linguistic and intellectual skill development. Useful evaluation instruments include those that reflect the intricate interweaving of reflexes and early voluntary movements and more traditional instruments based upon the normal stages of development.

A major challenge to be met by educators, therapists, and medical personnel during the last years of this century will be to provide adequate programming for young children whose developmental stages are suspect or lagging behind normal infants and children during the first 3 years of life. The more familiar interventionists are with all developmental phases—language, motor, social, cognitive—the better able they will be to employ strategies and assistance that will aid the child's total development.

REFERENCES

Astbury, J., Orgill, A.A., Bajuk, B., & Yul, V.T.H. (1983). Determinants of developmental performance of very low birthweight survivors at one and two years. *Developmental Medicine & Child Neurology, 25,* 709-716.

Balster, R.L. (1980). The effects of PCP and three analogues on motor performance in mice. *Pharmacology, 20,* 46-51.

Bayley, N. (1984). *Bayley scales of infant development.* New York: Psychological Corp.

Bower, T.G.R. (1974). *Development in infancy.* San Francisco: W.H. Freeman.

Brazelton, T.B. (1973). *Neonatal behavioral assessment scale.* Philadelphia: Lippincott.

Bricker, D.D. (1982). *Intervention with at-risk and handicapped infants.* Baltimore: University Park Press.

Brigance, A. (1977). *Inventory of early development* (2nd ed.). North Billerica, MA: Curriculum Associates.

Bromwich, R.M. (1977). Stimulation in the first year of life? A perspective on infant development. *Young Children, 14,* 71-83.

Campbell, S.K., & Wilhelm, I.J. (1985). Development from birth to three years of age of 15 children at very high risk for central nervous system dysfunction. *Physical Therapy, 65,* 463-469.

Chasnoff, I.J. (1983). Phencyclidine effects on the fetus and neonate. *Developmental Pharmacology Therapy, 6,* 404-408.

Cratty, B.J. (1986). *Perceptual development in infants and children* (3rd ed.). Englewood Cliffs, NJ: Prentice-Hall.

Ellison, P., Browning, C.A., Larson, B., & Denny, J. (1983). Development of a scoring system for the Milani-Comparetti and Gidoni method of assessing neurological abnormality in infancy. *Physical Therapy, 63,* 1414-1423.

Eng, G.D., Koch, B., & Binder, H. (1979). *Infantile hypotonia: Diagnostic dilemma* (Monograph). Washington, DC: Children's Hospital, Dept. of Medicine & Rehabilitation.

Frankenburg, W.K., Dodds, J.B., & Fandal, A. (1975). *The Denver developmental screening test.* Denver: Ladoca Publishing Foundation.

Freedman, D., Boverman, H., & Freedman, N. (1966). *Effects of kinesthetic stimulation on weight gain and on smiling in premature infants.* Paper presented at the meeting of the American Orthopsychiatric Association, San Francisco.

Gesell, A., & Amatruda, C.S. (1947). *Developmental diagnosis:* New York: Paul B. Holder.

Golden, N.L. (1982). A practical method for identifying angel dust abuse during pregnancy. *American Journal of Obstetrics & Gynecology, 142*, 359-360.

Harris, S.R., Halty, S.M., Tada, W.L., & Swanson, M.W. (1984). Reliability of observational measures of the movement assessment of infants. *Physical Therapy, 64*, 471-475.

Hoskins, T.A., & Squires, J.E. (1973). Developmental assessment: A test for gross motor and reflex development. *Physical Therapy, 53*, 117-126.

Koontz, C.C. (1974). *Koontz child development program.* Los Angeles: Western Psychological Services.

Korner, A.F., Ruppel, E., & Rho, J. (1982). Effects of water beds on the sleep and motility of therophylline-treated premature infants. *Pediatrics, 70*, 864-869.

Milani-Comparetti, A., & Gidoni, E.A. (1965). Pattern analysis of motor development and its disorders. *Developmental Medicine & Child Neurology, 9*, 631-638.

Noller, K., & Ingrisano, D. (1984). Cross-sectional study of gross and fine motor development. *Physical Therapy, 64*, 308-313.

Pasamanick, B., & Knobloch, H. (1966). Retrospective studies on epidemiology of reproductive causality: Old and new. *Merrill Palmer Quarterly, 12*, 7-26.

Rice, R.D. (1977). Neurophysiological development in premature infants following stimulation. *Developmental Psychology, 13*, 69-76.

Rose, S.A., & Bridger, W.H. (1979, March). *Enhancing visual recognition memory in pre-term infants.* Paper presented at the meeting of the Society for Research in Child Development, San Francisco.

Rossett, H.L., & Sander, L.W. (1979). Effects of maternal drinking on neonatal morphology and state. In J.D. Osofsky (Ed.), *The handbook of infant development.* New York: Wiley.

Thelen, E. (1981). Kicking, rocking and waving—Contextual analysis of rhythmic stereotypies in normal human infants. *Journal of Animal Behaviour, 23*, 3-11.

Thelen, E., & Fisher, D.M. (1983). From spontaneous to instrumental behavior: Kinematic analysis of movement changes during very early learning. *Child Development, 54*, 129-140.

Ulrich, B.D. (1984). The effects of stimulation programs on the development of high risk infants: A review of research. *Adapted Physical Activity Quarterly, 1*, 68-80.

ADDITIONAL REFERENCES

Cratty, B.J. (1986). Evaluation of movement qualities. In B.J. Cratty, *Perceptual and motor development of infants and children* (3rd ed.) (ch. 10). Englewood Cliffs, NJ: Prentice-Hall.

Uhlig, G.E., & Krantz, M. (1976). *Research on the psychomotor development of young handicapped children.* Washington, DC: U.S. Office of Education.

QUESTIONS FOR DISCUSSION

1. What are stereotypies, and what is their role in the motor stimulation of infants?
2. In what ways might a hypotonic infant and a hypertonic infant differ in appear-ance and movement characteristics? In what different ways might a therapist work with each of the two types of infants?
3. How might the asymmetrical tonic-

neck reflex be used in therapy?

4. What general principles might be formulated to guide parents through a home-applied program of infant stimulation?

5. How might an infant who lacks the ability to sit be placed so that the hands are free to manipulate objects in the environment?

6. How can objects be used to stimulate infants' movement characteristics and developmental goals?

STUDENT PROJECTS

1. Visit a program of infant stimulation. Try to ascertain what general principles are being employed and the role of movement experiences within the program.

2. Either through library research or through interviews with experts, formulate an assessment program helpful in the early identification of motor problems in infants and pre-school children.

3. Construct a program of infant stimulation to incorporate early cognitive experiences. Be specific.

RESOURCES

American Alliance for Health,
   Physical Education and Recreation
1201-16th St., N.W.
Washington, DC 20036

Division for Early Childhood
Council for Exceptional Children
1290 Association Dr.
Reston, VA 22091

26 Self-Control and Attention

The most pervasive characteristics of populations of children and youth with special needs are distractibility, lack of self-control, and poor attention. Typically these problems occur because the individual is overactivated or too excited to function normally, or underactivated or too "dreamy" to pay proper attention to important parts of the environment. These problems can be manifested in (a) poor assimilation of a lesson, (b) social abrasiveness and aggression toward peers, parents, and teachers, and (c) physical danger to the child or youth himself or herself.

Over the years many professionals have suspected that hyperactivity and inattention have a familial basis. Data from a recent study suggest that hyperactive children may or may not have family members who are similarly afflicted (August & Stewart, 1983). These same investigators found that a child, one of whose parents may have been hyperactive, is likely to display a greater variety of behavioral disturbances than a child whose family members are free of hyperactive tendencies. Usually, hyperactivity in a child is caused by organic (neurological) problems combined with environmental and social-emotional factors. Educators promoting physical activity have a special obligation to understand the root causes of distractible behaviors and provide techniques and methods by which these undesirable aspects of behavior may be adjusted in positive ways. A useful tool has been developed by Torrey (1981) to help parents and others identify hyperactive-hypertensive children in need of various kinds of intervention. This Hyperactivity Behaviors Identification Questionnaire is beginning to be used in various research studies (Brandon, Eason, & Smith, 1986). The questionnaire asks the rater to rank a child on a 5-point scale ranging from 5—always through 3—sometimes to 1—never. Thirteen statements are rated in this manner. For example: "My child gets into things" . . . "My child is easily upset" . . . "My child is impatient."

For several decades various medications (usually stimulant drugs) have been used in efforts to reduce hyperactive/inattentive behaviors. For the most part, however, medications have not significantly improved test scores, they produce highly variable individual reactions, and they may not have long-term positive effects extending into adulthood. Recent reviews of this kind of therapy suggest that some behavioral interventions, including cognitive-behavioral techniques such as those described here, are superior (Gadow, 1983).

In the last several decades, methods of activation adjustment have involved changing physiological behaviors (muscular relaxation, deep breathing, and the like), imagery (e.g., "Imagine yourself by a quiet stream"), and, more recently, helping people to *think* differently and thus aid in self-control (e.g., "Tell me how you should plan this lesson before starting it"). Some of these methods have been inspired by mystical-religious strategies dating back for centuries; others are the product of modern psychologists who are interested in cognitive adjustment. Physical education teachers who can call upon several of these techniques when appropriate can be far more effective than those who cannot or will not.

And children and youth who learn and are able to apply methods of self-control often acquire heightened feelings of self-worth and self-effectiveness (Meichenbaum & Goodman, 1969).

DIMENSIONS OF THE PROBLEM

Hyperactivity and lack of attentiveness have numerous facets. Indeed, a case may be made that hyperactivity is in the eye of the beholder! Hyperactive children at times have been found objectively to be no more active than students judged "good" by their teachers; their movements simply occur at socially inappropriate times.

With that note of caution, hyperactivity may be classified into at least three broad categories: (a) *visual hyperactivity*—displayed by children whose bodies remain in place (in their classroom seats) but whose eyes dart from place to place; (b) *bodily hyperactivity*—demonstrated by children who do not remain in one place and are seldom in their seats or in proper positions for participation in planned activities; and (c) *manipulative hyperactivity*—exhibited by children whose hands are constantly moving although the body remains relatively fixed. Of course, some individuals evidence all of these behaviors in various combinations.

Theories and models that try to explain hyperactive behavior abound. These generally focus on any of three sets of variables: (a) *neurological health* of the individual, or causes arising within the person; (b) *behavioral make-up* of the person together with the make-up of the social environment in which the person must function; and (c) *learning-teaching environment*. To some extent, the acceptance of a given model or theory—particularly as it relates to a specific child or youth—tends to guide remedial strategies.

For example, an explanation or diagnosis of a child as having a neurological problem (usually related to brain stem function) may prompt the prescription of a medication to correct the problem. On the other hand, a more environmental or behavioral orientation toward a given youngster's distractibility encourages the use of psychotherapy coupled with adjustment of learning and social variables.

Finally, hyperactivity and related attentional disorders sometimes are situational. A child may have relatively controlled behavior in one setting (in the home, while watching TV) while at school he or she may be judged as highly impulsive and difficult to teach. Therefore, a thorough diagnosis of a so-called hyperactive child should involve assessments of that child in a number of the life settings in which he or she must function.

PRINCIPLES, GUIDELINES, AND TECHNIQUES

The remainder of this chapter contains straightforward techniques that have been found useful in reducing hyperactivity and improving attention and self-control, with emphasis on the principles and general guidelines underlying them. No hyperactive child is like another; most have unique problems. Therefore, professionals involved with the child should work closely as a team and should apply individually designed programs to a given child or youth. The interventions covered here are limited to those appropriately applied by a physical educator. Although medication, diet control, and other strategies often are used in conjunction with the movement strategies to be discussed, the former should be supervised by professionals who are competent in their use.

Muscular Relaxation

Edmund Jacobson (1938) has been credited with introducing techniques involving muscular relaxation in the English language texts almost 50 years ago. This approach is based on two major premises:

1. Individuals can learn, usually with the help of others at first, to adjust muscular tension.

2. The control or reduction of excess muscular tension is likely to produce parallel and positive adjustments of an individual's emotional state.

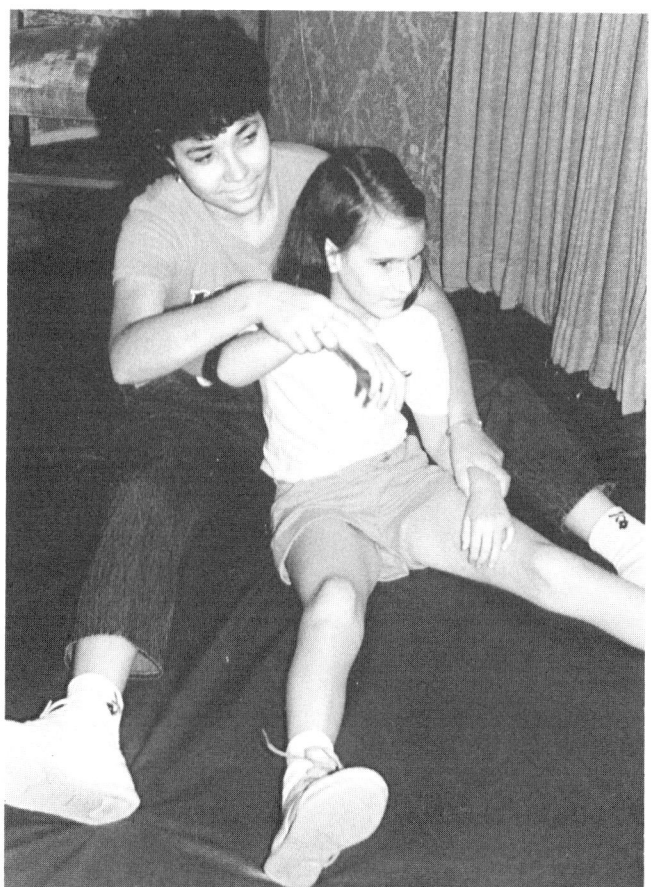

In the puppet game the instructor works from behind the child, encouraging her to relax completely so the instructor can move the child's arms.

Typically a session involves talking an overly tense individual through successive stages of relaxation, together with imagery that is likely to induce better perceptions of excess tension and of consecutive stages in relaxation. Capable, mature persons often can adopt the technique after a few sessions. With atypical individuals, however, the program is supervised by a therapist or instructor. Effective relaxation specialists are able to conjure up effective relaxation imagery through appropriate words and phrases. The following lesson might take place after the youngster has been placed in a comfortable position, as seen in Figure 26.1.

First, see how hard you can tighten the muscles in your face by closing your eyes tightly and tightening the muscles of your cheeks. . . . Now try to relax these same muscles completely—first the muscles of your forehead . . . now those around your mouth . . . and now the jaw muscles and cheek muscles.

Now let's move down your body and do the same thing with the muscles in the front of your neck. Pull your chin down toward your chest, and tighten the muscles in your neck . . . harder. . . . Now relax your neck completely, and slowly move your head up and down to see if you have done so. (Often the teacher/therapist will move the person's limbs and other body parts to see if tension and then relaxation have been consecutively achieved.)

Now let's go further down your body and tighten the muscles in the front of your chest as hard as you can. Roll your shoulders slightly inward to do this. Now take a deep breath and relax your chest muscles completely . . . more . . . more. . . . Take another breath and let it out.

Next we will work on your arms. Tighten your arms to your side and make hard balls of your fists. . . . Now release your hands, relax them in an extended position, and try to relax your arms and shoulders completely.

The stomach muscles might be alternately tightened and relaxed in the same way. Then the therapist/teacher might proceed downward to the hips, leg, and feet muscles and work up again from the feet to the head and face. During successive sessions, finer and finer discriminations of muscle tension might be promoted. For example: "Now you have tightened your muscle as hard as you can. See if you can tighten it half that hard . . . now half-again as hard as you did last time."

Relaxation training often is accompanied by visual imagery and helpful breathing exercises. For example: "Imagine yourself beside a quiet stream as you lie there relaxing." Tightening muscles often is paired with breath holding. Relaxation may be heightened if the student attempts to exhale completely or to breathe rhythmically with complete inhalation and exhalation.

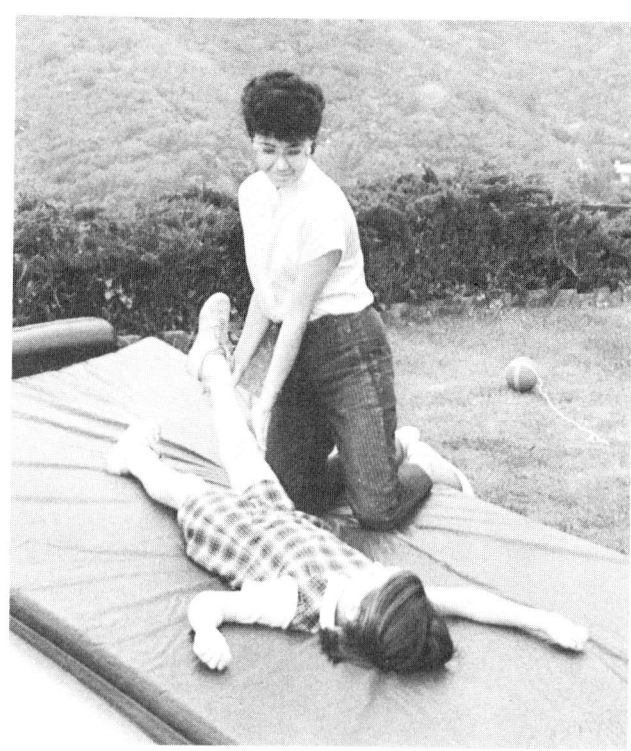

*Lifting the leg and letting it
drop encourages relaxation.*

Figure 26.1   A Position Conducive to Relaxation Training

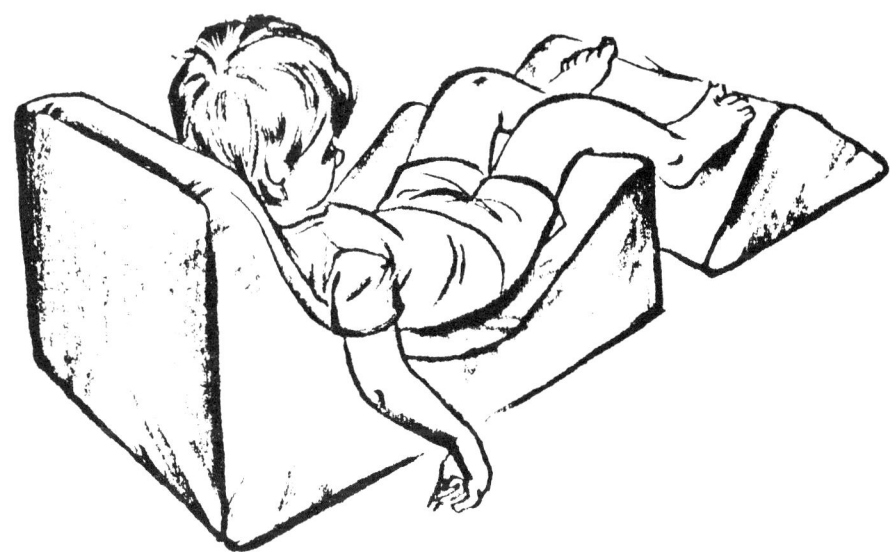

Jacobson's traditional methods are constantly being refined and improved. For example, Herson and Barlow (1976) have developed a technique they have labeled *behavioral relaxation training* (BRT). It involves directing training in 10 postures that have been found to be maximally relaxing, based upon electromyographic verification. This method has been used in several recent studies (Brandon, Eason, & Smith, 1986; Poppen & Maurer, 1982; Schilling & Poppen, 1983) with both adult and child subjects, achieving positive results. And Jacobson also applied his techniques to children (Jacobson, 1973). At times relaxation training administered through tapes has resulted in behavioral and academic improvement in children and youth (Dunn & Howell, 1982).

Relaxation training has had many recent applications with various kinds of special populations. For example, Glantz (1983) found that reading improved in adults with emotional problems when they received relaxation training together with breathing exercises. Hypertensive patients achieved significant reductions in both systolic and diastolic blood pressure following relaxation training; moreover, these effects were maintained after a 5-month period (Wadden, 1983).

In another study (Rickard, Thrasher, & Elkins, 1984), individuals within four IQ ranges were found to benefit from several types of relaxation training, including those involving imagery as well as suggestions to relax and to control breathing. Even the individuals in the lower functioning groups seemed to comprehend the instructions and benefit from the training. Brandon and his colleagues (Brandon et al., 1986) found that relaxation training improved the ability of learning disabled males to attend to a "demanding motor task." Relaxation training also has been shown to be effective in handwriting training, auditory memory, spelling, and oral reading (Carter, Lax, & Russell, 1979; Carter & Russell, 1980; Carter & Synolds, 1974).

Relaxation training has several advantages—and a few cautions. Advantages include the fact that it is easily applied, with a minimum of space, time, and expense. Emotionally "high" children may be aided by reducing muscular tension, leading to reduced emotional tension.

Two major cautions are: (a) At times children may be brought too far "down" and rendered too lethargic for subsequent participation (in a demonstration in Spain, a "helpful" volunteer put six children so far "under" that they could be awakened only with great effort and care on the part of onlookers!) and (b) the methodology may not work equally well with all people. Individuals have unique patterns of muscular tension that, while consistent within that person, vary greatly from person to person. Some children and adults have activated emotional states that are not accompanied by any discernible muscular tension. Thus, even though the techniques are practiced over time, positive results may not be obtained with all individuals.

Nevertheless, this method, and variations thereof, is potentially beneficial in arousal adjustment. Medication, if recommended by educationally sophisticated physicians, may be a helpful adjunct. When applied optimally, success in using this approach is probable over time.

In the early 1980s Schilling and Poppen (1983) developed a useful behavioral relaxation scale composed of 10 behaviors that purportedly reflect a state of relaxation, including "(a) body—no movement of the body trunk, (b) mouth-lips—slightly parted at the center of the mouth, (c) feet—pointed away from each other." In general these observational sign-posts correlate rather well with electromyographic evidence of relaxation (Poppen & Maurer, 1982).

Impulse Control Activities

Activities that encourage slow, controlled actions may be useful in adjusting tendencies to move too much, to move inappropriately, or to exhibit poor attention span. Historically, impulse-control exercises have been a part of oriental cultures, where they continue today. Middle-aged and elderly Chinese people often begin their day with Tai Chi.[1]

Two simpler impulse-control games are illustrated. Both involve using a well controlled peer as a model with whom the less controlled (hyperactive) child may identify by imitating well controlled movements. In one photo the hyperactive child is a closely following "shadow" to the model. In the second a tactile tracking game is employed, in which the hyperactive child replicates slow and fast movements of the model. Prolonged walking tasks like that illustrated in Figure 26.2 likewise may lengthen the attention span.

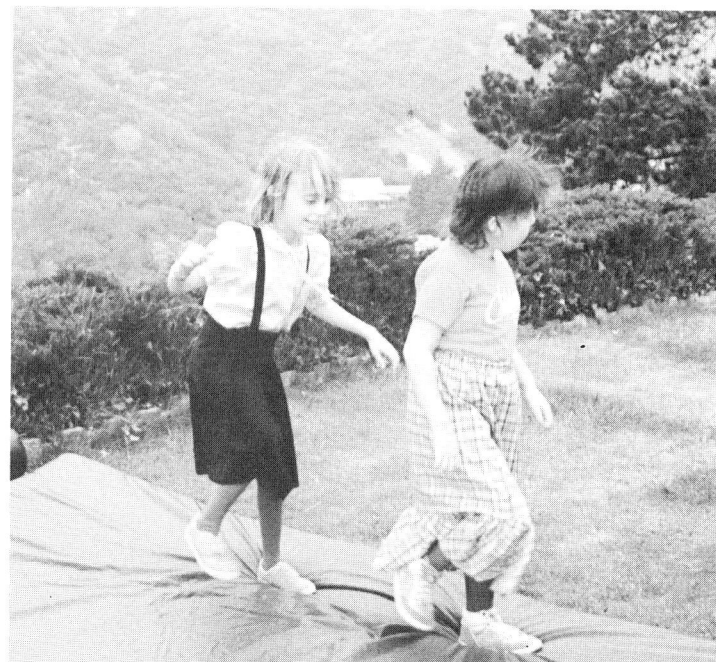

Playing "Me and My Shadow" helps the hyperactive child, who imitates the movements of a controlled child.

1. Positive physiological effects presented in research studies discussed at the International Congress of Sports Medicine in Beijing in 1985 include delays in deterioration of bones, as well as heightened flexibility.

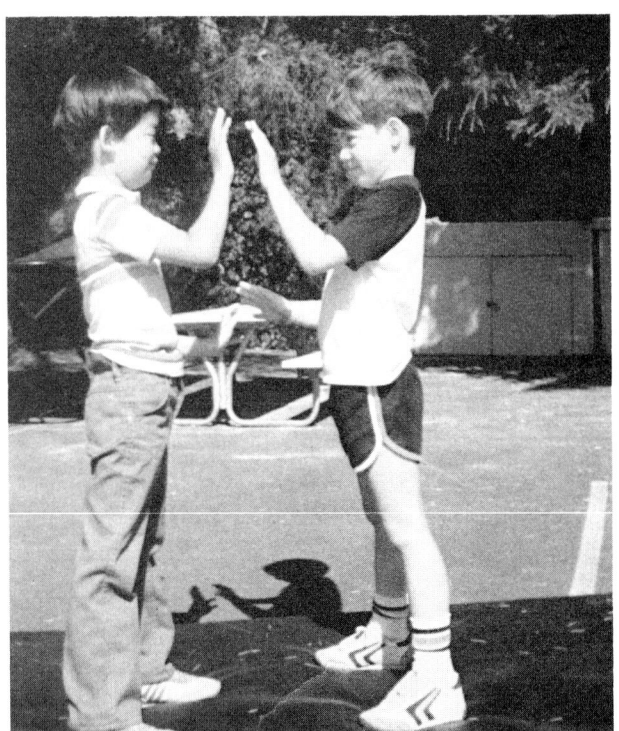

Hyperactive child follows movements of another child through tactile tracking.

These activities also may be used as evaluative tools, because rather precise scores may be obtained from requests such as, "Draw a line as slowly as you can" or perhaps, "Stand up (from a back-lying position) as slowly as you can." Furthermore, controlled movements of this kind may be encouraged by having students compete in tasks to determine which of them can *finish last* in activities such as line walking, slow drawing, and arising. These impulse-control activities may be reinforced by external rewards in programs of traditional behavior modification. Moreover, their use with techniques of muscular relaxation often is useful.

As the child gains control in these actions, results may be determined by, for example, first asking a child to move slowly and then activating the child ("Let's see how fast you can run in place!"). This activation period can be followed by tasks that determine whether the child can again place himself or herself under control.

Research that I and others have conducted indicates that these actions correlate moderately to highly with test-taking attention and with teachers' ratings of self-control in classrooms. Recent data further indicate that the ability (or inclination) to move slowly when asked to do so may be somewhat specific to the action requested. Thus, a training program should include a variety of tasks rather than focusing on one or two "slow-moving" techniques (Savelli, Cratty, & Pistoletti, 1985; Setterlind, 1985).

Figure 26.2   Prolonged Walking Tasks to Lengthen Attention Span

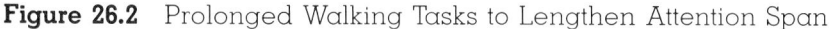

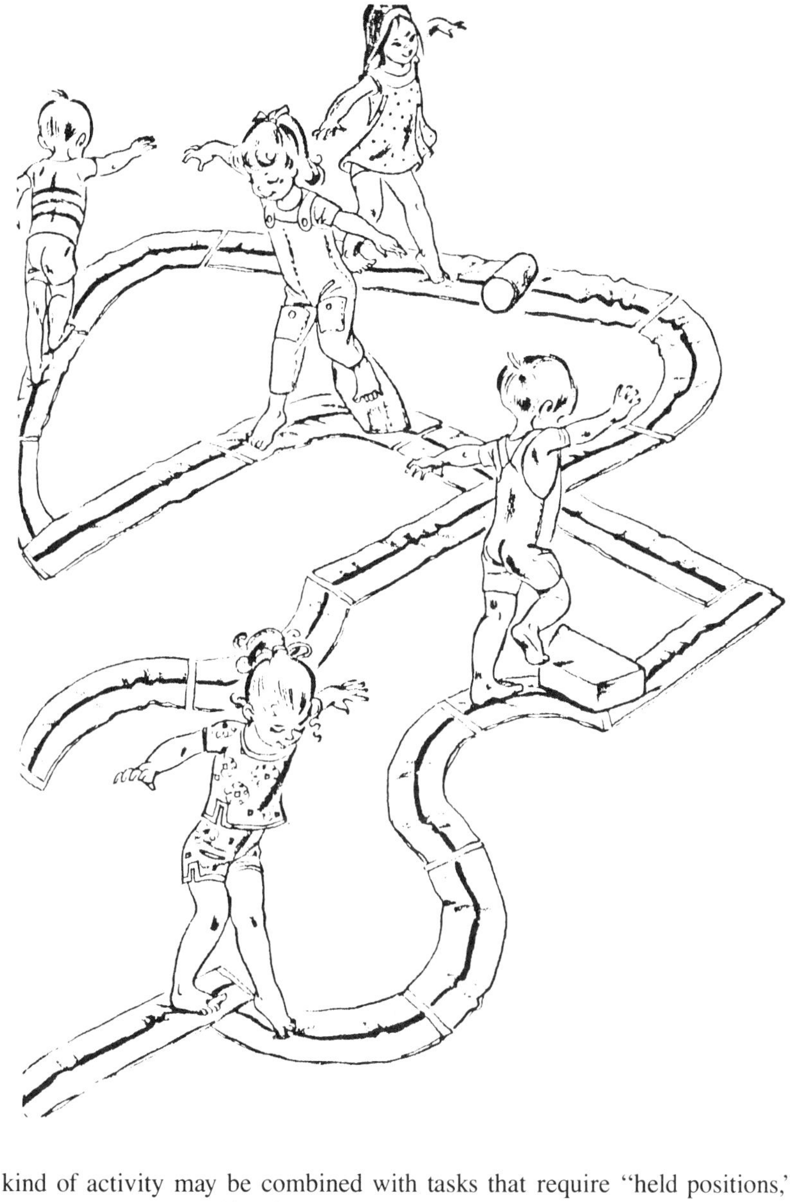

This kind of activity may be combined with tasks that require "held positions," as in typical yoga programs. Modifications of yoga have been found to be useful with special children, particularly those with excess tension and muscular and behavioral inflexibility. Classroom teachers and physical educators alike have used yoga successfully with various handicapped groups. If extreme positions are required and the yoga program is rigorous, however, the advice of physicians and therapists is essential.

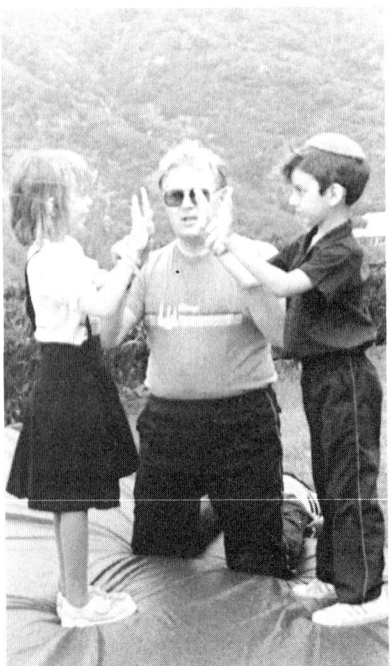 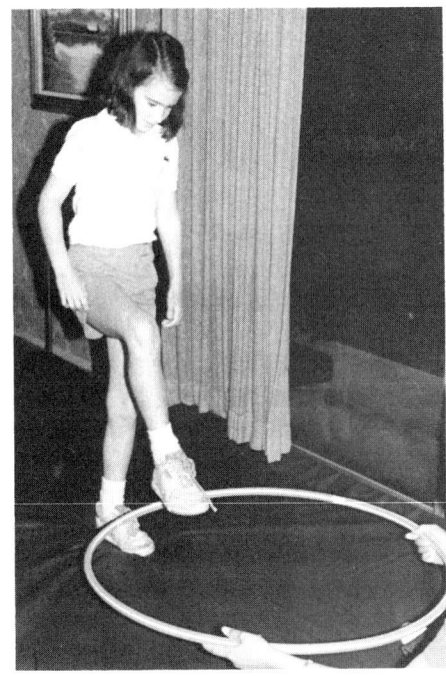

These activities encourage visual attention and self-control.

As is true with muscular relaxation techniques, impulse-control activities are successful to the degree to which the actions are incorporated in imagery and language palatable to immature persons. These types of actions often are best incorporated into "sensory-motor stories" in which characters' movements portray emotions and story content. Impulse-control activities may be used with individuals who have minimal expressive language, although receptive language (understanding verbal directions) is needed. For the most part, the next group of techniques requires at least minimal expressive language skills.

Cognitive-Behavioral Therapy

Cognitive-behavior theories and clinical models first appeared in the literature during the 1950s. During the 1970s their popularity and acceptance soared as more and more data emerged substantiating their worth. With this expansion of research came useful and precise ways in which this kind of therapy might be applied to groups as diverse as alcoholics, depressives, psychotics—and hyperactive children and youth with learning disabilities. Self-monitoring (self-talk) techniques aimed at improving hyperactive/distractible classroom behavior in learning disabled students have had positive results, for the most part (Hallahan & Sapona, 1983). This suggests that physical educators might take advantage of modern metacognitive strategies.

The rationale underlying this general approach is based upon the assumption that our behaviors and emotions do not emerge in unexplained reflexive ways but, rather, are controllable and guided by our thoughts. Acceptance of this idea further suggests that changes in behaviors and feelings may be elicited by helping people change how they think about events, others, themselves, and their work, as well as about emotions and thoughts themselves. Children who lack attentional skills, who "barge into" tasks without reflecting, are exhibiting poor intellectual skills surrounding task performance, including skills needed to plan approaches to tasks, thoughts that may accompany task execution, and thoughts present upon completion of school tasks. It follows that improvement in task performance will come about when children are helped to change how they think about tasks.

The main tool of cognitive therapists is called *self-talk*. It is hypothesized that the ways in which children talk to themselves (or fail to self-instruct) influence subsequent performance and, if improved, reflect improvement in school performance. A teacher applying this approach will in specific ways tell an impulsive child what to say before, during, and after assigned tasks. With repeated efforts it is assumed that the child will internalize (believe, or evidence a "cognitive click") and thus accept the valid pairing of improved self-talk and the thoughts it represents with changes in school-task effort and result. The scenario for such a lesson might be as follows:

Teacher/Therapist: Before you do this task, I want you to say, "I must think very carefully about the directions given to me." Now please say it.

Child: I must think about the directions given to me.

Teacher/Therapist   Now say, "I must remember what I am told and arrange my work carefully" . . . okay?

Child: I must remember what I am told and arrange my work carefully.

At this point, during these pre-task self-instructions (self-talk), even more task-specific directions might be encouraged—for example, "I must place my pencil at the proper starting point and hold the paper with the other hand."

Next come self-instructions appropriate *during the task:*

Teacher/Therapist: Now say, "While I do the task, I must watch carefully and avoid mistakes."

Child: While I do the task, I must watch carefully and avoid mistakes.

At this point the teacher/therapist might ask for self-talk that is specific to the kind of mistake the child might make in the task performed (e.g., "I should try to stay between the lines").

Finally the teacher/therapist should require self-talk appropriate *after the task is completed.* This talk may include phrases reflecting self-evaluation, rewarding statements, and information useful in the next try at the task. During this post-task phase the self-talk might consist of the following.

Teacher/Therapist:	Now say, "I made only a few mistakes. I did pretty well. Next time I will try harder to stay between the lines during the hard part of the maze."
Child:	I made only a few mistakes. I did pretty well. Next time I will try harder to stay between the lines during the hard part of the maze."

Various motor skills can be combined with this kind of training in appropriate self-talk. Physical tasks are useful in this context because they often take some time to complete and thus permit accompanying self-talk. Also, the relative success or failure (or score) of a physical task usually is apparent to both the learner and the teacher.

Careful attention should be paid to phasing out and transferring this kind of cognitive therapy. Transfer should be made from physical-motor skills to classroom activities, with the classroom teacher and physical education teacher working in concert. Task-specific self-talk should be phased out by reducing the vividness and detail of the self-talk, and it should be carried out by having the child move directly from a physical skill, in which better thought and self-control have been demonstrated, to a classroom task. At this point the self-talk may become more general, consisting of a pre-task statement such as, "Before I do a task, I must think about how I should do it and get and follow good directions." Phasing out vividness of self-talk consists of changing sentences ("I should evaluate myself after I finish a task to see how well I did and how I might improve") to sentence fragments ("Improve by thinking back to mistakes" or perhaps, "Mistakes help next time"), sentence fragments to whispers, and finally, whispers to gestures indicating silent internal self-talk (holding one's chin with the hand pensively).

Kendall and Finch (1979) have found that general self-instruction regarding task planning and execution behaviors is better than specific kinds of self-talk. These same researchers found that conceptual training of this type had positive long-term effects when applied to improving children's self-control.

The research clearly shows that this kind of training for *reflective* behavior (as contrasted with impulsive behavior) is most effective if a child model is used, as was suggested for the impulse-control activities. If a well controlled, thoughtful child is employed as a model, the child with low attention will improve more than if instructions and training pass directly from the teacher/therapist to the problem child without the mediating child model.

Cognitive-behavioral applications are most useful in relatively verbal children with attentional problems and concomitant learning disabilities. Extremely low functioning persons—those with obvious central nervous system deficiencies—are less likely to improve.

Training in self-talk is a positive improvement over simply teaching a child to relax or to move slowly. Becoming less muscularly tense or moving slowly in themselves are not components of academic learning. But organizing one's thoughts before, during, and after task performance is important to learning. Cognitive-behavioral therapy attempts to help children think about their thinking, or what is termed *meta-cognition*. Tasks in physical education programs can be either starting points or ending points in improving self-control. That is, the physical education teacher may use this approach to improve attention to the physical tasks in his or her program or use the physical education tasks and program to elicit higher levels of attention in the academic classroom.

OTHER CONSIDERATIONS

Among many other considerations when attempting to improve self-control:

1. The physical education teacher may be asked to help transmit information about a child's behavior to a doctor who is medicating the child. Indeed, if a medicated child evidences either undue drowsiness or exaggerated hyperactivity while on medication, the physical educator should inform those medicating the youngster, even if it is not requested.

2. The physical education program may be arranged so that the child's attention is better focused, by decreasing the size of the group (and thus the number of potentially distracting classmates). The size and complexity (stimulation) of the area devoted to physical education may be adjusted. The room might be partitioned and made smaller, and extraneous noise and decorations could be reduced to heighten students' attention.

3. Children may be encouraged to utilize the methods explained in this chapter themselves, within their limitations. Self-directed relaxation training is possible for many of the handicapped.

SUMMARY

Hyperactivity and impulsivity, as well as poor attention in its various forms, are encountered much more often in atypical populations, including the learning disabled. Many handicapped children display attentional difficulties or some kind of lethargic, dreamy state. These problems are amenable to treatment by physical educators who are knowledgeable and willing to apply specific techniques and methods.

Among the strategies useful in this context are: (a) *relaxation training*, in which an effort is made to reduce excess muscular tensions; (b) *impulse-control activities*, coupled with imagery, which encourage the child to move slowly and suppress the impulse to move inappropriately and excessively; and (c) *cognitive-behavioral strategies* employing movement tasks together with self-talk to reduce hyperactivity and help children manage their own thoughts more effectively. Thought-management is discussed throughout this book. It has been found useful to control seizures and to produce more effective classroom behaviors and learning as well.

Teachers should be aware of how a variety of conditions and factors contribute to or detract from pupil's attention. Management of the environment, specific techniques, and the teacher's own behaviors, postures, and voice combine to either heighten or reduce hyperactive, impulsive, and faulty attention behaviors in students.

REFERENCES

August, G.J., & Stewart, M.A. (1983). Familial subtypes of childhood hyperactivity. *Journal of Nervous & Mental Disease, 171*, 362-366.

Brandon, J.E., Eason, R.L., & Smith, T.L. (1986). Behavioral relaxation training and motor performance of learning disabled children with hyperactive behaviors. *Adapted Physical Activity Quarterly, 3*, 67-79.

Carter, J., Lax, B., & Russell, H. (1979). Effects of relaxation training on academic achievement of educable retarded boys. *Education & Training of the Mentally Retarded, 10*, 39-41.

Carter, J., & Russell, H. (1980). Biofeedback and academic attainment of learning disabled children. *Academic Therapy, 15*, 483-486.

Carter, J., & Russell, H. (1980). Biofeedback and academic attainment of learning disabled children. *Academic Therapy, 15,* 483-486.

Carter, J., & Synolds, D. (1974). Effects of relaxation training upon handwriting quality. *Journal of Hearing Disabilities, 7,* 235-238.

Dunn, F.M., & Howell, R.J. (1982). Relaxation training and its relationship to hyperactivity in boys. *Journal of Clinical Psychology, 38,* 92-100.

Gadow, K.D. (1983). Effects of stimulant drugs on academic performance in hyperactive and learning disabled children. *Journal of Learning Disabilities, 16,* 290-299.

Glantz, K. (1983). The use of relaxation exercises in the treatment of reading disability. *Journal of Nervous & Mental Disease, 171,* 191-195.

Hallahan, D.P., & Sapona, R. (1983). Self-monitoring of attention with learning disabled children: Past research and current issues. *Journal of Learning Disabilities, 16,* 616-620.

Herson, M., & Barlow, D.H. (1976). *Single-case experimental designs: Strategies for studying behavioral change.* New York: Pergamon Press.

Jacobson, E. (1938). *Progressive relaxation.* Chicago: University of Chicago Press.

Jacobson, E. (1973). *Teaching and learning: New methods for old arts.* Chicago: National Foundation for Progressive Relaxation. (ERIC Document Reproduction Service No. ED 097-295)

Kendall, P.C., & Finch, A.J., Jr. (1979). Developing nonimpulsive behavior in children: Cognitive-behavioral strategies for self-control. In P.C. Kendall & S.D. Hollen (Eds.), *Cognitive-behavioral interventions: Theory, research, and procedures.* New York: Academic Press.

Meichenbaum, D.H., & Goodman, L. (1969). Training impulsive children to talk about themselves: A means of developing self-control. *Journal of Abnormal Psychology, 7,* 533-565.

Poppen, R., & Maurer, J.P. (1982). Electromyographic analysis of relaxed postures. *Biofeedback & Self-Regulation, 7,* 491-498.

Rickard, H.C., Thrasher, K.A., & Elkins, P.D. (1984). Responses of persons who are mentally retarded to four components of relaxation instruction. *Mental Retardation, 22,* 248-252.

Savelli, M.D., Cratty, B.J., & Pistoletti, A. (1985). *Relaxation training effects upon classroom attention and impulsivity in youth 11-14 years.* Manuscript submitted for publication.

Schilling, D., & Poppen, R. (1983). Behavioral relaxation training and assessment. *Journal of Behavior Therapy & Experimental Psychiatry, 14,* 99-107.

Setterlind, S. (1983). *Relaxation training in schools* (Studies in Educational Sciences No. 43-335). Goteborg, Sweden: University of Goteborg.

Torrey, C. (1981). *The effects of progressive relaxation on a motor task with hyperactive children.* Paper presented at the Third International Symposium on Adapted Physical Activity, New Orleans.

Wadden, T.A. (1983). Predicting treatment response to relaxation therapy for essential hypertension. *Journal of Nervous & Mental Disease, 171,* 167-174.

ADDITIONAL REFERENCES

Barkley, R.A. (1981). *Hyperactive children: A handbook for diagnosis and treatment.* New York: Guilford Press.

Cratty, B.J. (1986). Self-control. In B.J. Cratty, *Active learning* (2nd ed.) (ch. 2). Englewood Cliffs, NJ: Prentice-Hall.

Hinshaw, S.P., Henker, B., & Whalen, C. (1984). Cognitive behavioral and pharmacological interventions for hyperactive boys: Comparative and combined effects. *Journal of Consulting & Clinical Psychology, 52,* 739-749.

QUESTIONS FOR DISCUSSION

1. What forms of hyperactivity and attentional difficulty might be seen in a classroom or within a physical education lesson?
2. Why might a parent not agree with the label "hyperactive" when applied by the child's teacher?
3. What reasons are given for the presence of hyperactive behavior, and what strategies might be indicated by each model or reason?
4. What are the advantages and drawbacks in using relaxation training with a group of youngsters? What are the drawbacks of using cognitive-behavioral therapy in a group of severely retarded adults? What might be the advantages of using cognitive-behavioral therapy with a group of learning disabled 10-year-olds?
5. What kinds of imagery games might be employed to reduce hyperactivity? What games of this nature do you know about that are not described in this chapter?

STUDENT PROJECTS

1. Assess impulse control by asking children in a classroom to draw a line as slowly as they can (use a chest-high channel of two lines, about 36″ long, to draw between). Without consulting with the classroom teacher, what might you find out about self-control and attention span from this test? Do your conclusions about the children you assessed correspond with the judgments of the classroom teacher relative to their hyperactivity or attention spans?
2. Observe a relaxation program intended to reduce hyperactivity. What principles seem to be used or violated in using these techniques?
3. Formulate, and try out if possible, an ideal program of hyperactivity control for a group of atypical children, youth, or adults, hyperactive learning disabled children, pre-school children with cerebral palsy, etc.

RESOURCES

American Association for the
  Advancement of Tension Control
P.O. Box 7512
Roanoke, VA 24019

National Foundation for Progressive
  Relaxation
55 E. Washington St.
Chicago, IL 60602

27 Rhythm, Dance, and Music

Rhythm is a universal human quality, manifested at work, at play, and while engaging in basic functions such as talking, walking, and breathing. Ever since the Europeans first attempted to work with the deaf and emotionally disturbed in the late 18th century, rhythm and music have been used to break through the barriers that surround the handicapped. Many universities and colleges offer majors in dance therapy. Music and dance have become increasingly used tools in institutions and classes for the retarded, the emotionally disturbed, the physically handicapped, and the sensory impaired. Even the deaf and near-deaf can communicate through rhythm and music; as sound is transmitted through the surfaces on which they stand, the vibrations ignite their impulse to move with the beat.

For years music educators and dance therapists rhapsodized over the positive effects that song and dance were having on various atypical populations. Yet not until the 1960s did we have a substantial body of literature delineating the effects of music and rhythm on the developmentally delayed, intellectually impaired, emotionally disturbed, perceptually handicapped, and other atypical populations. Since that time, music and rhythm have been found to aid social and emotional adjustment, proved to be an effective motivator and reinforcer, been helpful in changing a person's activity level, and even used to further learning in some academic tasks.

Background music with a regular beat has been found to facilitate the task performance of severely retarded individuals (Harrison, Lecrone, Temerlin, & Trousdale, 1966; Luckey, 1967). Dance has been shown to facilitate manual dexterity and improve gross motor skills in the learning disabled (Couper, 1981). Further study is needed to specify just how rhythmic experience may bring out the withdrawn emotionally disturbed, although it has been used successfully in many instances. More research with more varied populations, and in which the variables of music or rhythm are carefully defined and described, also would be helpful.

Approaches utilizing dance and rhythm are likely to accomplish the following objectives in work with handicapped groups:

1. Rhythm and dance encourage a variety of actions that contribute to improved motor functions and fitness.

2. Music, dance, and similar strategies often are used to break through the barriers that sometimes surround emotionally disturbed individuals who are removed from reality.

3. Rhythm and dance often encourage children and youth to express themselves creatively. This may be done through mime or simply as projections of a variety of movement patterns for their own sake.

4. Various movements, both passive and forceful, may aid a child with problems to vent feelings not easily expressed or dissipated verbally. Movement tasks done to music and rhythm also help children and youth communicate emotions to others, which may not be easy for them to do verbally.

5. When observed by a competent clinician, the quantity and quality of movements expressed may aid in diagnosing mental health problems.

6. Dance and recreation provide fun. The actions may be exhilarating for their own sake, independent of the objectives listed above.

7. Exposure to folk dance is not only an immediate social experience but also elicits appreciation for the cultural roots from which the dance has come.

Programs of dance and rhythm may be provided in an almost infinite number of forms. Variation occurs because of the marked influence of the dance teacher's or therapist's personality on technical and emotional experiences provided. The pages that follow survey the variety of ways in which movement experiences containing music, dance, and rhythm may be used with children and youth who have special needs.

The initial section contains guidelines and principles when attempting to introduce, motivate, and sustain a program of this nature. Ways to introduce rhythm and expressive movements instigated by music are included in this section, along with graduated sequences that may be employed when trying to encourage a child or group of children to engage in activities expressing creativity, energy, and exploration. The second section contains examples of specific types of rhythm and dance programs that may be used to aid various handicapped groups—simple and basic rhythmic experiences, as well as experiences incorporating more structured dance forms. The third section discusses movement as therapy and problems that may be encountered with special children.

We do not always realize the strong positive effects that music and rhythm may have. I have never gotten over an experience I had years ago when working as a movement consultant for the Special Education Branch of the Los Angeles City Schools. One of my weekly stops was at a school for the moderately retarded. Most of the pupils were children with Down syndrome. Upon arriving each time, I patiently worked with both children and teachers in relatively direct, simple movement experiences using balance beams, balls, and the like. My success was limited, and the children's motivation was not always high. In fact, the students often seemed impossible to change and awkward to the extreme.

One week, however, I arrived off-schedule and observed a student dance at the school in which popular music of the day was being played for the youngsters, who ranged in age from about 12 to 18. I was astonished! My apparently awkward charges had become as light as feathers. As the music blared, their formerly stiff bodies became flexible works of art, swaying precisely to each beat. The experience, although leaving me somewhat shaken, gave me insight into the powerful tool that rhythmic activities can be. This is an understanding many others had gained before me, an awareness I hope readers will act on fully.

Judging from the writings in contemporary journals of dance therapy, modern dance therapists are insightful, sensitive, and highly creative in their approaches to using movement with special populations. Their current interests range from younger brain-damaged children to senior citizens suffering from degenerative conditions in the central nervous system, joints, and muscles. Their efforts have been particularly fruitful when applied to the severely emotionally disturbed and the withdrawn. Dance and music seem to comprise one of the only ways (excluding medication) that can bring these individuals in touch with reality.

The "research" published in these journals, however, is more insightful and even self-congratulatory than it is scientifically rigorous. Even an effort made recently to formulate ways of evaluating various aspects of nonverbal behaviors in special groups is based more on subjective guesses than upon hard data obtained under scientifically acceptable conditions (Wolf-Schein & Cohen, 1985). Certainly the categories of nonverbal behaviors placed into this recently developed behavioral assessment, might prove to be starting points for more disciplined research. These include (a) communication and affective behavior, (b) vocalization and expressive speech, (c) sound and speech reception, (d) visual behavior, (e) motor behavior, (f) learning style, (g) reactions to food, (h) stereotyped behavior, and (i) ritualistic behavior. But, for example, the sub-categories under the heading "motor behavior" include "clumsy walking" and "clumsy with hands"—sub-divisions lacking precision, and from which little information might be obtained for recording improvement or for planning a program.

GUIDELINES AND PRINCIPLES

Introductory Experiences

Rhythms, and later dances, should be introduced gradually. Often the extremely withdrawn, the emotionally disturbed, and the retarded must be approached in an oblique manner. For example, they first may be permitted to listen to a beat or music without any obvious urgings to participate. This listening introduction often is allowed to go on for prolonged periods, during which time the children and youth may appear to remain out of contact with what is happening.

The situation should be nonthreatening. Even gradual changes in the children should be appreciated and praised. For example, their eyes may shift from a downward position, looking up from the floor to the source of the beat. This often is the first sign of improvement, which may lead toward full participation later.

After a beat or music with a beat has been used for a lengthy period of time and the children seem to be aware of the stimuli, models for movement may be provided. The teacher or a peer may begin to move in rather simple ways to the beat. The model's first movements might consist of only nodding the head or tapping the foot while seated facing the children. As the model continues, any child or youth who seems to catch the beat or the intent of the lesson may be gently encouraged to participate. To reach this phase may take minutes, hours, days—or even weeks, in the case of some extremely withdrawn populations of the emotionally disturbed.

Many music therapists believe that initially requiring children or youth to match a prescribed beat is not as good as watching the children's movements and keeping the beat with them! They seem to control the rhythm rather than being controlled by it or trying to meet another's notions of appropriate rhythm. Research indicates that both normal and atypical individuals have preferences for speed and rhythm that remain relatively fixed and constant over time and consistent within a given type of movement—foot tapping, for example. Thus, in a lesson involving rhythm and music, children should be encouraged to exhibit their personal rhythms, and the teacher should try to match the beat to these preferences.

Conformity and Variations

Many handicapped youngsters and adults—particularly the emotionally disturbed, perceptually handicapped, and some retarded—exhibit an extreme lack of variability in the ways they move. They are perceptually and even conceptually rigid, and they perseverate in their actions. One of the goals of an able music therapist or a physical education teacher using music and rhythm should be to encourage variety in the movement patterns of those they serve.

Variety in movement and rhythm may take place within several dimensions: (a) variations in beat, both regular and irregular; (b) variations in force exhibited, from passive, relaxed actions to extremely emphatic movements; (c) variations in the manner in which space is utilized (e.g., upward and downward movements); (d) movements involving the total body, as well as limb and hand movements; (e) movements that travel on a horizontal plane and those that are spiral or move through space in lateral "slashes" rather than in neat right angles; (f) movements that travel inward toward the center of the body and those that move outward; (g) movements that are primarily flexion versus those that are extension; (h) movements that are forward and backward versus sideways; and (i) a whole classification of movements that may be called rotary, involving rotations of the limbs or the total body.

Clever music and dance therapists are armed with verbal suggestions that elicit imagery in children and in turn tend to produce the variety of movement possibilities and combinations just listed. The therapist has to be sensitive to the emotional strengths and limitations of the children or youth, the impact of the therapist's own personality on those being served, and the possible threat inherent in "moving children along too fast" in terms of difficulty of movements and rhythms they are being encouraged or requested to make.

Most therapists believe that developmentally the easiest movements to bring out of children are those in which they move freely; the beat or music follows the child. Variations in force (e.g., "Stamp your feet") are easier to elicit than extreme variations in direction of movement. Directions of movement that require the child to move back and forth in a horizontal plane are easier to obtain in younger or developmentally delayed children than are movements that require them to move up and down in a vertical plane. Spiral-shaped movements—those traveling laterally in space—are the most difficult. Even normal children usually do not perform these movements well until middle childhood.

Children might be encouraged first to follow a beat using a single part of the body—one hand or a hand and arm. Later they may be able to make bilateral movements, alternating their hands in back-and-forth actions. Rhythms of the total body (e.g., jumping in place) also are relatively easy starting points. Rhythms in which both limbs and the total body are active are the most difficult of all. These latter types require some exposure to lessons in which a beat (or music) and movements are combined in various ways.

Special devices and aids that may be useful in stimulating participation in rhythmic experiences include the following:

- Hand-held flags that ripple when moved up and down and in all directions add visual stimuli and sound to the beat. Using a flag, the reverse also may be at-

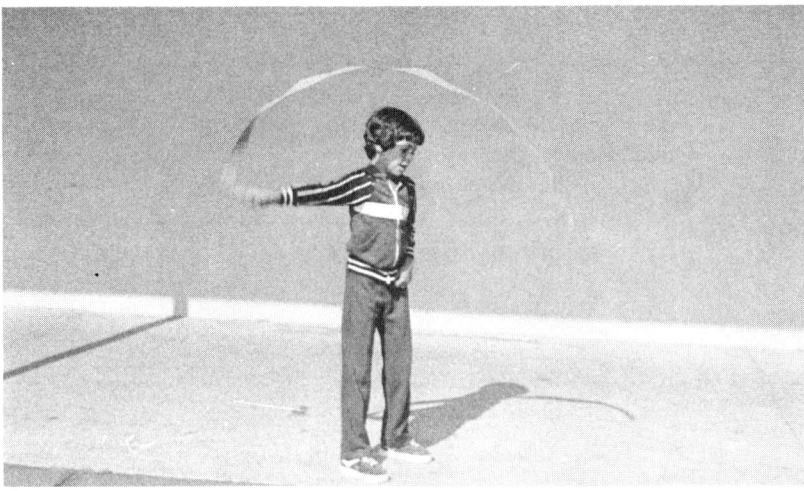

Flowing streamers are useful in rhythmic activities.

tempted—first having the child swing the flag and then installing a musical beat
or rhythm (e.g., knocking two sticks together) to accompany the rhythm the
child has established.

- Hand-held flowing streamers, as illustrated, indicate vividly where a child's
  limb has traveled, its direction and velocity. The sight of the trailing streamer
  is motivating and aesthetically pleasing. Length of the streamers may be adjusted, and they may be varied in color, of course, for visual appeal.
- Balloons kept aloft through head and hand pushes are a happy accompaniment
  to rhythmic activities. Again, the children may attempt to match their "hits" to
  some prescribed beat, or the beat can vary as the children touch the descending balloons.
- The traditional hoops, balls, and ropes may be used—similar to those employed
  in modern gymnastics. The variety inherent in these pieces of hand-held equipment is endless. For interested readers, the Additional References at the end of
  this chapter describe some of the techniques involved.
- Bands about 3"-4" wide that stretch to 2'-3' are useful in encouraging children
  to explore the directions in which they may move. They also stimulate force
  patterns and variations. Long latex bands such as those sewn in the waists of
  pants may be used.
- Large parachute-like pieces of cloth may be helpful when used in group activities carried out to music or rhythm, with the children holding and moving the
  cloth to produce interesting patterns.
- Many devices afford the opportunity to create music and rhythm patterns. The
  Orff-Schulwerk (Orff, 1969) program, for example, details how instruments can
  be employed when working with the handicapped, including the retarded and
  emotionally disturbed. Often, instruments may be modified. As examples, a

drum stick might be tied to a child's hand, and the components of marimbas could be enlarged to accommodate a motorically deficient child.

- Large three-dimensional shapes—cubes, traffic pylons, and the like—may encourage children and youth to instigate motor patterns in space. They may run to, get into, skip around, or otherwise deal with this type of equipment.

FORMS OF RHYTHMIC AND MUSIC EXPERIENCES

Rhythm and music may be employed in an infinite number of ways with both atypical and normal children and youth. Modifications of the forms discussed next, as well as the quality of progressions leading from them, are dependent primarily on the experience and creative dimensions of the teacher and on the teacher's perceptions of and sensitivity to what is occurring within the clients.

Rhythm, Listening, and Variations

First experiences consist of little more than having the children listen to a beat and then encouraging them to replicate it. Then the beat is changed—made faster and slower. If the children react properly by slowing and speeding up their own movements (e.g., walking, running, hand clapping), the instructor may try irregular beats of various kinds to determine whether the youngsters can move in rhythm to these.

Force Variations

Force variations are usually next to be acquired. While marching to a rhythmic beat, a child model or the teacher may emphasize one beat or another by stamping the foot hard while walking. The children first are encouraged to imitate these force patterns and then to determine their own ways of providing emphasis in their movements ("Can you think of and show me other ways to 'hit hard' when you move?"). The children can stamp while walking or "hit" outward into the air for emphasis and force.

Horizontal Variations

Movements in a horizontal plane usually are taught next. Starting with walking patterns, the children are encouraged to walk in all directions, including backward and sideways, to music or to a rhythmic beat. Later, horizontal movements may be combined with force and speed changes ("Can you run backward or sideways?"). And variety in horizontal movements—skipping, galloping, hopping, jumping, and the like—may be tried.

After the concept of horizontal movements has been acquired, the children may be encouraged to exhibit movements in this plane using just limb, hand, and head movements, as pictured ("Can you move your arms sideways, fast and slow?" "Can you make other sideways movements with your arms, head, knees, and other parts of your body, including your feet?").

Up-and-Down Movements in a Vertical Plane

Vertical movements usually explored next. When using the total body, these sometimes require leg and trunk strength, as children may be encouraged alternately to bend, squat,

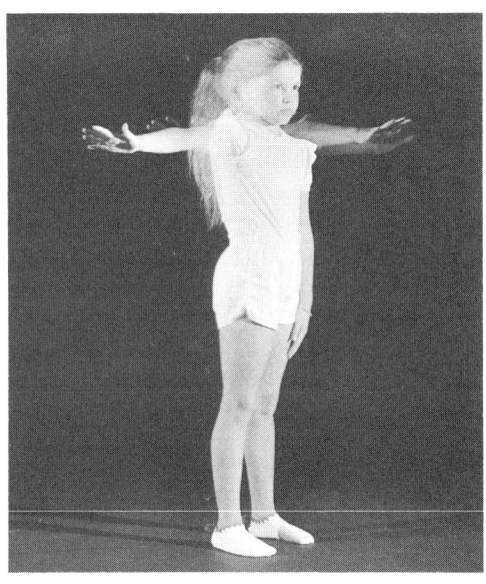

This strobe picture illustrates movement in the horizontal plane, using only the arms, hands, and head.

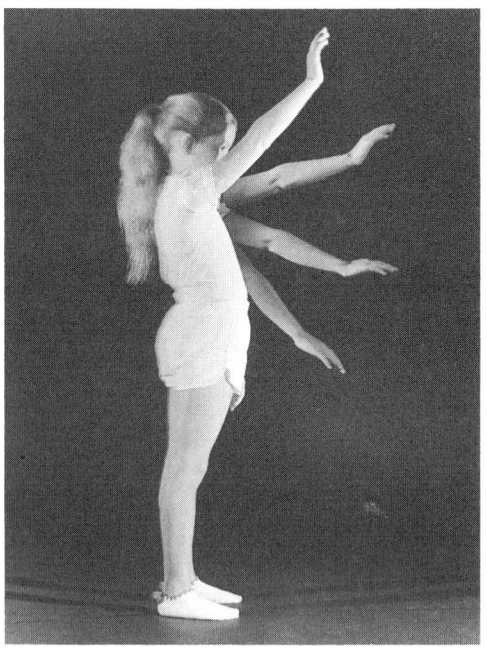

Movement in the vertical plane can be executed using just the hands and arms.

Reprinted from *Perceptual and Motor Development in Infants and Children* (3rd ed.) by B.J. Cratty, 1986, with permission of the publisher, Prentice-Hall.

and then rise, both rapidly and slowly. Vertical movements of the body are encouraged by imagery ("Can you make yourself small and then tall?") Following vertical movements of the total body, limb movements may be expressed in a vertical plane, as pictured, and then a combination of total body and limb movements in total patterns ("Rise slowly like a tree, your arms waving like branches reaching toward the sky").

Circular and Lateral Movements

Circular and lateral movements tend to be more difficult than vertical and horizontal movements, in which relatively right-angled or straight movement lines are called for. One way to promote a spiral-shaped movement is to ask children to duplicate the throwing pattern of a big-league pitcher, bringing a hand from behind one leg, over the shoulder, and finishing in front of the other leg.

Circular movements are simpler and might begin by simply spinning the total body in place—an action that is exhilarating but should be avoided if the child has balance problems or perseverates. It also could prompt seizures in children who are prone to them.

Circular and lateral movements, inscribing spirals, can be most graceful. Their pleasing execution often depends on the skill and motivating qualities of the model who demonstrates the movements. Most important, these movements should involve a total flow of chained-together motions of the legs, trunk, shoulders, arms, hands, and head. Cues might begin with, "Lead with your wrists and elbows," as the arm starts from a flexed position across the waist and moves to an extended (and supinated) position up and over the head, as pictured.

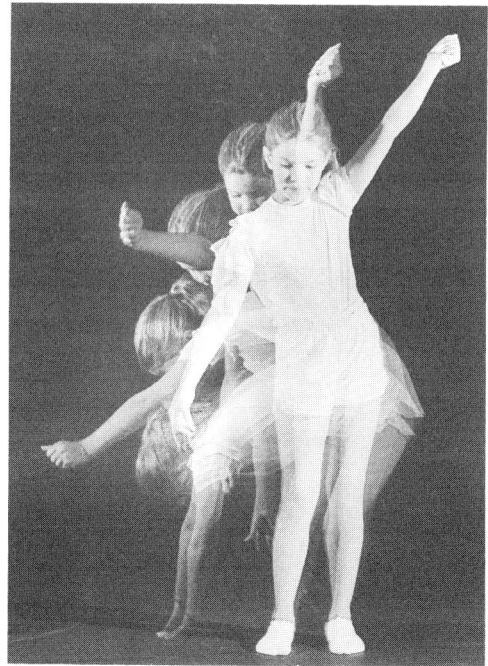

Lateral movements usually are more difficult than horizontal or vertical ones.

Reprinted from *Perceptual and Motor Development in Infants and Children* (3rd ed.) by B.J. Cratty, 1986, with permission of the publisher, Prentice-Hall.

Imitation and Mime

Many movement qualities may be encouraged by using music and stories to portray people, places, things and ideas, and emotions with the body and body parts. These experiences can be done in a group or in isolation and carried out to suggestions such as, "Make your body seem happy, without laughing or making a noise" or "Pretend you have just had a sour lemon—use your mouth and your entire body to portray this."

Mimes may reflect parts of stories being told. Children may be asked to "pretend you are castles" when a castle is mentioned in a fairy tale. Characters in stories ("Be the witch") as well as emotions ("The king was *angry* at the messenger") can be used as stimuli to instigate these creative movement experiences.

Children may be asked to imagine themselves in various situations. For example, they may be asked to break out of a box—an idea that might elicit forceful outward movements as they pantomime the action.

More rhythmic actions may be elicited as children are asked to pretend they are "raindrops, now falling harder and harder" or perhaps "the king's horses." Blocks, two sticks, or other noisemakers can be introduced during breaks in the story to accompany children's attempts to present ideas and things in rhythmic ways. The photo shows children in this type of "pretend" situation.

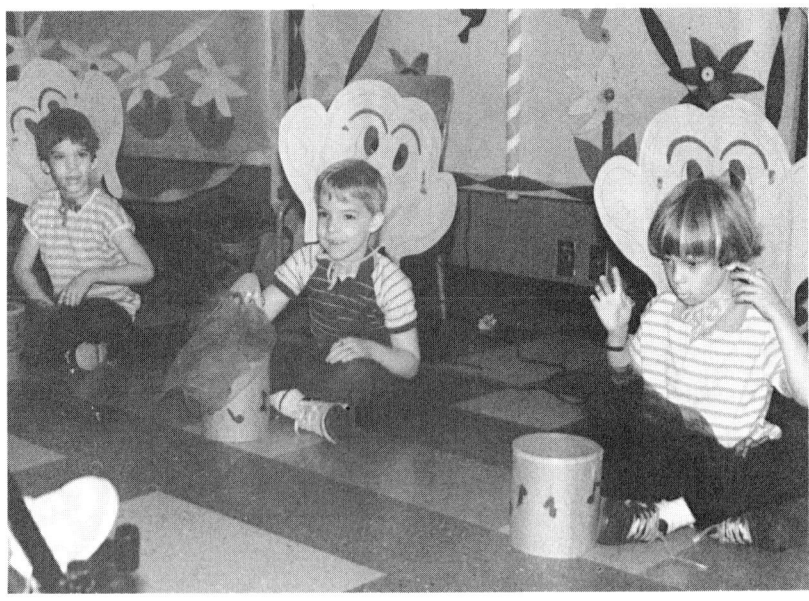

Children use rhythm in imaginative ways while acting out a story.
Courtesy, Special Education Branch, Los Angeles City Schools

Dance Routines

Conceptual qualities, both short- and long-term memory, and divergent thought production ("How many different ways of doing this can you think of?") may be encouraged in children who are capable, by asking them to formulate their own creative dance routines, singly or as a group. In doing this, some do's and dont's are:

1. Spend enough time—weeks or months, if necessary—giving the children movement experiences they can draw upon in constructing their routines.

2. Don't expect sequences to be too long or too sophisticated, particularly with the developmentally and intellectually less able.

3. Don't make too many suggestions for the routines. The ideas and movements should be the children's own.

4. Don't envision the final performance to be in front of an audience—unless the children want this. The goal in any case should be to encourage the children to develop, memorize, and perform the routine as a personal goal, with only the teacher observing.

5. Do permit and expect variations in the routine from performance to performance rather than insisting on precision and exactness.

Routines of this nature can incorporate various equipment and devices that have been described, for part of or for the entire composition. The length of a routine could vary from 30 seconds to 5 minutes or more, depending on the youngster's capabilities and motivation. With proficiency, filming the routine may bring the children pleasure.

Folk Dances and Current Dances

Rhythmic experiences can include folk dances and contemporary dances. When employed with the handicapped, these can be highly motivating. Older handicapped youngsters often are closely attuned to current musical fads and want to act like their normal peers in this respect. The dance sequences used, however, should not be too difficult or complex for the youngster's abilities.

Dances in which the child moves independently of others are easier than those in which interactions with others are a requisite (e.g., square dancing). Dances initially should require only one or two basic steps, and the children should overlearn these basics before proceeding to variations and combinations of the rudimentary movements.

MOVEMENT AS THERAPY

As has been suggested in other portions of this text, the physical education teacher should not attempt to fill all professional roles, to be all things to all people. When introducing music, rhythm, and dance as stimuli for helping children with special needs, professionals whose backgrounds have prepared them for this kind of intervention should be consulted.

Sometimes, by accident, the emotions triggered by this form of therapy are negative rather than positive. Disturbed children often act out their problems when exposed to rhythmic and music experiences. This should be expected and should not be met with undue alarm or attention. Using dance as a medium, physical educators should be sensitive to unusual behaviors and attempt to increase the chances for eliciting positive behaviors and emotions (kindness, cooperation, self-control) and reduce the potential for undesirable emotions (aggression, hostility, withdrawal). Consultation with a psychologist, psychotherapist, or psychiatrist who is familiar with the total dynamics of an emotionally disturbed child is imperative.

SPECIAL PROBLEMS WITH SPECIAL CHILDREN

Special problems may arise when using music and rhythm with special children. Representative of these unusual problems, together with possible solutions, are the following:

Problem: Rhythmic experiences may overexcite a child who is hyperactive or has emotional problems.

Proposed Solutions: Work on a continuum when introducing the rhythm and music, beginning with stimuli and tasks that cause minimal excitation before attempting activities that are likely to elicit too much or too strong emotion. Virtually all groups of handicapped and normal youngsters require a calming-down period following stimulating experiences. Rhythm and movement provide an ideal vehicle through suggestions such as, "Try to be a puppet on a string—all floppy and loose" or "Lie down and be like a heavy stone, sinking onto the mat" or "Act like spaghetti and slowly become a little pile on the floor."

Problem: Limitations in movement prevent some children from performing all of the movements and suggested actions.

Proposed Solutions: Do not call attention to these children as they begin to explore what they can do. When they attempt something, praise them quickly and unobtrusively. Permit them to rest and just to think whenever indicated, and never force them to be in constant motion. As a helpful motivator, take pictures of their actions after they have achieved some success.

SUMMARY

Rhythm, music, and dance have long been ways of approaching and alleviating problems in individuals with special needs. The emotionally disturbed, in particular, have been found to be amenable to the therapy inherent in rhythm. Music and rhythm encourage children to express themselves emotionally, as well as to exercise vigorously, improving their fitness and strength.

Simple, direct movements are easiest to pair with music. Later, lateral, spiral-shaped movements and even dance routines can be practiced. Initially it may be easiest to encourage movement of *any* kind and then to insert rhythm to match the child's own movements. Various kinds of implements, including hoops, balls, ropes, streamers, and flags, can be used to heighten the impact of the rhythmic experience. And models have proved to be an effective means of eliciting advantageous movements in children and youth.

REFERENCES

Couper, J.L. (1981). Dance therapy: Effects on motor performance of children with learning disabilities. *Physical Therapy, 61,* 23-25.

Harrison, W., Lecrone, H., Temerlin, M.F., & Trousdale, W.W. (1966). The effect of music and exercise upon the self-help skills of non-verbal retardates. *American Journal of Mental Deficiency, 71,* 279-282.

Luckey, R.E. (1967). Severely retarded adults: Responses to rhythm band instruments. *American Journal of Mental Deficiency, 71,* 616-618.

Orff, C. (1969). *Basic musical forms for Orff-Schulwerk classes in the elementary school.* Bellflower, CA: Bellflower School District. (Mimeograph)

Wolf-Schein, E.G., & Cohen, I.L. (1985). A study of the use of non-verbal systems in the differential diagnosis of autistic, mentally retarded, and fragile X individuals. *American Journal of Dance Therapy, 8,* 67-80.

ADDITIONAL REFERENCES

Alvin, J. (1976). *Music for the handicapped child.* London: Oxford University Press.

Dickinson, P.I. (1972). *Music with ESN children: A guide for the classroom teacher.* Windsor, England: NFER Publishing Ltd.

Gaston, E.T. (Ed.). (1968). *Music in therapy.* New York: Macmillan.

Hibben, J., & Scheer, R. (1982). Music and movement for special needs children. *Teaching Exceptional Children, 14,* 171-176.

Reardon, D.N., & Bell, G. (1970). Effects of sedative and stimulative music on activity levels of severely retarded boys. *American Journal of Mental Deficiency, 75,* 156-159.

Ross, D.N., Ross, S.A., & Kuchenbecker, S.L. (1973). Rhythm training for educable mentally retarded children. *Mental Retardation, 11*(6), 20-23.

Seale, T.F. (1969). Success in small doses: Music for the retarded. *Music Journal, 27,* 26-27.

Stevens, E.A. (1971). Some effects of tempo changes on stereotyped rocking movements of low-level mentally retarded subjects. *American Journal of Mental Deficiency, 76,* 76-81.

QUESTIONS FOR DISCUSSION

1. With reference to chapter 9 (emotional disturbance), what specific conditions are most likely to be improved through what kinds of rhythmic experiences?

2. What kinds of special equipment may help the handicapped move with more fluidity and joy when exposed to music and rhythm?

3. What kinds of rhythmic experiences might be enjoyed by those in wheelchairs?

4. What kinds of teaching cues and imagery might be used to advantage with a severely emotionally disturbed adolescent through rhythmic activity designed to be motivational?

5. What kinds of movement experiences would be useful to stimulate a moderately retarded 6- to 8-year old?

6. How might rhythmic experiences be used to aid counting and similar academic tasks?

7. How might music and rhythmic activities adversely affect a hyperactive child? A distractible child?

STUDENT PROJECTS

1. Consult the research literature to determine which kinds of attributes may be improved on the part of which kinds of handicapped individuals through rhythmic experiences.

2. Trace in the literature the history of using dance, music, and rhythm with the handicapped.

3. Design and create a special device or piece of equipment for use in rhythmic activities.

4. Collect instruments (real or junk) that make noises. Form an "orchestra" of children and perform a number.

5. Observe the first and last of series of dance lessons. What motivational devices are used? What seems to work well? What does not? What changes did you note between the first and last sessions? To what extent do you believe the dance instructor's personality and experience influenced the outcomes?

6. Formulate an evaluation tool for both physical and psychological changes that might result from participation in a program of music or rhythm. Consult a dance therapist about the validity of the instrument; then modify it if necessary and apply it in a real situation.

RESOURCES

American Dance Guild
1133 Broadway, Room 1427
New York, NY 10010

American Dance Therapy Association
1000 Century Plaza
Columbia, MD 21044

Congress on Research in Dance
   (CORD)
Dance Dept., Education 675 D
New York University
35 West Fourth St.
New York, NY 10003

Dalcroze School of Music
161 East 73rd St.
New York, NY 10021

Dance Horizons
1801 East 26th St.
Brooklyn, NY 11229

Dance Notation Bureau
8 East 12th St.
New York, NY 10003

Laban Institute of Movement Studies
133 West 21st St.
New York, NY 10011

National Dance Association
1900 Association Dr.
Reston, VA 22091

28 *Locomotion and Variations*

Many static postures and dynamic positions reflect preparation for and variations of locomotion. These provide the bases for more complex sports activities, as well as for other movements needed in daily living (Peiper, 1963; Wickstrom, 1970). Frequently, handicapped children and youth lack precision in these fundamental movement patterns. As they try to walk, run, jump, and otherwise manage their bodies, they may lack efficiency; their balance is often disturbed; and the mechanical efficiency with which they perform basic, as well as more specific, skills is often less than optimal.

This chapter presents sequences reflecting these basic movement patterns, as well as techniques for teaching them. Thorough knowledge of how these movements should be performed, their relative difficulty, and the times when they normally appear in the life of a child should enable physical education teachers to help children move in fundamental and important ways. Teachers also should understand the role of reflexes in promoting, but sometimes later inhibiting, development in standing and walking.

Initially, the sequences that lead to upright gait and initial walking attempts by normal infants are reviewed. Awareness of these stages is essential because many handicapped children need help in attaining these static postures and action patterns. With special help, handicapped children who learn basic walking skills then can begin to experiment with variations in gait, such as hopping, skipping, and galloping. A more thorough look at the pre-walking stages, together with intervention efforts, is found in chapter 25, dealing with infant stimulation.

REFLEXES IN THE INFANT

The infant at birth may seem to the uninitiated to be a confusing symphony of constantly changing movement patterns. To the well trained, careful observer, however, these apparently aimless writhings constitute a kaleidoscope of *deep-tendon reflexes* involving the larger muscle groups, which provide a basis for acquiring later voluntary movements and postures, and represent, at times, non-useful evolutionary remains of movement patterns of our primate ancestors.[1]

Some reflexes seem useful for the later acquisition of an upright gait; others have to be subordinated by the higher centers or somehow phased out before the infant can engage in useful voluntary movements. For example, a number of reflexes in normal infants indicate that they are somehow unconsciously aware of the upright and are seeking to overcome the pull of gravity so that they may sit, stand, and walk. These are called *labyrinthine reflexes*. Others, including *prehensile* and *plantar flexion reflexes* (the tendency for the hand to close when the palm is stroked, and of the feet to flex and curl when the soles are touched) may in the first case interfere with smooth voluntary grasping and in the second case, if continued, interfere with a stable foot base as the child tries to stand for the first time. These reflexes are illustrated in Figure 28.1.

---

1. Other reasons for reflexes are to maintain life in the infant. In the sucking and rooting reflex, for example, the head turns and sucking begins when the cheek is stroked.

Figure 28.1   Three Infant Reflexes

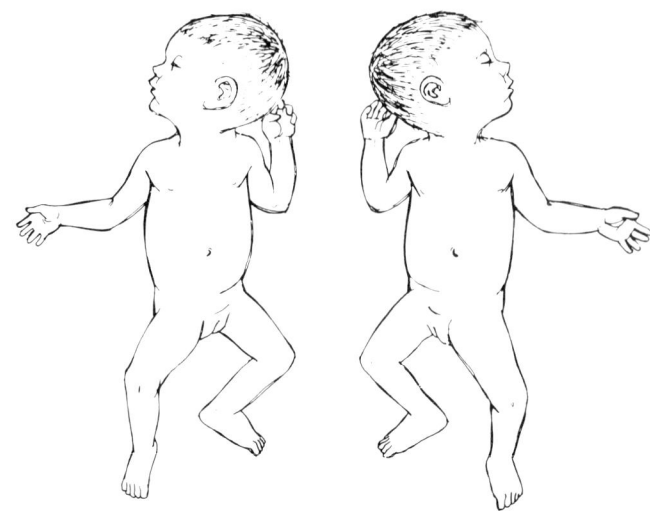

Labyrinthine reflexes

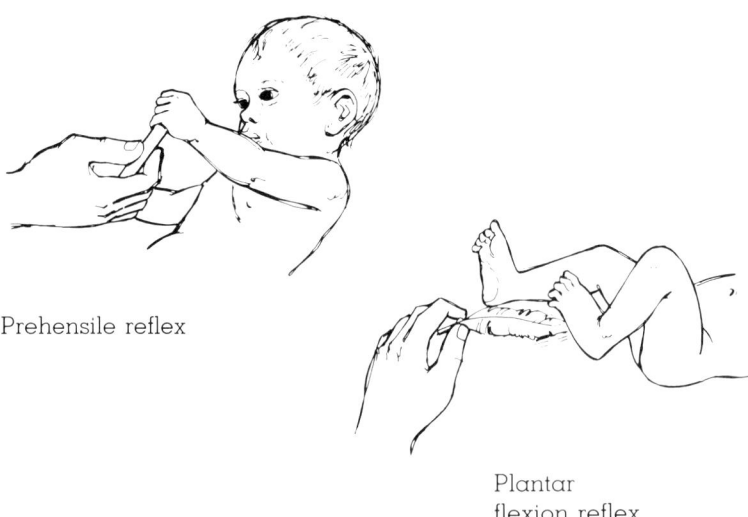

Prehensile reflex

Plantar
flexion reflex

Note. Figures 28.1-28.5 from B.J. Cratty, *Perceptual and Motor Development in Infants and Children,* 2d ed., © 1979, pages 51, 55, 56, and 61. Reprinted by permission of Prentice-Hall, Englewood Cliffs, NJ.

Some reflexes seem to have mixed effects on the child's acquisition of helpful voluntary movements. For example, the *asymmetrical tonic neck reflex*, also shown in Figure 28.1, tends to place one hand in a position where the child can look at it as the head is turned to one side. If this reflex persists, the continually outstretched hand on the side toward which the head turns prevents the infant from rolling from back to front efficiently.[2] Thus, at times therapists have to "tease out" this reflex, at least momentarily, while helping the neurologically impaired child execute the basic roll on the longitudinal axis of the body. This may be done by stretching the arm extensors until contraction is obtained in the biceps.

Other reflexes, when chained together, produce useful sequential actions, which apparently evolve into voluntary movements. For example, infants soon support themselves in an arms-extended position on their front, with the stomach still in contact with the floor. Figure 28.2 illustrates this *supporting reflex*. Then, as an object passes across the visual field, the head reflexively turns, causing the hips to turn in the same direction involuntarily. Thus the first turns from the stomach to the back are made. Later this turn is initiated voluntarily in normal infants.

A number of reflexes resemble variations of voluntary locomotion. For example, if, soon after birth, an infant is held upright or upside down against a surface, stepping motions will be observed—the *walking reflex*. Figure 28.3 shows this reflex. For some years it was assumed that this reflex phased out well before the onset of voluntary walking. But more recent findings indicate that if this reflex is continually triggered by appropriate conditions, the infant will engage in voluntary walking sooner. Other locomotor-like reflexes include a *swimming response* if the infant is held on or over water and a *crawling reflex* if the bottoms of the feet are alternately touched while the child is on his or her stomach.

Figure 28.2 Supporting Reaction   **Figure 28.3** Walking Reflex

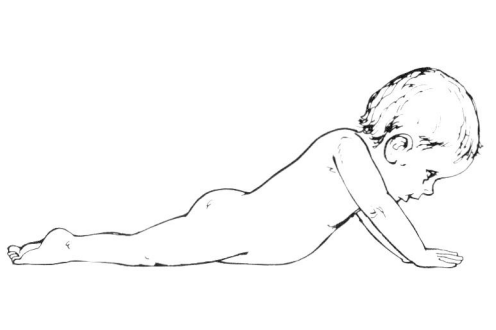

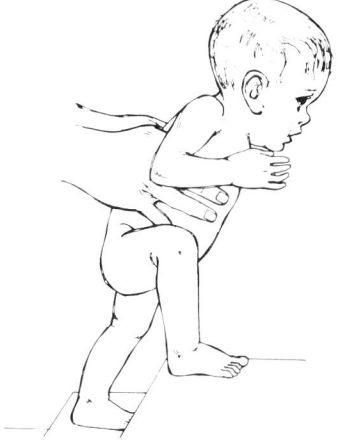

2. A contemporary look at these reflexes, early voluntary movements, and rhythmic stereotypies is found in chapter 5 of *Perceptual and Motor Development in Infants and Children* (3rd ed.) by B.J. Cratty, 1986, Englewood Cliffs, NJ: Prentice-Hall.

EARLY POSTURES AND MOVEMENTS

Sometime after the 4th month, and usually by the 7th month, the infant will begin to rise in a hands-and-knees position. At first this is difficult for the normal infant. As strength and balance are achieved, the position becomes more stable. This posture along with a seated position and a standing position represent the three key balance positions. They are difficult, and therapists dwell on them extensively when working with brain-injured and developmentally delayed children.

Movement from the all-fours position begins to occur when the child starts to reach out with one hand for an object. The first attempt usually results in a fall to the chin, but with further practice the first crude movements occur, with feet and hands moving in a rather random order. Then a more refined crawling pattern emerges, as shown in Figure 28.4. A cross-extension pattern is the final result, with the right hand and left knee moving forward in concert. This movement sometimes must be aided in atypical children, as pictured. At times the ability to maintain a hand-knee position is thwarted if the child's asymmetrical tonic neck reflex is too strong; the child tends to suddenly flex the arm at the elbow on the side toward which the head moves.

Later the normal child, on falling from a hands-and-knees position or being supported and encouraged by parents, gains a seated position, freeing the hands for increased manual activity. Maintaining this position, as well as those previously discussed and those to follow, is partly dependent on head control. If the child's head is not well controlled and may suddenly move forward, backward, or in either direction, maintenance of a seated posture and other static postures is difficult. In both prone and supine positions most normal infants begin to gain control of head movements. Motor-handicapped children, however, may

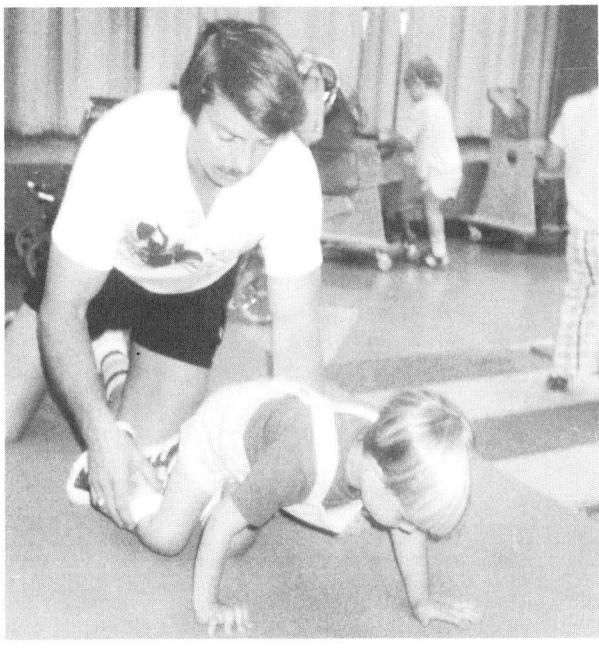

Creeping sometimes must be aided.

Courtesy, Special Education Branch, Los Angeles City Schools

Figure 28.4 Cross-Extension Crawling

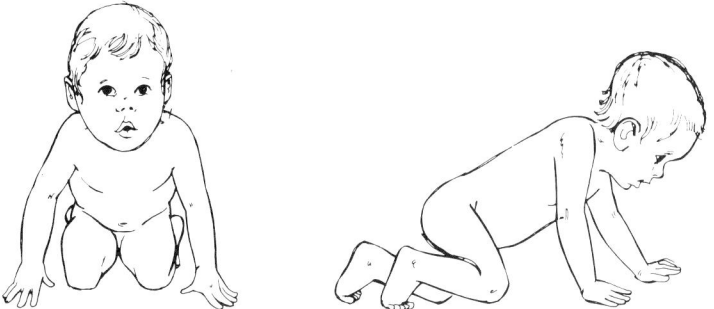

need constant work on head control. In a seated position the child also may make attempts to move backward, pushing with the legs in a scooting action.

Two thirds of the way through the first year, the normal infant has a variety of postures and movements that are precursors to later standing and walking. For example, when placed in a standing position and held by the hands, the child tends to regain the upright if gently pushed backward or from side to side, as shown in Figure 28.5. This is called a *pull-up reaction*.

By the end of the 8th, 9th, or 10th month, children will seek the assistance of an adult or an object to pull themselves to upright positions. This usually occurs slightly earlier in girls than in boys. Handicapped children in particular should have access to apparatus that permits them to pull themselves to their feet if they cannot already do so.

Gaining a momentary position, even with assistance, and maintaining it for increased periods, is dependent on (a) suppression of the plantar flexion reflex, previously described, because suppression of this reflex permits flat and solid bases of support from the bottoms of the feet, and (b) a group of movements called *parachute reactions*. These latter reactions, as illustrated, enhance the ability to fall from a standing position without undue trauma.

Figure 28.5 Pull-Up Reactions

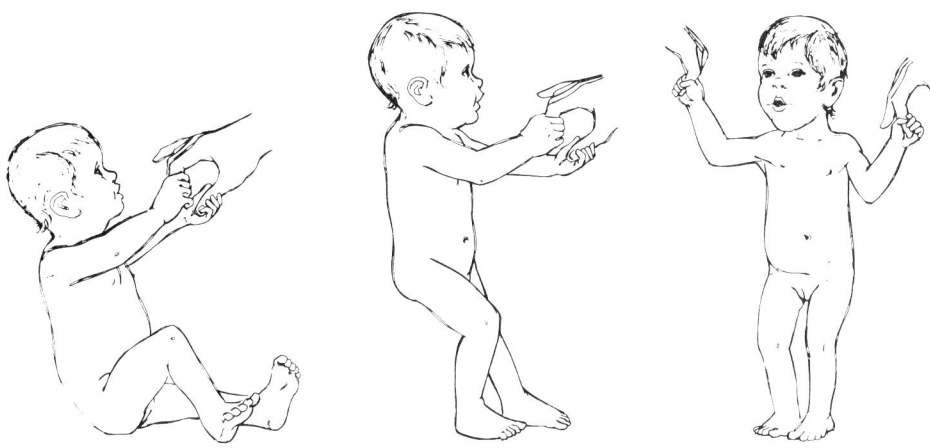

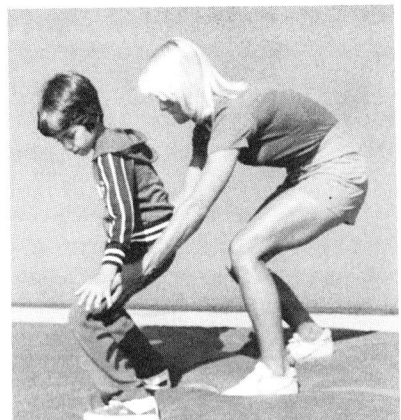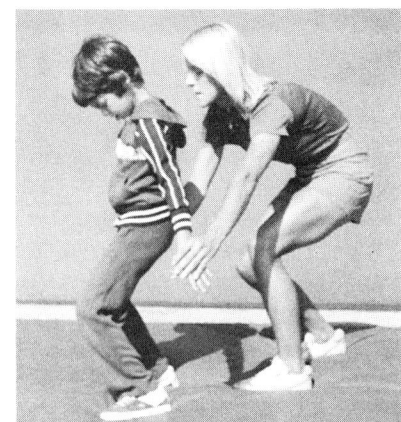

Awkward or palsied children may need help learning parachute reactions to minimize trauma from falling.

They consist of a quick knee-bend while reaching out with one or both hands. If the child is about to fall backward, the head leans forward, the hips bend forward, and the hands reach out and back to break the fall. A fall forward also requires a quick knee-bend and a reaching out to the front to stop the fall. Therapists working with children who are awkward or have cerebral palsy may spend considerable time eliciting these safety reactions.

Usually, after a child gains an upright stance, the next achievement is *cruising*. The child moves laterally to one side, holding onto a low table top or some other means of support. Finally, at about the end of the first year, the child begins to evidence a true walk, first with aid, then alone. This occurs, on the average, slightly earlier in girls than in boys and earlier in thinner children than in heavier children.

The first walking steps pose difficult balance problems. If the child leans forward too far, he or she falls forward (hopefully with a correct parachute reaction). The feet are spaced wide, and balancing the large (and not always cooperative) head is still a problem. The arms are usually in flexion in front of the body and do not evidence cross-extension with the legs until later.

If the child's arms do not coordinate (move in a cross-extension pattern) with the legs into the fourth year, several types of actions may be practiced. *Knee-walking* with assisted movements of the arms is helpful. The arm opposite the knee moving forward should be gently moved forward, as shown in photo A. Cross-extension walking with the knees high on a soft, thick mat or on a trampoline may be helpful. This can be exaggerated if the child reaches across the body, touching one hand to the opposite knee as it comes upward and forward (see photo B).

As walking is mastered, the child tries variations, including a fast walk—not a true run, because at no point is the child's body entirely clear of the ground—and then jumping, both feet at the same time. The first jumping actions usually are asymmetrical, one or the other foot slightly ahead, with no accompanying arm action. In these early attempts the child may not even leave the ground. By the 4th year, the child should be jumping and landing several times in succession—two-foot takeoffs and landings. By this time both the running and walking patterns should evidence fair to good arm-leg opposition.

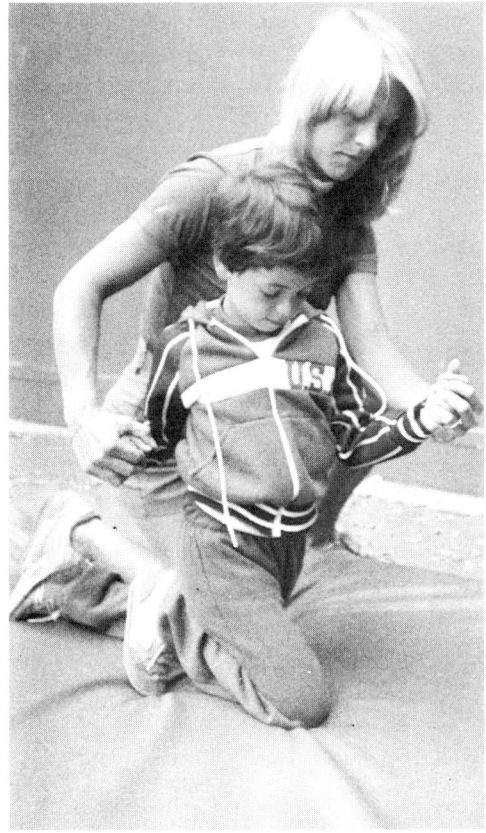

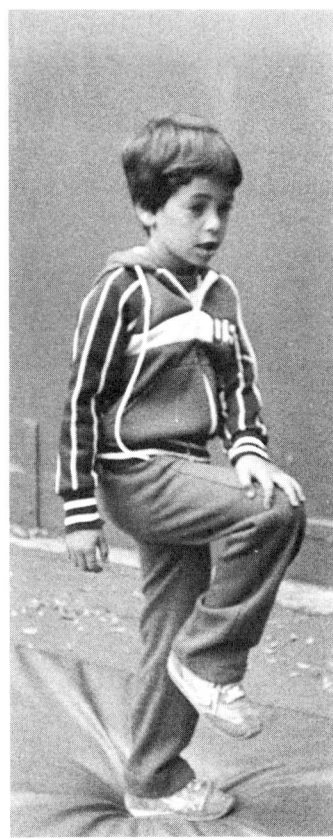

Handicapped children may need to learn and practice cross-extension and walking patterns.

A   **B**

ATYPICAL PATTERNS

Several atypical gait patterns are seen in children with various handicaps. Children who display these patterns should be referred to a pediatric neurologist and receive a thorough evaluation of their motor competencies. Among these often subtle problems are (a) a flat-footed, feet-turned-out gait and run (*pronated feet*), accompanied by incorrect or absent arm action (arms in flexion and immobile across the chest); (b) a *shuffling gait* (which also may involve pronated feet), in which knee-lift is minimal and arms are either too tense and immobile or floppy and out of control; and (c) an *asymmetrical gait* in which one side seems always to precede the other side of the body during movement. Usually in children with an asymmetrical gait, the stronger side (or leg) is pushing the weaker side (leg) ahead.

Among the pathological conditions that may be reflected in atypical gaits are the *scissored gait*, discussed in chapter 13 (cerebral palsy); a *staggering gait*, resulting from brain tumor and similar conditions; and a *stiff-kneed gait*, in which the support phase is followed by an extension pattern instead of normal flexion at the knee (a positive supporting reflex)—an indication of mild ataxia or some other condition that damages the spinal cord. Excessive foot drop may be caused by paralysis or weakness in the muscles in the front of the calf (anterior tibial muscles). An extremely asymmetrical gait reflecting paralysis or weakness of the gluteus medius muscle on one side results in excess weight shift to the strong side when walking. This is called the *Trendelenburg gait*.

Another atypical pattern is the *waddling gait*, caused by weakness in both gluteus medius muscles. An extremely asymmetrical gait in which both the arm and leg on one side maintain a flexed position may reflect hemiplegia. Victims of Parkinson's disease also display an inappropriate gait, usually walking in a stiff, shuffling manner, with much constraint in their movement patterns. Some developmentally delayed children have to be helped to learn where their feet are, as pictured. All of these atypical patterns should be referred for thorough diagnosis and treatment.

OTHER MOVEMENTS

Between the end of the 2nd year and the 5th and 6th years, many types of locomotor activities appear almost simultaneously if children are allowed and encouraged to move freely. These movements gradually become refined, especially when they are combined in culturally valued sports and games. Dance and rhythm also promote variations in locomotion such as galloping and skipping.

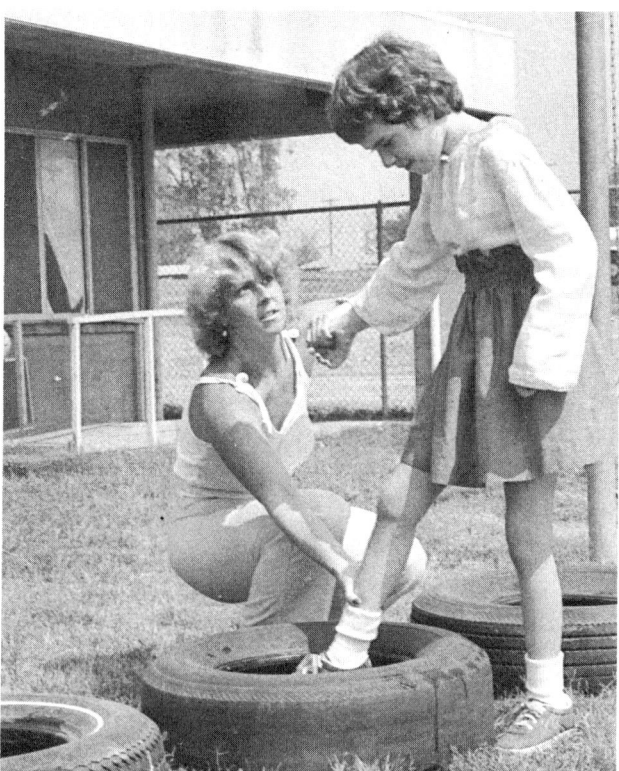

Older, developmentally delayed youngsters sometimes need help learning the location of their feet.

Courtesy, Fontana, California Public Schools

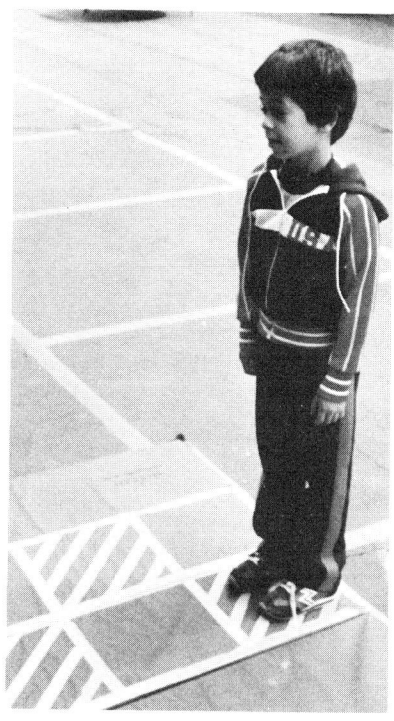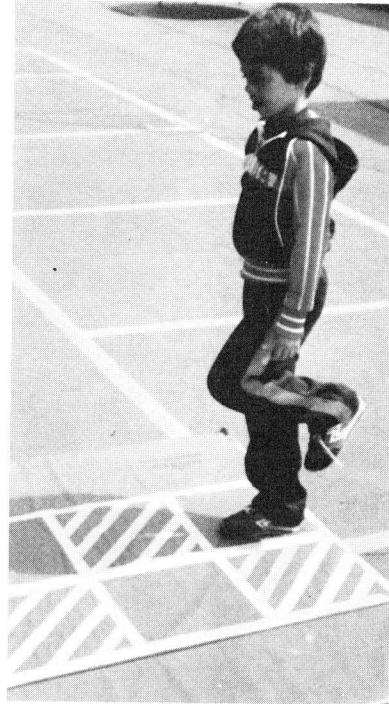

Normal children usually are able to hop and jump precisely by about age 6.

Leaping and Hopping

At about the time children begin to run—toward the end of the 2nd and the beginning of the 3rd year—they experiment with ways to leave the ground in addition to jumping. Usually seen next is an unsupported step or leap, taking off on one foot and landing on the second. This is typically attempted first from a slightly raised platform to a lower surface, and later on a level surface.

Hopping is more difficult. It is seen by the 3rd and beginning of the 4th year in most normal children. Many neurologically impaired children, including those found in some retarded populations, such as children with Down syndrome, never evidence a true hop. Precise hopping into a 1′ by 1′ square, as illustrated, usually is acquired about age 6 in normal girls and slightly later in normal boys.

Lateral Movement

Moving to the side is an imperative skill in ball games. Initially young children do it tentatively, and at times asymmetrically, moving better to one side than to the other. Soon, as balls are rolled to them, children must decide whether to remain facing the ball and move a step to the side to intercept its pathway or to cross over one foot and run to the side for a short distance before facing the ball again. Lateral movements to retrieve a ball are

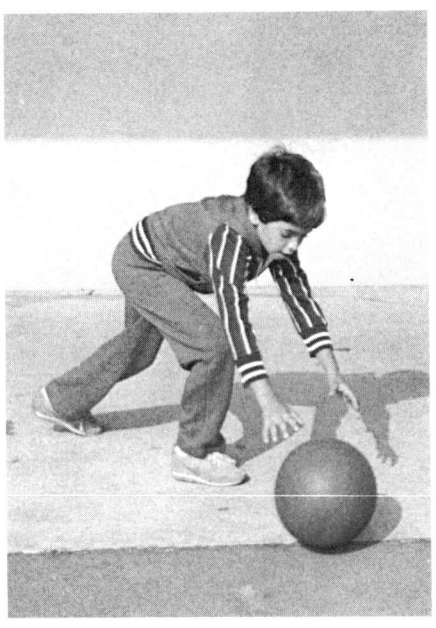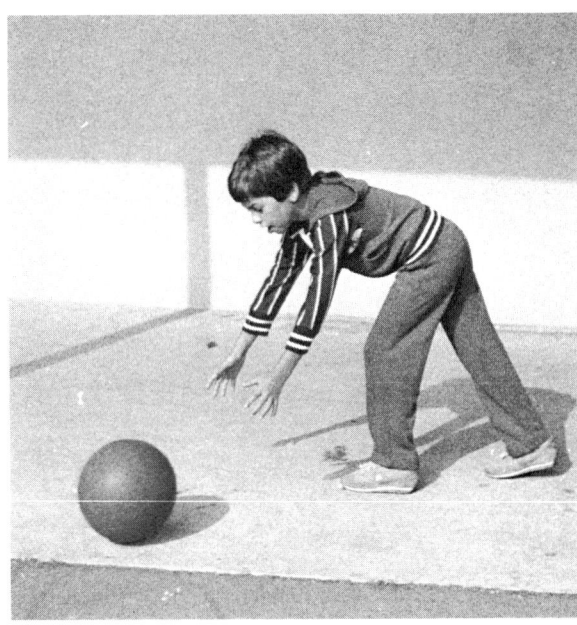

Lateral movements may be necessary to retrieve a ball.

illustrated. Some children make this decision unconsciously, after some exposure to incoming missiles; others have to be taught to make a conscious decision as to how and when to make the movements.

Just as when moving backward (a much more difficult skill), children must either learn or unconsciously acquire the ability to suddenly terminate their momentum and make a stop. Often, awkward children will think "stop" but make no changes in their body mechanics. Some must be taught to lower their hips suddenly to facilitate stopping, as illustrated. Otherwise they may cease leg actions but may remain upright and eventually stop in a stiff-legged position several feet from where they wanted to. "Shuffle drills" are helpful prior to introducing a child to sports activities such as basketball and tennis. In these drills children are taught to move laterally, not crossing their feet, and to bring the body to a quick stop by quickly lowering the center of mass (i.e., bending at the hips). This shuffling lateral movement is most efficient if the child maintains contact with the floor or ground most of the time. High leaps to the side generally are less efficient as children are unable to make changes in direction and speed while floating through the air between landings.

Backward Movement

Soon after achieving reasonably secure forward walking, normal infants experiment with sideways and even backward walking. Moving backward at any speed is an extremely dif-

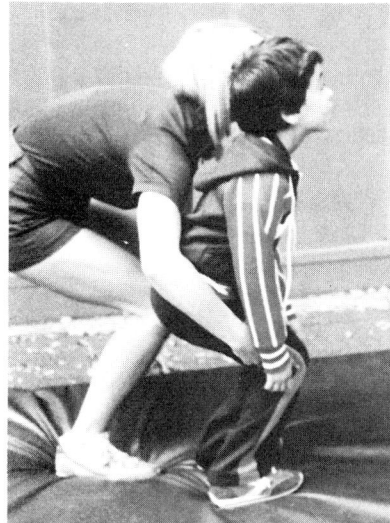 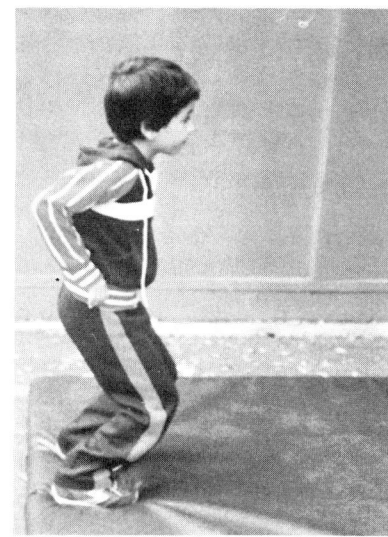

Children may have to be taught to lower their hips to facilitate stopping.

ficult undertaking and, at times, even dangerous. Although the movement is required in mature ball games, the moderately awkward child is in danger of falling if encouraged to walk, jump, or run backward too rapidly. Backward running must be accompanied by drills and lessons that elicit efficient stopping, and initially the surface over which backward exercises are practiced should be soft (mats or grass). The children all should have good parachute responses before attempting any backward speed.

In addition to moving directly backward, practice should be given in moving backward and laterally to the left and to the right. These movements are also required in ball games. Drills eliciting sideways, backward, and backward-and-sideways movements may be used. Later, balls may be rolled to various positions, requiring effort to intercept the pathway of the missile in the ways described.

Galloping and Skipping

Galloping usually appears before skipping, at about age 5 to 6 (slightly earlier in girls).[3] The movement involves keeping one foot in front of the other at all times while moving forward in a shuffling manner. It usually requires less integration of both sides of the body in rhythmic action than is required in skipping. Some children, however, may become able to skip before learning to gallop, because of available peers to imitate.

Skipping with one foot only appears at about age 5. Normal children may know what the body is required to do but cannot elicit the necessary dynamic balances plus the step-slide alternations to effect a true skip. Thus, the 5-year-old may take a step with one foot and then execute a regular skipping-like step-slide with the second. Practice in alternating the stepping foot in this one-foot skipping action is a good lead-in to true skipping while holding onto something.

---

3. A shuffling-like gallop can appear a couple of years earlier, however.

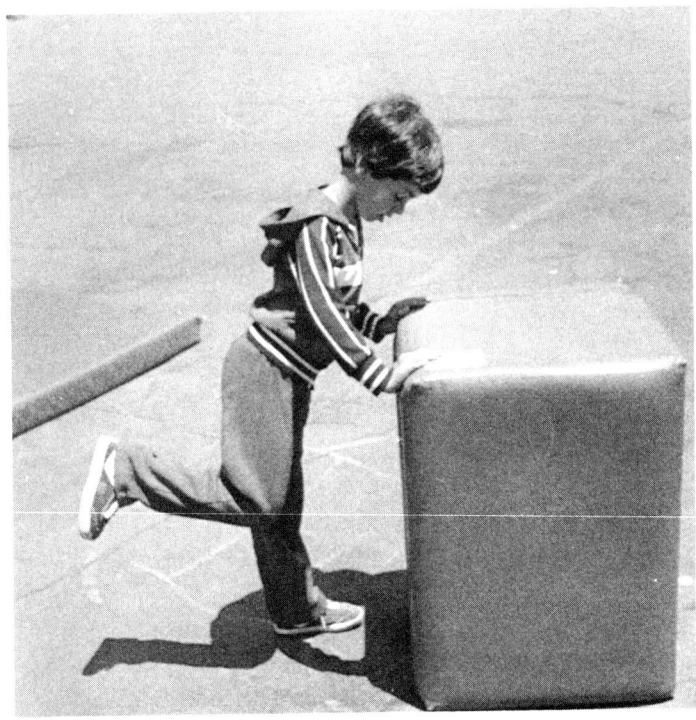

Learning to skip may
be facilitated by
holding onto something.

Usually skipping is accomplished by 60% to 80% of all girls by age 7, and over half of the boys of 7 exposed to the task usually accomplish it well. If a child has difficulty skipping by the age of 9 or 10, some motor problem involving integration of the body parts should be assumed to be present.

As in running, some children have excess overflow in the upper limbs and even in the face and mouth when skipping and galloping. The arms may be held tightly across the chest, fists clenched. In others the arms may dangle in a floppy manner. These faults should be corrected, if possible, through exposure to correct demonstrations, verbal suggestions, or moving the child's arms to stimulate the correct movements and degree of relaxation desirable.

Stair Walking

Ascending stairs in a crawling position is seen in infants if the stairs are well padded with carpet. Not until a reasonably stable walking pattern is achieved, in the 2nd or 3rd year, however, is the child confident in both ascending and descending stairs, even with the help of an adult or guide rail. Formulating norms for stair walking is virtually impossible because of the variation in the height of the risers, width of stairs, and height and type of bannisters, as well as the amount of help received from adults. In general, the following sequence prevails:

1. Initially, the child is comfortable ascending stairs with an adult holding one hand. The child usually places one foot (probably the dominant one) on a step and then brings the second foot to the same step before proceeding.

2. Next the child ascends the stairs in the same manner, unaided.

3. If each stair is not too high, the child ascends one foot at a time, with each foot reaching a different stair in the normal manner.

4. Descending stairs is more difficult and anxiety-producing to children than is ascending them. At the age when they can ascend one foot at a time, they often descend by bringing both feet to the same stair before proceeding downward. The sequence is the same as ascending, with the withdrawal of help initially and then (about age 4 to 5½) descent of stairs in a mature manner, lowering each foot to a different level.

Children with motor development problems may benefit from spending a considerable amount of time on practice stairs each week. Various combinations of movements may be attempted while moving up and down the risers backward, forward, and sideways. This kind of developmental exercise not only aids balance but also aids the integration of body parts (the legs on both sides of the body), adds to self-confidence, and improves leg extension strength.

Jumping Upward and Forward

After children learn to jump forward in a controlled manner for a short distance, they should be encouraged to experiment with ways of jumping that elicit either a high-jump or a broad-jump. Standing broad-jumps and high-jumps are good leg developers and lead into various track-and-field events (e.g., triple-jump and broad-jump) in middle childhood, as well as developing leg strength and power for innumerable sports. Broad-jumping is an event in the California Special Olympics, for example.

The normal child's first efforts to give impetus to jumping through use of the arms may be ineffectual. The arms move neither upward (extending at the shoulders) nor forward, as appropriate. Later the child may show a slightly upward and backward motion of the arms, elbows lifting up in back, while jumping. This may or may not occur at the same time as the knees extend. An example of this kind of immature jumping action is pictured.

As the child reaches the 4th, 5th, and 6th years, the manner in which the arms extend at the shoulders to give impetus to both the high-jump and broad-jump should be demonstrated, explained, and manually directed. A good lead-in activity is to have children experiment with jumping in various ways. Effort should be made to have them feel for themselves the ways in which the arms may or may not assist the total jumping action. A first jump or two with the arms and hands held stiffly to the sides might be tried, as pictured.

Were the children able to jump well or high this way? If the answer is no, children then might be encouraged to determine just what they might do with their arms, and when, so they can jump further or higher. Some might discover that throwing the arms upward at the same time the legs extend at the knees and hips may enhance an upward jump. The children then might experiment with upward jumping and forward jumping with arm actions that involve both upward and forward motions, as pictured.

Assistance from behind may help a child propel the arms properly and at the correct time. Once the child discovers the principle of assistance of the arms, a common fault is to either lift or throw the arms forward, but at the wrong times, before or after the legs extend at the knees and hips. The photo shows the instructor helping the child to extend his arms at the proper time.

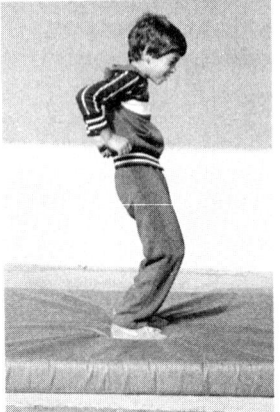
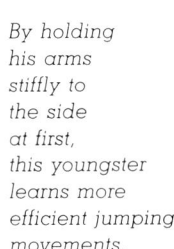
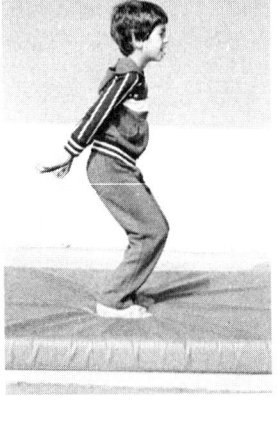

Immature arm and leg movements may be seen in initial jumping efforts.

By holding his arms stiffly to the side at first, this youngster learns more efficient jumping movements.

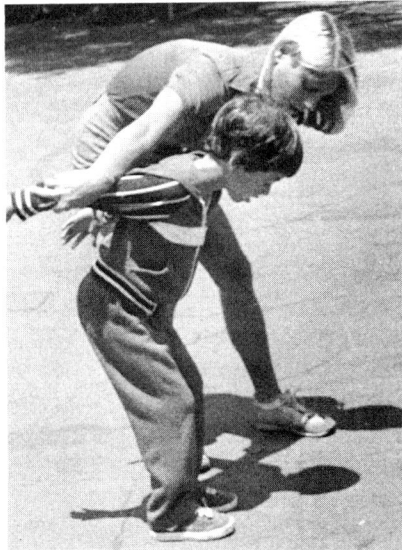
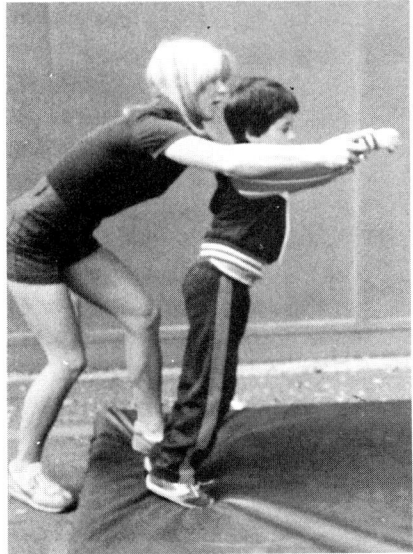

Upward and forward motions of the arms can enhance the height and distance of a jump.

In jumping, the arms must be extended at just the right time.

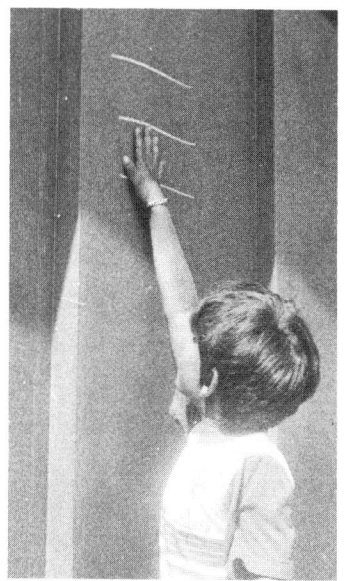
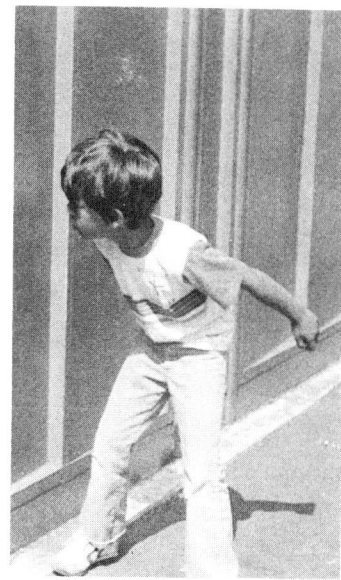

After determining their standing height plus reach (A), children may try to exceed that measure by jumping as high as they can (B).

After simultaneous movement of the arms and legs, extension begins to occur in both upward and forward jumping. To encourage this, a line may be marked out to determine whether children can exceed their distance in a broad jump. Also, a vertical linear measure may be placed on a wall, and after the children stand against it, reaching upward to determine their standing height plus reach, they turn to the side and with a rhythmic swing or two, accompanied by a knee-bend, swing the arms upward, touching as high a point as possible with hand and fingertips, as shown.

Rhythmic Hopping and Rope Jumping

Alternate hopping patterns are often used as (a) evaluative criteria, and (b) components of various drills and dances. Generally, not until children are 7 or 8 years old can they successfully transfer a three-to-three or two-to-two hopping pattern from one foot to the other (two hops on foot, followed immediately by two on the opposite foot, repeated several times). A hopping pattern involving a three-two count is even more difficult.

One of the more difficult skills for awkward children to acquire is rope jumping. Not only must they learn jumping patterns, which include an abbreviated half-jump (between a full jump), but also the mechanics of turning the rope. Usually the first teaching steps consist of jumping from one side of a line to another using the jump/half-jump action—a true jump followed by a knee-bend pseudo-jump during which the feet do not leave the ground, another jump to the opposite side of the line, and a pseudo-jump in the same manner, repeated over and over again. When this is accomplished, a real rope may be used, swung gently in only a half-swing.

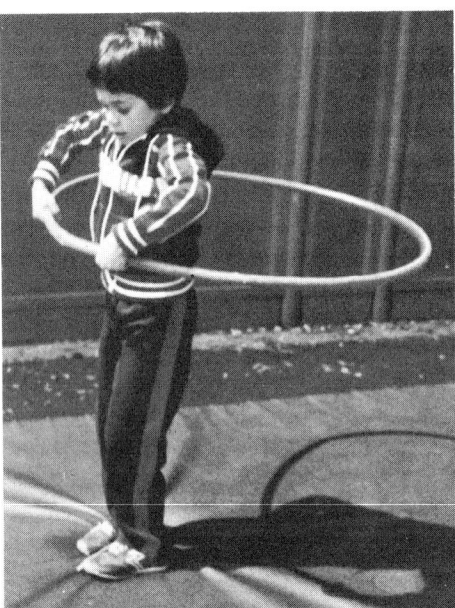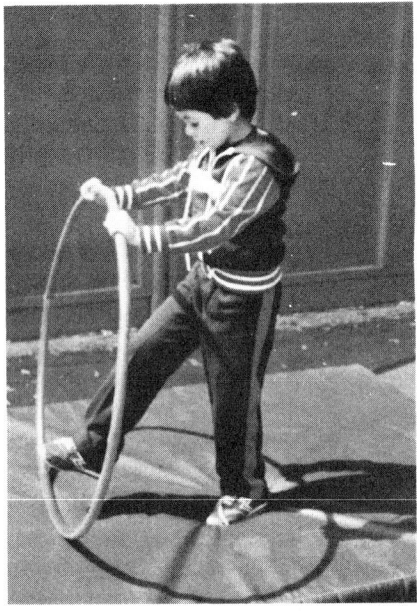

A hoop may be used as an intermediate step in learning to jump a self-held rope.

Finally, children may be introduced to holding and jumping a rope at the same time. Initially the rope should be swung to one or the other side of the feet to establish the required rhythm, including the speed of the rope and the jump. Then the rope may be opened up in the usual manner, with children encouraged to jump over their own hand-held rope. A hoop may be used as an intermediate step in learning to jump in this manner, as its position in space is much easier to maintain than that of a rope, and therefore more predictable as it passes under the jumper's feet. Uses of the hoop are pictured.

CHECKLIST FOR EFFICIENT LOCOMOTOR BEHAVIORS

The following checklist follows the normal developmental sequence of movement in infants and developmentally delayed individuals. It might be used as a guideline for therapists and others who work with children to achieve these actions.

1. *Good head control.* The child is attracted to and moves the head and eyes to a source of interest, such as an object or a noise, without undue stress or extraneous head movements. This is seen in both supine and prone positions.

2. *Turning over.* The child is able to turn from front to back, first, and then back to front when desired and does not get stuck during the rollover or become frustrated by being unable to roll on all occasions.

3. *Seated balance.* Balance is stable; head control does not disrupt seated balance, and the child is able to reach out, grasp, and manipulate objects without undue disruption of balance.

4. *All-fours balance.* The child is able to posture steadily in an all-fours position, maintaining good head control and not evidencing sudden flexion of the arm opposite to that toward which the head is turned.

5. *Creeping (crawling).* The child is able to move in a cross-extension pattern toward an object without losing balance.

6. *Standing with support.* The child pulls up to a standing position when desired and when reasonable supports are available, maintaining the position by holding onto the support.

7. *Immature walking, assisted walking, and falling.* The child makes stepping movements, feet relatively flat and in alternating order, while being helped. Later, steps are taken, feet wide apart and arms in flexion, with a low knee-lift, for a few steps before falling. Falling evidences appropriate parachute reaction so that the pelvis does not contact the walking surface with too hard an impact.

8. *Mature walking.* Walk assumes rhythmicity; arm opposition is beginning; steps lengthen; and knee-lift becomes more pronounced. Arms move in a forward-and-backward motion instead of across the body. Shoulder rotation is not excessive; the knee bends in a relaxed manner after the contact-support phase of each step is completed. The child experiments with variations in velocity and the force of gait.

9. *Running.* Arm action opposes leg action appropriately. The child leans more and more to "get off balance" at each running step. Hands are held in a relaxed, cupped position rather than tightly in fists or too loosely. The child learns to lean more when more speed is required, depending more on toe drive, and leans back more when slowly jogging, permitting the heel to contact the ground first, with proper knee give.

10. *Jumping.* Feet leave the ground and contact the ground at the same time, knees giving at the completion of the jump. Arms lift forward or upward (depending on the action required) at the same time the knees extend. Knee-bend becomes more pronounced and knee-extension more forceful as the vigor of the jump increases, either upward or forward.

11. *Leaping, unsupported step.* Take-off is with foot straight ahead; ending is on opposite foot with proper give of the knee to take the landing shock. Arms swing upward as the take-off leg is extended. The child is able to execute unsupported step (leap) in a variety of situations and from a variety of take-off points (lower or higher than the landing point).

12. *Hopping.* Foot is straight ahead and is accompanied by arm-lift when leaving the ground. Descent is followed by a relaxed give of the knee as the same foot contacts the ground, foot straight ahead. Variations in upward and forward distance of the hop are achieved with changes in vigor of the arm thrust and leg extension.

13. *Lateral movement.* Movement to the side is relaxed and as rapid as the task demands, involving one or more cross-over running steps, or side steps during which the feet do not cross. Arms are not stiff. Facility in moving to either side is equal. The side movement chosen is appropriate to the situation.

14. *Galloping.* The movements are rhythmical, feet straight ahead and knees relaxed and bent following each contact phase of the movement. Directional change is possible when galloping and when skipping. Movements are not accompanied by uncontrolled arm movements across the body causing or reflecting excess hip rotation. Children are able to adjust speed and height of movements varying knee-lift and arm-thrust to obtain more vigor. Movements are modified to music beats and interpolated with other movements.

15. *Rhythmic hopping.* By age 8 or 9 the child is able to demonstrate rhythmic hopping in various patterns, continuously moving from one foot to the other in a two-two, three-three, or two-three pattern. Arms are held in slight flexion but without undue tension. These patterns are incorporated into games, folk dances, and the like. Modified hopping and jumping should lead to rope-jumping activities by late childhood.

SUMMARY

Many reflexes and voluntary movements contribute to children's ability to move through space by their own efforts. Problems in static positioning, as well as dynamic efforts arising from these positions, often beset various types of handicapped children and youth.

Numerous reflexes support later postures, locomotion, and voluntary movements. Various labyrinthine reflexes (reflecting the infant's relationship to gravity and to the upright) are precursors of voluntary sitting, standing, and walking. Locomotor reflexes, including a stepping reaction and crawling and swimming reflexes, resemble the voluntary counterparts.

If they persist too long in the child's "motor personality," some reflexes can inhibit standing and walking. Among these are the plantar flexion reflex, which results in an unstable foot position as the child tries to stand, and the asymmetrical tonic reflex, which may prevent assumption of the stable hand-knee position needed for crawling.

With good therapy hands and knowledge of locomotor development, physical educators and therapists can lead children through the developmental sequences of movements that culminate in an upright, unassisted gait. Following the acquisition of walking, normal children begin to refine the walking pattern to include a coordinated cross-extension pattern of the arms and legs in the action. They also begin to experiment with gait variations including backward and lateral movement, rapid walking, and then running, hopping, jumping, galloping, and skipping.

Atypical children may need special help in any or all of these skills and sub-skills. And they, along with normal children, may be trained to gain additional power in jumping upward and forward and to learn the intricate movements exhibited in alternate rhythmic hopping and dance steps.

The following detailed checklist may be used to formulate an assessment/screening tool reflecting the sequential acquisition of various locomotor behaviors discussed in this chapter. This is followed by some suggested variations.

Locomotion and Pre-Walking Behaviors

    1. Turns head in supine position to follow visual stimuli.

    2. Shows positive support reflex (push-up position) with stomach in contact with bed in prone position.

    3. Turns from stomach to back.

    4. Turns from back to stomach.

5. Evidences head control in supported sit.
6. Sits without support.
7. Scoots (pushes, back first, in seated position).
8. Balances in all-fours position, legs collapsing.
9. Reaches in all-fours position, legs collapsing.
10. Crawls (rudimentary), legs dragging and uncoordinated with arm action.
11. Crawls (random), arms and legs not synchronized and not in cross-extension pattern.
12. Crawls (coordinated) with cross-extension pattern.
13. Pulls to standing position.
14. Stands with support.
15. Cruises (moves laterally in standing position, holding onto support).
16. Stands momentarily without support; shows good parachute reaction when falling (knees bending, arms reaching out).
17. Stands well without support.
18. Walks with assistance.
19. Walks (rudimentary), nonrhythmic, for a few steps.
20. Walks (sustained), nonrhythmic.
21. Walks (rhythmic), arms in flexion; cross-extension pattern.

Variations in Locomotion

1. Hurried walk, non-run.
2. Slow, lateral movement, feet not crossing.
3. Backward walk without falling.
4. Rudimentary run; both feet clear ground at same time.
5. Rudimentary asymmetrical jump, one foot in front of the other on take-off or landing.
6. Asymmetrical jump, both feet in line on take-off and landing, for one to three jumps.
7. Precise jump into one-foot squares, over lines, etc.
8. Unsupported step, take-off on one foot, a nonsupport phase, landing on the other foot.
9. Assisted (hand-held) hop, one or more times.
10. Jump and turn (half-turn, both feet at once).
11. One or two unassisted hops (one foot to the same foot, clearing ground).
12. Run with proper arm-leg coordination (cross-extension pattern).
13. Run and stop, with some control; quick knee-bend.
14. Three to five unassisted hops.
15. One-footed skip (step on one foot, skip-like motion on the other).
16. Assisted skip (holding onto a chair).
17. Simple gallop (both feet not leaving the ground at once).
18. Gallop, one foot advancing in front of the other, both feet off the ground at the same time.
19. Alternate hopping from foot to foot in a two-two pattern.
20. True skipping, unassisted.
21. Alternate hopping on a two-three pattern from foot to foot.
22. Rapid lateral movement.

REFERENCES

Cratty, B.J. (1986). *Perceptual and motor development in infants and children* (3rd ed.). Englewood Cliffs, NJ: Prentice-Hall.

Peiper, A. (1963). *Cerebral function in infancy and childhood.* New York: Consultant's Bureau.

Wickstrom, R.L. (1970). *Fundamental motor patterns.* Philadelphia: Lea & Febiger.

QUESTIONS FOR DISCUSSION

1 What are some infant reflexes? What purposes do they have?

2. What is the parachute reaction, and how does it relate to standing and walking behavior?

3. What are some chains of reflexes involved in various voluntary actions?

4. What are the terms for reflexes involved in seeking the upright position?

The hand to close when the palm is touched? The feet to curl when the sole is touched?

5. How might a child be trained to skip? Be specific.

6. What is the order of difficulty for skills involved in a walking gait?

7. What are the normal ages at which crawling begins? Standing? Galloping?

STUDENT PROJECTS

1. Observe an infant a few weeks of age. What reflexes do you see? What seems to trigger these reflexes?

2. Ask a boy and girl 5 years old and another boy and girl 7 years old to broadjump as far as they can from a standing position. What differences, if any, do you see in the integration of movements?

3. Develop a 12-item checklist of locomotor activities and variations specific to a certain age group, and apply it to a group of normal children. Arrange the tasks in order of difficulty after observing the children. Do the same for a group of children of a wider age span.

4. Observe and classify on a 1- to 4-point scale (from poor to good) the efficiency with which children labeled motorically handicapped perform a group of locomotor skills. Contrast the scores obtained with those earned by a group of normal children. What tasks revealed the greatest differences in skill level? Why?

29 *Balls and Other Missiles*

Skills involving balls are ingrained in the cultures of virtually all modern and primitive societies. When first attempting to further physical skills in their children, parents most often begin by throwing them a ball. If the youngster cannot meet parents' expectations at this feat, frustration and tension may ensue—particularly if the child is developmentally behind agemates or awkward in this regard. Yet throwing and catching balls and other missiles (frisbees, beanbags, balloons, and the like) are relatively difficult skills involving coordination and precision of both the hands and the feet. Normally, children cannot predict until late childhood where a small ball thrown from a distance will arrive.

Catching requires accurate movements of the hands and feet together. Throwing is an equally difficult task, requiring a summation of forces, starting with positioning of the feet, continuing up the legs, where a rotary motion is initiated and the trunk is stabilized. A twist of the shoulders and, finally, the ballistic throw of the arm itself terminates in the release of the sphere at just the right time in the arc made by the arm. Needless to say, many children who are handicapped are not equipped physically to exhibit such a complex and forceful skill pattern.

Society also suggests that proficiency is desirable in sports in which an extension of the body is used to contact and otherwise deal with missiles. Tennis, field hockey, paddle ball, and golf require participants to locate their bodies properly to contact missiles with racquets, sticks, and clubs of varying weights, lengths, sizes, and materials. Needless to say, these sports can pose quite a challenge for some handicapped people without careful progressions and patient teaching.

This chapter obviously cannot cover all of the many ball games in which children and youth might participate. Rather, it presents sequences and activities that help youngsters gain the confidence to participate in games requiring them to come to terms with objects (and people) whizzing toward and away from them at various speeds.

Basic lead-in activities are presented first, followed by drills and games preparatory to some of the traditional sports. As when teaching all skills, the child or youth should experience a good deal of success in ball tasks before undertaking more difficult skills. The results of careful teaching can be rewarding. As a boy in my program stated one day, "I spent 10 years not catching a ball, and today I did. I feel very good!"

LEAD-IN ACTIVITIES

Normal children's first experiences with balls and missiles come almost by accident; they may swing a hand through the air in which there is an object that pulls away from the hand because of centrifugal force. This experience, when finally done voluntarily, represents the genesis of a throwing movement, which is satisfying to the person who does it.

Catching is usually very rudimentary at first, consisting merely of trapping rolling objects as they slowly approach. The following activities can be applied with the very young or the handicapped. They represent first experiences with balls.

Touching

Experiencing the feel of things in the hand is a first task. This can consist of merely passing balls and other objects from hand to hand, from child to child, as the children sit in a circle. The shapes, weights, and textures of the objects may be felt and discussed as the objects are passed around. Cubes and spheres made of clay, cardboard, and styrofoam may be used. The more variety, the better. The children's first experiments may be to place the objects on the floor to determine (with a hand push) which of them roll and which do not.

Trapping

Following tactile experiences, children, still seated, may attempt to stop or trap balls that are slowly rolled toward their outstretched legs (photo A). When this has been accomplished, the activity may be made more difficult by placing the children around a table and asking them to "keep the ball on the table" by pushing. Then, standing, they may attempt to trap balls rolled at them, first slowly, then faster and faster. Variations may be achieved by rolling the ball slightly to the child's left or right side, requiring lateral movement to intercept the rolling missile (photo B).

B

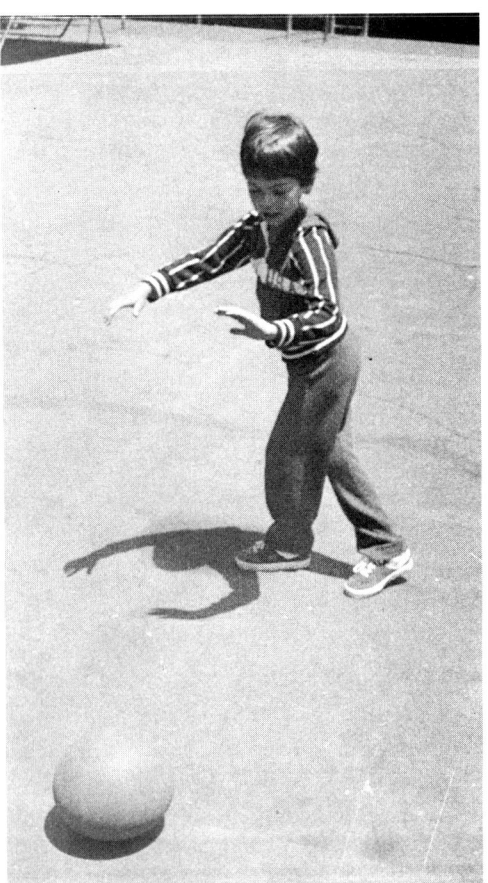

A

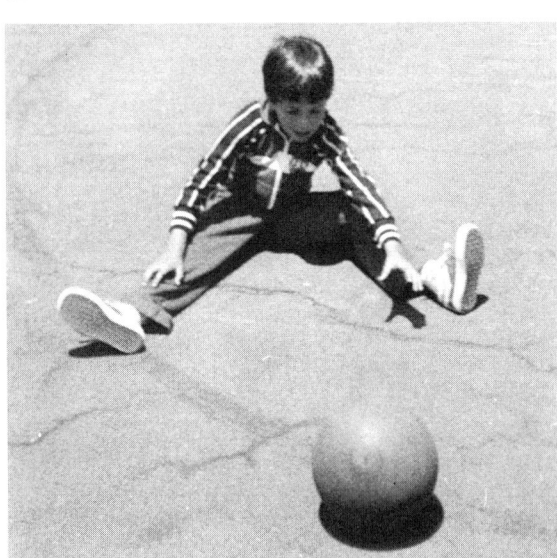

Trapping balls slowly rolled toward their outstretched legs is a good lead-in activity for the handicapped (A). Later they may practice moving to either side to trap balls rolled to them as they stand (B).

Rolling

During the previous activities children should be encouraged to impart varying velocities to the ball as they roll it. Different ways of starting the ball may be attempted. First, children might push the ball with both hands at once, as pictured, then with one hand, and then with an elbow or a foot. A slight incline up which children must roll the ball presents a challenge. Children later may be asked to roll a ball accurately into a garbage can placed on its side or onto targets painted on the playground, or to roll and trap a ball on a table top, as pictured.

Developmentally, releasing objects is a more difficult task than grasping them or pushing them. In some of these initial exercises (the seated tactile drill is a good place), children should be encouraged to release various objects until they learn a well coordinated volun-

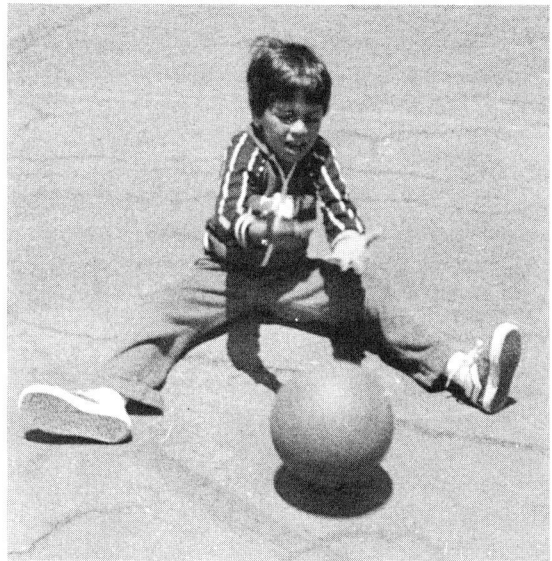

As a prelude to throwing balls, children may practice rolling a ball along the ground.

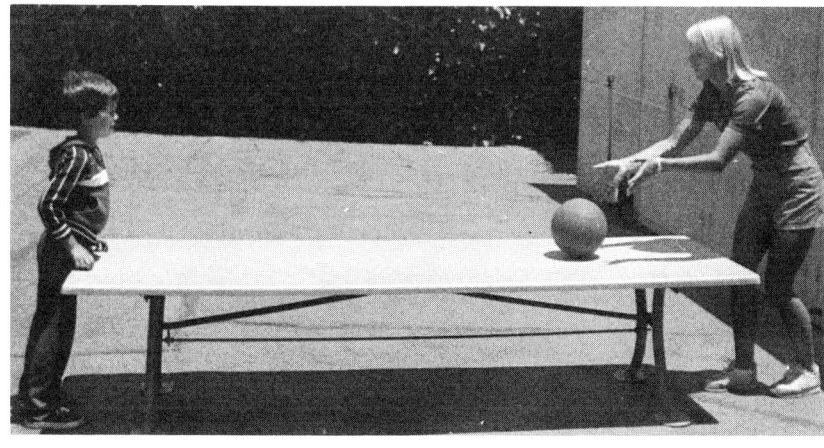

Rolling and trapping a ball on a tabletop requires some ball control and accuracy.

tary release. This is important initially, as an inappropriate release later will foil children's best efforts to throw a ball properly and efficiently. Objects of various sizes, shapes, and weights should be experimented with in these releasing drills.

Early Throwing and Catching

First attempts at throwing and catching are usually simple, direct, bilateral actions involving arms and hands at the same time. After the children are able to execute some of the initial skills reasonably well, they should be exposed to bilateral throwing and catching exercises and activities.

The Cradle   Initial attempts at catching should guarantee success. A child standing and facing the person with the ball, arms held out in front, elbows slightly bent and a few inches apart, presents a good target. The ball first may be bounced gently from about 10′ to 15′ away so that it lands in the cradle made by the catcher's arms with little effort or adjustment. This activity is pictured.

Two-Handed Overhead   A first crude throw that may be encouraged is a two-handed overhead throw, using a ball about 8″ in diameter of soft rubber. Accuracy should not be required at first. Initial efforts, no matter how variable, should be applauded. This kind of throw may be used to impart distance first and accuracy later. Force may be varied by asking children to "make the ball bounce one (two, three) times before getting to me." More advanced efforts should be accompanied by a weight shift and a step forward. This two-handed throw taken over one shoulder, with one hand in front on the ball and the other in the back, is the next developmental step in learning a one-handed throw with a smaller ball.

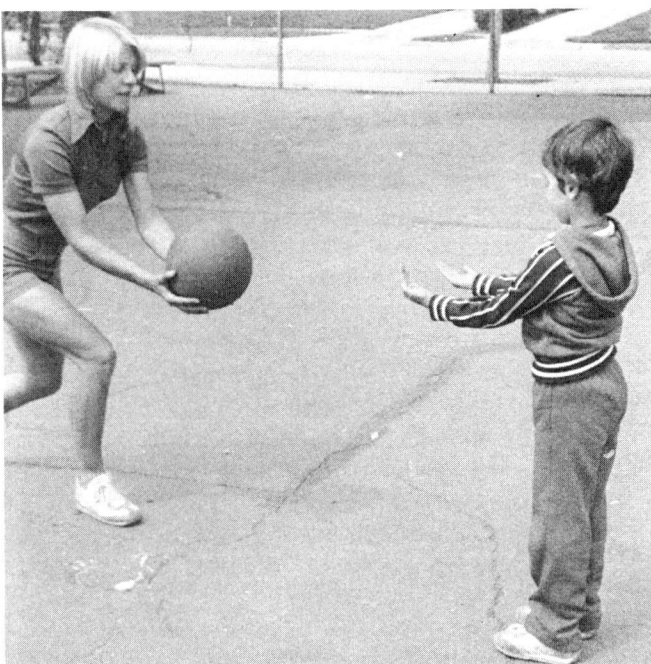

Catching the ball in a cradle made with the arms is an early catching experience.

SWINGING OBJECTS AND PRECISION CATCHING

The flight patterns of balls coming at a child via the throwing efforts of others are often highly unpredictable. Swinging a ball on a string as an initial task (a) results in a ball traveling a relatively predictable pathway, and (b) facilitates its interception when it almost stops at the end of the string. At first children should be placed at the end of the pendulum so the ball almost stops in their hands. Later they may be asked to dodge the ball, intercept it during faster parts of the swing, hit it with another ball on a string swinging at right angles to the ball to be hit, catch and throw balls of various sizes and shapes attached to strings, or play various group games using swinging balls (described in chapter 19, on orthopedic impairments).

Gradually children should be encouraged to intercept balls in this manner by using less arm action and more precision gripping (fingers and thumbs closing over the ball). In general, if a ball approaches a child chest-high or higher, the fingers should be pointed and spread upward in awaiting the catch.

Faulty catches result from closing the hand too soon (fingers may be jammed if the ball is thrown too hard), too late (the ball will bounce out), not "giving" enough as the ball arrives at the hands, or simply not placing the hands at the point at which the ball arrives. The concept of cushioning the shock with the hands as the ball arrives may be demonstrated to children by first throwing a ball at a hard-surface wall and watching it rebound off ("as it will do if your hands are too stiff") or throwing a ball against a relaxed surface (e.g., a large curtain) ("See how the curtain catches the ball?" Your hands must be relaxed like the curtain, when the ball gets to them").

Smaller balls may be first bounced toward children and later thrown on the fly from increasing distances. Until children reach middle childhood and later, they normally will not be able to run quickly and accurately to the spot where a small ball will arrive after being thrown from a distance of 20' or more. Younger children, or delayed youngsters whose developmental age is 6, 7, or lower, should not be expected to engage in ball games in which the balls are much smaller than 8" in diameter and the balls are to be caught from distances of 20' to 30'.

ADVANCED THROWING AND CATCHING

Throwing Strategies

As ball throwing and catching maturity is reached, children should be exposed to throwing patterns that involve the total body, both rotating and summating forces, starting from a push from the feet and ankles and terminating with a ballistic action of the arm accompanied by a weight shift as the hand releases the ball. When making a regular throw, a step is taken with foot opposite the throwing arm. This must be done simultaneously with a shift in weight. The weight shift may be magnified and accentuated by having the child stand on a tipping platform with the non-throwing foot ahead of the other. During the throw the platform tips forward with the weight shift and provides an additional noise cue as the front of the platform hits the surface of the playground or gym.

One-handed throws may be practiced for distance and accuracy. Force of the throw may be varied by asking the child to throw at targets at differing distances and to vary the number of bounces the ball takes from one point to another. Variations of force are particularly difficult for cerebral palsied children who are spastic. Children with mild cerebral palsy also have problems varying the force. Many times these children, to soften their throws, shorten the arc through which they move the arm rather than vary the speed of the limb prior to releasing the ball. They start a throw with the ball in front of the shoulder if they wish to throw a short distance and draw the arm back farther to throw a longer distance.

Children who are unable to kinesthetically perceive the location of their body parts tend to throw a ball by keeping it and their hand in front of the body where they can gain additional visual information about the location rather than drawing the arm and hand and ball back behind the throwing shoulder. Some help in front of a mirror or manual guidance may help relax this restricted throwing pattern.

Subtle differences in throwing methods should be pointed out to children. For example, when a basketball is thrown in a baseball pass, the foot opposite the throwing arm should be advanced as the weight is shifted. When making a one-handed basketball push shot, however, the foot directly under the shooting arm and hand is ahead.

Catching Strategies

In general, intercepting balls on the fly or after a bounce is harder for many handicapped children than throwing them. Not only must children judge (perceptually anticipate) where a projected ball will arrive, but they also must get their bodies to that position and then prepare their hands to close at exactly the correct time. A mistake in any one of these complex processes will result in failure.

Children first may be asked to throw a ball gently to themselves. Cradling a ball in their hands and arms, children may be shown how to straighten their knees and lift their arms at the same time, raising the ball for a short distance in the air and recatching it. This activity gradually may be made more difficult, using smaller balls and only the hands, instead of the hands and arms held in the simpler cradling position.

Next the ball may be dropped, allowed to bounce once, and then recaught by the same child. When trying this task, a common error of handicapped youngsters is not to come under the ball with their hands but instead to trap the large ball by gripping it above its "equator." The children must be helped to scoop under the ball and to try to recatch the ball at the top of the bounce, where momentarily it seems to hesitate, making its interception easier.

A circle game may be played in which someone (child or teacher) stands in the center and throws a ball in the air while calling the name of a child on the periphery. The child whose name is called attempts to catch the ball after one or two bounces and, if successful, assumes the middle position for the next round. Some handicapped children may have difficulty simultaneously throwing the ball in the air and remembering a name to call. A first tendency also may be to throw the ball at the child whose name is called instead of straight up in the air at the center of the circle.

When teaching handicapped children to catch, the actions initially may have to be broken down in parts. The children might first be exposed to shuffle drills in which they are encouraged to move laterally, not crossing their feet, as well as backward and forward, without worrying about intercepting balls. Emphasis should be placed on bending the knees slightly when moving, and then executing a more pronounced "stopping" knee-bend when the actions (lateral or forward and backward) are terminated. Likewise, children should be taught to make a cross-step initially and then run with their side toward the incoming ball, looking at it over their shoulder before facing it again in preparation for intercepting it.

Moving backward and laterally at the same time while watching balls (which need not at first be intercepted) is also a helpful drill. Most youngsters move better in one direction than the other. Teachers should give children extra help when children are required to move in a direction opposite from the one they favor.

When working on ball-catching skills, children also can be given tips on the basic physics of moving objects. If, for example, children are late in placing themselves in a position to catch a descending ball, the teacher might point out that a ball thrown from a distance drops faster as it approaches, so early positioning under it is necessary.

Beanbag Activities

Beanbags often are used to aid younger and atypical youngsters in throwing and catching habits. Beanbags are easily caught—they almost stick to the hand—and are relatively easy to throw. Also, children who are hit by a beanbag are not hurt. Beanbags are fun and may be employed in a variety of ways. They could be thrown at targets, for example, or attached to strings so that children in wheelchairs may reel them in after throwing them.

Beanbags may not be as useful as one might think, however, when trying to teach children to catch balls. The two activities are similar insofar as the child gains experience with tracking incoming missiles, and the throwing actions are not dissimilar. But the entire catching action is different when using beanbags and when using balls, particularly when the balls are hard and are thrown from some distance. The hands do not have to give with the catch when the beanbag arrives, as they do with ball catching. Therefore, beanbag activities can be enjoyable in their own right, but positive transfer from beanbag activities to ball skills might not occur, so the two types of activities should be viewed as independent from each other.

Simple Ball Games

A number of simple ball games may be attempted after children gain some control of balls. In one, a large box is filled with balls and the teacher throws (or rolls) the balls out in all directions. The children's task is to intercept the missiles and return them to the box.

Ball control may be gained by simply having children roll balls down lines while moving in a bent-over position. Variations of this activity may be incorporated into drills or relays.

One lead-in game for basketball simplifies the "basket," as pictured. Another calls for stationing a child in the center of double circles—one 2' in diameter and the other 4' in diameter. Two children on the outside of the circle attempt to get the ball to a teammate within the smaller center circle while two opponents standing within the ring between the outer and inner circles attempt to prevent the ball from getting to the "inside man." This drill teaches teamwork both offensively and defensively.

Games of a volleyball nature may be found in Blake and Volp's (1964) book. The object in these games is simply to throw the ball over the net (or a string placed at any height

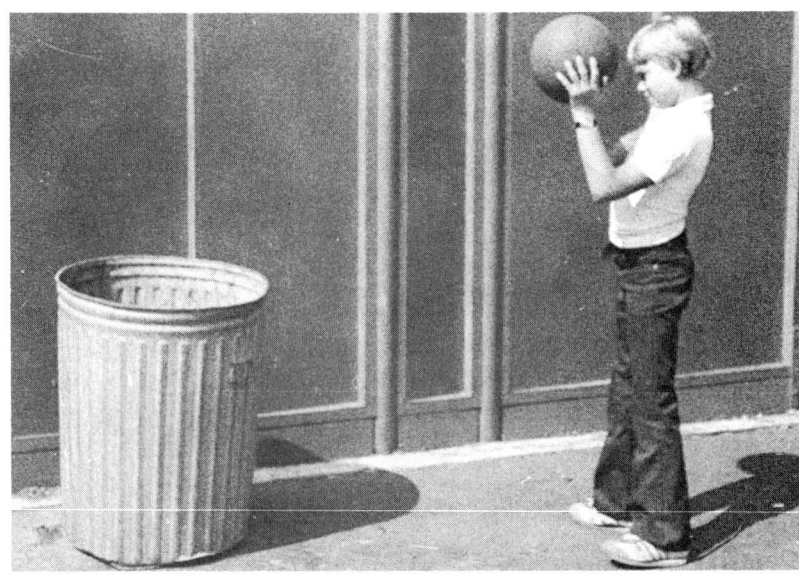

Garbage cans make easy targets for simple lead-in games to basketball.

deemed appropriate). Opposing players catch and rethrow the ball rather than hit it as would be true in a regular volleyball game. Additional simple ball games have been described in Schurr (1975).

BOUNCING AND DRIBBLING

Bouncing a ball in a repetitive manner is extremely difficult for many mildly to moderately physically handicapped youngsters. The feel of the ball is not always quickly translated into a second pushing action, as their kinesthetic-tactile perception of the ball in the hand may be faulty. The complex program of repetitive downward pushes may be difficult for the child to project into action. The child's hand may be either too tense or too flaccid as it contacts the ball.

When dribbling, the tips of the fingers should maintain the primary contact with the ball. A common error is slapping the ball with the palm of the hand as one attempts to bounce it. Initial bouncing is probably best tried with two hands at the same time. One-handed bouncing is more difficult and should be attempted only after two-handed bouncing is accomplished. In initial efforts at bouncing, the youngster should simply drop the ball, touch it once as it rises, and then attempt to catch it on the next bounce. Later the child may try to bounce the ball in a repetitive manner without catching it between bounces.

Of course, stationary bouncing and dribbling should be attempted before asking the child to move while controlling a ball in this manner. Later the child may be asked to walk while dribbling, then to jog a straight line and finally a zigzag pattern. Devices may be obtained or made that strap to the hand and project from the palm directly, eliminating the problem of palm-slapping the ball.

KICKING

Attempting to kick a round ball on the ground can be an extremely difficult undertaking for handicapped youngsters. Children with obvious balance problems should not be exposed to this kind of activity except in modified forms. For example, kicking should be done with a stationary ball at first, and with one of the child's hands on a support so that a fall is not likely to occur. If this seems successful, the ball may be rolled slowly and the hand removed from the support. When playing on hard surfaces, some children may need protection by wearing helmets and maybe foam pads in the pants to protect the end of the spine or other weak body areas.

Teaching points should include (a) the necessity of kicking below the "equator" of the ball to acheive some loft; (b) kicking through the ball rather than punching at it; (c) keeping the ankle rigid when making contact with the ball; and (d) achieving a stable position with the non-kicking foot (taking a short step) prior to shifting the weight through the ball. Emphasis also should be placed on a weight shift forward at the time the ball is contacted, for maximum power and distance. After gaining some proficiency, the children may be taught to direct the ball by positioning the foot on contact and to guide the ball along straight, and then angular, pathways, using the inside of the foot.

The sport of soccer utilizes kicking. It has been found to be excellent because of the continuous play, which creates a good overload on the cardiovascular system, as well as the many opportunities to be in contact with the ball. Soccer has been a particularly popular sport among the handicapped.

STRIKING WITH HANDS, RACQUETS, AND BATS

Striking the ball either with the hand or an implement is a relatively difficult skill, not mastered by some normal children until middle childhood or later. Striking a hand-held ball is difficult because of the necessity of holding the hand with the ball still while moving the other hand with vigor. Handicapped children with residual overflow of movements are unlikely to accomplish this without extensive practice. First attempts to strike a ball with the hand held in a fist should be done from a tee rather than from the child's other hand. This tee may be a large rubber traffic cone or the instructor's hand. Later the child may attempt to strike a self-held ball. When striking a ball, as in throwing, the emphasis should be on shifting one's weight as the ball is contacted. The ball should be hit below its middle to achieve loft. Directing the ball hit by the hand is an added refinement.

Handicapped children and youth sometimes are rushed into hitting balls with bats, golf clubs, and racquets long before they are ready. Many atypical youngsters are never ready for these difficult undertakings, and exposure to them may only lead to frustration and withdrawal from all similar physical activity. Exposure to hitting balls with racquets, bats, and the like should be attempted only if children have achieved coordination of the legs and feet to effect weight shifts when throwing balls without an implement and can throw and catch balls with reasonable facility.

Initial attempts to strike balls with a bat should be with a large, stationary object, such as a volleyball, placed at the feet of the child who is swinging the bat. The sound that such an impact makes is extremely satisfying in itself, and the task is not too difficult. Later the volleyball may be teed up off the ground, then rolled, bounced, and finally thrown

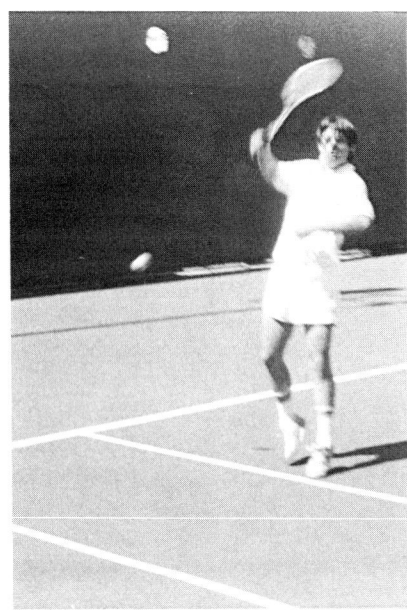

*Special Olympics programs of tennis for the
retarded began in 1982.*

toward the child, who attempts to hit it with the bat. The next obvious step is to reduce
the size of the ball until it approximates the diameter of a regular softball, going through
the same steps: stable, teed up, rolled, bounced, and thrown.

Tennis balls may be stabilized at first on tees and then suspended on strings before
children are asked to hit balls against a backstop and later on a tennis court. Racquet games
of this type, including paddle ball and badminton, should be taught to handicapped children
by a patient teacher who gradually builds in the sub-skills, including correct foot and body
actions and striking actions. In any case, these games are within the realm of possibility,
and Special Olympics programs of tennis for the retarded began in 1982. One of the participants is pictured.

Frisbees are fun, and proficiency in throwing them carries high status in some peer
groups. Catching and throwing this missile is not easy. The first attempts to catch one probably should be made with two hands—one hand above and the second hand below, in a
trapping motion.

Large and small foam plastic balls and cubes are also used in work with children whose
abilities may not be up to par. A large hurl ball made of a covered piece of round foam
plastic is thrown with a two-handed motion similar to the motion used in the hammer throw
but without the number of turns in this event. With proficiency the hurl can be thrown
some distance with satisfying results. The child simply faces the direction of the throw,
at first with both hands on the straps, and throws the ball. Later, if the child gains proficiency, some turns may be incorporated into the action.

A CHECKLIST OF BALL SKILLS

The following list might serve both as an assessment device and as a guideline for planning programs that involve skills with balls and other missiles.

Intercepting balls
(8" playground ball)

1 Watches rolling ball briefly.

2 Watches rolling ball for several seconds or longer.

3 Watches path of thrown ball.

4 Moves limbs, reflecting activation and agitation at ball rolled or thrown in visual field.

5 Attempts to stop rolling ball while in seated position.

6 Uses bilateral stop on ball rolled directly to child in seated position.

7 Adjusts hands to stop ball not rolled directly to child in seated position.

8 Attempts to stop rolled ball by leaning down from standing position.

9 Stops ball rolled directly, using both hands and leaning down from standing position.

10 Adjusts standing position a short distance to stop rolled ball.

11 Catches ball in arm cradle (arms extended slightly apart, elbows slightly bent) when ball is placed directly in cradle; may use body to cradle ball.

12 Adjusts cradle to catch ball thrown on one bounce from 10' directly at child; uses body to trap ball.

13 Catches ball in arm cradle without trapping ball against body.

14 Assumes proper arm-hand catching position, while standing.

15 Makes bilateral catch of ball, using arms and hands.

(Rubber playground ball, 4" diameter)

16 Traps rolled ball from standing position.

17 Catches ball bounced from 10' away, using arms and hands.

18 Catches ball bounced from 10' away, using hands only.

19 Catches ball thrown from 10' away, using hands only.

20 Catches ball thrown from 20'-30' away, using hands only.

21 Adjusts body position to catch ball thrown from 20'-30' feet away; catches ball, hands only.

Propelling and throwing balls
(8" playground ball)

1 Watches with interest as others throw balls.

2 Swipes inaccurately at ball in front of self in seated position.

3 Pushes at ball inaccurately with one or two hands, in seated position.

4 Pushes ball accurately with one or two hands, in seated position.

5 Pushes ball accurately in standing position.

6 Throws ball overhead with two hands, in standing position; no weight shift.

7 Varies two-handed throw of ball in standing position (from side, underhand, etc.; no weight shift).

8 Throws ball overhead with two hands, in standing position, with weight shift; little accuracy.

9 Throws ball overhead with two hands, in standing position, with accuracy for about 10'.

10 Throws ball one-handed over shoulder with one hand on front, dominant hand at rear of ball; no weight shift; no accuracy.

11 Throws one-handed as above but with weight shift and moderate accuracy to 10' (4" playground ball).

12 Throws one-handed with weight shift and steps with same foot and opposite foot.

13 Propels ball inaccurately (erratic release; no accuracy; no weight shift).

14 Varies one-handed throw with moderate accuracy to about 10' (underhand, overhead, etc.; no weight shift).

15 Throws one-handed with weight shift; fair accuracy.

16 Throws one-handed with weight shift and steps with foot on same side as throwing hand.

17 Throws one-handed with weight shift at same time, foot opposite throwing hand; fair distance and accuracy.

18 Throws one-handed accurately and with good distance, using proper weight shift and step.

Racquet and batting skills

1 Tennis racquet
  a Holds and moves racquet but does not contact ball.
  b Holds racquet and contacts teed-up ball.
  c Contacts ball swinging on string.
  d Contacts ball bounced from short distance.
  e Contacts ball in simple rally.
  f Contacts ball during game.

2 Light baseball bat
  a Holds and swings bat without releasing it.
  b Hits large ball placed on ground in front of self.
  c Hits ball (volleyball) rolled along ground to child.
  d Hits softball on tee.
  e Hits slowly pitched softball.
  f Hits regularly pitched softball.

SUMMARY

Many activities having prestige among peers with and without handicaps require basic bat skills. Handling balls, throwing and catching them, often requires greater visual-perceptual and motor ability than youngsters with various handicaps have. To help children acquire these skills requires carefully sequenced experiences of gradually increasing difficulty in tasks ranging from very simple to complex.

Initially children should be exposed by simply imparting force to balls and trapping rolled balls. Later, beanbags, bounced balls, and more complicated tasks may be introduced. When catching and throwing, proper foot movements should be taught before adding a ball to the action. Kicking balls and imparting force to balls with bats, racquets, and so forth present even more formidable tasks. Often, special equipment is needed to help the more physically handicapped youngsters propel and intercept balls and other missiles.

REFERENCES

Blake, O.W., & Volp, A.M. (1964). *Lead-up games to team sports*. Englewood Cliffs, NJ: Prentice-Hall.

Schurr, E.L. (1975). Skills and lead-up games for team sports (ch. 12) and Skills and lead-up games for individual sports (ch. 13). In E.L. Schurr, *Movement experiences for children*. Englewood Cliffs, NJ: Prentice-Hall.

ADDITIONAL REFERENCES

Cratty, B.J. (1986). Visual perceptual development (Ch. 11). In B.J. Cratty, *Perceptual and motor development in infants and children* (3rd ed.). Englewood Cliffs, NJ: Prentice-Hall.

Dauer, V.P., & Pangrazi, R.P. (1975). Manipulative activities (Ch. 15). In V.P. Dauer & R.P. Pangrazi, *Dynamic physical education for elementary school children*. Minneapolis: Burgess.

QUESTIONS FOR DISCUSSION

1. What developmental stages are seen when a normal child first learns to catch and to throw balls? Why might detailed knowledge of these sequences be helpful when working with a developmentally delayed youngster?

2. What sub-skills may motorically awkward youngsters need to master to learn to run and catch a ball thrown from 30' away?

3. How might catching beanbags hinder youngsters from later learning to catch balls?

4. What special safety precautions should be taken when asking a child with a balance problem to kick a ball while standing on asphalt or cement?

5. What sequential tasks might lead up to hitting, with a light bat, a softball thrown from some distance?

6. What kinds of teaching aids or cues might help a child execute a mature one-handed throw involving a weight shift and a simultaneous step with the foot under the non-throwing hand?

STUDENT PROJECTS

1. Help a group of handicapped children construct their own balls out of various materials, such as foam rubber, balled-up newspapers, and the like. Use these in simple games.

2. Develop an evaluation tool outlining sequences and sub-skills needed in throwing and catching. Use it with a group of children, and present the results to the physical education teacher.

3. Observe handicapped children throw-ing and catching balls and other missiles. What special problems do you note? What strategies or variations do they adopt? Which seem to be effective? Ineffective?

4. Teach a motorically handicapped child to throw a ball. What special problems occurred? What modifications, if any, did you permit the child to use?

5. Construct charts as visual aids for teaching how to catch and trap balls.

30 *Body Awareness and Tumbling*

For the most part, tumbling activities to which handicapped children and youth are exposed are simply less difficult modifications of tumbling activities found in regular education classes. The lessons may be not helpful developmentally, too difficult or dangerous, or not helpful with the child's movement problem. Sometimes the activities (e.g., prolonged rolling along the long axis of the body down a mat) have only a cursory relationship to the developmental patterns of the normally maturing child. Much of the time, these activities are carried out in a "mindless" manner; the minds of the children are not engaged in the execution of the stunts. They patiently and doggedly roll, fall, and otherwise contort themselves without really thinking about what is happening to their body or its parts.

The following activities are meant to be suggestive rather than all-encompassing. The multitude of activities that may be helpful to handicapped children in a gymnasium would take a "cookbook" many times the size of this text. Rather, examples of gymnastics activities scaled down for handicapped children and developmental actions that may help some motorically delayed children are presented. This chapter is organized as follows: (a) a movement vocabulary and body awareness; (b) getting up and down tasks that help children fall properly and move upward against gravity; and (c) rolling and turning movements, including simple, safe beginning steps for introducing rotation on both the long and short axes of the body. Individual, paired, and group activities are included. Finally, a model of body-image development is presented.

When implementing the following tasks, children should be encouraged to think about what is occurring, when possible and feasible. The activities are presented in sequential order, from simplest to most difficult. Readers who are interested in more complex, advanced gymnastic tricks and stunts appropriate for many handicapped children should consult the Additional References at the end of the chapter.

DEVELOPING A MOVEMENT VOCABULARY

When beginning to teach youngsters to move their bodies in space, a great many problems may be circumvented by ascertaining what movement terms the children may not be familiar with, and teaching these concepts before introducing the actual movements. New concepts can be added to each lesson, as appropriate. In groups, teachers should ascertain (a) which children are capable of understanding a concept (e.g., "lie down") but physically have trouble doing so, (b) those who are able to carry out the instruction but do not understand the verbal direction and concept, and (c) those who have little difficulty either understanding or executing the movements as instructed. Each of these requires a different approach within the group program.

As an assessment device, the various movements and positions may be listed, and beside each one a checkmark made when children have difficulty understanding or performing the action, or both. For example:

504

	Difficulty understanding	*Difficulty executing*	*Can both execute and understand, with practice*
1 Stand	_____	_____	_____
2 Sit	_____	_____	_____
3 Squat	_____	_____	_____

Aids to teaching the following concepts and movements include the teacher's demonstration and verbal explanation; a mirror in which children may watch their movements and positions; stick figures whose limbs and trunk positions may be changed to correspond to various movement commands; and demonstrations by children in the class. At times, manual manipulation of a child's limbs or trunk may be necessary for them to assume various positions or to move in various ways. Additionally, children's attempts to do specific movements (e.g., bend their legs) should be practiced in different positions (e.g., lying on the back with eyes closed, sitting, standing) so they will learn the concept independent of their orientation in space and the positions of other parts of their bodies.

Basic Static Orientations of the Body in Space

Several basic concepts about the orientation of the body in space are essential to facilitate a tumbling lesson:

1. Sit down.
2. Stand up.
3. Lie down (on back, on front).
4. Lie down (with feet nearest me, with head nearest me).
5. Stand with your side (back, front) toward the mat.
6. Stand on the mat. Stand on the edge of the mat.

Reactions to these directions first may be recorded on a checklist and then incorporated into a formal lesson. More difficult instructions include:

1. Lie down on your left side (on your right side).
2. Stand with your left (or right) side toward me (teacher).
3. Stand facing another child. Stand with your back to another child.

Other basic, static orientations of the total body in space may be encountered in later lessons. At these junctures, the lesson should be interrupted while the concept is introduced and mastered.

Dynamic Movements of the Total Body

If lessons on the mat are to be successful, many dynamic movements of the body must be acquired. Instructions for some of these movements are:

1. Turn toward me (teacher).
2. Turn away from me, with your back toward me (teacher).
3. Roll (on the long axis of the body).
4. Move sideways to the left (right).

5. Move away from another child.
6. Move toward (closer to) another child.
7. Lie down quickly (slowly).
8. Walk toward me (teacher).
9. Move away from me (teacher).
10. Bend backward.
11. Jump upward.
12. Squat downward.
13. Walk backward.
14. Get up slowly (rapidly).
15. Jump as high as you can.

Using a large cardboard box, the following actions might be initiated:

1. Get into the box.
2. Stand on the box.
3. Get under the box.
4. Stand with your left (right) side toward the box.

Sequence of Body-Part Identification

The sequence of the acquisition of body-part labels in Table 30.1 may be used as a guide when planning various body image games and activities:

Table 30.1   Guide for Sequence of Body-Part Identification

Age	Acquisition of Concepts
2–3 years	Names stomach, arms, legs, hands, fingers (as a whole), feet, and back.
4 years	Places left and right body parts on opposite sides of the body only about 50% of the time—no better than chance.
5 years	Names the body's joints—knee, elbow, shoulder. Points to the side of the body when asked. Names first finger, little finger, and thumb.
6–7 years	Names left and right body parts better than chance (about 75% of the time). Learns parts of limbs—forearm, thigh, and calf. Places objects correctly on left (right) side of the body.
7–8 years	Locates body in various left-right ways (e.g., responds correctly to "lie down on your left side"). Makes various "crossed judgments" (e.g., responds correctly to "touch your left shoulder with your right hand").
8–9 years	Moves within another's reference system and points correctly to left and right (hands, etc.) of someone facing self.

The development of body vocabulary is likely to parallel closely the emergence of the child's vocabulary as a whole and may not be closely correlated with the youngster's ability to use the body parts that are named correctly. The body-image abilities listed above are reasonably well developed at age 7. These abilities continue to improve until about age 12, when they approximate those of adults.

Figure 30.1 illustrates a tactile activity that can heighten awareness of the body, its parts and surfaces. Figure 30.2 illustrates a body-image game in which the children lie on a surface and another child or the teacher draws a line around the configurations for the child to see and match.

Figure 30.1   Tactile Experiences to Heighten Body Awareness

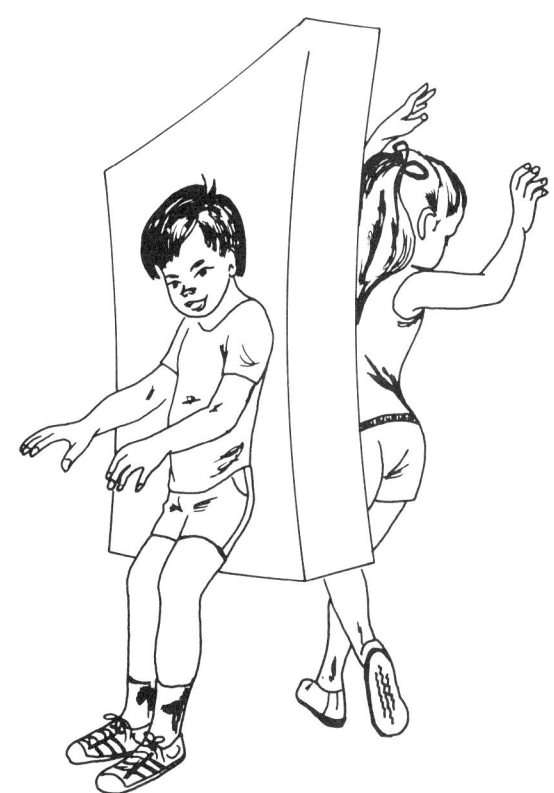

Figure 30.2   A Body Image Game

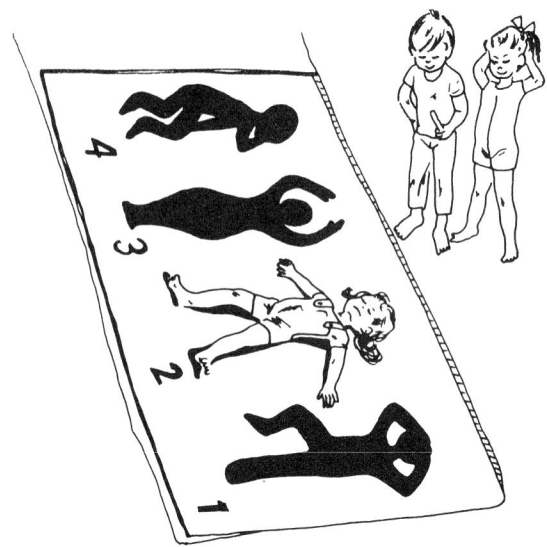

Static and Dynamic Limb Positioning

Investigations by Roach and Kephart (1966), Berges and Lezine (1965), and others have shown that duplication of static and dynamic limb positions helps children gain awareness of the body and its parts. Some of the more important static limb positions are:

1. Stand with hands on hips and legs straight.
2. Stand with arms to the front, side, and up above head.
3. Squat down with knees half bent.

Dynamic limb movements are critical when teaching tumbling and related skills. Some of these positions are:

1. Straighten arms.
2. Bend arms.
3. Straighten one arm (left or right).
4. Bend one arm (left or right).
5. Bend both legs.
6. Straighten both legs.
7. Lift both legs at hips while in a back-lying position.
8. Straighten one leg (left or right).
9. Turn arms (palms) upward (outward).
10. Turn arms and hands (palms) downward (inward).
11. Lift hands and arms high over head.
12. Touch toes with hands.

GETTING UP AND DOWN

Working against gravity while maintaining balance, as well as moving upward against gravity, is one of the more difficult tasks for many handicapped people. Some children and youth spend years, with the help of therapists, merely trying to rise alone and maintain a standing balance. Others may be able to get up and down but with considerable difficulty. The following activities are of two types: (a) those that encourage children to move in various ways vertically, and (b) those that help children fall down while maintaining control.

Turning and Rising

Children in physical education classes often are asked to roll like logs along mats on the long axis of the body. Because the circumference of most children's hips is smaller than that of their shoulders, they roll off onto the floor. Rolling, although helpful in gaining control of the muscles around the waist, does not constitute a natural skill in children as they develop locomotor ability. Better, children might be helped to execute a half-turn and rise from their back or from their front. This task may be varied by asking them to rise from the back without turning first, or to rise from the front while maintaining the same direction. These ways of getting up (from back and front, with and without a half-turn first) may be done at the child's own speed, assisted (moderately), done "as slowly as you can" to encourage impulse control, or "as fast as you can" to encourage ballistic strength of the leg extensors and other anti-gravity muscle groups. If the children are not too excitable, they also may compete to see who can get up fastest or slowest.

Motor planning may be encouraged (and evaluated) if a demonstrator first shows children ways of getting down and up and then asks the children to copy them. For example, while facing a child, the demonstrator descends first to one knee and then to the other, and then

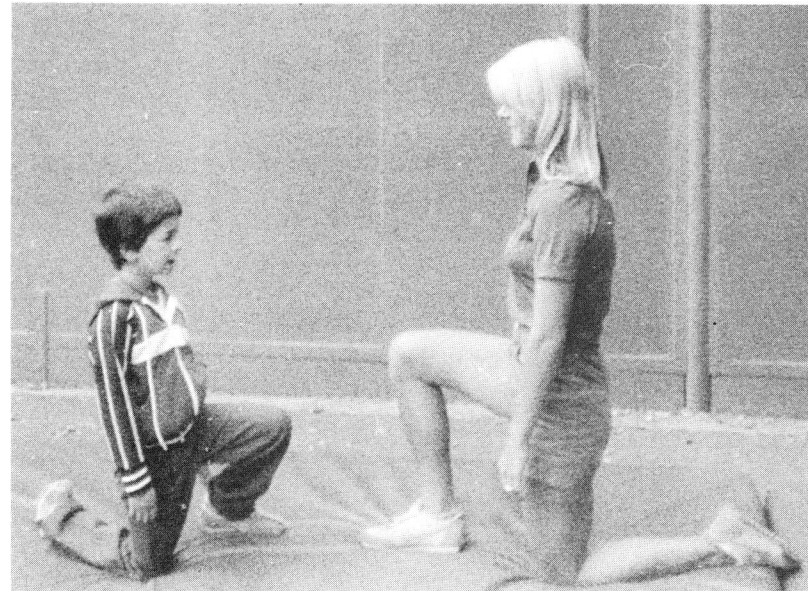

Imitation of rising sequences is a good initial motor planning activity.

rises, one leg at a time. The child tries to copy this four-count movement in the same manner, first descending to one knee then the other, then to one hand, leaning forward, and then to the other hand, ending on all fours. Finally, the demonstrator arises, one movement at a time, reversing the sequence. This activity is pictured. Using these and other movements, creative teachers may think up other activities that move the child upward, against gravity—which aids motor planning and duplicates components of normal motor development.

Getting Down/Falling Safely

As important as rising is descending properly and safely. This skill carries over into safe falling responses in other settings. The four actions described below do not exhaust the possibilities; the creative teacher may think of more. The movements should be carried out in a controlled manner and should be mechanically correct, or corrected by the teacher. For example, as the child leans forward, the head and shoulders should bend slightly backward so that the child maintains balance over the feet as long as possible before the knees touch the mat. If a front fall is being practiced, the knees should land quietly rather than sharply, with the body in control.

Front Descent   While standing at the edge of a soft mat (at least 3"-4" of foam), the child lowers one knee and then the other to the mat, leans forward on both hands, and ends in an all-fours position. The child, as pictured, slides his arms forward so that he ends in a front-lying position. This should be first demonstrated, then assisted by holding the child's head and shoulders back slightly as the knees touch the mat. After successful practice, this serial movement can be speeded up.

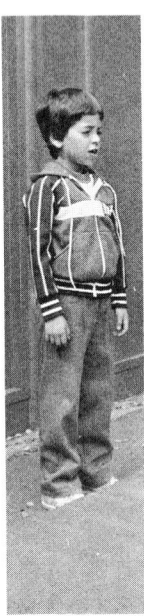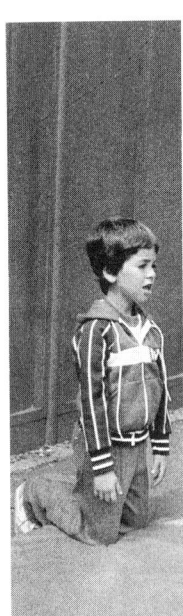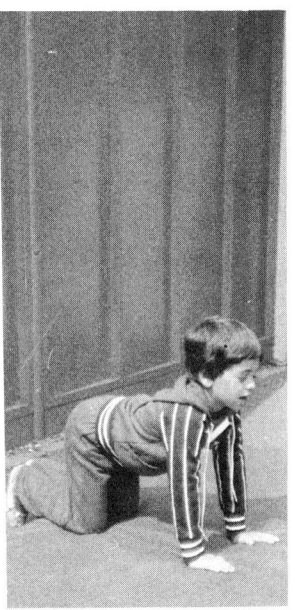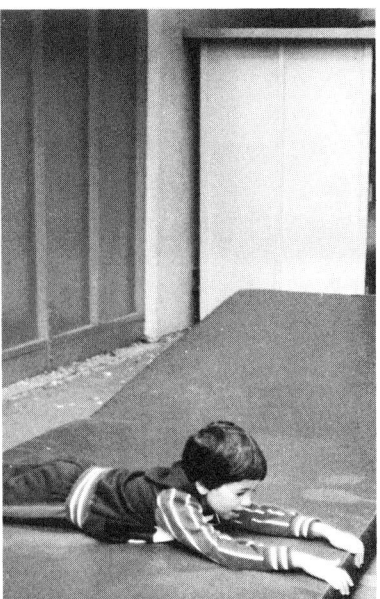

Children should practice front descent movements correctly and slowly several times before speeding up the activity.

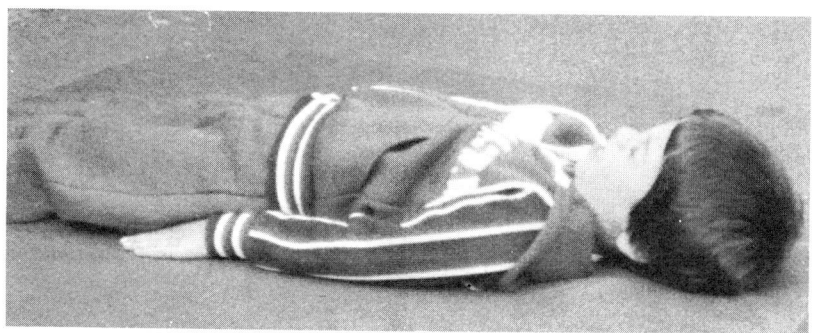

At the end of the back descent, the body should be positioned as shown.

Back Descent Back descent should begin in a squat, with the child's hips over the mat and then touching the mat in a sit. Next, the hands go down, fingers facing forward, and then the child should lie back flat, as pictured. Again, this should be done slowly at first until the mechanics are mastered (lean forward at first so that the hips touch, not hit, the mat), then speeded up.

Side Descent Turning with one or the other side to the mat, the child slowly, under control, places the knee nearest the mat on the mat. The hand on the same side of the body is placed in the middle of the mat, and then the hand is slid away from the body until the side is resting on the mat. This is done slowly. One side, then the other, is practiced, before adding speed ("Get down as fast as you can").

Variations and Games Developmental games and variations of front, back, and side descents may be employed with children after the movements have been mastered. For example:

1. Children face a "caller," who calls out left, right, back, or front, to see if the children can descend to the correct plane of the body. Other children may act as observers to determine whether classmates have descended to the correct position.

2. A child slowly walks down the mat, listening for a command from another child (back, front, left side, or right side). The child then descends to the position indicated. Evaluators can inspect for correctness. Children who have been performers then become callers.

3. A series of descents is called out (back, front, etc.), and children assume each position, arising between each movement. Instructions may include "fast" or "slow."

4. Ways of ascending are alternated with ways of descending. Student evaluators determine whether verbal commands are being followed correctly.

5. Prescribed falls are used between movements on an obstacle course, interspersed with crawling under and over obstacles, jumping over lines or into hoops, and so on. One child may demonstrate a series of movements, and children try to repeat those actions in the proper sequence.

ROLLING

The Long Axis

Even moderately awkward children sometimes have problems when trying to execute a front roll. They may lack arm strength for the momentary support required and lose awareness of their body and its parts as they look through their arms at the beginning of the roll. During the roll itself, they may lose the sense of where their body is and open up in an extended position (stopping the rolling action) rather than maintaining a tucked-in position. The following variations of rolling on the long axis of the body are safe ways to begin to give children the experience of turning over and managing their bodies in space.

Short Log Rolls   Like all rolls, these may be started on an incline, then executed on a level surface, and finally performed uphill. To help children conceptualize about their body parts and planes, a slow roll is sometimes helpful, with children stopping after each one-quarter turn and saying whether they are on their side, back, or front. The arms may be held in various positions.

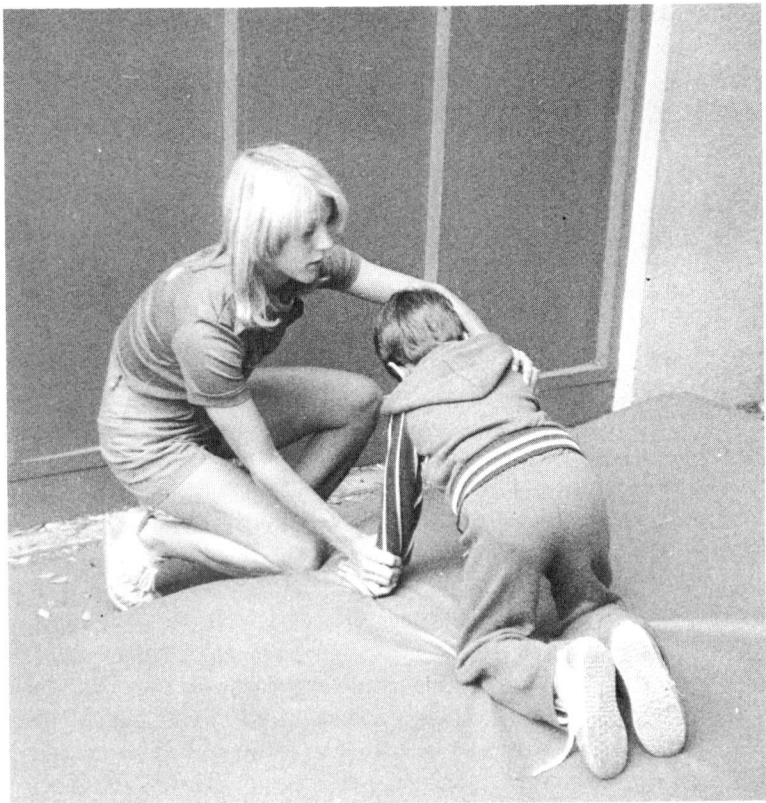

Floppy children may need help from a spotter to begin a long-axis roll.

Hand-and-Knee Rolls   Beginning in an all-fours position, hand-and-knee rolls are made over the shoulder in the direction in which the roll is executed by "breaking" the arm on that side and reaching across to the opposite wrist to begin the roll. Floppy children may need assistance, with the spotter taking the wrist of the arm-support, which has to be removed to start the roll, and placing it across the child's chest, as pictured. These rolls may be done in both directions. Several children may be lined up at the same time and asked to roll to the left or to the right. Each roll should be completed with children in a hand-knee position.

Tuck Rolls   The child is asked to lie on the back, grasping the knees tightly against the chest in a bent-knee position. The roll is initiated by the child, or with the help of the teacher, and the child remains in a tucked position throughout, as pictured. Care should be taken on this roll and others to stay on the side toward which the head is facing so that if children roll off an inclined surface or mat, their heads are protected by the teacher's hand and they are manually "straightened out."

Straddle Rolls   Using a bolster, as pictured, the child grips it with the legs and knees, and with the arms. The roll is initiated by the child or by the teacher.

Crooked Back and Front Rolls   Back and front shoulder rolls are of intermediate difficulty and should precede regular front and back somersaults. Both may be started on downhill mats and should be carefully spotted and carried out slowly at first. These rolls may be combined with regular front rolls and side rolls as children gain proficiency.

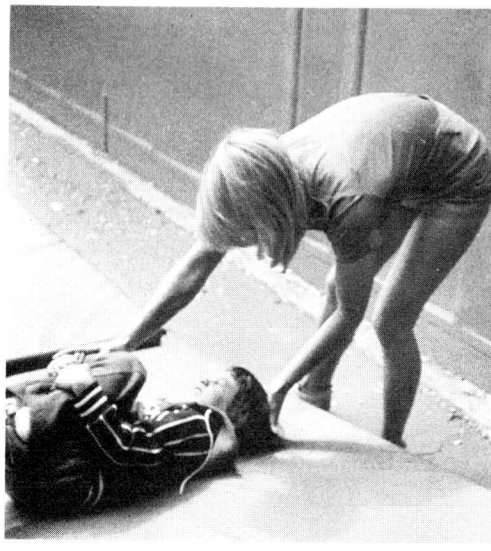
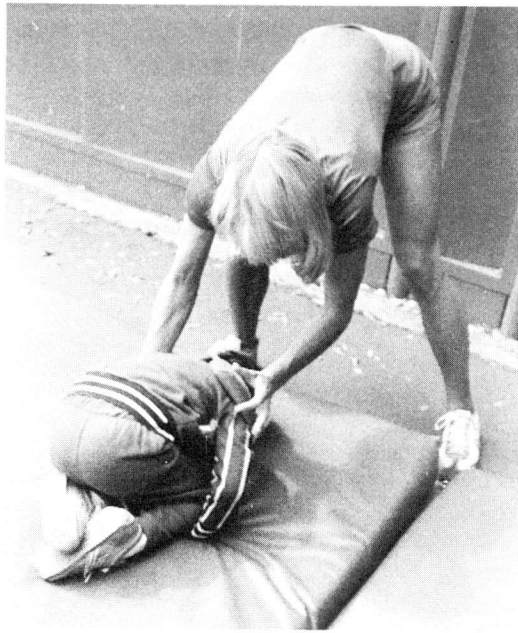

The teacher should protect the child's head while executing a tuck roll.

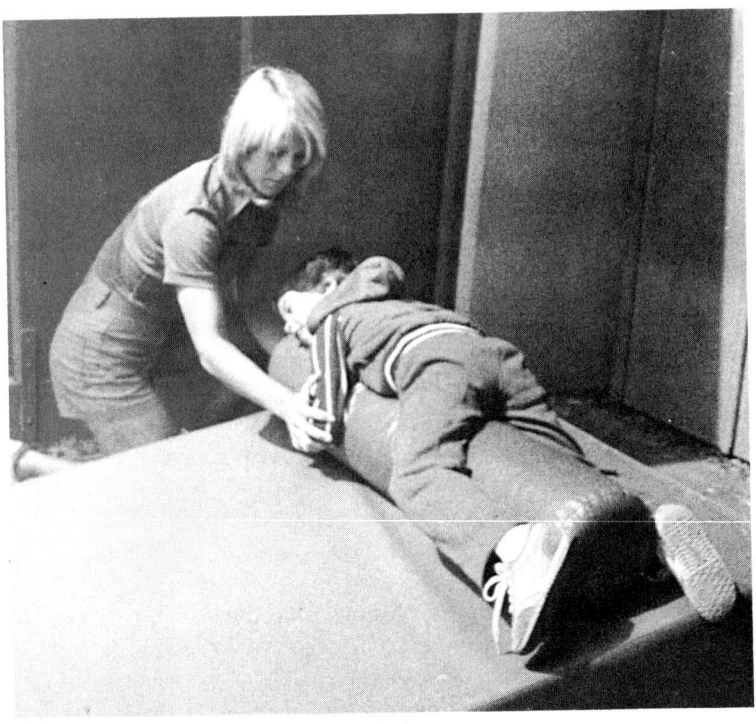

Straddle rolls are performed using a bolster.

Numerous modifications and variations of these and similar rolls may be employed in series, or as parts of obstacle courses. Using inclines, children may roll uphill and then fall off the high end onto another mat. Children may play roll tag on a large, square mat, attempting to tag each other while maintaining a tucked position and rolling to avoid being tagged or to tag others. The hand-and-knee roll may be made more difficult, and more balance may be required, by starting and ending the roll in the higher hand-foot position. The knees should be lifted from the mat in a four-point support (both feet and both hands) at the beginning and at the end of the roll. These rolls are but some of the many that may be employed as children and handicapped youth first attempt to turn over in space.

The Short Axis

Front Shoulder Rolls   The child, as pictured, starts in a crouched position, facing the direction in which he is to roll. Next the hand of the shoulder over which he intends to roll reaches for the opposite ankle. Children should not start from their knees, and the hips should be high preceding the roll. Children should then crouch more and place that shoulder, with the head turned to the side, on the mat and proceed to roll over the shoulder and recover their feet. The teacher or spotter initially may place one hand on the wrist

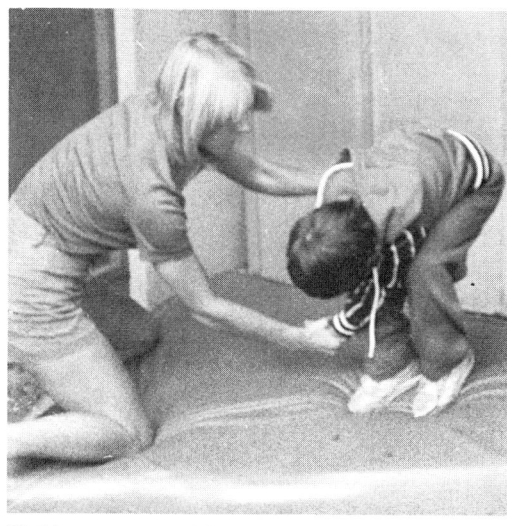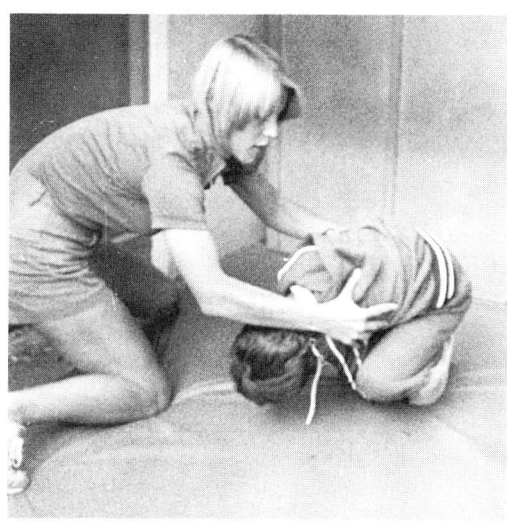

Children may need help from the teacher to learn the correct position for starting front shoulder rolls.

of the hand going across and the second on the shoulder over which the child is to roll. As the roll is competed, the teacher's grip may be retained on the wrist to facilitate recovery.

These rolls may be done with less and less help and more and more momentum. When learned, using both shoulders, they may be used to heighten left-right concepts ("Roll over your left shoulder, and then your right").

Back Shoulder Roll The child in the photo first sits with knees bent and then lays back, bringing the bent knees over the shoulder over which he intends to roll. The head is turned slightly in the opposite direction so that it does not get "stuck" and cause some minor

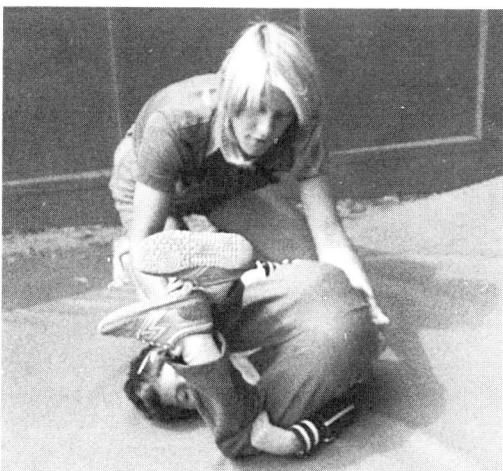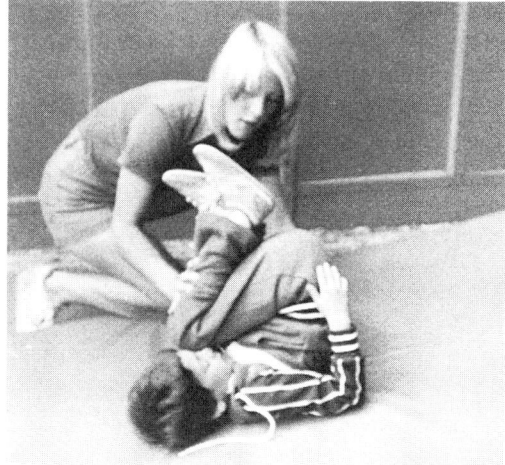

Back shoulder rolls may be executed over either shoulder.

neck trauma. With practice, rolls can be done over both shoulders with increasing speed and less guidance. Children are asked to "stay in a ball" until the roll is completed, and then push to their feet, using both hands. The hands and arms do not take a very active part in the turning movement itself. Again, left-right concepts may be practiced by varying directions as to which shoulder to roll over.

Regular Front and Back Rolls   Regular front and back rolls, as has been pointed out, require some minimal arm strength and some awareness of where the body is when turning. If not done properly, rolls can result in injury to the neck—a muscle strain, or worse. Children should not be rushed into doing rolls before they have learned the previously described activities and the teacher has ascertained that they have adequate arm strength.

Front Roll   The front roll is started in a crouching position (difficult for some atypical children to maintain because of weak leg extensors), with the knees not on the mat. The hands are flat and shoulder-width apart, relatively close to the body. Common problems with handicapped children are failure to place the hands flat, premature buckling of the knees, and a tendency to try to do the roll from the knees. A too low starting position does not permit the roll to be executed efficiently because the child's center of mass is not high enough to permit the turn.

The teacher should offer assistance at the upper back (not the head, because undue flexion of the neck can occur). The child should be assisted during the turn, to prevent stopping while resting on top of the head and risk twisting the neck. Upon completion of the roll, the child should be helped to recover to the feet (as is true of all such movements). The initial spotting technique is pictured.

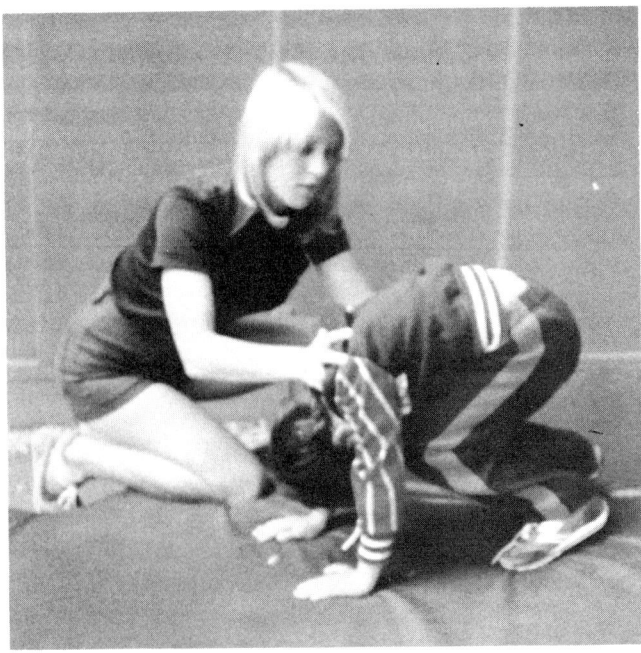

Children must learn not to rest on the head or neck while doing front rolls.

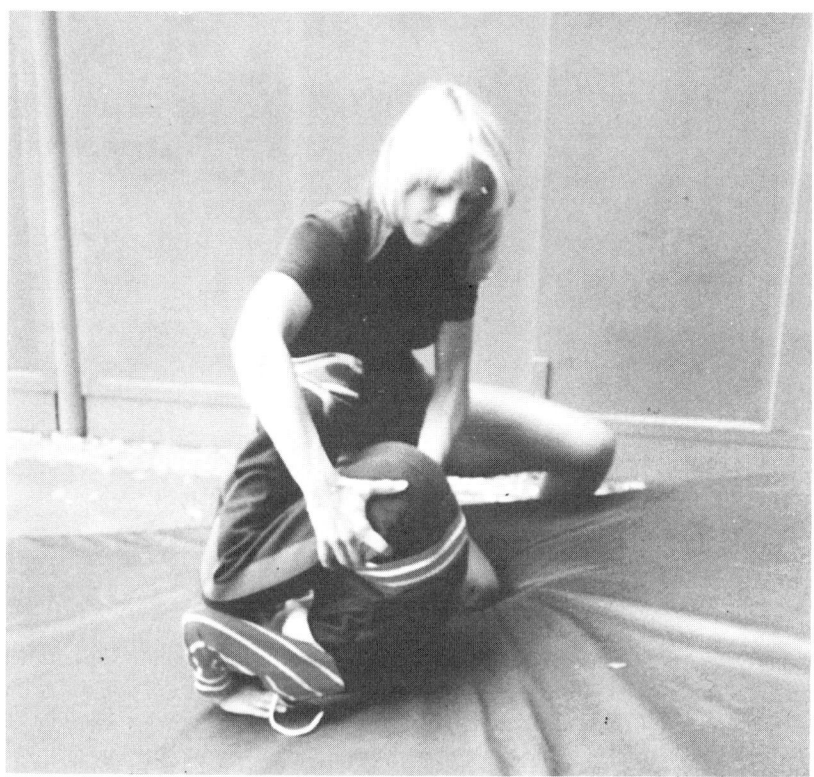

The teacher lifts the child during a back roll to take weight off the neck.

Back Roll The child starts with the back to the mat, in a squat, hands (fingers leading) held over either shoulder, palms up. The head should be down, chin on chest, with the back and rear of the head presenting a smooth curve to the mat's surface. As the child starts the backward movement, the knees are bent and the head is not thrown backward—which would disrupt the curve of the roll. As the child reaches the point at which pressure is likely to be exerted on the head and neck, the teacher should reach inside the "ball" that the child is making with the body at the waist and lift upward, taking the weight off the neck, as pictured. Excess weight on the rear of the head can cause injury.

Later, children may start from a standing position and learn to sit back with greater speed. Completion of the roll is successful when the hands are moved quickly in position to push off the mat and help gain a standing position.

Physical educators may wish to explore intermediate and advanced tumbling tricks and stunts with more able children. Books describing advanced tumbling activities for use on apparatus and mats are readily available. Some are listed in the Additional References at the end of the chapter.

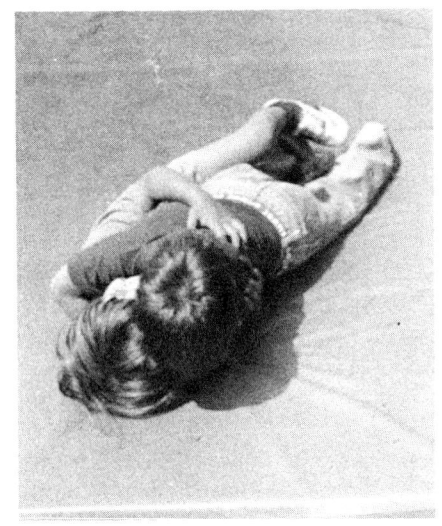

Two children perform a simple log roll together.

Paired Rolls

Many simple and advanced stunts may be performed by more than one child. These range from the simple roll in a bundle, pictured, in which two young children simply do a log roll together, to more sophisticated pyramid work and tumbling activities.

Only children with sufficient arm strength and those who have mastered a front roll by themselves with no problems should attempt paired front rolls. One child lies on his or her back, legs up in the air; the second child stands by the head of the first child. Each grasps both ankles of the other (photo A). The standing child then places the feet of the second child close to the hips, shifts body weight to the hands (still holding the second child's ankles) (photo B), and tucks the head down in a front roll (photo C) while the child on the ground is pulled to a standing position, still holding the ankles of the child who has just completed the front roll (photo D). This sequence is continued.

SPRINGY SURFACES

Springy surfaces can aid children and youth in learning to jump and in building leg strength and control. These can be made from a large rubber tire with a webbed material in the center, or from a wide board 2″ × 8″ × 6′-10′ in length whose ends are rigidly supported. These devices offer exhilarating exercise, and balance may be improved as the child tries to maintain equilibrium. Trunk strength, as well as strength of the other anti-gravity muscle groups, is heightened as these muscles are called upon to become rigid when the youngster lands and then rebounds from the springy surface.

One type of springy apparatus, the trampoline, should not be utilized unless the risks are fully understood and proper cautions are taken. Preferably, the trampoline should be set into the ground. If used properly, it can have a positive effect on locomotor skills, agili-

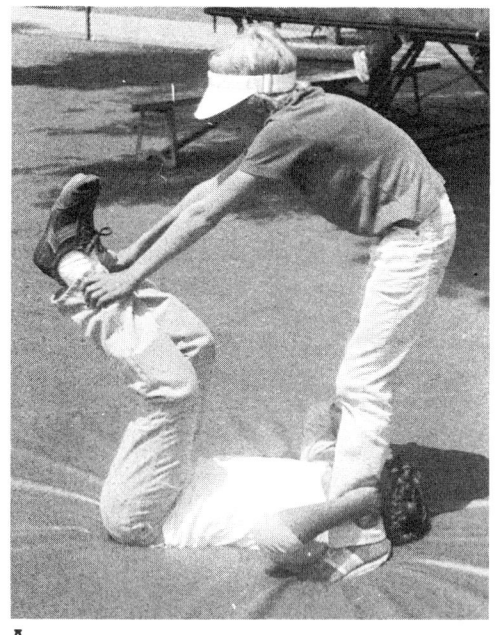

A

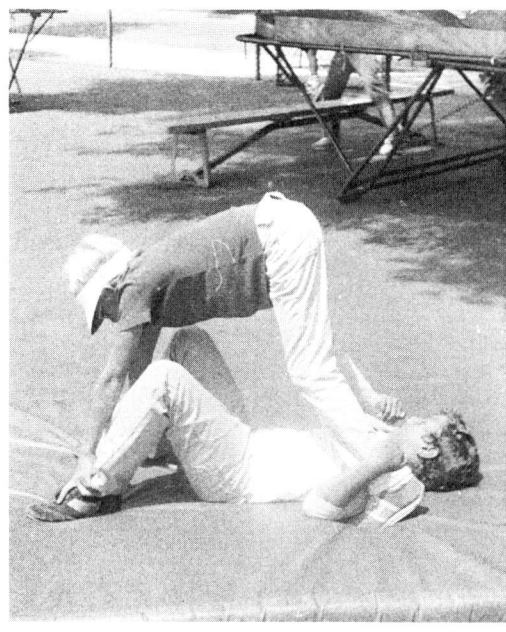

B

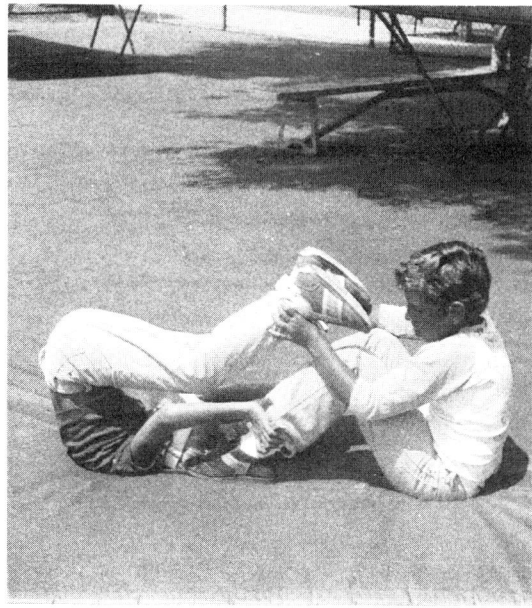

C

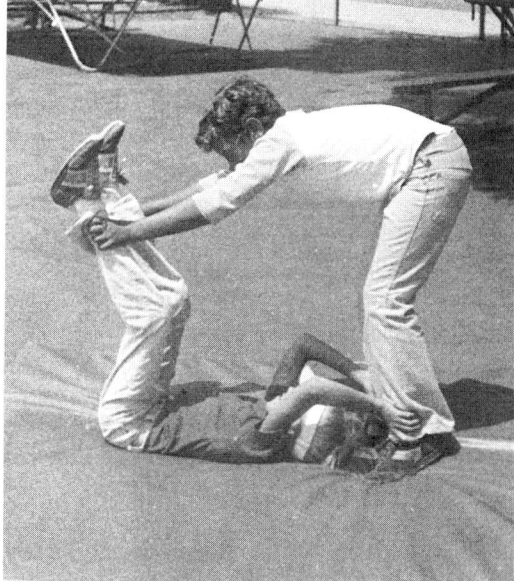

D

Children with sufficient arm strength may enjoy paired front rolls.

ty, strength, and other physical qualities. If used improperly, injury can result. The surface, while seemingly soft and supple, actually does something that the ground or flooring does not: It snaps back at the participant. If the body is not well aligned (if the back is too arched, for example), the misalignment may be suddenly exaggerated, with accompanying injury to the joints, tendons, ligaments, or bones. Teachers should insist that (a) children bounce low and under total control, and (b) contact with the surface does not engender unnatural stress to any body part. Under no conditions should difficult or daring stunts be attempted. Also, some emotionally disturbed children tend to perseverate on the apparatus, getting into a rhythm that is almost "hypnotic" to them. Not all children are suited for physical activity using this type of equipment.

A MODEL OF BODY-IMAGE DEVELOPMENT

The three-dimensional model depicted in Figure 30.3 was developed to depict how the child's body image might be developed and to aid in formulating objectives. The three dimensions are (a) *objectives,* consisting of a variety of goals possible within a physical education context; (b) *strategies* or methods that may be employed by physical educators, including touching children, assisting them, affording them resistance, permitting them to move under their own initiative and with mechanical aids, and verbal encouragement to engage in some act (usually, a combination of these); and (c) *space fields* in which the child may move, arranged in developmental order proceeding from simple turning movements expected of an infant (or a profoundly retarded child) to complex, mixed movements occurring in more than one space field at a time, exemplified by a child running to catch a ball and preparing the hands to catch it.

The model has several benefits such as encouraging teachers/therapists to consider an expanded number of therapeutic strategies, rather than to concentrate on a "pet" remedial approach, and aiding in the formulation of specific objectives, many of a subtle nature, that are appropriate for the individualized education program. Also, the model helps one to think developmentally—to proceed from activities of a primitive, basic nature to more complicated activities in which the child may be working within two or more space fields at the same time.

Space Fields

Figure 30.4 depicts the spatial dimensions that are occupied by the body and its parts. Consideration should be given first to the "cones of space" that the arms and legs occupy. Within these cones the child may be encouraged or aided to move in many ways, including flexion-extension, grasping, and rotation. Later, objects may be introduced and contacted within these cones of space.

Next, "horizontal cylinders" are explored. The child turns over and begins to move forward (creeping/crawling), elongating these cylinders of space. The child learns to organize and occupy "vertical cylinders" of space as he or she begins to sit up and later to stand in an elongated vertical cylinder. The child then begins to occupy a "hallway of space" as locomotion commences. A "compartment of space" must be conquered as the youngster becomes able to move in all directions.

Figure 30.3 A Model for Development of Body Image Via Sensory-Motor Experiences

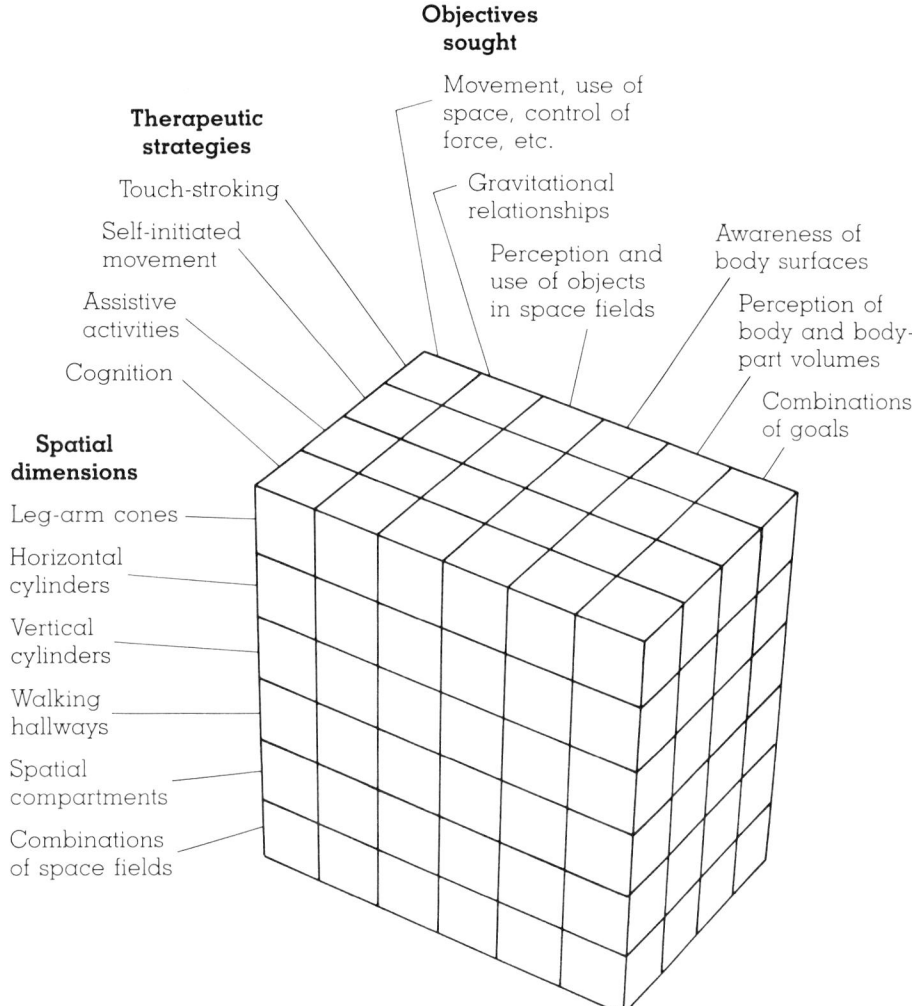

Many of life's activities involve the child's organizing and occupying more than one space field at a time. For example, the child must balance in a vertical cylinder while engaging the arms and hands in a horizontal cylinder of space.

Therapeutic Strategies

Helpful strategies involve not only the traditional ones used by physical therapists (assistive, voluntary, and resistive activities) but also more subtle ones that incorporate verbiage and encouragement requiring the child to think. Other parts of this dimension include various kinds of sensory input—touch, sound, heat/cold, smell, and kinesthetic imagery.

Figure 30.4   Spatial Dimensions of Body

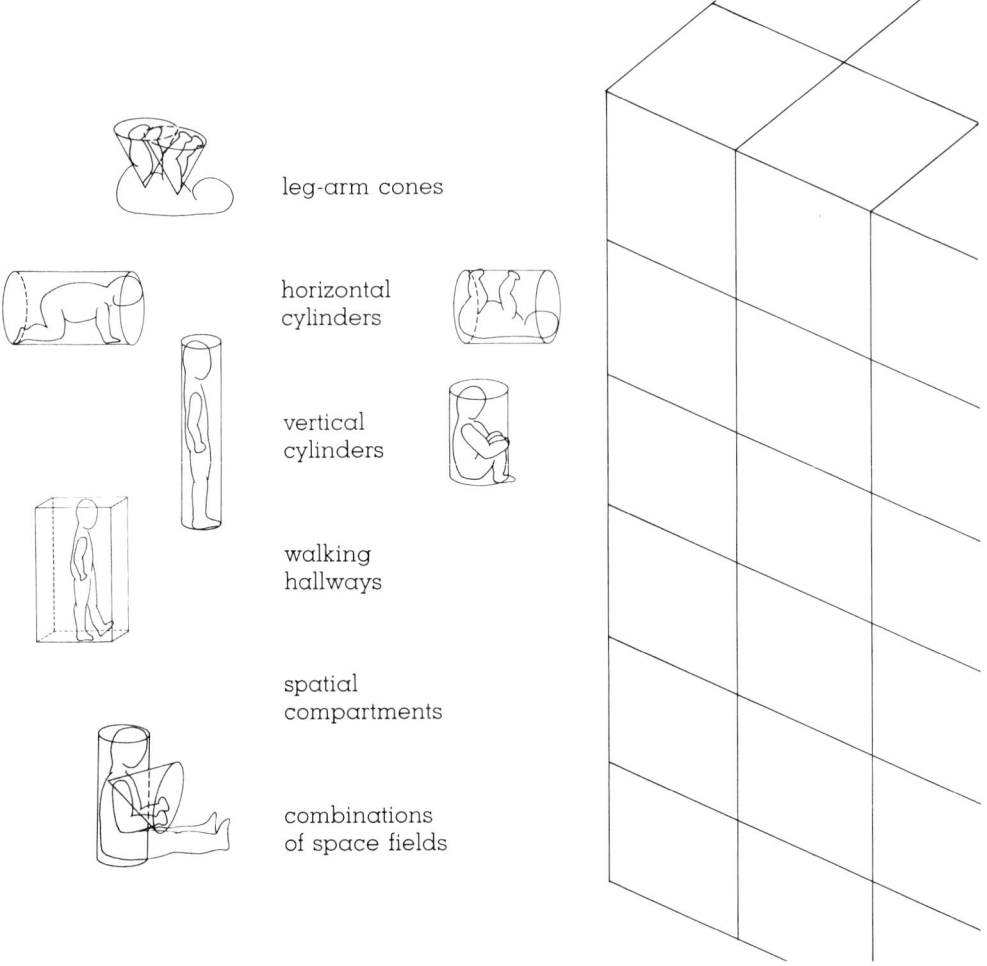

leg-arm cones

horizontal
cylinders

vertical
cylinders

walking
hallways

spatial
compartments

combinations
of space fields

Objectives

Objectives include the more obvious ones, such as helping the child to move more accurately and with force, and subtle perceptual tasks, such as (a) learning that body parts have thickness and volume, (b) discovering the body surfaces, (c) relating to gravity and balance, (d) varying tension and learning to relax, and (e) dealing with objects in the various space fields.

The model thus has several applications:

1. Task analysis may take place by first deciding upon a given child-teacher "interact" and then tracing just what therapeutic strategy or strategies are involved, together with the space fields used and the objectives the interact represents.

2. In a given program with a given type of disability, the teacher/therapist might consider a "slice" or two of the model. The program might concentrate, for example, on how a child learns to sit and focus attention and strategies on the ways this might be accomplished.

3. The model encourages thought about subtle perceptual qualities. For example, a blind child might be led to discover how the body extends and then is discontinous with space and other objects.

SUMMARY

Carefully sequenced movement activities offer excellent ways for atypical youngsters to learn about the body and its potential for movement. Children should learn about body parts and the corresponding movement vocabulary before proceeding to more complex tasks. Simply getting up and down in various ways affords experiences that enhance basic body concepts. Pairing simple movements against gravity with verbal commands can aid both expressive and receptive language, as well as the movement qualities inherent in the tasks at hand.

Rolling and tumbling activities initially should consist of actions employing the long axis of the body. Only when sufficient arm strength is achieved should traditional front and back rolls be attempted, using the short axis of the body. Springy surfaces—inner tubes, springboards, and the like—may be employed, but with caution. These may aid balance, agility, and strength in various anti-gravity muscle groups including those that extend the back, muscles in the upper back and the rear of the neck, the muscle groups extending the legs at the knee, and the hip extensors.

A model of body-image development that may be helpful in planning programs has three dimensions: (a) objectives, (b) therapeutic strategies, and (c) spatial dimensions. These facets can be combined in many ways to fit the unique needs of an individual child.

REFERENCES

Berges, J., & Lezine, I. (1965). *The imitation of gestures* (trans. Arthur H. Parmelee). London: Spastics Society Medication Education and Information Unit/Wm. H. Heinemann Publishers.

Roach, E.G., & Kephart, N.C. (1966). *The Purdue perceptual-motor survey.* Columbus, OH: Charles E. Merrill.

ADDITIONAL REFERENCES

Cratty, B.J. Physical growth and the changing body image. In B.J. Cratty, *Perceptual and motor development in infants and children* (3rd ed.). Englewood Cliffs, NJ: Prentice-Hall.

Drehman, B., & Holdahl, A. (1967). *Head over heels—Gymnastics for children.* New York: Harper & Row.

Johnson, B. (1966). *A beginner's book of gymnastics.* New York: Appleton-Century-Crofts.

Mosston, M. (1965). *Developmental movement.* Columbus, OH: Charles E. Merrill.

O'Quinn, G. (1970). *Gymnastics for elementary school children.* Dubuque, IA: Wm. C. Brown.

QUESTIONS FOR DISCUSSION

1. How may tumbling tasks be used to heighten the verbal-cognitive awareness of body parts and the body's left-right dimensions? Give some examples of tasks used in this manner.

2. What are critical safety procedures to follow prior to attempting more difficult gymnastic tricks, including front and back rolls?

3. What is a logical sequence to learning a front shoulder roll?

4. How should a front roll and a back roll be spotted? What kinds of injuries may occur if these and similar exercises are not properly spotted?

5. How might mats be arranged to assist the learning of a simple log roll? How might they be arranged to make the maneuver increasingly difficult?

STUDENT PROJECTS

1. Prepare a bibliography of pamphlets and books containing beginning tumbling skills. Which activities might be used with various handicapping conditions?

2. Referring to equipment catalogs, what kinds of tumbling mats and shapes might be purchased to optimize a tumbling program?

3. Prepare a checklist of tumbling skills appropriate for normal children of 6 years.

4. For the same population prepare a listing of body parts and movements of the body arranged in order of difficulty on which to base an initial evaluation and a follow-up testing program after the children have engaged in a program of tumbling and body-awareness activities.

5. Using the list in project 4, test a group of children and rearrange your list of tasks in order of difficulty, based on the percentage of correct reactions to each of the commands on your list (''Touch your left arm,'' etc.).

31 *Aquatics/ Swimming*

In the 1930s, hydrotherapy was popularized as a way of treating and exercising the physically handicapped. Methods of teaching swimming to the retarded are now discussed in many monographs and books. The swimming pool is the only place where some handicapped youngsters can change their positions in space in any way. Released from the confines of their wheelchairs, straps, and braces, they find joy in wiggling from place to place (perhaps with some guidance) in warm therapy pools. Not only is this activity physically helpful, particularly for the muscle and heart-lung systems, but improvement is highly measurable.

Competitive swimming is another type of water skill in which many handicapped people excel. Success is often satisfying to participants who might be unable to exhibit proficiencies in other forms of physical or academic endeavors.

Water ballet and related skills in the water have attracted the attention and participation of many handicapped children and youth over the years. Water polo and variations on water polo (using inner tubes) are also wholesome, enjoyable recreational activities.

Exposing handicapped children and youth to swimming and related experiences, however, can pose special concerns:

1. Care must be taken with some children not to overload their muscular or cardiovascular systems.

2. Some handicapped groups (e.g., the deaf) seem to be susceptible to infections when in the water. Other handicapped groups are potential carriers of infections to the water and the people in it.

3. Highly anxious individuals must be carefully introduced to the perceived traumas of learning to swim and related experiences. Some of these youngsters relate death by drowning to the very sight of water. They thus need adroit teaching, with gradual introduction to every sub-phase of the processes.

4. Although some authorities have claimed that exposure to water, and immersion of the body when learning to swim, heightens the body image, the reverse may be true. On entering the water, children with any kind of coordination problem may act as though their bodies have disappeared! The absence of the usual information from receptors in the muscles, joints, and tendons as these children suddenly become almost weightless in the swimming pool gives them this feeling. Being in the water makes it difficult for them to locate their various body parts as they try to kick their feet or move other body parts.

The primary focus of this chapter is on activities, sequences, and methods specifically suited for the handicapped. Detailed skill acquisition in some of the aquatic specialties is not dealt with extensively; the reader is directed to handbooks listed at the end of the chapter for this type of information.

Initially, principles and techniques appropriate when teaching young children or beginners to become familiar with and propel themselves through water are described. The second part deals with survival skills in the water—ways in which children or youth may

525

maintain position and survive if suddenly exposed to dangerous situations. The chapter concludes with a discussion of special health problems to be considered and pool facilities and equipment for the handicapped.

Aquatic activity for handicapped youngsters may be subdivided into several categories:

1. Familiarization with the water, water play, having fun, and simple games.

2. Elementary forms of floating and propulsion, simple strokes, and gliding (including modifications for the handicapped and for amputees).

3. Survival skills in the water, including bobbing and proper breathing.

4. Hydrotherapy and exercises in the water to remediate handicapping conditions, both physical and emotional.

5. Competitive swimming strokes, starts and turns, and training regimens.

6. Variations and modifications, water polo games, water ballet and modifications, simple and competitive diving.

Some handicapped children may not progress beyond water play. Simply having fun in the water can be a logical and laudable objective for many. At the same time, even the most severely physically handicapped emerge, after some work, exhibiting various elementary forms of locomotion. This is the only way some can transport themselves from one place to another, so it is a satisfying experience indeed.

Many handicapped children and youth are exposed to various forms of hydrotherapy to relax spastic muscles, to reeducate damaged tissue, or to habilitate poorly functioning muscles and muscle groups. The emotionally disturbed, too, may be able to relax and achieve better psychic health through various exercises and activities in the water. Competitive swimming—a highly measurable skill—is possible for many handicapped children, including the deaf and retarded. In some cases, the handicap is erased and these children have no disadvantage when compared with normal peers.

WATER GAMES AND LEAD-IN ACTIVITIES

Before the Pool

A number of activities may be used to familiarize and otherwise prepare a reluctant or developmentally delayed child to enter the water and participate in activities that will lead to water fun and perhaps ultimately to swimming.

1. Relaxation training on mats may be helpful. Placing tense youngsters in comfortable positions and aiding them to relax muscles with verbal suggestions (chapter 28) often helps them enter the water in a more relaxed mood.

2. Basic arm and leg movements may be practiced without the unfamiliarity and stress of being in water. The simple pull-back movement used in the breaststroke may be practiced out of the water so that the children can see the action required. Kicking movements practiced with children on their backs so that the legs may be watched, or with their sides to a mirror so that visual inspection of the legs is possible, may be helpful in promoting similar movements in the water. These out-of-water movements do not replicate the feel

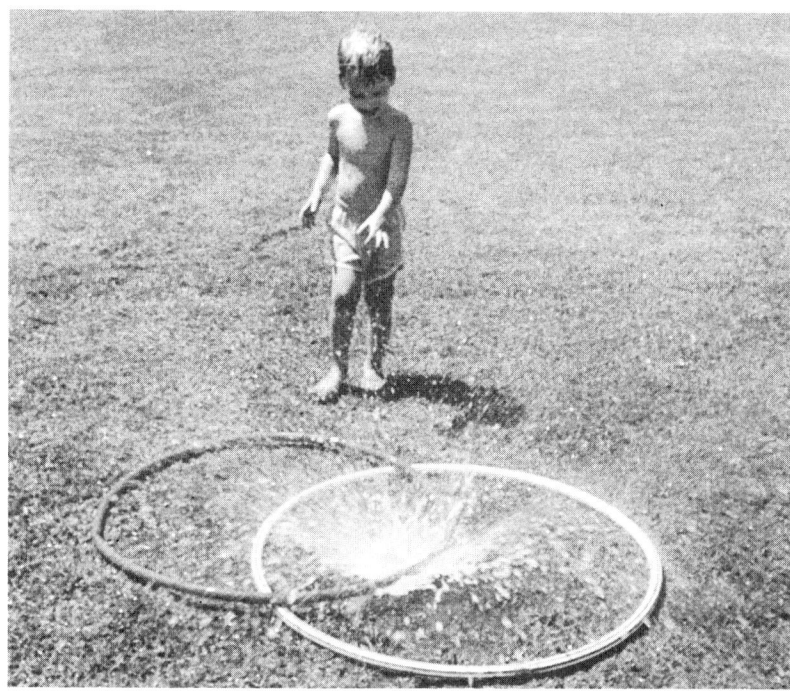

Just getting wet is fun!

Courtesty, Special Education Branch, Los Angeles City Schools

of these same movements in the water, of course, because of the difference in forces on the limbs in the water as contrasted to a gravity-present situation on land.

3. Splashing the face may be done out of the water, using a small pan of water. Other ways of just getting wet on land may be tried. One way—the garden hose—is pictured.

4. Strength exercises, particularly for the stomach and lower back (bent-kneed sit-ups and arch-ups from a front-lying position), may be employed to help children develop a stable and strong trunk base from which to later kick and pull the water, using the various strokes.

Playing in the Pool

Often, atypical youth and children must be given considerable time to become accustomed just to standing in water of various depths. Innumerable water games may be played, including some that resemble ball games on land. Large, square sponges, about $4'' \times 4''$, may be used for throwing and catching games. Objects such as these, which will not sink, are best.

Games that require simple locomotion in waist-deep or shallower water also may be used. Circle games in which the children hold hands and move to the left or right, changing directions when requested, are examples of this kind of game. Water relays in which running is required also may be introduced.

Actions that require jumping and bouncing off the bottom in waist-deep water are also helpful and give the children the first verification that the water may indeed hold them up. As they slowly descend from a vertical jump in the air into shallow water, they experience brief periods of weightlessness. This kind of jumping game may be played in water of increasing depth as the children gain confidence.

Splashing-the-face games may be played in the water also. Because of fear, children initially may take a sharp breath inward suddenly as water touches the face—an action that can suck water into the nose, causing choking and coughing. Relieving the fear through time and familiarity will generally relieve this reaction.

The children may be asked to place the mouth close to the water and blow gently, which will make ripples on the surface. This blowing action might be translated into games in which sponges or ping-pong balls are blown across the surface. As the children become accustomed to this activity, their mouths may be placed closer to the water, even touching it.

Some handicapped children may go no farther than the elementary play stage in their water experiences. Many, however, advance to the point at which they recognize that: (a) the water is a friendly place if the proper things are done, and (b) after feeling the water's support, they may propel themselves through it.

Lead-In Activities

For children to gain the feeling that water will support them, a number of gradual steps must be taken. These steps should terminate in a prone glide, during which the face is submerged and the child is watching the bottom with the eyes open. A glide in a prone position with the heavy head held high will simply pile too much "cargo" on the "boat" of the body rather than contributing to the "hull of the ship" and will displace the child's weight in the water. A head-up glide will make the child feel insecure and result in a frightening loss of support and sinking.

Children should be encouraged to place the face in the water for increasing periods of time while holding the breath, and later to open their eyes while the face is submerged. Next they may begin to reach for objects on the bottom. Finally, they may leave their feet for a prone glide along the surface.

Attempts to get children to place the face under water should be made very gradually. Out-of-water face splashing is a good initial step. A second step could consist of the splashing that normally occurs while children are participating in water games. Further steps in the water may include:

—a nose-held, quick submersion, with the eyes closed. The instructor should not use physical force but instead should encourage the child to go under voluntarily. Water should be wiped from the eyes as the child emerges. This kind of quick submersion should be prolonged after some practice. This submersion should not be done with the head in a vertical position, as water may rise up the nose, causing choking. The children should be in water shallow enough to permit them to bend forward at a 90° angle at the waist and to place the whole face in the water at the same time. In this way, water will not rise up the nose as easily.

—a longer nose-held submersion with one or both eyes open. This may be checked by having the child later retrieve objects from the bottom or count fingers held up by the instructor. As the children's eyes are able to remain open longer under water, a great deal of tension will be dissipated. The child will become oriented to this environment, and their fear should begin to go away.

—objects retrieved in water of increased depth. After an eyes-open (nose-held) action is accomplished, children should be taught to tighten their stomachs, creating a column of air in the nose and permitting the hand to be released from the nose as they submerge. Water is less likely to rise up a nose in which a column of air is pushing the other way. Practice in this kind of stomach tightening may be done while the child is standing, and then practiced with the face submerged.

A usual problem at this point is for a child, because of fear, suddenly to "snort" in the nose as it descends into the water, causing choking. Practicing maintenance of a column of air in the nose is helpful. A slow humming out of the nose may also be tried at this point, first out of the water and then in the water. The teacher should ascertain whether air is really coming out of the nose. The child at first will have problems timing the duration of the hum to coincide with the time the face is submerged. The humming out may stop as the child suddenly breathes in while the face is still under the water. Once this humming-out action is accomplished, however, it may be used later in prone glides, again preventing the child from sucking up water.

LEARNING TO SWIM

Assisted Front Glide

After the children become accustomed to submerging their faces, looking at things under water, and retrieving objects in deeper water, thought may be given to achieving a prone glide. First it may be done with assistance, and then without. As children attempt to go down and get things from the bottom in waist-deep water, they will experience the pressure upward of the water against their bodies and then begin to realize consciously or unconsciously that the water is trying to hold them up!

Most handicapped children and those under age 5 or 6 need another person in the water with them when attempting to leave their feet for the first time in either a front prone glide or a back-lying position (assuming a position for a back float). Initial attempts at these difficult, but critical, intermediate steps should be made with a single instructor working with just one child at a time.

When attempting to encourage the child to execute a face-under front glide, the following steps should be taken:

1. With the instructor facing the child, both of the child's hands should be held (and straightened in one of the instructor's hands, as shown in Figure 31.1(A). The instructor's second hand should be on the child's upper chest or stomach, keeping the child's arms extended at the elbows.

Figure 31.1   Steps in Teaching the Prone Glide

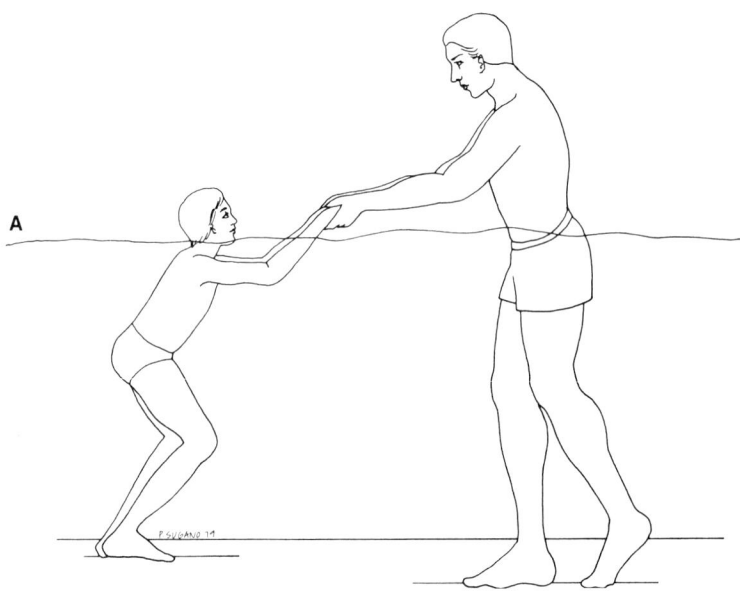

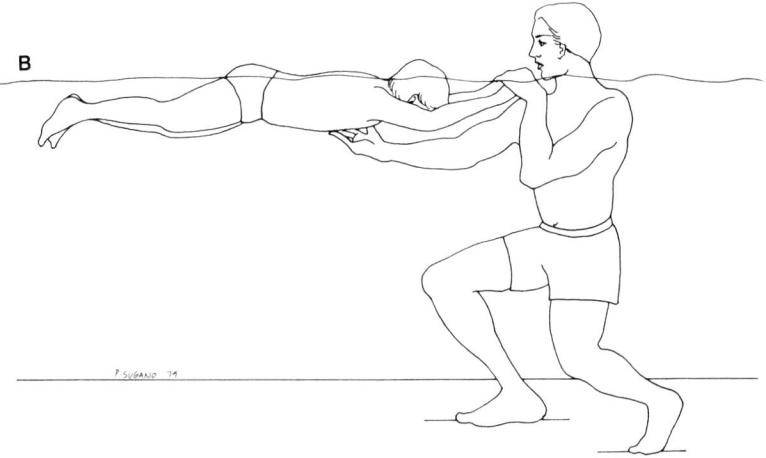

Figure 31.1 (Continued)

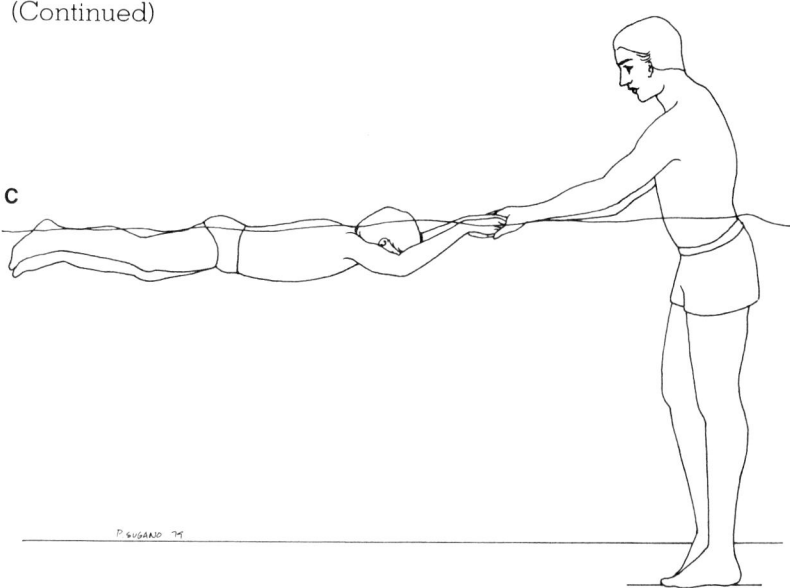

c

P. SUGANO 74

2. Once this support position is gained, the child should start with the chin in the water and simply turn the face downward, rather than charging into the water with head and shoulders initially well above the water. This latter action will plunge the child well under the water and may cause fear.

3. As the instructor gently pulls, the child should attempt to jump gently from the bottom, turn the face down, eyes open toward the bottom, and assume the prone glide (B). The hydraulics involve water passing under the child's body, providing additional lift upon leaving the feet. The arms should be held straight, as this tends to keep the child's body extended at both the hips and the knees. These assisted glides should be practiced with less and less help from the instructor. If the child becomes fearful, the instructor should give additional assistance or go back to an object-retrieval game that reminds the child of the "water is trying to hold me up" sensation.

4. The assisted glides should proceed until the instructor's hand is removed from the child's stomach (C). Less and less assistance also is given the child's hands. Finally, only one hand may be assisted.

5. Instructions on how to recover one's feet on completing the glide may be simply, "Bend your knees." This tends to make the child's feet touch the bottom as the knees extend. This causes children to feel more secure in the gliding position because they know they are able to get out of the prone glide and thus do not feel helpless in the face-down position. The instructor may have to reach back and manually assist children to perceive the knee-bend as some physically handicapped children may not feel the positions and even the presence of their lower limbs in the water.

6. Breathing instructions also should accompany the glides: "Hold your breath" or "Breathe out gently through your nose . . . hum" or "Let's hear you do it in the air before coming to me."

7. Finally the moment of truth arrives: The child is urged to "try it yourself." When this is accomplished and repeated sufficiently, the child may be taught simple ways of achieving propulsion. But propulsion is not advisable, or even possible, without first attaining a relaxed, self-initiated glide.

Back Glide: Positioning and Support

Also in waist-deep water, and at times alternating with practice in the front glide described, an instructor, working with one child at a time, may encourage the child to lean backward slowly and gently (to avoid suddenly plunging under the water). Again, proper hand positions are required of the instructor, as shown in Figure 31.2. One hand should be on the child's neck, permitting the rear of the head to displace water, and the second hand on the back. The child should be supported and encouraged to lean back as shown; arms should be extended at a 90° angle at the shoulders, with the arms supinated and thumbs rotated backward, lifting the rib cage.

As was true with the prone glide, the back glide should begin with the child's neck already on the water, so that the lean back is not followed by submersion, as would occur if the child were to charge into the movement from well above the surface of the water.

Prior to going into this position, the child should be taught how to expel water that may inadvertently splash into the mouth or nose. The child's face should not be allowed to go under water. If the instructor suddenly releases the head, trust will evaporate and further lessons may be impossible.

Figure 31.2   Assisted Back Glide

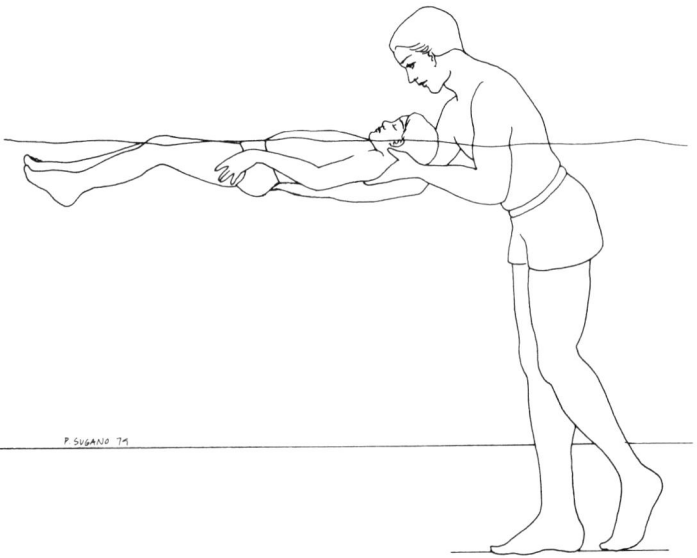

P. SUGANO 79

As with the prone glide, the child should be gently pulled toward the instructor as the instructor backs up, so that a gliding action is experienced. The instructor should say to the child first, "I'm going to back up." The child's neck should be gently palpated, to dissipate tension. The instructor should not encourage propulsion until the back glide position is achieved.

Just prior to having the child attempt a back glide alone, the instructor may encourage practicing the hand movements of an elementary backstroke, hands drawn up the sides of the body until they reach under the armpits and then extend outward, with a quick press of the hands toward the feet. This hand movement may be practiced first with visual inspection out of the water, then in an eyes-closed position out of the water, then with assistance in the water, the instructor's hands on the child's wrist, and finally unassisted in the water, with the instructor backing up while holding the rear of the child's head.

In this back-gliding position, the goals are (a) to show how simple propulsion is possible, (b) to lead toward an unsupported float position, hands well back (feet may or may not drop toward the bottom), and (c) to have the child achieve unassisted floats and propulsions using a elementary backstroke or a back crawl, or some combination (e.g., hands doing an elementary backstroke with the feet executing a flutter kick).

Continuing the Front Glide

Meanwhile, the unsupported front glide may be molded into several actions, such as, first, a simple, simultaneous pulling-back action of both hands, similar to a breaststroke arm action, then accompanied by a relaxed flutter kick (heels should break the top of the water). Also, prone glides may be accompanied by a bubbling-out action so that the child experiences some of the loss of buoyancy that occurs with exhalation during cycles of a regular crawl stroke.

In each lesson these front glides should be frequent and varied and, if the child is able, gradually made more difficult—e.g., a single downward and backward arm action with one arm at first, simulating a regular crawl stroke, then adding a breaststroke kick after achieving the bilateral arm stroke. Two arm strokes may be added to the glide, one at a time, duplicating a regular crawl arm stroke. A flutter kick then may be introduced, together with a slow, bubbling-out for the short duration of the glide.

For the most part, the instructor should stand a few feet (not more than 10') away and assist children to recover their feet and explain what may have gone wrong or right. The instructor should never back up without telling children in advance. To maintain their confidence while attempting to teach them to swim, one should never deceive them, particularly in an anxiety-provoking situation such as a swimming lesson.

A number of useful progressions may be attempted:

1. A relatively lengthy swim, while holding the breath, consisting of arm and leg movements duplicating a breaststroke or crawl stroke.

2. One assisted stroke, with attempts to raise the head to the front (as in the breaststroke) or to the side (as in the crawl stroke) for the first breath—a real accomplishment! The latter is depicted in the photograph.

3. Small breath-held half-circle swims around the instructor, perhaps while both instructor and child are near the edge of the pool. These half-circle swims, as pictured, are

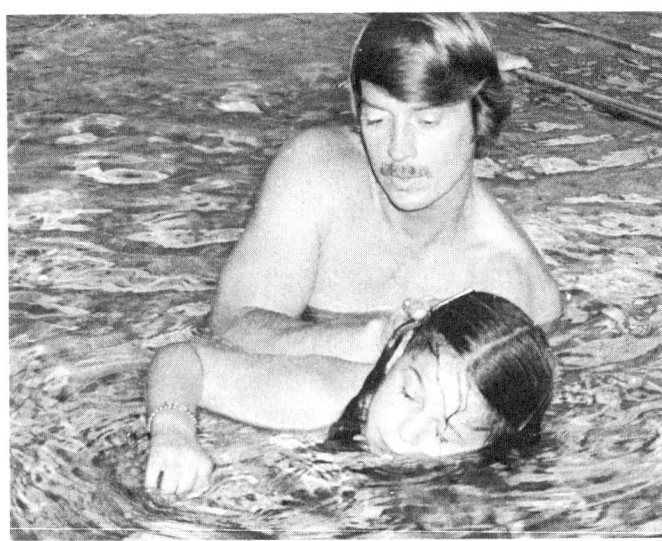

This girl is learning to take one stroke and a breath, with assistance.

Courtesy, Special Education Branch, Los Angeles City Schools

more important prior to achieving regular breathing than are swims in a linear direction. A child who somehow falls in a pool during the course of the lessons will become able to swim quickly in a half-circle and get out again rather than trying to swim in a straight line to the far side of the pool. Half-circle swims should be terminated by an assisted hand-reach for the edge of the pool, and then preceded by sliding into the pool from a seated position.

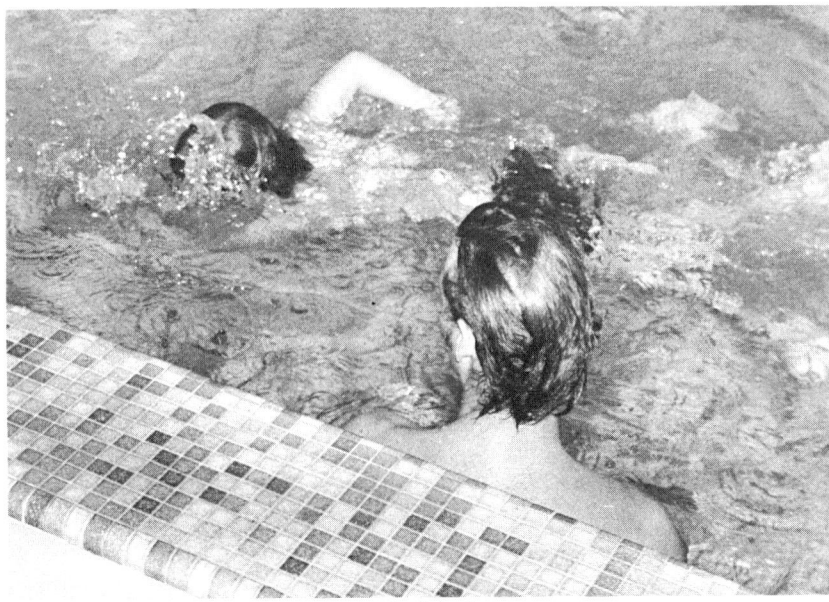

Learning to swim in small half-circles at the edge of the pool builds confidence.

Courtesy, Special Education Branch, Los Angeles City Schools

Figure 31.3   Walking Down a Ladder into Deep Water

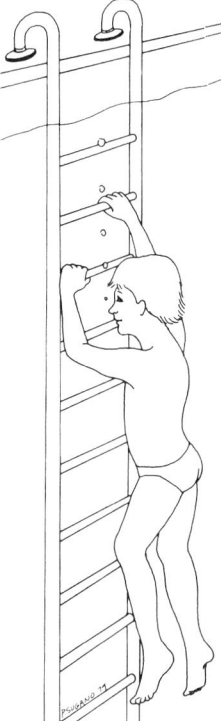

4. Additional confidence that the water will not "let me down" may also be gained at this point by having the child walk down a vertical pool ladder, under the water, to a comfortable depth. Then the child should release the rungs of the ladder, permitting the body to rise to the surface. This is illustrated in Figure 31.3.

BREATHING

Rhythmic breathing is essential in all swimming strokes, whether the swimmer is on the back or on the front. Regular intake and output of breath promotes relaxation and places reasonable demands on the cardiorespiratory system. Undue breath holding is not helpful, particularly for the handicapped, and may aggravate a heart condition or at least make attempts at movement through the water inefficient.

While on the back, a regular breath should be taken at some time during the stroke. In the case of the back crawl, it may be taken in with one arm stroke and expelled with the next. In this stroke, like others, continued exhalation may result in a less than fixed abdominal region and make the stroking actions less vigorous than they otherwise might be. Elementary backstroke breathing also is usually an intake as the arms recover and an exhalation as the arms press. In these strokes, and others that will be described, breathing rhythm and various techniques should be experimented with until breathing is relaxed and comfortable.

When swimming on the front, breathing is more of a problem. If the head is turned to the side or upward, as much of the head as possible should remain in the water, displacing weight and preventing the swimmer from using undue force to get the head out of the water. When breathing to the left side, for example, the opposite ear should remain in the water.

Among the methods used when experimenting with a comfortable breathing pattern are the following:

1. After breathing in on one stroke, slowly bubble out both the mouth and nose continuously while the face is under water, running out of air just before the next breath is to be taken.

2. After an inhalation, hold the breath and then explode it quickly out both the nose and mouth just prior to the next breath. This method, while keeping swimmers tenser in the water, may keep them more buoyant during most of the stroke, as a column of air is trapped in the chest instead of being gradually exhaled.

3. After an intake of breath, start bubbling only through the nose, in a humming action, with the lips tense and close together. This method has the advantage of not scooping water in the mouth as the head is turned or held upward, for all outgo of air is through the nose. All intake is through the mouth, when the face is not submerged.

4. Explode the breath just before the next intake, through the nose only. Do not exhale at all below the water, but make a quick burst out, breathing air outward just as the head rises into the air, and then take a quick inhaled breath as the head submerges again.

In general, the methods that involve slow exhalation in a continuous manner result in a more relaxed trunk and shoulder, and thus a more relaxed stroke. When the breath is held, the swimmer may remain more buoyant, but the stroke is likely to appear forced and tense. Various methods may be experimented with as the swimmer first simply stands and practices breathing and bubbling in a regular manner while the head is to the side or to the front (as in the breaststroke), prior to adding the arm stroke and leg kick to the total swimming pattern.

VERTICAL BOBBING

As children gain confidence in the water, feel it hold them up, and begin to propel themselves through it, at least one critical survival skill should be introduced. Vertical bobbing is only one of the several skills that may be incorporated into a survival swimming training program. Because acquisition of this skill enables children to remain relaxed in water over their heads, it is a big step toward becoming water-safe. The technique should be first taught in water that may be over the head of the learner but shallow enough for the instructor to stand in.

A good preliminary activity is walking down the ladder into deep water (Figure 31.3) and then letting go and ascending to the surface. Next the child should be told to assume a vertical, face-down position in the water and to hold the breath. First attempts may be in water shallow enough to permit the toes to touch bottom.

As the child needs air, the head should be slowly rolled backward, and as the mouth and nose break the surface, the child should take a breath and hold it. This usually causes the child to submerge again, then slowly rise to the surface. Again, after the back of the neck and head have broken the surface and after a breath is needed (this may not be immediately), the child quickly expels a breath in the water in the face-down position. Then, as the head and face are rolled back above the surface, the child takes another breath. These actions may be repeated until the child is tired or has been in the water a specified period of time. These periods could range from 5 to 30 minutes, perhaps.

To review, the segments of the sequence, also depicted in Figure 31.4, are:

(A) Assume vertical face-down position, and hold the breath; the body will submerge.

(B) Roll back the head and upon breaking the surface of the water, take a breath and hold it.

(C) Allow the body to submerge and expel air.

(D) Allow the body to again rise to the surface, whereupon the cycle is repeated.

Common errors include:

—Taking breaths too rapidly, without waiting for complete ascent of the body and without needing another breath.
—Taking in water when a breath of air is needed, either because of bad timing (not waiting for the face to clear the surface) or because of a small wave hitting the face. This can be corrected by alerting the child to the possibility and quickly sniffing out (if in the nose) or blowing out (if in the mouth) the excess water.

Figure 31.4 The Sequence for Vertical Bobbing

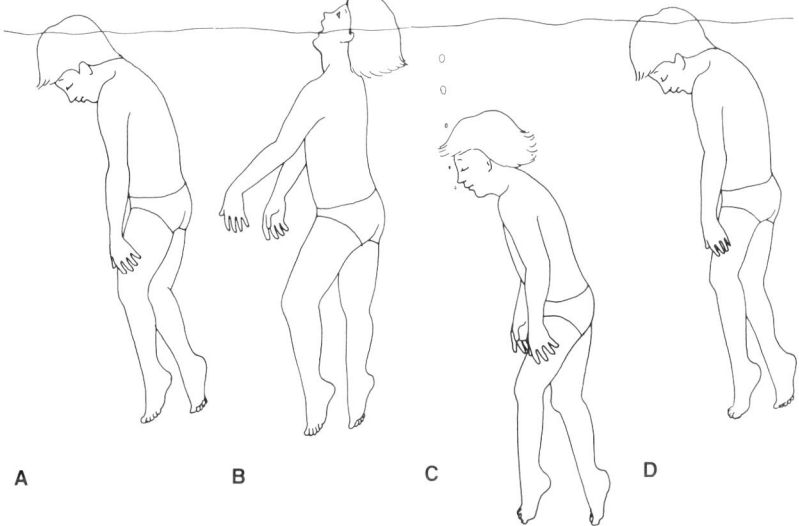

A   B   C   D

—Not remaining as relaxed as possible throughout the sequence, particularly
   when the body rises to the top and is at the top.

Once the bobbing has been mastered, relaxation in all the swimming strokes usually
follows. Drills combining the following skills should be used to thoroughly "waterproof"
a child.

1. Push off from the side into deep water, swim a short distance, let the feet drop,
vertically bob for 1 minute or longer, regain a horizontal position, and swim to the side.

2. Jump feet-first into deep water, bob in the vertical position, level off in a horizontal
position, and swim for the side.

3. Push off from the side, bob in the vertical position for a minute or more, then swim
in a semi-circle around a float or the instructor and back to the side.

Jumping and Diving

Learning to jump and to dive into water over the head can provide recreational fun. It also
is a safety skill in the event of sudden, unexpected falls or pushes into water over the head.

Jumping into the water should be accompanied by a sharp exhalation of air through
the nose, counteracting the force of water forced up the nose. This may be practiced out
of the water. It consists of a short half-breath accompanied by tightening of the diaphragm.

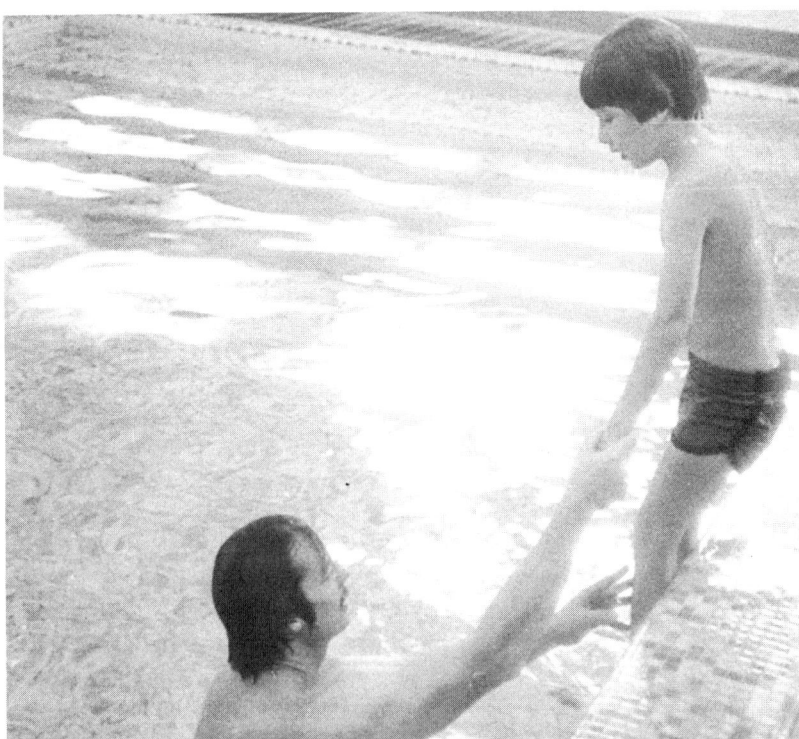

*When first jumping
into the pool,
the child should
be guided.*

Courtesy, Special Education Branch, Los Angeles City Schools

Both jumping and diving may be taught using the following progression. Common to both is that initially the jump and dive are from short distances above the water, and as proficiency is gained in both, the height is gradually increased.

When first jumping, the child actually should be guided from a seated position at the edge, with the instructor holding the child's hands, as pictured, and guiding the child to the surface. Gradually this should be done from higher positions and with less guidance from the instructor, until all help is phased out. The skills of bobbing and walking down the ladder, previously described, are useful preparations.

First dives should be from a seated position. Again, the child's hands should be held by one of the instructor's hands, with the child's arms by his or her head. Next a kneeling position should be taken, as pictured. In the final step before a real dive, one of the legs should extend straight up and back, tipping the child into the water. Finally, the child should get off-balance, bending the legs, and then straightening them when approaching the water. As a further step in either jumping or diving, the child could jump over a stick held 4″–6″ above the deck and near the edge.

Diving is more difficult than jumping because the head goes deeper. It causes more anxiety because more time is needed to ascend to the surface. When guiding the child initially, the instructor should be careful not to somersault the child's body into the water. Also the child's chin should be down on the chest. In more advanced standing dives the hands should reach the water first, breaking the surface for the body to follow.

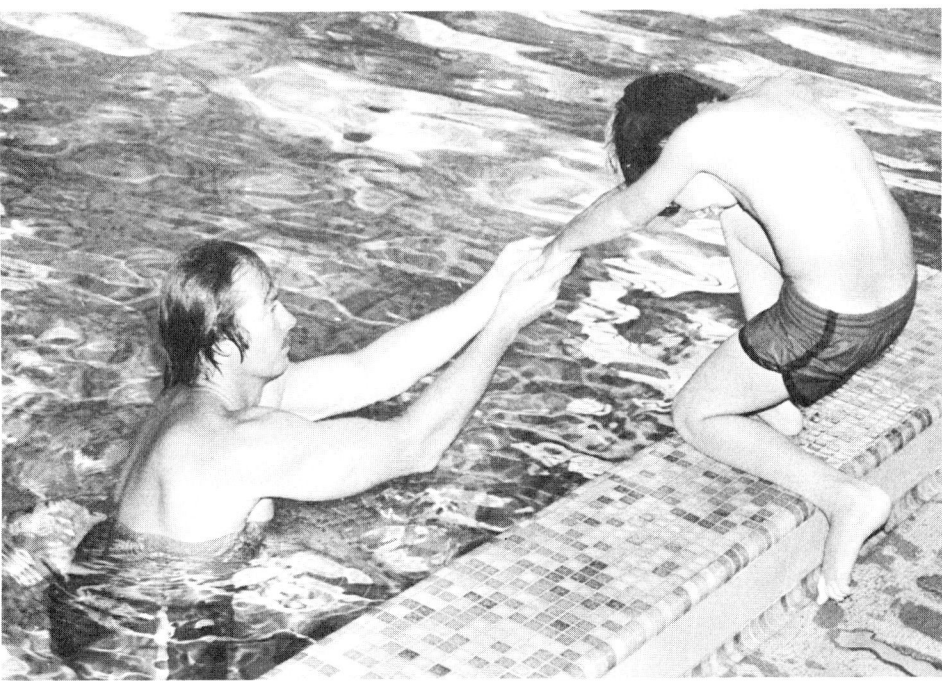

When teaching a child how to dive, the hands are guided into the water.
Courtesy, Special Education Branch, Los Angeles City Schools

SWIMMING STROKE ADAPTATIONS

Every handicapped individual has a most comfortable and efficient way to move through the water and gain pleasure doing so. Children should be helped to find that way and receive that pleasure, despite so-called "correct" ways to accomplish "accepted" strokes.

Some strokes, although simple, may not be helpful for a given kind of handicapping condition. For example, the elementary backstroke, whose kick depends heavily on the strength of the adductors of the legs, may not be good for a child with cerebral palsy. Many of these children are attempting therapy to correct overaddiction of the legs (which causes the legs to scissor when the child attempts to walk).

For the most part, so-called power strokes (breaststroke, sidestroke) are more useful for many handicapped people than are the speed strokes (butterfly, back and front crawls). Also, emphasis on a rapid leg kick, especially the flutter kick in the back and front crawl, does not pay off in terms of ratio between energy expended and movement achieved. A mechanically correct arm stroke should be emphasized, as this creates a propulsive effort that depends on the smaller muscles of the arm and shoulder and thus requires less energy by the swimmer.

When teaching handicapped people, relaxation and proper balance in the water (in a horizontal or near-horizontal position), rather than rapid propulsion, should be emphasized. Urging a child with mild or moderate spasticity (or mild or moderate anxiety) to "kick your feet harder" may "tie the child in knots," preventing any kind of propulsion.

The following strokes and stroke modifications are often taught to individuals with handicapping conditions. The stroke or modification used should be based on the specific disability, body structure, prior swimming experiences, and preferences of the swimmer.

1. Amputees with one upper limb missing totally or partially often use a sidestroke, taking a powerful underwater pull while swimming with a scissor kick on the side of the intact arm.

2. Hemiplegics, spastics, and others with one-sided involvement also may effect a sidestroke with the involved side on top and the good side on the bottom of the stroke. When using a crawl stroke, these individuals invariably breathe more easily when turning to the side opposite the good arm.

3. Amputees with one leg missing can engage in both back and front crawl strokes and in elementary backstrokes and regular breaststroke. At times stroke components are combined. For example, a dolphin-like action of the body may accompany a breaststroke and an arm stroke with both pull and recovery under the water.

4. Amputees with both legs missing or individuals with both legs inoperative also may do a front crawl, a breaststroke, or an arm stroke, breathing every second or third stroke, as needed. A back crawl and an elementary backstroke may be done by some lower-limb amputees.

5. Individuals with both arms missing or inoperative may move through the water with a flutter kick, on their faces, thrusting up periodically to breathe. They also may use a dolphin-like action of the legs and trunk to gain propulsion.

The amputee's center of balance and center of gravity may be displaced to one side or the other. Thus, extensive practice in turning and floating on the back and front and in vertical positions is necessary before attempting propulsion. For example, if the right arm is missing, the center of balance is displaced toward the left; the reverse is true if the left arm or leg is missing.

SPECIAL HEALTH PROBLEMS IN WATER SPORTS

The following are just some of the many health problems that may be particularly prevalent within handicapped populations. The instructor should be aware of these:

1. Skin infections and the propensity for infections may be particularly prevalent among the handicapped. Participants should be inspected each day for new skin conditions that may have developed overnight. Children with dry skin or a tendency to develop rashes should have their skin creamed after getting out of the water.

2. Bowel control is a problem for some handicapped children. They should not be permitted in the water or should be placed in small therapy pools (that may be easily cleaned) for water play and preliminary swimming skills. Rubber pants may reduce the possibility of contaminating the water.

3. Children with chronic ear infections, allergies to water or chlorine, osteomyelitis in the active stage, joint inflammations (including rheumatoid arthritis), severe cardiac conditions, and possible venereal diseases should not participate in swimming or water-play programs.

4. Swimming may or may not have a calming effect on hyperactive children. Some hyperactive children may become calmer for the remainder of the school day if permitted a swimming lesson or vigorous water recreation early in the day. Each child is different, and each child's reaction to the water and the relationship of the water experience to distractible behaviors should be individually assessed before prescribing aquatic activity to reduce hyperactivity.

5. Diving and other acitivities that involve striking the head on the surface of the water or going under the water for several feet are not usually indicated for children with anomalies of the facial region and head, or children with arrested hydrocephalus, hemophilia, and cerebral palsy.

6. Individuals who are susceptible to seizures should approach water activities with caution and medical advice. One of the first symptoms of an impending grand mal seizure is rapid evacuation of air from the lungs, so these persons may imperil their lives if this happens when they are under water. Sometimes they do not inform supervisors of their condition, as they enjoy water programs and become more relaxed. Mandatory physical examinations are especially applicable to aquatic programs.

7. Children and youth should be carefully watched for signs of undue fatigue and excessive chilling (such as blue lips), in which case the lesson should be terminated. Children should not be permitted to wait in wet suits or in a draft prior to entering the water or between tasks.

FACILITIES AND SPECIAL EQUIPMENT

The following are some ideas for facilities and special equipment needed by handicapped children.

1. Flotation devices may be employed but should not be used at the expense of the child's gaining strength or exercise from aquatics. Rings, life jackets, and so forth help a child have fun in the water, but they may not be useful (a) if they are not carefully monitored for safety (e.g., a child might slip out of a ring, or a life jacket could become inverted); (b) if they create a dependency that impedes achievement; or (c) if they engender a false sense of security in a child. One flotation device is pictured.

2. The bottom of a pool (particularly pre-construction) could be planned to contain inlaid tiles with interest factors, such as pictures of animals, to encourage diving and looking at the bottom. Shallow teaching pools likewise could contain visual guidelines on the bottom on which children can stand or from which they can move.

3. Pool temperature should be at about 88°–90° optimally. These higher temperatures, however, bring on fatigue more quickly. More than an hour or so of exposure may be enough for the instructor as well as the children.

4. Teaching pools should have ramps for entry and, preferably, lifts to permit severely handicapped individuals to participate in aquatic programs readily. These are pictured.

5. Teaching pools may be subdivided into smaller teaching sections by using rods that move in either direction, as pictured.

6. Pool depth should be indicated incrementally, by a chart on the wall against which a given child can be measured.

7. The acid balance or pH of the water should be monitored frequently.

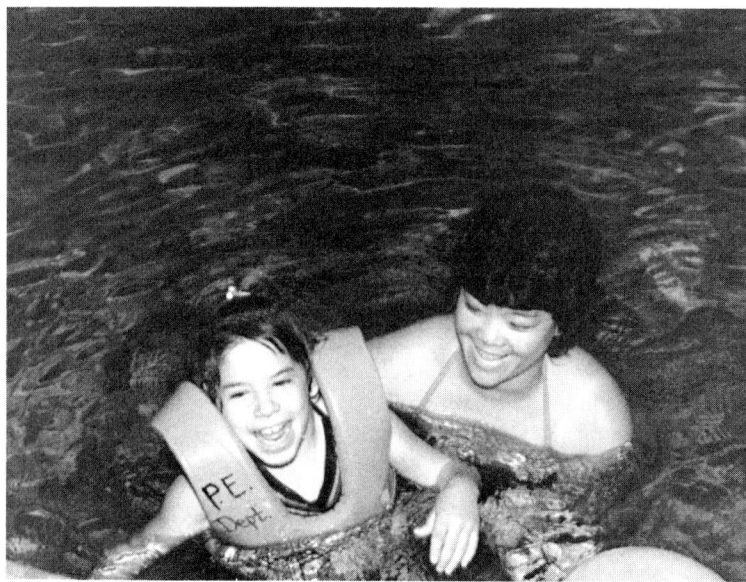

A flotation device may be beneficial if used wisely.

Courtesy Special Education Branch, Los Angeles City Schools

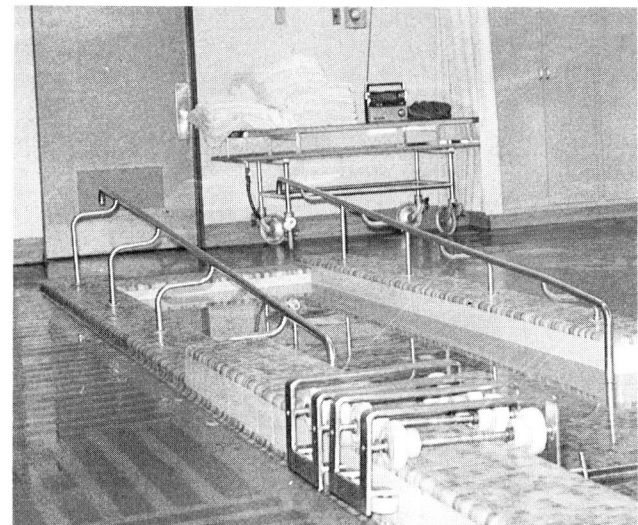

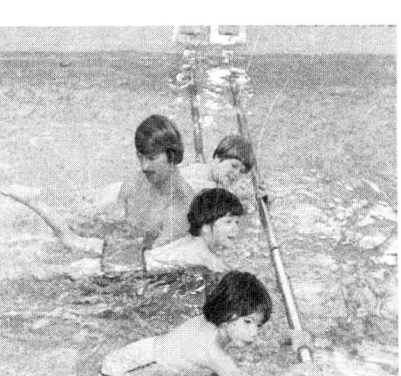

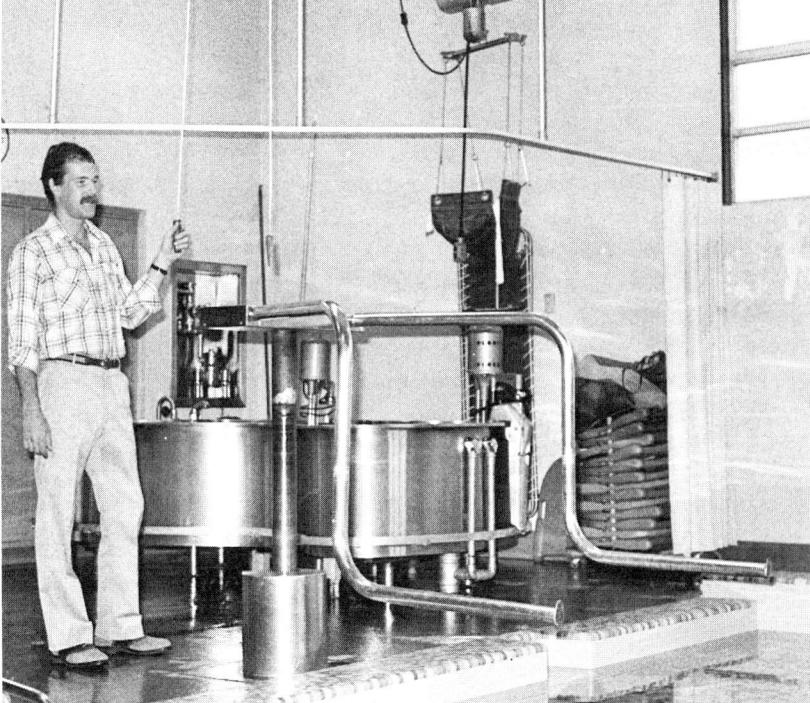

*A well equipped teaching pool for the handicapped will have a gradually sloping
ramp (A), pool dividers (B), and lifts for lowering children into and raising them out
of the water (C).*

Courtesy, Special Education Branch, Los Angeles Schools

A checklist of these ideas and more is provided below:

- Tile walls (not painted)
- Built-in temperature gauges (for air and water)
- Pool flooring—in solid color, not confetti pattern
- Ramp from 3″ depth to gradual slope
- Movable horizontal bars across length (width) of pool
- Non-skid decking
- Hydraulic lift with gurney
- Steps into water
- Wall depth markers
- Deck (floor) drains in enter and exit areas
- Dressing rooms with built-in hair blowers
- Clothes dryer for wet suits, and clothes washers, if possible
- Plenty of cupboards and shelves
- Large bulletin boards for group achievement charts
- Grab rails around pool/water surface and along ramps into water
- Telephone
- Built-in benches in pool area and locker rooms
- Clothes bags and hooks in dressing rooms

SUMMARY

Various forms of aquatic activity are potentially useful for virtually all handicapped groups. The experiences may be as simple as merely getting one's face wet, ranging all the way to competitive swimming and water ballet. Often the only way severely handicapped children can move their limbs or their total bodies is through water, and this can be an emotionally satisfying experience indeed.

As when presenting any type of activity to both normal and atypical youngsters, aquatic activities must be presented in sequences that are achievable, from the simple to the more difficult. This kind of analysis, breakdown, and gradual presentation of tasks is even more imperative when working in water because of the fear many youngsters, particularly the emotionally disturbed, feel when in the water.

Many severely and profoundly handicapped children need not be led toward swimming for water experiences to have a positive effect on their welfare. They may engage in simple water games as ends in themselves.

Several handicapped groups need special attention, activities, and equipment when working in the water. The deaf sometimes are susceptible to ear infections. Amputees must be taught special ways of swimming. Physically handicapped youngsters often must have special equipment.

The water may be employed as a place where children not only gain a heightened awareness of their bodies and their movement potentials but also can exercise. For centuries, forms of hydrotherapy have been used to exercise and relax the handicapped.

QUESTIONS FOR DISCUSSION

1. What special precautions should be taken when introducing the deaf, blind, and physically handicapped to a swimming pool for the first time?

2. What muscle groups are exercised by participation in the crawl stroke, the elementary backstroke, the breaststroke? What strokes might contribute to a postural abnormality? What strokes might aid various postural abnormalities?

3. What sequence would you take children through to get them to leave their feet and swim a simple stroke, face down?

4. How would you teach a child to dive in the water head first?

5. What water safety skills would you teach moderately retarded 10-year-olds who could move through the water for about 15'?

6. What emotional advantages might success in a competitive swimming program have for a handicapped child? What stresses in such a program should be considered?

7. What special lead-in activities might help a child learn to breathe in a relaxed way when swimming the front crawl? What are some modifications in breathing you might experiment with?

STUDENT PROJECTS

1. Reviewing the literature, compile a list of water games that are recreational in themselves. Compile another list of water games that lead toward the sub-skills of the front crawl; the breastroke.

2. Work for a month in an attempt to teach a handicapped youngster to swim or to have fun in the water. Keep a diary of your daily problems and progress. What did you discover after lessons were underway that might have aided you earlier?

3. Arrange, in order of difficulty, aquatic skills leading toward a front crawl stroke with breathing. How can you be sure that the skills are arranged in proper order? If possible, try out your sequence with a novice swimmer.

4. Discuss with a physical therapist how hydrotherapy is used to work with various kinds of handicapping conditions.

5. What special equipment might be needed when designing a pool for the physically and mentally handicapped? Draw your conception of such a pool, showing this kind of special equipment.

RESOURCES

American Association for Health, Physical Education and Recreation. (1968). *A practical guide for teaching the mentally retarded to swim.* Washington, DC: Author.

American Red Cross. (1975). *Swimming for the handicapped—Instructor's manual.* Author.

Canadian Red Cross Society. (1970). *Manual for teaching swimming to the disabled.* Ontario, Canada: Author.

Hackett, L. (1975). *Water learning.* Palo Alto, CA: Peek Publications.

Reynolds, G.D. (Ed.). (1973). *A swimming program for the handicapped.* New York: Association Press.

United Cerebral Palsy Association. (1970). *Swimming for the cerebral palsied.* New York: Author.

32 *Games That Teach Things*

Ever since the rise of humanism in Renaissance Europe, it has been speculated that permitting children to move in natural ways within the educational environment contributes to their total development. The earliest kindergartens were established with this premise in mind. At the turn of this century, practitioners such as Maria Montessori explored multisensory approaches to education. This gifted Italian educator taught arithmetic operations, for example, by permitting children to group themselves and then count how many were present in each cluster. Many pre-school experiences in contemporary America are designed to help infants explore and learn through the medium of movement.

Coupled with contemporary scientific concern with human thinking processes, intelligence, cognitive psychology, problem solving, and creative thinking has been a parallel interest in the way in which movement activities may enhance thinking. The objectives range from simple perceptual discrimination, through academic operations, to abstract thinking. In general, experimental work giving validity to the use of an active approach to learning is of two types:

1. Studies attesting to the role of movement in the acquisition of basic conceptual operations and concepts. For example, Saltz (1982) found that the enhancement of memory for objects, as well as for sentences, occurred if movements accompanied memorization efforts. If objects to be remembered are also handled, retention will be improved. Likewise, a series of sentences can be retained better if the child acts out the sentence (Saltz & Donnenwerth-Noland, 1981).

2. Movement in a standard academic context, noting differences in improvement from that of children exposed to a passive, traditional approach. Studies of this type have been summarized by Cratty (1985) and also appear in works by Van Osdol, Johnson, and Geiger (1974), Thornburg and Fisher (1970), and others.

In recent years active games have been used to meet an expanded list of goals: (a) to enhance foreign language learning (Asher, 1969); (b) to fulfill the goals of mainstreaming children in physical education (Salend, 1981, 1982); (c) to improve the social interactions of both normal and aggressive emotionally disturbed children (Edmondson & Han, 1983); and (d) to improve conversational skills and assertiveness (McGee, Krantz, & McClannahan, 1984). Movement also provides a useful tool in a behavioral-therapeutic approach to the improvement of self-control (Cratty, 1985; Meichenbaum & Asnarow, 1979).

Movement and thought may be paired in direct ways. The following reflects several of my personal biases:

1. If one is to aid a child in learning something through the use of movement, one must pair a movement experience with a cognitive or an academic operation in rather precise and obvious ways.

2. Movement is a powerful motivating tool in the academic setting.

3. Children might well learn best through active participation. Some of these youngsters are found in special populations, including the deaf, retarded, learning disabled, and emotionally disturbed.

4. When a child moves and thinks and at the same time is visually engrossed in a task, the result is a high level of attention to that task.

5. When a child acts out academic operations and intellectual processes, the quality of the result is apparent immediately. Future adjustments may be made by making the task harder, by lessening its difficulty, or by modifying the experience in some way.

In employing the various activities presented in the following pages, several cautions should be remembered:

1. Some physical educators substitute good physical education and motor development activities for so-called learning games in an effort to engender more respect for their program. Rather, these activities should be used as adjuncts to learning experiences that usually are initiated by a classroom teacher and completed within a classroom setting. Motor development is a laudable goal independent of possible intellectual carry-over.

2. Learning games often require special playground markings or equipment. These factors should be considered and weighed when contemplating an active learning approach.

3. The use of learning games requires teachers who are flexible enough to adapt and modify their curricula and lessons—which not all teachers are willing to do. Before it can be successful, teachers must be willing to embrace the philosophy behind the approach.

4. The approach may not work with all children. If it does not, the teacher should accept that eventuality and not impose it if it does not suit an individual child's needs or learning style.

The activities that follow are only examples, drawn from my own experiences and writings and those of others. Readers who are intrigued by the possibilities inherent in this approach to learning are urged to consult other sources, some of which are given in the Additional References at the end of this chapter. In the next few pages are activities representing ways to (a) teach about directions in space, (b) help children translate signs into meaning and movement (coding games), (c) teach them about shapes and geometric figures, (d) teaching reading and mathematical concepts and operations, (d) instill problem solving skills and creativity, and (e) illustrate psychological and social concepts through movement games. Requisite to acquisition of the five sets of qualities listed are good attentional skills. Movement experiences to improve attention are explored in chapter 26.

TEACHING ABOUT DIRECTIONS IN SPACE

Large-muscle activities may be employed to teach spatial concepts and to teach children to correctly draw lines and shapes that may be gradually molded into letters and numbers. To a 4-year-old entering school or to a developmentally delayed child, a spoon is a spoon, whether it is hanging on the wall, lying on the floor or on the table. A fork is a fork regardless of its orientation in space. On being introduced to printing and similar skills, children are suddenly confronted with the fact that society (i.e., their teacher) is not happy unless one draws lines in prescribed directions. Thus, the child must grasp important spatial concepts, some of which are extremely hard to learn. For example, a line drawn away from the child on a page may be called "up" by the teacher!

To make more vivid some spatial concepts that later may be used to transcribe words onto paper, large-muscle activities may be used to act out ideas about space. Using the total body, children can learn about a horizontal line by holding a jump rope parallel to the ground and running back and forth along its length. After this is accomplished, they may be asked to go to the classroom and draw the shape of the rope as they remember it (the rope may be brought in as a reminder). When this has been mastered, these same horizontal lines may be drawn on a piece of paper while the paper is anchored with the elbow. This sequence is pictured, showing tasks that range from the gross-motor activity of throwing a ball, to intermediate motor activity (the limb movements used on the black-board or on a large piece of butcher paper), to the fine-motor activity represented by the arm-wrist movement needed to draw a horizontal line with a pencil on a small piece of paper.

The concept of a horizontal line may be further refined to include the idea that one may travel along the line from left to right and from right to left (directionality). This is a more difficult concept. Therefore, the rope (as well as the drawings) might have ends of different colors—e.g., red for the right (stop) end of the line and green for the left (start)ing end.

Vertical lines and directions also may be explored on the playground. Examples include throwing a ball directly up in the air and inspecting a flagpole. This concept, too, can culminate in drawing lines on a piece of paper, first toward the body (easier) and then away from the body, with an anchored movement.

Next in difficulty is the concept of circles and half-circles. These are relatively easy to find and simulate on the playground. Children may run around circles drawn with chalk or around the half-circle of a basketball court "key." Again, the circle and half-circle may be translated into intermediate and fine-motor activities.

Slanted lines are more difficult. Slanted ropes and sliding boards, viewed from different angles and directions, provide two possible props involving total body movement. Intermediate motor activities may utilize butcher paper or the chalkboard. Finally, the child may be asked to draw slanted lines on a piece of paper (fine-motor). Right-handed children will find slanted lines from upper left to lower right easiest to draw. Then they may practice drawing lines from lower right to upper left. Finally, they may be asked to draw slanted lines that require them to cross the body (e.g., from upper right to lower left and lower left to upper right).

Lines that cross are difficult for some children to master. When walking a line on the playground, they may at first veer off and walk along a crossing line. In any case, the procedure is the same: Introduce children to lines that cross on a playground, duplicate the movements and concepts through intermediate motor activity, and refine it in fine-motor drawing. Some special playgrounds for handicapped children contain tricycle "roads." These should cover a small enough area so that the child can perceive the configurations of the path.

The length of time to cover each spatial concept is dependent upon the perceptual and motor abilities of the child, as well as developmental age. One child might grasp the idea immediately and translate it at once from a total body movement experience on the play-

A

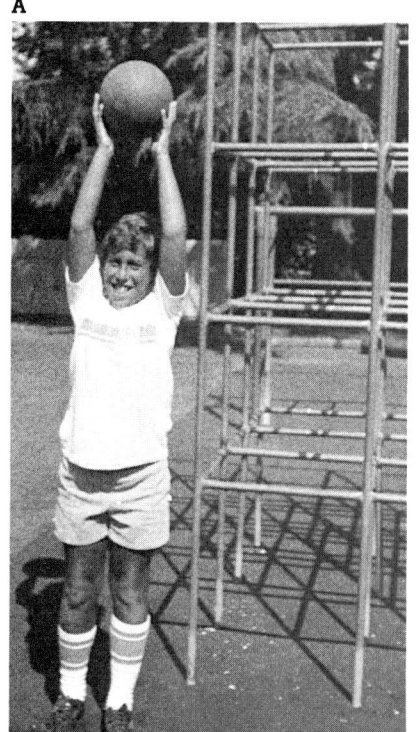

B

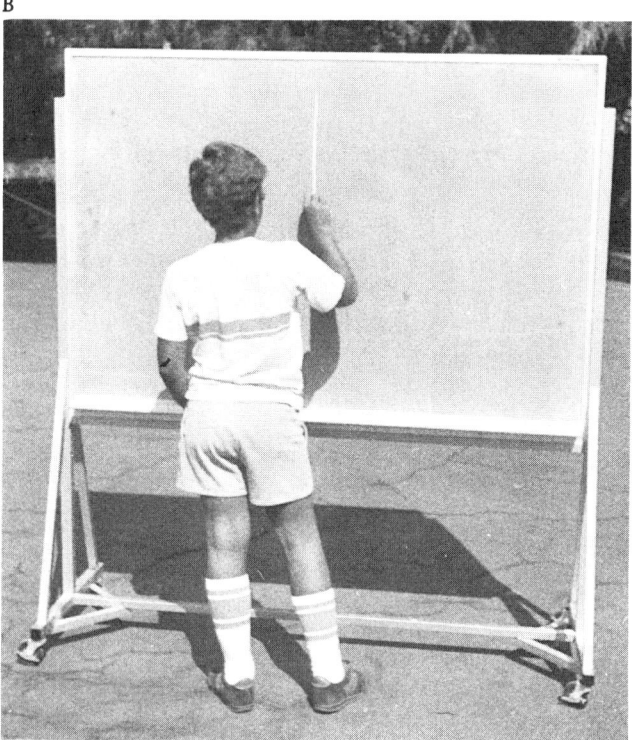

C

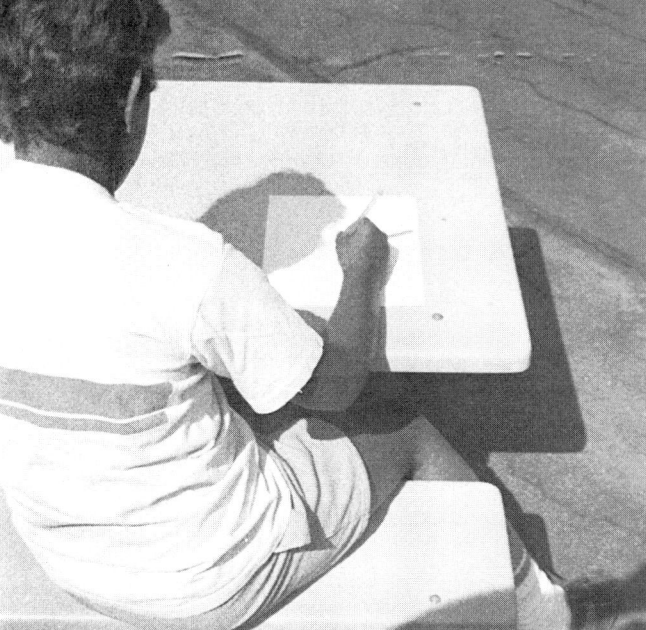

*Spatial concepts may be taught
through activities ranging from the
gross body movements of throwing
(A), to the intermediate limb movements of writing on a chalkboard (B),
to the fine muscle movements of
drawing on paper (C).*

ground to the written page. Another may require a week or a month to learn the concept. This kind of lesson is a helpful accompaniment to some of the other lessons that follow, including coding games, to help children identify letters and numbers.

CODING GAMES

The basic premise on which the use of coding games is based is that to learn many basic academic skills, children must decipher a number of cultural codes composed of intrinsically meaningless, nonsense shapes representing quantity (numerals), as well as ideas, people, places, things, words, and actions. The concepts that coding games can potentially help to teach range from the simplest idea for retarded children to complex concepts for the gifted.

Initially, children are introduced to the idea that some kind of mark may represent some action. They are first shown an X, for example, and told that X means "clap your hands." The X is shown again, and the children are asked to demonstrate what it means. This may require more than one exposure if the child is developmentally delayed, but once this simple concept (that something written can stand for something else) is learned, a world of possibilities presents itself.

1. More than one symbol may be introduced, representing more than one action (e.g., X = clap, / = stand up).

Figure 32.1   A Coding Game

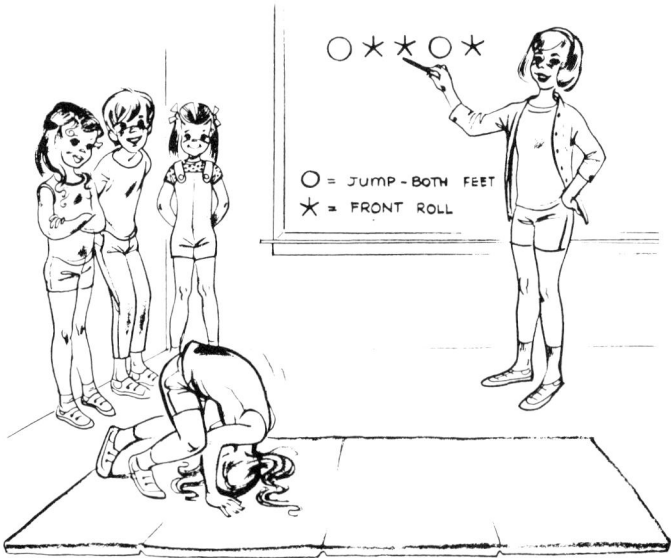

Note. From *Intelligence in Action* by B.J. Cratty, 1973, Englewood Cliffs, NJ: Prentice-Hall. Used by permission of the publisher.

2. Symbols may be presented in various combinations, and children asked to "read" the symbols via their movements. The teacher is able to confirm the quality of the "translation" by observing the children's movements. Figure 32.1 illustrates one possible sequence.

3. Nonsense shapes may be replaced by the initial letters of actions. Children may be told, for example, that *G* means "go around your chair" and *J* means "jump." After these and similar verb-symbol combinations are learned, the letters may be stretched into words. *G* may be changed to *GO*, and *S* may be changed first to *SND* and finally to *STAND*. At that point, the children are actually reading!

4. Children's names may be added to the game. *M* might represent *MARY* who is asked to *STAND*, while *G* (Gary) is asked to *RUN*. Again, the initial letter of a name may be expanded gradually until the child recognizes the symbol that society uses to represent his or her name.

5. This kind of game may be expanded to include location. For example, *W* might indicate *WINDOW*, where *MARY* has been asked to *WALK*. The locations, too, may be stretched into the real words—in this case, *WNDOW* and, finally, *WINDOW*.

The main clues children use as they first learn to recognize words are the first letter, then the last letter, and finally the shape of the total word. When stretching words, this should be kept in mind.

Uses of coding games are almost infinite. For example, more able physically handicapped children may be asked to make up their own symbol-to-movement code, or perhaps a code in which a symbol represents a classification of movements. These and other coding games are included in a book by that title by Cratty (1981).

GEOMETRIC FIGURES

As the next set of activities, children may be asked to walk around and otherwise interact with large geometric configurations painted or chalked on the playground. In Figure 32.2, the children are naming the figures as they jump onto them. In games involving counting, the children could say the number of sides of an angular shape while standing on it. Or youngsters could modify them into letters and numbers. A triangle, when modified, may become an A; a single line and two half circles make a B. After learning about geometric figures in this manner, children may cut out templates containing the same shapes and translate their knowledge about shapes onto paper. Finally, these shapes may be changed into words.

LETTER AND NUMBER RECOGNITION

Physical responses may be used as aids to learning about both letters and numbers. Children may jump onto or throw objects at grids containing letters or numbers, while saying aloud the letter or number. These grids can be chalked on a playground surface or, if children are to throw objects (such as beanbags) at the letters or numbers, placed vertically on the classroom wall.

Figure 32.2   A Geometric Shape Game

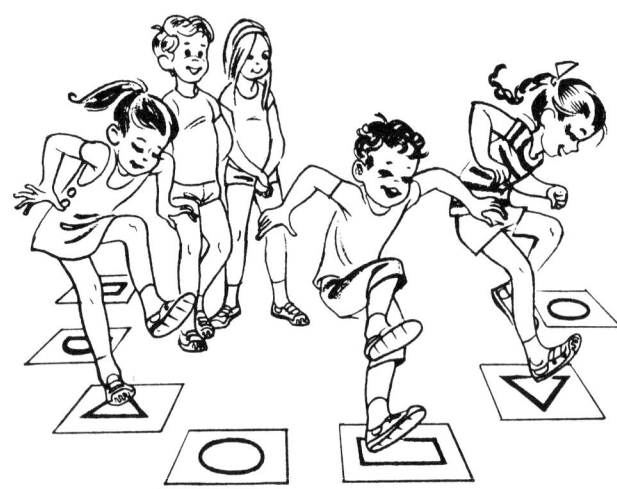

Note. From *Active Learning* by B.J. Cratty, 1971, Englewood Cliffs, NJ: Prentice-Hall. Used by permission of the publisher.

Figure 32.3   A Game Matching Lowercase and Uppercase Letters

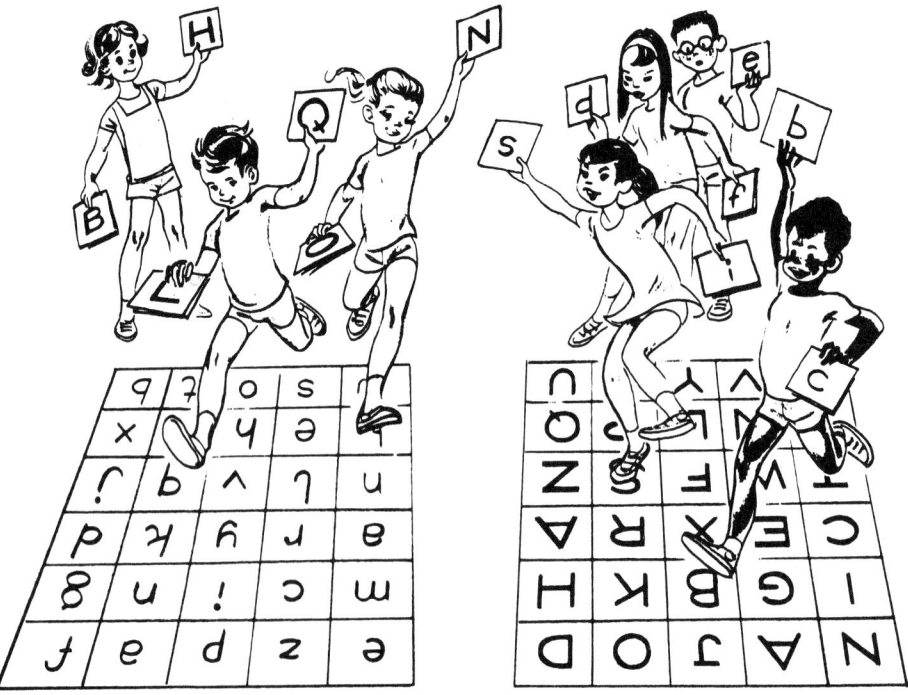

Note. From *Active Learning* by B.J. Cratty, 1971, Englewood Cliffs, NJ: Prentice-Hall. Used by permission of the publisher.

The size of playground grids should be about 6 feet square and contain 36 one-foot squares. This size permits easy jumping from one letter to another in squares that the children's feet fit easily. Each row of the grid should contain at least one vowel, so that a child using a line of six letters may construct a number of words. Or upper and lower case letters may be matched, as shown in Figure 32.3.

Children may be involved in different roles—recorders, jumpers, evaluators, and so forth. These roles should be rotated from time to time. The grids also should be produced on a chalkboard so children can see the relationship between the letters, the total lesson content, and the school program. A mathematics grid might contain not only numbers but also =, +, −, and ÷ signs. Pictures of animals may be a helpful adjunct (e.g., "3 rabbits plus 4 rabbits equals how many rabbits?") Details of these and other grids and games can be found in books such as Cratty's (1985) *Active Learning*.

Two other types of configurations are especially good with mentally and otherwise handicapped children. By running along an oversized series of shapes, children gain knowledge about the letters and numbers the configurations represent. This type of activity has been used successfully with the visually impaired, mentally retarded, and physically handicapped. The book *Educational Games for Physically Handicapped Children* (Cratty & Breen, 1972) contains modifications of these games for children with physical disabilities. And an interesting activity based on a line having various configurations can be devised as shown in Figure 32.4. The children place letters printed on cards besides parts of the line that correspond to that letter.

Figure 32.4 Configuration Matching Letter Shapes with Cards

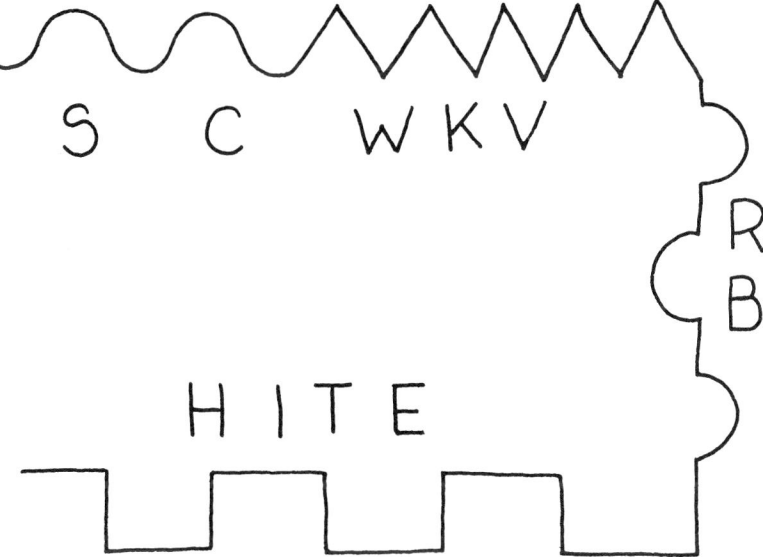

Combining letter recognition games with phonics training has been used with success over the years. For example:

1. Jump, or throw an object, into the letter square beginning the word *apple.*

2. Jump, or throw an object, into the letter square for the *br* sound.

3. Jump, or throw an object, into the letter square containing the ending sound in *tent.*

4. Jump, or throw an object, into the letter square containing the middle sound in the word *bag.*

READING GAMES

Reading games have been used for centuries, according to the historical review by Humphrey and Sullivan (1973). The easier games of this type use words that contain the actions called for—action verbs. Games containing other parts of speech may be employed also. Examples of some reading games are:

1. Obstacle courses, with a card at each obstacle stating how to negotiate the obstacle (jump, hop, etc.). Peer "teachers" and peer evaluators can be used with games of this type. Competition between two teams also is possible.

2. Modifications of games that require progression through space (e.g., base games). Children may hit a ball and then gain an extra base if they read a word on a card flashed by a member of the opposite team. Croquet also may be modified in this manner, as may goal games such as soccer (an extra stroke or point added if a word is read correctly).

3. Relay races. A team is required to read a word after each leg of the relay. The participants may be required merely to read the word, or to use the word in a sentence, or to define the word.

4. Steal-the-bacon type games. Two children from two facing teams simultaneously run and try to be first to pick up a card containing the word called out.

5. Combined spelling and reading games. Cards containing a letter apiece are placed in a pile, and children from opposing teams run to the pile and see how fast each can construct a word from the available letters.

6. Noun games, using pictures of people, things, and animals. Children must either jump on, run and touch, or throw an object at the correct picture when its written name is held up. The opposite of this game is also possible; children physically respond to the written word when its picture is flashed or drawn, as shown in Figure 32.5.

MATHEMATICS GAMES

Virtually all sports require score keeping, a mathematical operation in which all team members may participate. For younger children, counting, grouping, and the like may be taught by having the children place themselves in groups and then count the number making up the group. (They may have to be reminded to count themselves!). Older children may use number and symbol grids to jump on or throw an object at their answers to mathematics problems, as illustrated in Figure 32.6.

I recently attended the "grand opening" of a playground specially designed to enhance the mathematical abilities and operations of deaf and hard-of-hearing youngsters. The

Figure 32.5   A Reading Game

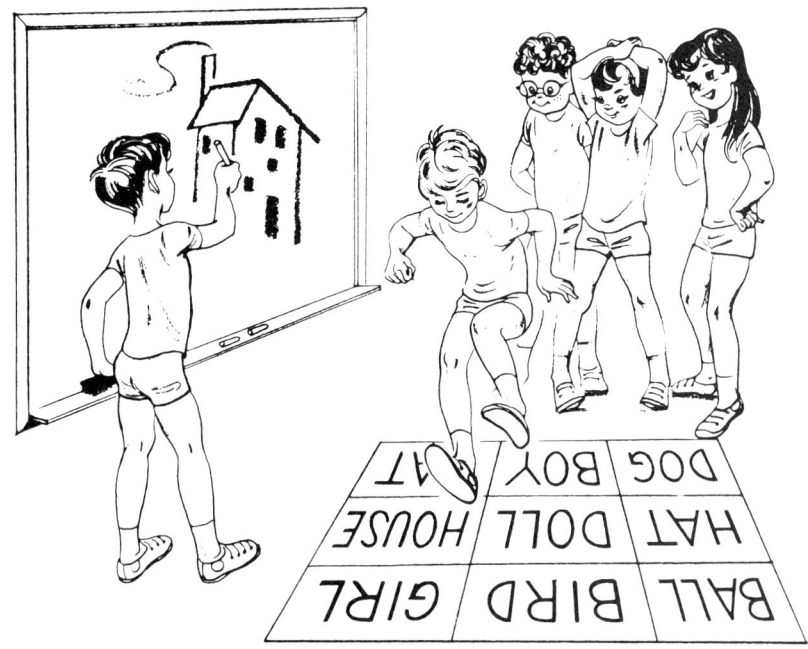

Note. From *Active Learning* by B.J. Cratty, 1971, Englewood Cliffs, NJ: Prentice-Hall. Used by permission of the publisher.

Figure 32.6   A Math Game

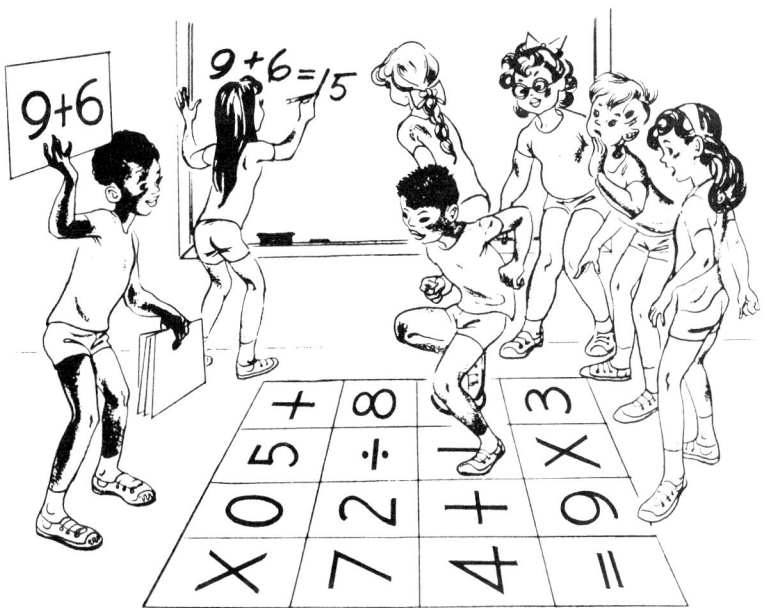

Note. From *Active Learning* by B.J. Cratty, 1971, Englewood Cliffs, NJ: Prentice-Hall. Used by permission of the publisher.

playground, located at the California School for the Deaf (Riverside), contains several stations. Four of these are pictured. Examples are a large clock into which children may insert their bodies, acting as "hands," in order to begin to tell time; "computer keyboards" that help children, by jumping from key to key, understand spatial and numerical concepts; large grids containing various representations of quantity (numbered dots, arabic and roman numerals, etc.), to help children transfer numerical and quantitative concepts. A large "mathematical mountain" also is included, with steps through which children may learn to count as they ascend the promontory.

Track meets and similar activities afford chances for dealing in mathematics, as (a) distances are computed for a team or for three broad jumpers (addition); (b) individual legs of relays are figured (subtraction and addition); (c) distances in parts of the triple jump are calculated (addition); and (d) training procedures are checked (e.g., heart rate is counted in 10-second intervals and multiplied by 6 to determine heartbeats per minute immediately after 1 minute and 5 minutes after termination of exercise).

Courtesy, California School for the Deaf, Riverside

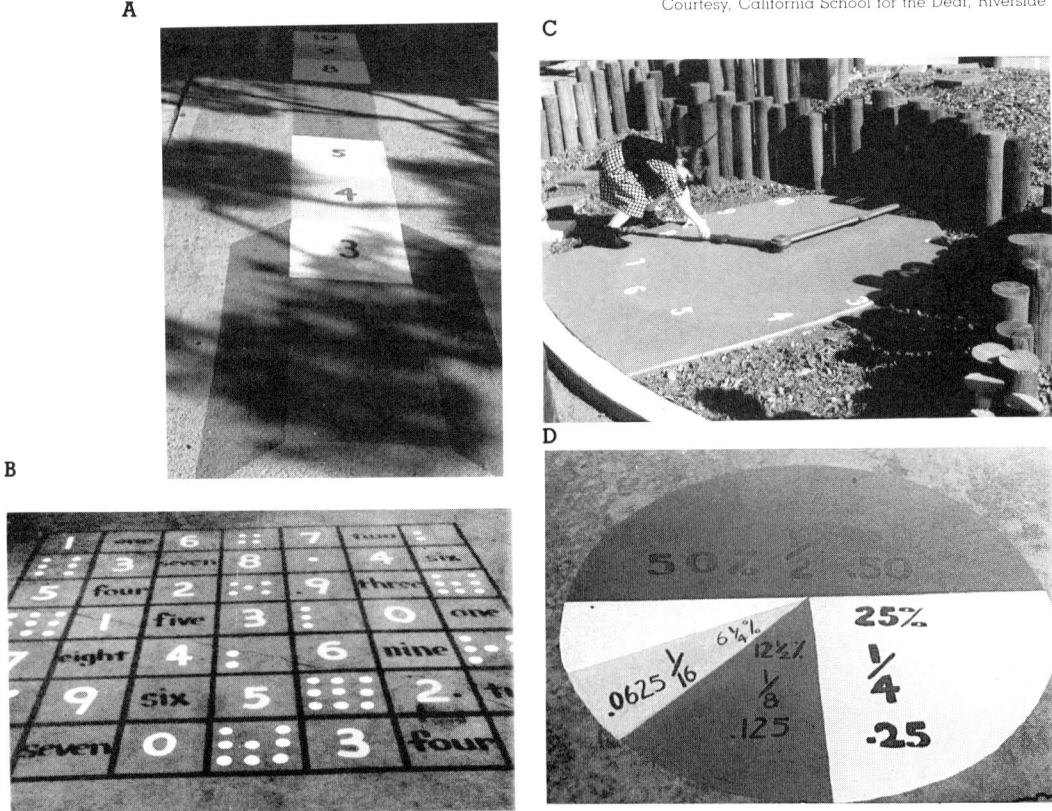

Four of the many activities in the mathematics playground at the California School for the Deaf are: (A) number "rocket," (B) grids displaying quantity, (C) life-size "clock," and (D) percentage/fraction/decimal "pie."

PROBLEM SOLVING AND THOUGHT

Most conceptual operations can be translated into movement tasks. Many of these are too abstruse for retarded children, but other handicapped groups can benefit from activities that require intellectual operations. In addition to the activities presented below, readers may wish to consult books such as *Intelligence in Action* (Cratty, 1973) to gain further insight into the integration of thought and action.

Divergent Thought Production

The production of divergent thought is an intellectual operation that is usually found in movement education programs. It is recognizable by the preface to each command—"How many . . . ?" For example: "How many ways can you jump over the line?" "How many ways can you enter the hoop?"

   This approach purportedly helps children become flexible and innovative, creative in their approach to movement experiences. When well conceived and involving a variety of movement experiences (e.g., throwing, jumping, running, tumbling), divergent thought activities can constitute a productive part of any program for younger children and those who are developmentally delayed in various ways. Using this approach, instructors should (a) be prepared to wait for children's responses and not to impose their will on the children; (b) be accepting of *any* (safe) responses children may initiate, if the responses truly represent their efforts; and (c) not expect children to invent something out of nothing; a lesson requiring a child to formulate "new" ways of going over a vaulting horse probably should have been preceded by lessons in which some data have been fed to the children via various teacher-instigated ways of vaulting a horse.

Convergent Thought Production

Convergent thought production is the formulation of a single or best way of accomplishing something, within limitations imposed by instruction or physical conditions (equipment, etc.). Asking children to get over a line, left foot first, with a half-turn, hopping in the air and landing on the right foot, is such a problem, for there is only one solution called for. "Move down the mat with your back to it and with only one foot and two hands touching it, backward" poses a similar problem.

   A lesson can alternate problems involving convergent and divergent thought production so that children become alert, reflective thinkers, thinking in precise, as well as free, creative terms. A task can be gradually changed from one that requires divergent thought ("How many ways can you get down the mat?") to one that requires increasingly convergent solutions ("Can you show me some hopping ways to get down the mat, using half-turns each time you hop on your left foot?").

Analysis and Synthesis

Analysis means taking apart, inspecting, and interpreting the components of something. In contrast, synthesis means building up, putting together, and forming wholes from parts. Both of these operations may be conducted in innumerable physical game settings. The concepts may be too difficult for some handicapped groups to grasp consciously, but they may help others.

Marlow (1980) has written about the manner in which a games-analysis approach may be employed in an educational context. Based upon ideas by Morris (1976), Marlow has suggested six categories into which games may be broken down: (a) players, (b) equipment, (c) movements, (d) organizational patterns, (e) purposes, and (f) limitations. For example, variables that influence how a ball (equipment) might be used could include its size, weight, color, and so forth. The three processes that children are encouraged to engage in are (a) shared decision making, (b) problem solving skills important in analytic processes, and (c) discovering variations in movement skills and the individual differences and variations in other children's capacities.

Learning these concepts via movement experiences is meant to be only a bridge to their application to other aspects of academic study and to life itself. The rationale for incorporating these and other concepts into movement experiences is to make them more vivid and interesting.

An example of a game in which synthesis might be employed would be to have each of four children individually demonstrate a movement (e.g., hop, turn, roll, jump) to a group of other children. The observing group combines the four movements into a continuous action having some flow into it. A smooth end result synthesizing the four sub-movements might be achieved with more facility through music. The children also might try to demonstrate various ways in which the four sub-movements might be combined.

An example of analysis might be the children's demonstration of a game—dodge ball, for example. The observing children then determine what sub-skills are employed in the game (throwing the ball, moving laterally, etc.). Another example might be a teacher demonstration of a complicated movement (e.g., hopping backward on the left foot six times in a straight line). Children then might be asked to determine what single words might act as cues for a child who has not witnessed the movement to copy it exactly (hopping left, straight line, six times, etc.). A child who has been excluded from the demonstration then may return and synthesize the other children's analysis by trying to execute the total movement after being given word cues, one at a time. This is illustrated in Figure 32.7.

Classification and Categorization

One game previously outlined in this chapter involves placing letters of various shapes beside a line having a number of different shapes that correspond to the letter shapes (Figure 32.4). Other games that might be played with more children include those in which children are asked to "Show me all of the jumping things you can do," or "Show me all of the hopping things that are possible" or, "Can you do something that combines hopping and jumping?"

Original Thinking and Creativity

Creativity has been defined by some as placing together two or more "things" that previously had not been associated. The following games may tap the creative abilities of both normal and atypical children and youth.

1. From a large box with various athletic equipment and junk (a bent wastebasket, a length of hose, etc.), select two or three items and construct a game that no one has played before.

Figure 32.7 A Game Involving Analysis

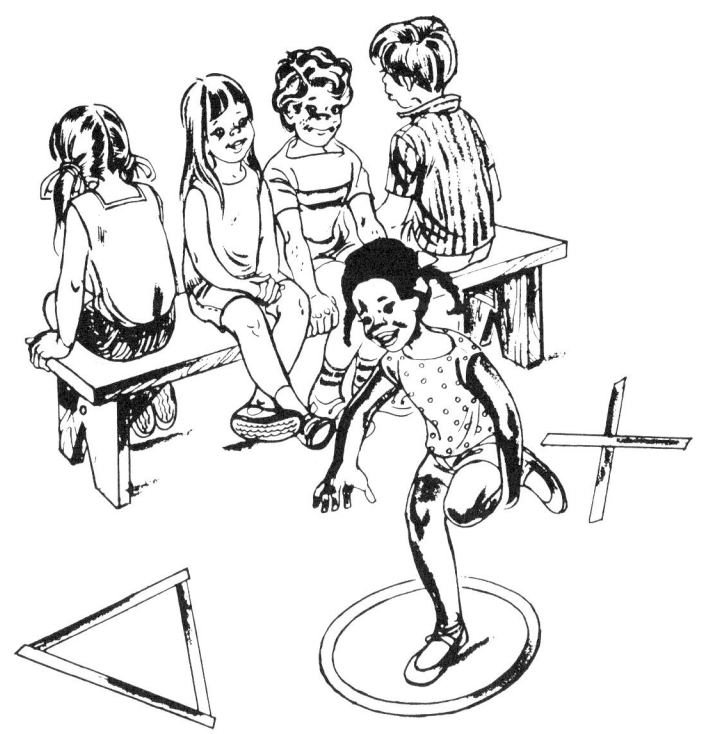

Note. From *Learning About Human Behavior Through Active Games* by B.J. Cratty, 1975, Englewood Cliffs, NJ: Prentice-Hall. Used by permission of the publisher.

2. Using a pack of cards, each containing a game rule (e.g., only one may hit the ball), select three cards and construct a game that meets the demands of the rules.

3. Think up games that are cooperative instead of competitive. Games of this nature are found in a publication by Orlick and Botterill (1975) and others. These sources give teachers suggestions with which to stimulate children's thoughts. Noncompetitive games are excellent for the emotionally disturbed, the awkward, and the retarded—all groups that may have had a great many bad experiences at being last and losing in games. An example of a game in which the object is to cooperate instead of compete is a handball game with a large ball thrown against a backboard. The object of the two players is to see how long (by the clock) they can keep the ball in play, rather than beat each other.

Creativity may be enhanced in a number of movement contexts. Dalke (1984) and others have written about the use of large, life-size gameboards of various types. These boards, expanding the size of smaller board games such as checkers, chess, and monopoly, have great possibilities in the movement and cognitive education of children and youth. The mathematics playground for the deaf, previously discussed, is ringed by a large monopoly board; after rolling large dice, children leap into spaces. An entire group of games resembling video games is presented in *Active Learning* (Cratty, 1985). These include "missile interception" concepts, as well as "chase" ideas.

PSYCHOLOGICAL AND SOCIAL CONCEPTS

A book entitled *Teaching about Human Behavior through Active Games* illustrates how various ideas in psychology and sociology might be introduced to young children in contrived games followed by structured discussions. One example is illustrated in Figure 32.8. Some of these games, if carefully handled and presented, may be useful in work with the retarded, the emotionally disturbed, and other atypical groups. Among the ideas contained in the games are those that have to do with working together, honesty, trust, cooperation, and competition.

Figure 32.8   A Game to Teach Psychological Concepts

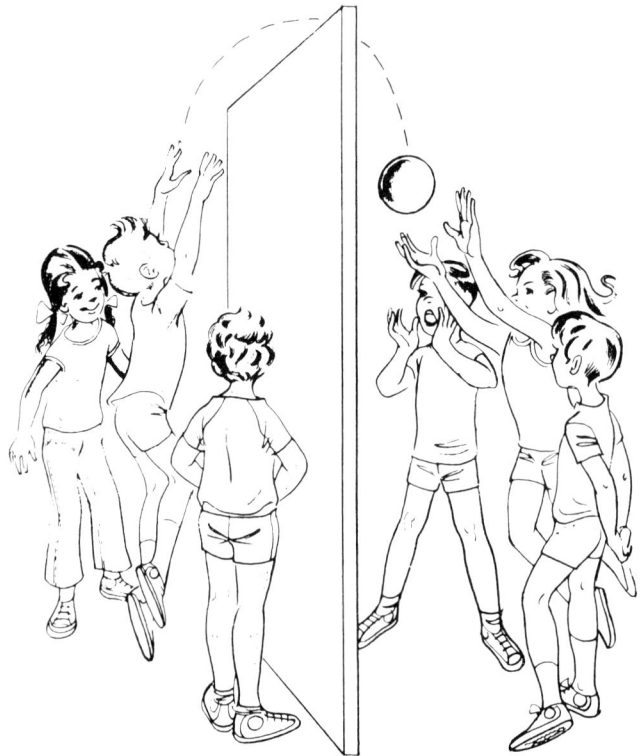

Note. From *Learning About Human Behavior Through Active Games* by B.J. Cratty, 1975, Englewood Cliffs, NJ: Prentice-Hall. Used by permission of the publisher.

Salend (1981) and others have proposed various games to assist in the social interactions of children mainstreamed in physical education situations. These games, Salend suggests, pass through four phases: (a) a foundation stage, during which information is collected; (b) a formulation stage, when the game is being devised; (c) an experimentation stage, during which various modifications may be experimented with; and (d) an evaluation phase, during which both children and teachers stand back and assess the results of the game or activity.

Games of this nature may be employed as part of a getting-along-together lesson in the classroom. They also may be employed when applicable problems arise.

Through exposure to this type of game, emotionally disturbed children who have trouble getting along in a regular physical education class might be helped to determine why they are having problems.

SUMMARY

Virtually every academic task or cognitive operation may be translated into a movement experience. Heightening the attractiveness of an academic task is only one of the properties of pairing movement with thought. Another benefit is the opportunity to observe and assess the quality of youngsters' movements and the manner in which they become focused on an academic or intellectual operations as they are required to move, speak, and look at the task at hand.

Preacademic movement experiences should help focus attention and lengthen the attention span. Others utilize large configurations painted on the playground to teach pattern recognition, which in turn may be translated into letter shapes. Physical responses, including jumping, hopping, and throwing, may be employed in a number of games that teach letter and number recognition, as well as reading and mathematical operations.

Various cognitive operations, including analysis, synthesis, divergent and convergent thought production, and flexibility and reversibility in problem solving, may be acted out in motor tasks. Additionally, concepts of psychology, social psychology, and sociology may be made more vivid through the use of contrived games followed by precise and meaningful discussions about human qualities, emotions, social interactions, and values.

REFERENCES

Asher, J.J. (1969). The total physical response technique of learning. *Journal of Special Education, 3,* 45-52.

Cratty, B.J. (1973). *Intelligence in action.* Englewood Cliffs, NJ: Prentice-Hall.

Cratty, B.J. (1975). *Teaching about human behavior through active games.* Englewood Cliffs, NJ: Prentice-Hall.

Cratty, B.J. (1981). *Coding games: Active ways to encourage reading and thought.* Denver: Love Publishing.

Cratty, B.J. (1985). *Active learning* (2nd ed.). Englewood Cliffs, NJ: Prentice-Hall.

Cratty, B.J., & Breen, J.E. (1972). *Educational games for physically handicapped children.* Denver: Love Publishing.

Dalke, B. (1984). Life size learning games. *Teaching Exceptional Children, 16,* 106-109.

Edmonson, B., & Han, S.S. (1983). Effects of socialization games on proximity and prosocial behavior of aggressive mentally retarded institutionalized women. *American Journal of Mental Deficiency, 87,* 435-440.

Humphrey, J.H., & Sullivan, D.D. (1973). *Teaching slow learners through active games.* Springfield, IL: Charles C Thomas.

Marlow, N. (1980). Games analysis: Designing games for exceptional children. *Teaching Exceptional Children, 12,* 48-51.

Meichenbaum, D., & Asnarow, J.R. (1979). Cognitive-behavioral modification and metacognitive development: Implications for the classroom. In P. Kendall & S. Hollon (Eds.), *Cognitive-behavioral interventions: Theory, research, and procedures.* New York: Academic Press.

McGee, G.G., Krantz, P.J., & McClannahan, L.E. (1984). *Journal of Autism & Developmental Disorders, 14,* 319-323.

Morris, G.S.D. (1976). *How to change the games children play.* Minneapolis: Burgess.

Orlick, T., & Botterill, C. (1975). *Every kid can win.* Chicago: Nelson Hall.

Salend, S.J. (1981). Active academic games: The aim of the game in mainstreaming. *Teaching Exceptional Children, 12,* 3-6.

Salend, S.J. (1982). Cooperative games promote positive student interaction. *Teaching Exceptional Children, 13,* 76-79.

Saltz, E. (1982). Let's pretend: The role of motoric imagery in memory for sentences and words. *Journal of Experimental Child Psychology, 34,* 77-92.

Saltz, E., & Donnenwerth-Nolan, S. (1981). Does motoric imagery facilitate memory for sentences? *Journal of Verbal Learning & Verbal Behavior, 20,* 323-332.

Thornburg, K.R., & Fisher, V.L. (1970). Discrimination of 2-d letters by children after play with 2 or 3-dimensional forms. *Perceptual & Motor Skills, 30,* 979-986.

Van Osdol, R.M., Johnson, D.M., & Geiger, L. (1974). The effects of total movement on reading achievement. *Australian Journal of Mental Retardation, 3,* 16-19.

ADDITIONAL REFERENCES

Bentley, W.G. (1970). *Learning to move and moving to learn.* New York: Citation Press.

Cratty, B.J. (1973). *Physical expressions of intelligence.* Englewood Cliffs, NJ: Prentice-Hall.

Gerhardt, L.A. (1973). *Moving and knowing.* Englewood Cliffs, NJ: Prentice-Hall.

Gilbert, A.G. (1977). *Teaching the three R's through movement experiences.* Minneapolis: Burgess Publishing.

Mosston, M. (1972). *Teaching: From command to discovery.* Belmont, CA: Wadsworth.

QUESTIONS FOR DISCUSSION

1. In what ways might movement experiences heighten and lengthen attention span?

2. In what ways might you help a child gain awareness of the sounds associated with various letters and letter combinations in the English language, using movement as a modality?

3. How might number recognition be heightened through movement activities?

4. How might children be encouraged to engage in divergent thought production using movement activities? Be specific; give concrete examples.

5. What contrived game might bring to children's attention the concept of cooperation? Of competition? What concepts might arise in a discussion following such a game?

STUDENT PROJECTS

1. Design on paper a playground containing configurations to optimize academic learning and problem-solving behavior using movement tasks. If possible, implement a simple configuration in cooperation with school personnel.

2. Outline a lesson in which you hope to teach a group of moderately retarded 7-year-olds to recognize common geometric shapes, using their total bodies as a learning modality. What kinds of coding games also might be used to teach these same youngsters that action verbs may be represented by various initials? Finally, change these initials to the full words (action verbs) they represent.

3. After consulting books that contain games to teach about human behavior, what do you think might be the drawbacks of using experiences with disturbed youngsters? What might be the advantages? How might you optimize these experiences for the emotionally disturbed child or youth?

Appendix: Resources

In addition to the organizations listed at the end of specific chapters, many resources are available to serve the handicapped, parents of the handicapped, and physical educators in more general ways. Some of these publications and organizations are listed below.

Adapted Physical Activity Quarterly
Human Kinetics Publishing
Champaign, IL

Academic Therapy Publications
200 Commercial Blvd.
Novato, CA 94947

Adapted Sports Association
    Communications Center
6832 Marlette Rd.
Marlette, MI 48453

American Alliance for Health,
    Physical Education, Recreation
    & Dance
1900 Association Dr.
Reston, VA 22091

American College of Sports Medicine
1440 Monroe St.
Madison, WI 53706

American Occupational Therapy
    Association Blvd.
Rockville, MD 20852

American Physical Therapy Association
1156-15th St., N.W.
Washington, DC 20005

American Psychological Association
1200-17th St., N.W.
Washington, DC 20036

American Red Cross
17th & D Streets, N.W.
Washington, DC 20006

American Thoracic Society
1740 Broadway
New York, NY 10019

Breckenridge Outdoor Education
    Center
Programs for Handicapped
P.O. Box 697
Breckenridge, CO 80424

Handicapped Flyers International
1117 Rising Hill
Escondido, CA 92025

National Handicapped Sports and
    Recreation Association
4105 East Florida Ave.
Denver, CO 80222

National Inservice Network
Indiana University
2853 East 10th St./Cottage L
Bloomington, IN 47405

Longman Group, Limited Periodicals
    and Directories Division
43/45 Annandale St.
Edinburgh, EH7 4AT
Scotland

National Center for Health Statistics
Public Health Service, HRA
Rockville, MD 20852

National Council of YMCAs
291 Broadway
New York, NY 10007

National Rehabilitation Association
1522 K Street, N.W.
Washington, DC 20004

National Therapeutic Recreation
    Society
1601 N. Kent St.
Arlington, VA 22209

National Wheelchair Athletic
    Association
40-24 62nd St.
Woodside, NY 11377

People-to-People Committee
    for the Handicapped
1522 K Street, N.W., #1130
Washington, DC 20005

Physical Educator
Special Populations Issues
Publications Office
9030 Log Run Dr., N.
Indianapolis, IN 46234

President's Committee on Employment
    of the Handicapped
1111 20th St., N.W.
Washington, DC 20036

Special Education Programs (SEP)
400 Maryland Ave., S.W.
Donahoe Bldg.
Washington, DC 20016

Sports 'n Spokes
5201 N. 19th Ave., Ste. 108
Phoenix, AZ 85015

Telephone Pioneers of America
Beep Ball Information
195 Broadway
New York, NY 10007

U.S. Department of Health
    & Human Services
Public Health Service
Office of Health Research, Statistics,
    and Technology
National Center for Health Studies
3700 East-West Highway
Hyattsville, MD 20782

U.S. Olympic Committee
57 Park Ave.
New York, NY 10016

Author Index

Subject Index